TO OUR PATIENTS

WHO HAVE TAUGHT US

ALL WE KNOW

DISORDERS OF
THE SMALL INTESTINE

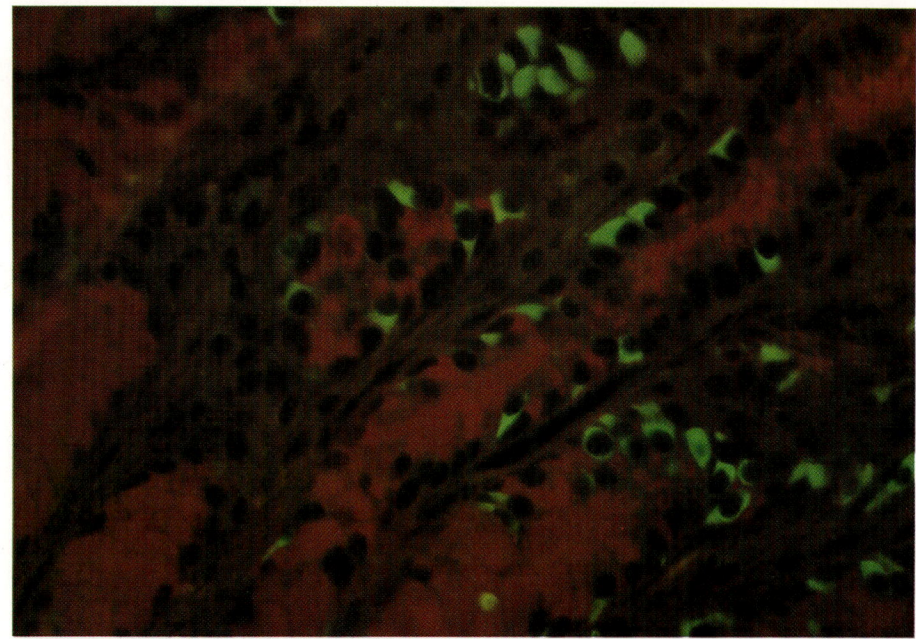

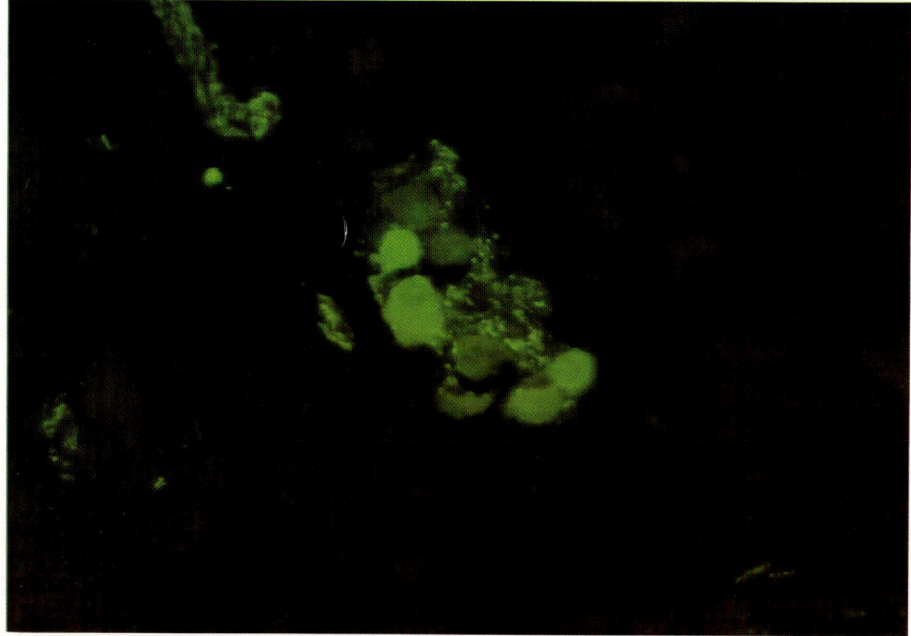

Frontispiece (Top) Endocrine cells of the gastrointestinal tract demonstrated by the technique of indirect immunofluorescence. The tissue was counterstained with haematoxylin and periodic acid-Schiff's reagent ($\times$ 5600). (Bottom) Submucosal perikarya and fibres of the intestine immunostained for vasoactive intestinal polypeptide using the technique of indirect immunofluorescence ($\times$ 5600). (Courtesy of Professor Julia Polak.)

DISORDERS OF THE SMALL INTESTINE

EDITED BY

Christopher C. Booth
MD, FRCP
*Clinical Research Centre,
Northwick Park Hospital, Middlesex*

AND

Graham Neale
BSc, MB, FRCP
*University of Cambridge and
Medical Research Council,
Dunn Nutritional Laboratory,
Cambridge*

BLACKWELL SCIENTIFIC PUBLICATIONS

OXFORD LONDON EDINBURGH

BOSTON PALO ALTO MELBOURNE

© 1985 by
Blackwell Scientific Publications
Editorial offices:
Osney Mead, Oxford, OX2 OEL
8 John Street, London, WC1N 2ES
23 Ainslie Place, Edinburgh, EH3 6AJ
52 Beacon Street, Boston
　Massachusetts 02108, USA
744 Cowper Street, Palo Alto
　California 94301, USA
107 Barry Street, Carlton
　Victoria 3053, Australia

All rights reserved. No part of this
publication may be reproduced, stored
in a retrieval system, or transmitted,
in any form or by any means,
electronic, mechanical, photocopying,
recording or otherwise
without the prior permission of
the copyright owner

First published 1985

Printed and bound at The Alden Press,
Oxford

DISTRIBUTORS

USA
　Blackwell Mosby Book Distributors
　11830 Westline Industrial Drive
　St Louis, Missouri 63141

Canada
　Blackwell Mosby Book Distributors
　120 Melford Drive, Scarborough
　Ontario M1B 2X4

Australia
　Blackwell Scientific Book Distributors
　31 Advantage Road, Highett
　Victoria 3190

British Library
Cataloguing in Publication Data

Disorders of the small intestine.
　1. Intestine, Small—Diseases
　I. Booth, *Sir* Christopher C.
　II. Neale, Graham
　616.3'4　RC860

ISBN 0-632-01059-2

Contents

Contributors, ix

Preface, xi

Introduction, xiii

1 Assessment of Small Intestinal Disease, 1

   A Clinical Assessment, 1
   A.J. Levi and Christopher C. Booth

   B Radiological Examination, 5
   Robert Wilkins, Conall Garvey and Gerald de Lacey

   C Small Intestinal Biopsy, 12
   Ashley B. Price

   D Intestinal Function Tests, 21
   M.G. Rinsler and Christopher C. Booth

   E Nutritional Assessment, 29
   Graham Neale

2 Congenital Anatomical Abnormalities, 43
   John Walker-Smith and Vanessa Wright

3 Congenital and Inherited Defects of the Enterocyte, 52
   J. T. Harries, D.P.R. Muller and P.J. Milla

4 Motility and its Disorders, 78
   D.G. Thompson and D.L. Wingate

5 Effects of Gastric Operations, 93
   J. Alexander-Williams and I.A. Donovan

6 Intestinal Resection and Bypass, 101
   Christopher C. Booth

7 Food-Allergic Disorders, 118
   Anne Ferguson

8 Immune Deficiency, 135
   A.D.B. Webster

9 Coeliac Disease, 153
   Anthony M. Dawson and Parveen Kumar

10 Lymphoma and Alpha-chain Disease, 179
   William F. Doe

11 Crohn's Disease (Regional Enteritis), 195
   D.P. Jewell

12 Ulcerative Lesions, 209
   Christopher C. Booth and Graham Neale

13 Infiltrative Lesions, 218
   Graham Neale and Christopher C. Booth

14 Infections, 231
   Sherwood L. Gorbach

15 Bacterial Overgrowth, 249
   Soad Tabaqchali and Christopher C. Booth

16 Whipple's Disease (Intestinal Lipodystrophy), 270
   H.J.F. Hodgson

17 Parasitic Infection, 283
   G.C. Cook

18 Effects of Nutritional Deficiency, 299
   Devhuti Vyas and R.K. Chandra

19 Tropical Sprue, 311
   Andrew Tomkins and Christopher C. Booth

20 Vascular Abnormalities, 333
   Graham Neale

21 Intestinal Lymphangiectasia, 348
   Graham Neale

22 Tumours and Tumour-like Conditions, 363
   Gerard Slavin

23 Regulatory Peptides and Hormone-
secreting Tumours, 376
S.R. Bloom and Julia M. Polak

24 Drug-induced Disorders, 398
Charles F. George and Greg E. Holdstock

25 Radiation Enteritis, 413
Barry T. Jackson

Index, 425

Contributors

JOHN ALEXANDER-WILLIAMS, MD, ChM, FACS, FRCS,
19 Farquhar Road, Birmingham B15 3RA

STEPHEN R. BLOOM, MA, MD, DSc, FRCP,
Department of Medicine, Royal Postgraduate Medical School, Hammersmith Hospital, London W12 0HS

CHRISTOPHER C. BOOTH, MD (St. And.), LlD (Dundee) (Hon.), FRCP, FRCPE, FACP (Hon.), Docteur hon. causa (Paris VII, Poitiers)
Clinical Research Centre, Watford Road, Harrow, Middlesex HA1 3UJ

RANJIT K. CHANDRA, MD, FRCP (C)
Professor of Pediatric Research, Memorial University of Newfoundland, and Director of Immunology, Janeway Child Health Centre, St John's, Newfoundland, Canada

G.C. COOK, MD, DSc, FRCP, FRACP
Department of Clinical Tropical Medicine, London School of Hygiene and Tropical Medicine, London WC1E 7HT

ANTHONY M. DAWSON, MD, FRCP
Department of Gastroenterology, St Bartholomew's Hospital, West Smithfield London EC1A 7BE

GERALD DE LACEY, MA, MB, BChir, FRCR
Department of Diagnostic Radiology, Northwick Park Hospital and Clinical Research Centre, Watford Road, Harrow, Middlesex HA1 3UJ

WILLIAM F. DOE, MSc, FRCP, FRACP
Department of Medicine and Clinical Science, John Curtin School of Medical Research, Australian National University, Canberra, Australia

IAN ALEXANDER DONOVAN, MD, FRCS
University Department of Surgery, Dudley Road Hospital, Birmingham B18 7QH

ANNE FERGUSON, PhD, FRCP
Gastrointestinal Unit, Western General Hospital, Edinburgh EH4 2XU

CONALL J. GARVEY, MB, FRCR
Department of Radiology, Northwick Park Hospital, Watford Road, Harrow, Middlesex HA1 3UJ

CHARLES F. GEORGE, BSc, MD, FRCP
Clinical Pharmacology Group, Medical & Biological Sciences Building, Bassett Crescent East, Southampton SO9 3TU

SHERWOOD L. GORBACH, MD
Professor of Medicine and Chief of Division of Infectious Diseases, Tufts University School of Medicine, New England Medical Center, Boston, Massachusetts 02111, USA

The late JOHN T. HARRIES, MD, FRCP
Department of Child Health, Institute of Child Health, 30 Guilford Street, London WC1N 1EH

HUMPHREY J.F. HODGSON, DM, FRCP
Department of Medicine, Royal Postgraduate Medical School, Hammersmith Hospital, London W12 0HS

GREG HOLDSTOCK, DM, MRCP
Southampton General Hospital, Tremona Road, Southampton

BARRY T. JACKSON, MS, FRCS
St Thomas's Hospital, Lambeth Palace Road, London SE1 7EH

D.P. JEWELL, MA, DPhil, FRCP
Gastroenterology Unit, Radcliffe Infirmary, Woodstock Road, Oxford OX2 6HE

PARVEEN J. KUMAR, MD, MRCP
Department of Gastroenterology, St Bartholomew's Hospital, West Smithfield, London EC1A 7BE

A.J. LEVI, MD, FRCP, FRCP(E)
Northwick Park Hospital and Clinical Research Centre, Watford Road, Harrow, Middlesex HA1 3UJ

PETER JOHN MILLA, MSc, MBBS, MRCP
Department of Child Health, Institute of Child Health, 30 Guilford Street, London WC1N 1EH

DAVID P.R. MULLER, PhD
Department of Child Health, Institute of Child Health, 30 Guilford Street, London WC1N 1EH

GRAHAM NEALE, MA, BSc, MB, ChB, FRCP
Addenbrooke's Hospital, Hills Road, Cambridge CB2 2QQ

JULIA M. POLAK, DSc, MD, MRCPath
Department of Histochemistry, Royal Postgraduate

Medical School, Hammersmith Hospital, London W12 OHS

ASHLEY B. PRICE, MA, BM, BCh, MRCPath
Consultant Histopathologist, Department of Histopathology, Northwick Park Hospital and Clinical Research Centre, Harrow, Middlesex HA1 3UJ

M.G. RINSLER, MD, FRCPath
Department of Clinical Chemistry, Northwick Park Hospital and Clinical Research Centre, Watford Road, Harrow, Middlesex HA1 3UJ

GERARD SLAVIN, MB, ChB(Ed.), FRCP (Glas.), FRCPath
Professor of Histopathology, St Bartholomew's Hospital Medical College, West Smithfield, London EC1A 7BE

SOAD TABAQCHALI, MB, ChB, MRCPath
Reader in Medical Microbiology, St Bartholomew's Hospital Medical College, West Smithfield, London EC1A 7BE

DAVID G. THOMPSON, BSc, MD, MRCP
Medical Unit, The London Hospital, Whitechapel, London E1 1BB

ANDREW TOMKINS, MB, FRCP
Department of Human Nutrition, London School of Hygiene and Tropical Medicine, Keppel Street, London WC1E 7HT

DEVHUTI VYAS, PhD
Post Doctoral Research Fellow, Immunology Department, Memorial University of Newfoundland, St John's, Newfoundland, Canada

J.A. WALKER-SMITH, MD(Syd.), FRCP(Lond.), FRCP(Edin.), FRACP
Reader in Paediatric Gastroenterology, St Bartholomew's Hospital Medical College, West Smithfield, London EC1A 7BE

A.D.B. WEBSTER, FRCP
Division of Immunological Medicine, Clinical Research Centre, Watford Road, Harrow, Middlesex HA1 3UJ

R.A. WILKINS, BSc, MB, ChB, FRCR
Department of Radiology, Northwick Park Hospital, Watford Road, Harrow, Middlesex HA1 3UJ

D.L. WINGATE, MA, MSc, DM, FRCP
Academic Unit of Gastroenterology, The London Hospital, Whitechapel, London E1 1BB

VANESSA WRIGHT, MB, BS, FRCS, FRACS
Consultant Paediatric Surgeon, Queen Elizabeth Hospital for Children, London E2

Preface

Our aim in producing this book has been to give a comprehensive and up-to-date account of disorders of the small intestine. The authors of the various chapters were selected on account of their acknowledged expertise and contributions to scientific knowledge. The book starts with assessment and then deals with congenital abnormalities, the effects of surgical operations, immunological disorders, coeliac disease and Crohn's disease, microbial and parasitic infections, as well as with disorders of blood vessels and lymphatics. Malignant lesions and secreting and non-secreting tumours are then described. The importance of the newly discovered regulatory peptides in small intestinal disease is discussed in detail. Finally, there are chapters on the deleterious but usually inadvertent effects of drugs and radiation on the small intestine.

The book is intended primarily for postgraduate students and for practising gastroenterologists who may wish to include on their shelves a volume on the small intestine among those already available on other organs of the gastrointestinal tract. The undergraduate student, however, may also find much of interest in these pages, as may the physiologist or biochemist investigating small intestinal function.

We have found the editing of the book to be a rewarding experience and there are many to whom we are indebted. We first thank all who have contributed for their cooperation and forbearance during the editing of the volume. We also thank Professor Charles Haex of the University of Leiden for information about life in Holland at the end of World War II and for helpful discussions on the work of Professor W.K. Dicke. We are particularly grateful to Dr A.B. Price for advice on small intestinal pathology, to Dr R.A. Wilkins for radiological guidance and to Mr Richard Bowlby of the photographic department of the Clinical Research Centre at Northwick Park for illustrations. We also thank Dr Sue Barter, Dr Anne Hemingway and Professor David Allison (Department of Radiology at the Royal Postgraduate Medical School) and Dr Alan Freeman (Addenbrooke's Hospital, Cambridge) for contributing radiographs, Dr Lionel Fry (St Mary's Hospital) for illustrations of the skin in dermatitis herpetiformis, Professor M.S. Losowsky (St James's Hospital, Leeds) for the photomicrographs of the jejunal mucosa in systemic mastocytosis, Dr Paul Conn (Addenbrooke's Hospital, Cambridge) for photographs of lesions caused by vasculitis affecting the small intestine, and Professor Kristin Henry (Westminster Hospital) for the electron microscopic pictures of alpha chain disease. Dr J.S. Stewart (West Middlesex Hospital) has generously provided dissecting microscopic and histological photographs of the jejunal mucosa in normal individuals and in coeliac disease, and Dr David Levinson and Mr Peter Crocker of St Bartholomew's Hospital have contributed scanning electron microscopy in bacterial overgrowth. We thank Dr Anthony James (Hillingdon Hospital) for providing us with illustrations of the clinical features of Peutz–Jegher's syndrome. We are particularly indebted to Dr P.E.C. Manson-Bahr for allowing us to review the slides of the original autopsy carried out on a patient with tropical sprue by his father, Sir Philip Manson-Bahr, in Ceylon in 1913, and to Dr Margot Shiner for the first peroral jejunal biopsy in tropical sprue. We were greatly helped during our years at the Royal Postgraduate Medical School and Hammersmith Hospital by many colleagues but we particularly thank Professor D.L. Mollin, Mr R.H. Franklin,

Professor R.E. Steiner, Dr J.W. Laws, Dr G.R. Thompson, Dr Vinton Chadwick and Professor R.H. Dowling for their helpful collaboration in the investigation and treatment of patients with disorders of the small intestine. We would also like to express our thanks to Mr Peter Saugman, Mr Jeremy Trevathan and Mrs Caroline Richards of Blackwell Scientific Publications for all their help in the production of this volume. Finally, we warmly thank Mrs Jane Greig for her unfailing support throughout and for typing virtually the entire manuscript.

C.C. Booth
G. Neale
January 1984

Introduction

It was the Swedish aeroplanes that heralded the new era. Towards the end of World War II, in response to news of the famine conditions under which the Dutch people were then living, the Swedish authorities despatched urgently needed supplies by air to relieve the starving population. The idea that bread might be harmful to children with coeliac disease had already been germinating in the fertile mind of Professor W.K. Dicke for he had noted, whilst working as a paediatrician in the Hague, that the children with coeliac disease for whom he cared appeared to improve during the disastrous food shortages of the latter part of the War. The Hague was the area of Holland worst hit by famine. There was no bread available and people were reduced to eating tulip bulbs and sugar beet. To Dicke's astonishment, the coeliac patients improved under these appalling conditions. Shortly before the end of the War, Swedish aeroplanes dropped bread which was eagerly devoured by the half-starved children. Soon after, Dicke noted that the children with coeliac disease relapsed and it was these astute clinical observations, made under the most adverse conditions, that convinced him that bread was harmful to sufferers from the coeliac condition, something he had suspected since the 1930s. His work was first published with characteristic modesty only in his MD thesis in 1950 and thereafter the role of gluten in inducing coeliac disease was clearly established by further work in Utrecht with his colleagues Weijers and Van der Kamer.

The decades that have passed since this epoch-making discovery have witnessed a remarkable expansion of knowledge of small intestinal physiology and disease. Techniques of intestinal intubation and biopsy and the use of radioactive tracers made possible for the first time detailed investigations in human subjects of the physiology and pathology of the small intestine. Advances in lipid and sterol biochemistry opened up exciting new vistas for those investigating fat absorption or bile salt metabolism in health and disease. Mechanisms of intestinal transport were elucidated and disorders due to transport defects clearly defined. Techniques for the isolation of membranes made possible the demonstration of the brush border localization of the disaccharidases and at the same time clinicians recognized the clinical conditions associated with disaccharidase deficiency. The discovery that the absorption of vitamin B_{12} is a specific function of the ileum led to the realization that the small intestine, like the renal tubule, has different functions in different parts of its length. This was important in understanding how pathological processes in different parts of the small intestine affect intestinal function. In addition, the adaptive response of the small intestine to malnutrition, hormonal change, disease or resection has been investigated in detail.

It has been known for nearly a century that there is a remarkably rapid turnover of cells in the small intestinal mucosa, each adult epithelial cell absorbing no more than three or four breakfasts, dinners or teas before it is shed. Only recently, however, have investigators devised methods for measuring rates of cell production in experimental animals and in man. A terminology, which we have followed in this book, has been developed to describe the cells involved in this process, which so much resembles the production of erythrocytes by the bone marrow. The germinative cells in the crypts of Lieberkuhn are defined as 'enteroblasts' and the adult absorbing cells on the side of the villi, 'enterocytes'. The whole process can be described as 'enteropoiesis'. This terminology raises the question whether there is an 'enteropoietin' which stimulates enteroblasts in the same way that erythropoietin stimulates the bone marrow. Studies of adaptive responses by the small intestinal mucosa and of regulatory peptides are actively investigating this question.

Microbiologists have also played an important role, particularly with the recognition of the importance of the metabolic functions of anaerobic bacteria. The discovery of the role of enterotoxins elaborated by *V. cholera*, as well as *E. coli*, has made possible a dramatic improvement in the prognosis not only of cholera but also of childhood enteritis in recent years. In addition, a range of new viruses has been implicated in the pathogenesis of diarrhoea.

The revelation of the circulation of lymphocytes and their capacity for homing to the gut has been of fundamental importance in our understanding of the immunology of the small intestine, as has the demonstration of the secretory immune system. These discoveries have greatly stimulated studies of immune mechanisms in human small intestinal disease.

Endocrinology has also made a major contribution. Mutt and Jorpes first isolated and purified the known hormone, secretin, from intestinal mucosa and then went on to identify a new family of intestinal regulatory peptides, many of whose functions are not yet clearly established. Simultaneously, pathologists and electron microscopists have been able to identify the endocrine cell types in the intestinal mucosa responsible for secreting these substances.

These dramatic developments are by no means at an end. The impact of modern techniques of molecular biology on the diagnosis and elucidation of human small intestinal disease is only beginning to be apparent.

Clinical research has played an important role in all these developments. Although the application of knowledge gained in basic science to clinical problems has been of great importance, clinical investigation itself has also been vital not only in clarifying the problems of human disease but also in influencing the direction of basic research. Dicke's classical observations, for example, were a major stimulus to studies of gastrointestinal immunology. The investigation of the single patient with a tumour-secreting enteroglucagon (described in Chapter 23), encouraged investigations of the trophic effects of gastrointestinal hormones on the gastrointestinal tract. In addition, a galaxy of new disorders of the small intestine has been recognized and in many instances, as a result of careful clinical studies, effective therapy has been devised. Many problems remain, not least the enigma of Crohn's disease, a bane to the increasing number of young people who suffer that affliction.

This book is predominantly clinical in orientation. It seeks to bring together current knowledge of disorders of the small intestine, an area of the gastrointestinal tract which in the past tended to be neglected by gastroenterologists. Conditions such as megaloblastic anaemia and osteomalacia, so frequently associated with small intestinal disease, were thought to belong to the realm of the haematologist or metabolic physician. Today, however, small intestinal disease is a vitally important part of the work of the gastroenterologist who must understand not only those upper and nether regions of the gastrointestinal tract that he can so easily visualize, but also the vital area between, the small intestine. Growth, development, reproduction and mental activity ultimately depend on the satisfactory function of this essential organ.

In general, we have not sought to include acute surgical conditions in this book since these are covered adequately in most contemporary surgical texts. It is for this reason that disorders such as intussusception and volvulus are not described. We have also excluded ulcerative lesions of the duodenum. There is some degree of overlap in the text and cross references between chapters have been given where necessary. The editors, however, together with the authors of the various chapters, have sought to achieve both a reasonable balance and a uniformity of style throughout the volume.

Good clinical practice, no less than clinical research, depends on the accurate and careful analysis of single patients and their problems, and we have therefore not hesitated to include individual case reports which serve to illustrate particular principles or which have provided a specific stimulus to research. Since it is from our patients that we have learned all that we think we know, it is to them that we dedicate this book.

Chapter 1
Assessment of Small Intestinal Disease

A. CLINICAL ASSESSMENT
A. J. LEVI AND CHRISTOPHER C. BOOTH

Clinical history 1
Physical examination 3
Investigations 4

In all fields of medicine a close and sympathetic relationship between patient and medical adviser is essential. This is especially true in disorders of the small intestine for, if one excludes acute infections, many conditions such as coeliac disease require attention and advice throughout life. It is therefore vital that the medical adviser establishes an understanding relationship from the first interview. Sensitivity is particularly required in eliciting the clinical history and in carrying out the physical examination. Diagnostic investigations should be chosen with care and with the aim of causing the least amount of discomfort and inconvenience compatible with achieving an accurate diagnosis. The nature of the patient's disorder must be clearly defined and its importance assessed in relation to work and family as well as to physical and psychological well-being.

Clinical history

A detailed and careful clinical history, involving a review of all systems, is the first requirement in the assessment of a small intestinal disorder. At the outset, it may not be at all obvious that the patient has small intestinal disease. Symptoms may be non-specific and easily confused with those arising from other conditions.

The presence of aphthous ulceration in the mouth, for example, is most frequently a self-limiting condition of unknown cause, but it may also indicate coeliac disease, Crohn's disease or Behçet's syndrome. Soreness of the mouth and tongue and angular stomatitis may occur with deficiencies of iron, folic acid, vitamin B_{12} and vitamin B complex. These symptoms are relatively late indicators of nutritional deficiency. Dysphagia may occur as a result of obstructive lesions of the oesophagus which in turn may be complications of small intestinal disease. It also occurs in certain patients with scleroderma and, rarely, if there is a post-cricoid web due to long-standing iron deficiency. Anorexia occurs frequently in disorders of the small intestine and is often more important than malabsorption as a cause of loss of weight in such conditions. Vomiting is unusual even with obstruction unless this is high in the small intestine.

Abdominal pain is an important symptom. In gastrointestinal practice, it is more often an indicator of the irritable bowel syndrome than structural intestinal disease. Colicky pain associated with watery diarrhoea is an important feature of Crohn's disease of the small intestine and may occur with other obstructive lesions such as intussusception complicating coeliac disease. If the patient's sleep is disturbed, then organic disease is likely. A constant boring pain, unrelieved by analgesics and exacerbated by eating, signifies intestinal ischaemia or intra-abdominal malignancy. Severe abdominal pain of sudden onset alerts the clinician to the probability of an intra-abdominal catastrophe such as a perforation of the small intestine occurring as a result of an ulcerative or neoplastic lesion. A sense of vague abdominal discomfort with gurgling is often a feature of giardiasis.

Diarrhoea in patients with small intestinal disease is not invariably due to steatorrhoea. Conversely patients with steatorrhoea do not necessarily have diarrhoea. If there is significant steatorrhoea, the stools are more offensive than normal, pale, tend to float and stick to the side of the pan, necessitating repeated flushing of the toilet. This can be a cause of acute embarrassment to a sensitive patient visiting friends. As with pain, diarrhoea during sleep usually indicates the presence of organic disease. In Crohn's disease the stools are usually ill-formed and contain excess mucus. Overt bleeding is unusual. In many other disorders of the small intestine, including giardiasis, disaccharide malabsorption, ileal resection and lymphoma, watery diarrhoea may be a predominant feature of the illness. Voluminous watery diarrhoea (more than 1l/day) occurs as a result of bacterial enterotoxins (as in cholera) or in association with tumours of pancreatic or neural tissue producing vasoactive inhibitory polypeptide (VIP), or with purgative abuse.

Apart from gastrointestinal symptoms, the clinician should be aware of the effects of small intestinal disorders on other organs. The skin may provide useful clues. An itchy rash involving the extensor surfaces of the limbs may indicate dermatitis herpetiformis and gluten-sensitive enteropathy. The painful red lumps of erythema nodosum may indicate Crohn's disease. Recurrent 'hives' (urticaria) alerts the clinician to the possible presence of parasites in the gut. Painful joints are a frequent feature of Crohn's disease and Whipple's disease, and red eyes occur in both Crohn's disease and Behçet's syndrome. A history of bleeding, either into the skin or gastrointestinal tract, may indicate vitamin K deficiency, and melaena may be due to an ulcerative lesion of the small intestine, especially if the stomach and duodenum are endoscopically normal. Peripheral oedema due to hypoalbuminaemia is more frequent in inflammatory diseases causing protein-losing enteropathy such as Crohn's disease or radiation enteritis than in coeliac disease.

Deficiencies of iron, folic acid or vitamin B_{12} may occur singly or in association and produce pallor, breathlessness and oedema due to anaemia. Vitamin D deficiency frequently causes symptoms of weakness with a disordered gait due to myopathy rather than bone pain, which is usually present only in long-standing disease. Numbness and tingling in the fingers may be symptoms of tetany due to calcium or magnesium deficiency and should be distinguished from the neurological symptoms of peripheral neuropathy.

It is always important to enquire into the patient's previous history. Previous surgery may have led to resection or to the creation of blind loops in the small intestine. An adult coeliac patient may have a story of a diarrhoeal illness or a failure to thrive in childhood with remission in adolescence. A history of holidaying in certain areas of the tropics or of living in an area with a high incidence of parasitic disease may be important in recognizing parasitic infection or tropical sprue. Giardiasis is probably the commonest identifiable cause of persistent diarrhoea occurring in travellers returning from even short visits abroad. The history of drug ingestion should always be carefully assessed, in view of potential deleterious effects on the small intestine. The family history is also important, particularly in patients with disorders such as hypolactasia or coeliac disease.

The social history may throw considerable light on the patient's disorder and will influence its management. Diarrhoea is more incapacitating for a taxi-driver or market trader than for a housewife. The patient may have been exposed to an infective or toxic agent and in the catering trade infection with intestinal pathogens is liable to cause greater havoc than in other occupations.

An appreciation of the changing pattern of some diseases is also important. The incidence of Crohn's disease has been rising and this is probably the most intractable problem now facing the gastroenterologist in the Western world. Symptomatology is changing too. Although diarrhoea was a major presenting feature of coeliac disease a decade ago, most patients are now recognized early because of slow growth in childhood or a mild nutritional disturbance such as deficiency of folic acid.

Physical examination

Small intestinal disorders may be associated with abnormalities of a wide range of systems and for this reason a careful physical examination is essential. The general appearance of the patient should be noted, the height and weight measured and an overall assessment of nutritional status made. Restriction of growth in children, and in some cases infantilism, may be presenting features of small intestinal disease, particularly coeliac and Crohn's disease. Unexplained pyrexia is a feature of some patients with inflammatory lesions of the small intestine, such as Crohn's disease, and may be the presenting feature of Whipple's disease. On the other hand, patients with severe malnutrition may become hypothermic.

The skin should be carefully examined. There may be pallor due to anaemia, associated in severe cases of megaloblastic anaemia with a tinge of jaundice. Skin rashes, such as the bullous lesions of dermatitis herpetiformis (Fig. 1.1), are usually obvious but a careful search may be necessary to find cutaneous lesions in support of a possible diagnosis of gastro-intestinal angiomata. They should be particularly sought in the mouth, subungually or at mucocutaneous junctions. Subcutaneous haemorrhage may be a sign of vitamin K deficiency and may also be seen as an allergic reaction in conditions such as intestinal strongyloidiasis. Acute urticarial lesions of the skin may be a feature of other allergic reactions and occur in patients with C1-esterase inhibitor deficiency. Generalized pigmentation of the skin occurs in Whipple's disease and in occasional patients with coeliac disease in whom it may be severe enough to resemble Addison's disease. Localized pigmentation in the form of perioral and mucosal freckling is characteristic of Peutz-Jeghers syndrome. Erythema nodosum and pyoderma gangrenosum may both occur in inflammatory bowel disease and occasionally lesions resembling erythema nodosum may occur after intestinal resection or bypass.

Examination of the *mouth* may reveal aphthous ulceration, or there may be glossitis and angular stomatitis (Fig. 1.2) indicative of iron deficiency or avitaminosis. Evidence of scurvy, however, is rarely found in patients with small intestinal disease.

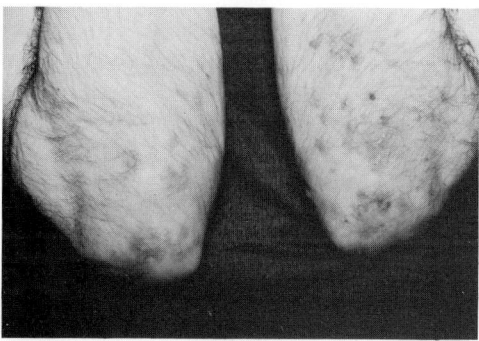

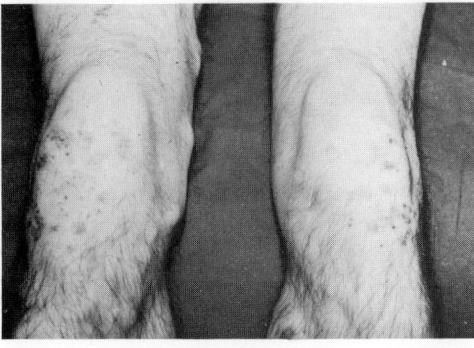

Fig. 1.1. Dermatitis herpetiformis in a patient with coeliac disease, showing lesions on elbows and knees. (Courtesy of Dr Lionel Fry.)

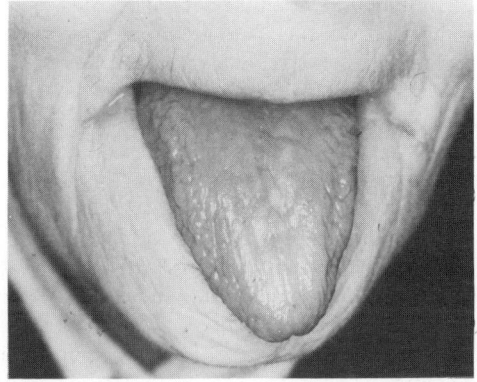

Fig. 1.2. Smooth tongue and angular stomatitis in a patient with a partial gastrectomy.

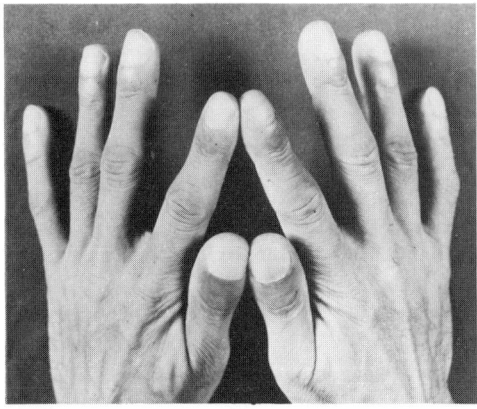

Fig. 1.3. Clubbing of the fingers in a patient with abdominal lymphoma.

Ocular lesions such as iritis and iridocyclitis may be a feature of Crohn's disease. The skeletal system should be carefully examined. Both *monarthropathy* and *polyarthropathy* occur in Crohn's disease, which may also be associated with the stiff rigid spine of ankylosing spondylitis. The diagnostic triad of arthritis, pigmentation and diarrhoea is characteristic of Whipple's disease. *Clubbing of the fingers* (Fig. 1.3) is frequently associated with many small intestinal disorders and may be particularly marked in intestinal lymphoma.

In many patients with small intestinal disorders, *examination of the abdomen* reveals few abnormalities. There may, however, be evidence of distension in patients with lesions such as strictures causing chronic obstruction. In such patients, peristalsis is frequently visible. The presence of visible peristalsis is so significant that it should be sought with considerable care, the characteristic sweep of contraction along a bowel segment frequently being produced by asking the patient to take a glass of water. The peristalsis of low grade intestinal obstruction should be carefully distinguished from normal contractions of the bowel which can often be seen through a thin abdominal wall or an old operation scar. Abdominal tenderness is a frequent finding in patients with inflammatory lesions and palpable masses may indicate Crohn's disease. Masses may also be found when there is an intra-abdominal neoplasm such as a lymphoma. Occasionally, the intra-abdominal lymph nodes of Whipple's disease may present as a palpable mass. The liver and spleen may be enlarged in such conditions. Rectal examination should always be performed, at which time the faeces can usefully be examined for colour, the presence of blood or mucus, and consistency.

Cardiovascular abnormalities usually only occur in the presence of severe malnutrition, when extrasystoles and other arrhythmias may be found. The *respiratory system* should be carefully examined, particularly in patients with coeliac disease, in view of the possible association with bird fancier's lung and allergic alveolitis. Examination of the *nervous system* may reveal evidence of peripheral neuropathy but signs of subacute degeneration of the cord are unusual in patients with B_{12} deficiency due to small intestinal disease. A positive Chvostek's sign (contraction of the labial muscles on light tapping of facial nerve) may indicate calcium or magnesium deficiency, and tetany and carpal spasm may be induced by cuff occlusion of the blood supply in the arm (Trousseau's sign). Tender bones and a waddling gait may indicate osteomalacia due to vitamin D deficiency.

Investigations

In the investigation of small intestinal disease, the gastroenterologist is particularly dependent on the expertise and advice of his radiological, histopathological, biochemical and microbiological colleagues. In acute diarrhoea, microbiological investigation may be paramount. In more chronic conditions, there are three main lines of investigation. First, the anatomical diagnosis should be established by careful radiology and biopsy of the small intestine when required. Secondly, it is necessary to establish whether or not there are nutritional deficiencies. Thirdly, tests of intestinal function may be carried out to establish the pathophysiological consequences of the intestinal lesion. Rarely, laparotomy may be required to clinch a diagnosis.

For carrying out routine jejunal biopsies,

we prefer the Watson modification of the original Crosby biopsy capsule (Crosby & Kugler 1957, Read et al. 1962). It can be rapidly guided to the duodeno-jejunal flexure with an 'overtube'; the procedure is well tolerated and easy to carry out. For research purposes, a multiple sampling tube may be required, in which case either the Quinton—Rubin tube (Brandborg et al. 1959) or one of its modifications should be used.

B. RADIOLOGICAL EXAMINATION
ROBERT WILKINS, CONALL GARVEY AND GERALD DE LACEY

Barium examination 5
Angiography 8
Isotope imaging 11

Despite recent advances in imaging techniques, barium examination remains the mainstay of radiological diagnosis. Plain radiographs contribute principally to the management of surgical problems. No place has yet been established for nuclear magnetic resonance or digital subtraction angiography, and the role of both computerized tomography and ultrasound is limited. However, angiography has an important role and isotope investigations are useful in some circumstances.

Barium examination

It is common practice for examination of the small bowel to be performed as an add-on investigation following a barium meal. This has been shown to be of doubtful use both clinically (Rabe et al. 1981, Fried et al. 1981, Herlinger et al. 1983) and because varying degrees of barium density and unreliable

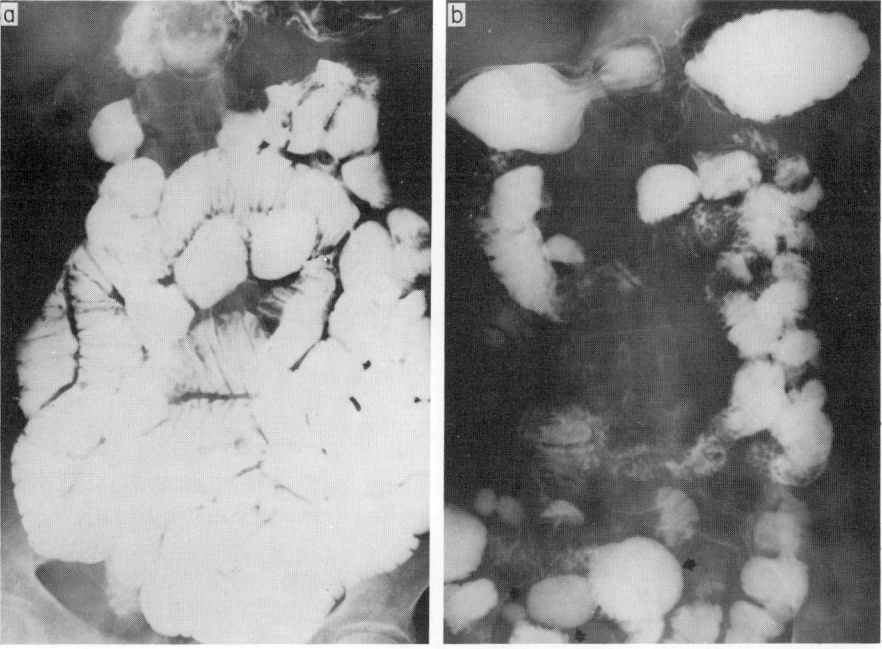

Fig. 1.4. (a) Add-on barium follow-through 15 min after a double-contrast barium meal using high-density barium. There is non-specific dilatation of small bowel loops. Two diverticula are seen with difficulty in the duodenal loop. (b) 10-min film from a subsequent small bowel meal in the same patient using dilute barium. Numerous jejunal diverticula are seen. These were obscured on the earlier high-density study.

coating detract from the quality of the examination. Moreover, this practice is even less desirable following a modern double-contrast meal as the dense barium will obscure much of the small bowel (Fig. 1.4). It is therefore recommended that barium examination of the small bowel be performed as a separate study, distinct from the barium meal, either by oral or intubation technique.

Oral administration (small bowel meal)

This procedure, tailored to the small bowel, differs from the add-on investigation in several important respects. The patient is fasted and the colon is cleansed as for a barium enema using a non-washout regimen (De Lacey et al. 1982). This preparation has been considered essential because a full caecum slows transit through the distal ileum (Nice 1963, Nice 1974), but this is questionable. A large volume (500 ml) of low-density barium, 30–50% w/v, is given by mouth. Metoclopramide (20 mg orally) is given to increase gastric emptying and promote intestinal peristalsis (Howarth et al. 1969). Other manouevres employed to speed up the examination include lowering the temperature of the barium which enhances peristalsis (Morton 1961, Sellink 1983), or adding 10 ml Gastrografin, a water-soluble contrast medium which produces a similar effect. Interval radiographs and fluoroscopic spot films are obtained and most examinations are completed in 1–1½ h (Howarth et al. 1969, Herlinger & Lintott 1983). In selected patients, air introduced per rectum when the barium reaches the caecum followed by intravenous glucagon may allow excellent double-contrast views of the terminal ileum (Figs 1.5 and 1.6).

Small bowel intubation (enteroclysis)

First suggested by Pesquera in 1929, this technique was refined by Sellink (Pesquera 1929, Sellink 1971). The patient is prepared as described for the small bowel meal. A small (12 French) PVC tube is introduced via the nose as far as the duodeno-jejunal flexure (Nolan 1979). Most examinations are single

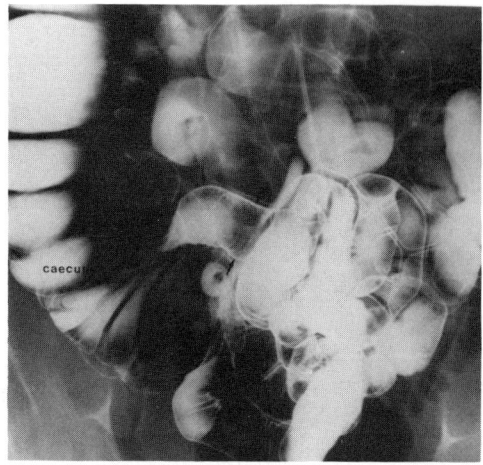

Fig. 1.5. Air introduced per rectum following intravenous glucagon shows the caecum and distal 3–4 ft of ileum (arrows) in double-contrast.

contrast and use dilute barium, 40% w/v, infused at a rate of 75–100 ml/min until the caecum is reached. High kilovoltage (120 kV) radiographs are necessary to penetrate overlapping loops. A modification of this technique enables double contrast images to be obtained. Two hundred millilitres of an 85% w/v suspension of high viscosity barium is injected at 100 ml/min. This is followed by approximately 2 l of a 0.5% solution of methylcellulose in water (Herlinger 1978) (Fig. 1.7). A similar technique using air instead of methylcellulose will provide excellent surface detail but the examination takes twice as long and success is very dependent on the experience of the operator (Herlinger 1983, Kobayashi & Nishiasawa 1976).

There is considerable disgreement concerning the relative merits of the small bowel meal and enteroclysis, even among those who have used enteroclysis widely (Marshak 1980, Pajewski et al. 1975, Dyet et al. 1976). Protagonists for the intubation technique prefer it to the small bowel meal on the grounds of improved accuracy (Sellink 1971, Fleckenstein & Pedersen 1975, Sanders & Ho 1976). However, it has disadvantages. The small bowel meal is simple, whereas enteroclysis may be uncomfortable for the patient, particularly during intubation. If

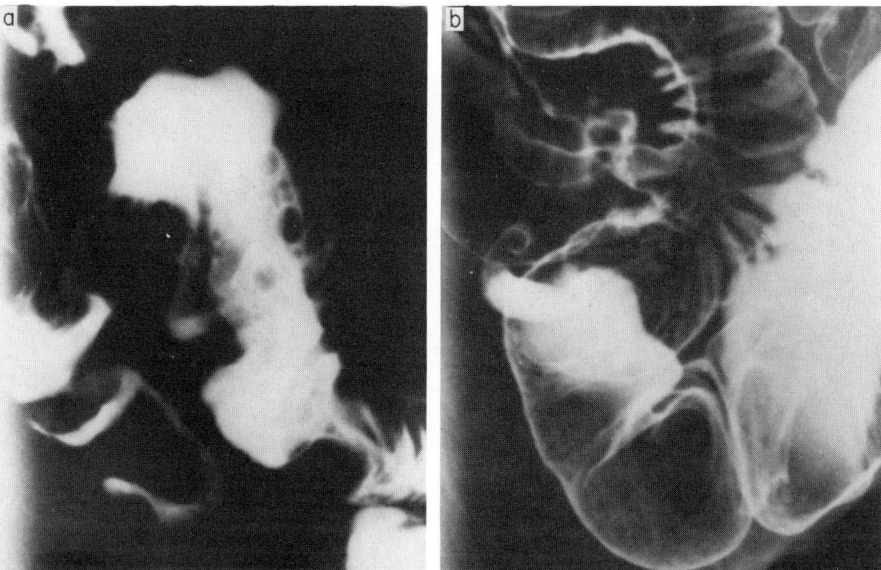

Fig. 1.6. (a) Single-contrast film of the ileo-caecal region shows distortion of the terminal ileum. The exact nature of the abnormality is unclear. (b) Same examination. Air was introduced per rectum. Eccentric involvement of the ileum with nodularity and spiculation causing distortion of folds are well shown. Proven ileocaecal Crohn's disease.

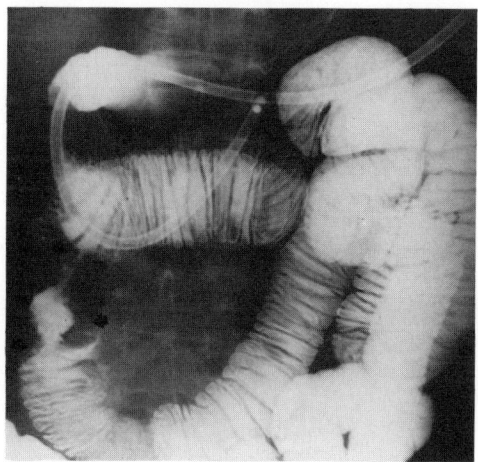

Fig. 1.7. Double-contrast enteroclysis with methylcellulose showing a markedly narrowed segment of jejunum (arrows) with shouldered distal edges due to circumferential infiltration by malignant melanoma. The jejunum on either side of the strictured area is well shown.

barium refluxes into the stomach during enteroclysis, this may cause vomiting. Though enteroclysis takes less time than the oral method, and is usually completed within 40 min, it is time-consuming for the radiologist as it requires his presence in the screening room throughout the examination. Another disadvantage is that although excellent distension and visualization of the jejunum and proximal ileum is routine with enteroclysis (Fig. 1.8), in some patients it can be difficult to show the terminal ileum due to dilution or hold-up of the barium column. Many radiologists have yet to be convinced that the intubation technique should replace the small bowel meal as the routine procedure at the present time. It is common practice to use the small bowel meal as the routine examination, reserving enteroclysis for difficult clinical problems. These include: known, complex small bowel disease; obstruction, where identification of the site and extent of the obstructing lesion is important; or a preceeding equivocal small bowel meal (Herlinger 1978, Dyet et al. 1976, Maglinte et al. 1984).

Other methods of visualization

Attempts have been made to improve small bowel visualization by other methods. Miller

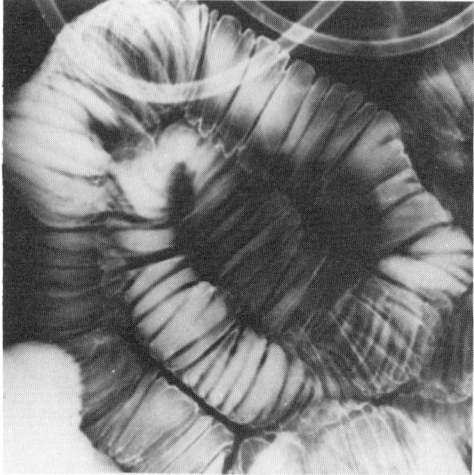

Fig. 1.8. Enteroclysis. Excellent demonstration of jejunum.

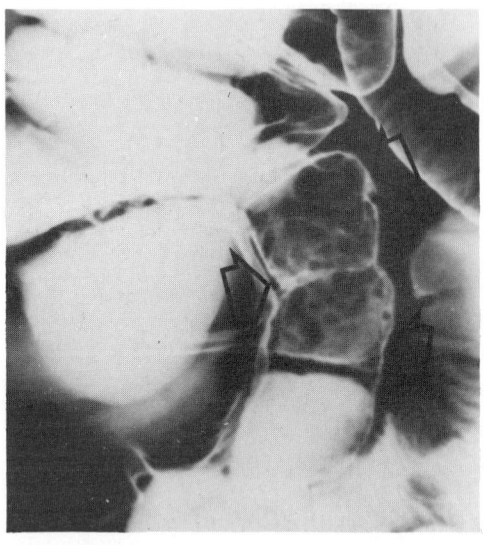

Fig. 1.9. Double-contrast view of the terminal ileum obtained during a barium enema examination in a 16-year-old boy showing the characteristic nodular appearance of lymphoid hyperplasia — normal at this age.

obtained retrograde filling of the ileum by introducing barium per rectum (Miller 1965). It is possible to examine the entire small bowel in this way though the technique has many technical disadvantages: the ileocaecal valve may remain competent preventing reflux of barium, overlapping colonic loops may obscure the small bowel, and the examination may be painful. However, a modification of this technique is to attempt, in the appropriate clinical setting, to visualize the terminal ileum during a barium enema. Reflux into the small bowel does not always occur but, with the use of intravenous glucagon, it is usually successful (Violon et al. 1981). This method gives excellent visualization of the terminal ileum (Fig. 1.9). Another interesting method of small bowel visualization includes the use of the synthetic C-terminal octopeptide of cholecystokinin. Given intravenously after the barium has left the stomach, it increases intestinal peristalsis to such an extent that the barium reaches the terminal ileum within 15 min (Efsing & Lindroth 1980). Until recently, however, this hormone has not been readily available and there have been insufficient large-scale studies performed to determine its usefulness.

Abnormal findings on barium studies of the small bowel are described in appropriate chapters in this text. A useful classification of abnormalities in small intestinal contour and calibre has been put forward by Goldberg & Sheft (1976). The appearances in inflammatory diseases of the small bowel are well described by Pringot & Bodart (1983). Normal and abnormal findings on enteroclysis are excellently described by Sellink (1976).

Angiography

The small bowel derives its blood supply from the superior mesenteric artery (SMA). This may be catheterized using a variety of pre-shaped catheters via a percutaneous transfemoral or transaxillary approach.

The main indication for angiography is gastrointestinal haemorrhage. Bleeding from the small bowel may occasionally be massive but it is often chronic or intermittent (Bookstein 1982). Haemorrhage may arise from tumours (Fig. 1.10), from arteriovenous malformations (angiodysplasias) (Fig. 1.11), from aneurysms (traumatic or mycotic), in association with ectopic gastric mucosa as in Meckel's diverticulum, or as a post-surgical complication. In acute bleeding angiography

Assessment of Small Intestinal Disease

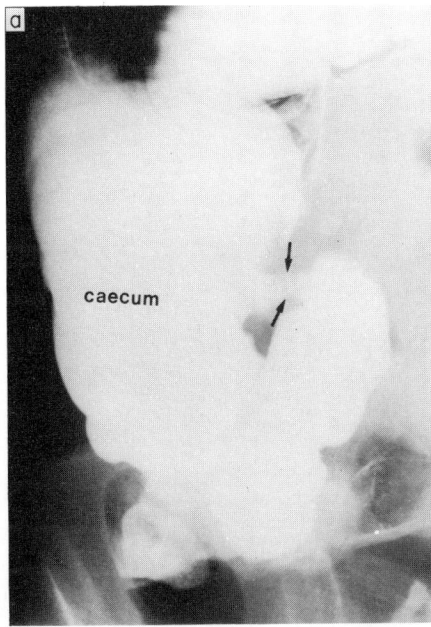
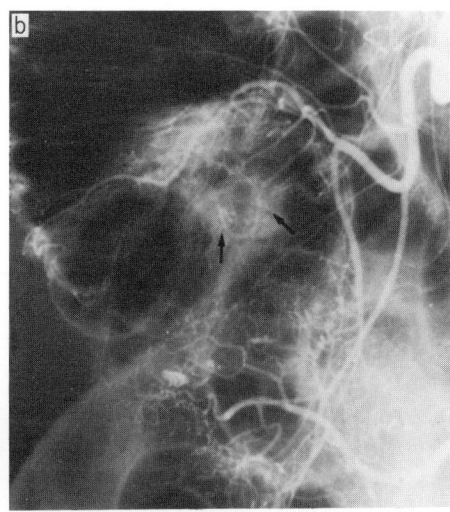

Fig. 1.10. (a) Retrograde filling of the terminal ileum during a barium enema reveals a short stricture immediately proximal to the ileo-caecal valve. (b) Same patient. Superior mesenteric angiogram showing an abnormal tumour circulation in the same area quite unlike the neovascularity of an angiodysplasia. This lesion proved to be an adenocarcinoma of the terminal ileum. Air was introduced per rectum to outline the caecum and distal ileum.

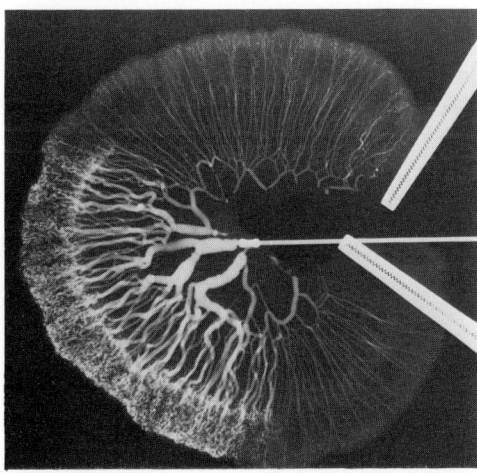

Fig. 1.11. Barium injected into a surgically removed section of small bowel reveals the characteristic appearance of a large angiodysplasia. (Courtesy of Dr J.J. Bookstein, San Diego.)

is not usually performed unless conservative management has failed or surgery is planned (Welch & Hedberg 1973). It is most likely to detect the extravasation if the bleeding is occurring at a rate greater than 0.5 ml/min (Baum 1983). In chronic bleeding, angiography is usually performed only after all other investigations have proved negative. This requires high quality studies with magnification or subtraction radiographs in order to show an abnormality such as angiodysplasia (Bookstein 1982).

In addition to its diagnostic role in small bowel bleeding, angiography can be used for treatment. Firstly, it may assist the surgeon. Using a side-winder catheter and a soft-tipped J-shaped guidewire, first and second order branches of the SMA can be selectively catheterized. A lesion such as an angiodysplasia, which can be extremely difficult to identify at surgery, may thus be accurately localized. Operative identification can be made easier by injecting methylene blue at superselective angiography immediately before surgery (Fig. 1.12). Secondly, therapeutic catheter embolization may be useful either as a palliative procedure before operation or as a permanent procedure in patients considered unsuitable for surgery.

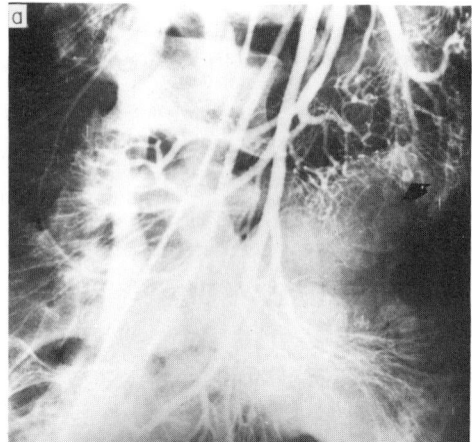

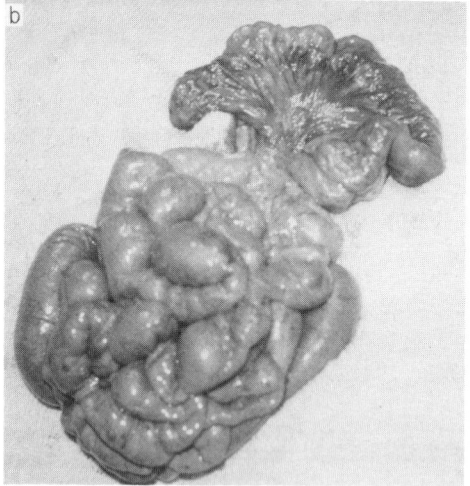

Fig. 1.12. (a) Superior mesenteric arteriogram showing a small bleeding lesion (arrow). As it was considered that this small lesion would be difficult to localize at operation, a catheter was selectively advanced into the branch supplying the lesion and the patient was taken to theatre with the catheter *in situ*. (b) Methylene blue injected at operation enabled the involved segment to be readily identified. A small ulcerated jejunal diverticulum was removed. A Meckel's diverticulum was also removed although this contained no gastric mucosa. The patient has remained well. (Courtesy of T.A.S. Buist, Edinburgh.)

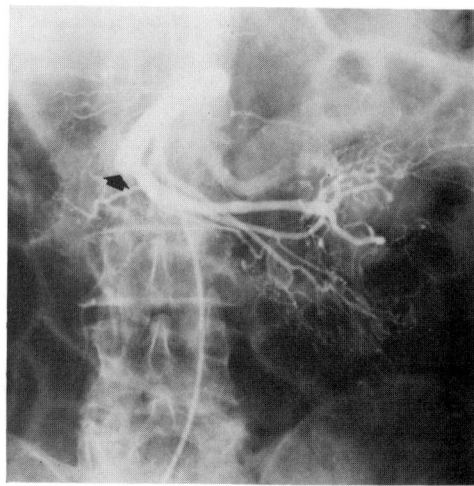

Fig. 1.13. A superior mesenteric angiogram showing a major occlusion (arrow). Only the proximal jejunal branches have filled with contrast.

The small bowel is poorly supplied with collateral vessels and the SMA can be regarded as an end-arterial circulation (Martin *et al.* 1982). Active bleeding may be stopped by selecting a small arterial branch and either infusing a vasoconstrictor (e.g. vasopressin) or embolization using particulate emboli such as Gelfoam or Ivalon (Bookstein 1982). Neither is without hazard and may lead to bowel infarction (Berardi 1974, Bookstein 1982). Particulate embolization should be considered as a primary procedure only in extreme circumstances.

Another role for angiography is in the preoperative demonstration of the site and extent of acute mesenteric occlusion (Fig. 1.13). Although an occlusion may be shown, 22–50% of all cases of ischaemic bowel disease are due to non-occlusive mesenteric ischaemia. This condition is associated with a high mortality, usually due to delay in diagnosis, but it can be recognized at angiography (Williams & Kim 1971). Arteriography shows generalized vasoconstriction with narrowing at the origins of multiple branches of the SMA, irregularity and beading of the intestinal branches, spasm of the intestinal arcades and impaired filling of intramural vessels. These changes may be reversible following infusion of a vasodilator (e.g. papaverine) (Siegelman *et al.* 1974). Finally in patients with chronic ischaemia due to stenoses of the coeliac axis, the superior or inferior mesenteric artery, it is possible to treat the lesions by balloon angioplasty (Furrer *et al.* 1980).

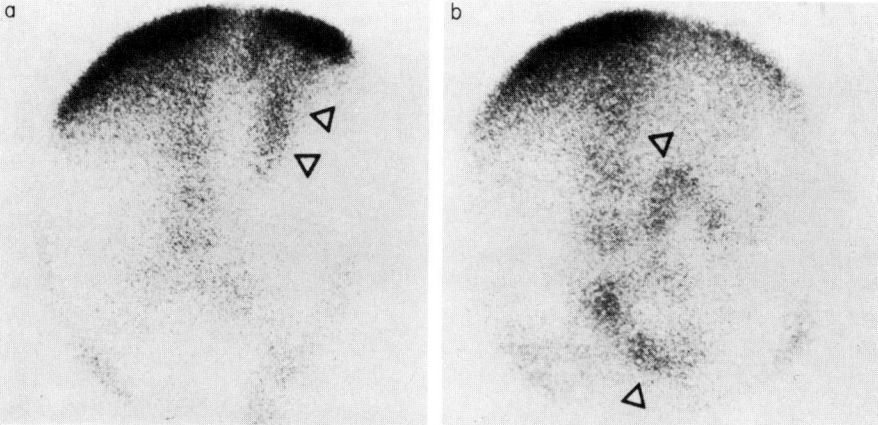

Fig. 1.14. (a) Gastrointestinal bleeding. Tc-99 m sulphur colloid scan. Area of increased uptake in the left upper quadrant at 10 min following injection. (b) The tracer has progressed through the bowel 30 min later. This bleeding lesion (an angiodysplasia) was thought to be in the proximal jejunum close to the duodeno-jejunal flexure. Angiography for precise localization was not undertaken. However, at operation, the lesion was eventually located 210 cm distal to the D–J flexure. Precise localization of the lesion can be difficult on isotope scanning.

Isotope imaging

Radionuclide scanning may be used in the investigation of chronic intestinal blood loss, acute haemorrhage and in the detection of inflammatory masses.

Chronic blood loss

In intermittent chronic bleeding, radionuclides including 99m-Tc or Indium-111 labelled red blood cells have been used (Ferrant et al. 1980, Winzelberg et al. 1979). In practice the results can sometimes be disappointing as small bleeding sites may be difficult to detect because of the high background activity that occurs with blood pool agents (Alavi 1980).

Acute haemorrhage

In acute haemorrhage, bleeding rates as low as 0.1 ml/min have been identified (Alavi 1980). A bolus injection of 99m-Tc sulphur colloid is rapidly removed by the reticuloendothelial system, principally the liver and spleen. If bleeding occurs during passage of the isotope through the circulation, a local area of increased uptake will be seen. Subsequent images will show change in position of the focal area of uptake indicating its intraluminal location (Fig. 1.14). Uptake in the liver and spleen may obscure bleeding sites in the upper abdomen which can lead to false negative scans (Winzelberg et al. 1979). Though theoretically more sensitive than angiography (Hattner 1983), isotope studies are not widely employed in Britain. In part this reflects the lack of availability of the technique but it is also because the precise site of bleeding, which may be critical at surgery, is often difficult to localize.

Pertechnetate is secreted by gastric mucosa, although the exact mechanism involved has been questioned (Spencer et al. 1983). Meckel's diverticula which bleed invariably contain ectopic gastric mucosa and this has allowed imaging with Tc-99m pertechnetate. The detection rate is high, and false negative rates as low as 10–20% have been reported (Cooney et al. 1982). However, the false positive rate may be as high as 50% though many of these patients will have other pathological lesions at operation (Cooney et al. 1982). Attempts have been made to improve the detection rate of the Meckel's scan by using either pentagastrin, glucagon or cimetidine (Spencer et al. 1983, Treves et al. 1978, Anderson et al. 1980, Petrokuli et al. 1978).

Protein-losing enteropathy

Protein loss into the small intestine may be detected by using Tc-99 Sb colloid (Soucy et al. 1983) or Indium-labelled transferrin (Saverymuttu et al. 1983a).

Inflammatory masses

Various isotopes have been used for localization of inflammatory masses within the abdomen. Indium-111 labelled leucocytes and Gallium-67 are the most widely used. Ga-67 has an affinity for inflammatory tissue but lack of specificity (Hoffer 1980) and the difficulty in differentiating normal faecal excretion from areas of diseased bowel has led to problems in scan interpretation (Kadir & Strauss 1979). The images obtained with In-111 leucocytes are easier to interpret than Ga-67 studies since no colonic activity is normally seen (Coleman et al. 1981). A study comparing In-111 labelled leucocytes and Ga-67 in patients with suspected focal infection found a high false negative rate (27%) with leucocyte scans in patients with foci of infection of longer than 2 weeks duration (Sfakianakis et al. 1982). A 10% false negative with Ga-67 occurred in patients with acute infections of less than 1 week duration, but no focal infection was missed when both studies were performed (Sfakianakis et al. 1982). This suggests that the labelled leucocyte scan is highly accurate in the detection of acute focal infection. Indium-III labelled leucocyte scanning may prove to be a valuable method of assessing inflammation in small intestinal Crohn's disease (Saverymuttu et al. 1983b). Gallium may be the more reliable when the clinical history suggests a low grade chronic infection, but, if the Gallium scan is positive, other causes of false positive scans, such as tumours, should be excluded.

Bowel viability

Finally, a somewhat speculative application of nuclear medicine studies of the small bowel is in the intra-operative assessment of bowel viability following gut infarction (Zarins et al. 1974, Moossa et al. 1974, Kressel et al. 1978). Reactive hyperaemia has been a consistent finding after revascularization of ischaemic muscle, and is also a good predictor of myocardial viability after coronary occlusion (Matthews et al. 1971) and of intestinal viability in animal experiments (Zarins et al. 1974, Moossa et al. 1974). Reactive hyperaemia can be assessed in theatre by the injection of 99m-Tc labelled albumin microspheres into the SMA during operation followed by imaging with a portable gamma camera. It is possible that in selected patients with small bowel infarction this technique could assist the surgeon during a revascularization procedure.

C. SMALL INTESTINAL BIOPSY
ASHLEY B. PRICE

Introduction 12
Handling the biopsy 13
Dissecting microscopy 13
Normal mucosa 14
Assessment of abnormalities 15
Morphometry 19
Special techniques 19
Transmission electron microscopy 19
Scanning electron microscopy 20

Introduction

The intestinal villi are delicate structures and a biopsy is easily damaged to a degree that makes interpretation difficult. Care in handling and processing the specimen is therefore critical and forms the foundation of an accurate clinico-pathological assessment. Apart from technical failures, other reasons for poor interpretation of small intestinal biopsies are either failure of the clinician to provide adequate information or failure of the pathologist to appreciate either the spectrum of normal histology or the significance of his observations (Perera et al. 1975). The clinician must also realize the limitation of the questions biopsy can answer. Furthermore the sampling error restricts its value in focal lesions and in those whose major impact is deep to the mucosa.

Before the biopsy the clinician should pause to consider the likely need for special techniques beyond routine light microscopy, such as immunofluorescence or scanning electron microscopy. It is too late to initiate such investigations with the biopsy already in a formalin fixative or processed to a paraffin block. Good communication will prevent most pitfalls and this is best achieved by regular clinico-pathological meetings between pathologist and gastroenterologist.

Handling the biopsy

The biopsy should be gently teased out of its capsule onto a suitable flat surface with the minimum of trauma and the villous surface uppermost. Orientation is commonly onto card, glass or Gelfoam. The most readily available is card which needs to be of good quality for otherwise its fibres adhere to the specimen which then damage the microtomist's knife and consequently the section.

Dissecting microscopy

At this juncture many clinicians examine the biopsy with the dissecting microscope but if this is done the biopsy must not be allowed to dry. A drop of saline, or fixative, if not contra-indicated by subsequent techniques, is adequate. The appearances of jejunal mucosa seen with the dissecting microscope can be graded as shown below (Lee & Toner 1980):

Grade	Appearance
I	Finger villi only (Fig. 1.15a)
II	Leaf villi only, or leaf and finger villi (Fig. 1.15b)
III	Leaf villi with some fusion to form small ridges or convolutions
IV	Convolutions or ridges with no recognizable villi (Fig. 1.15c)
V	Notable flattening of the mucosa, often with mosaic pattern (Fig. 1.15d)

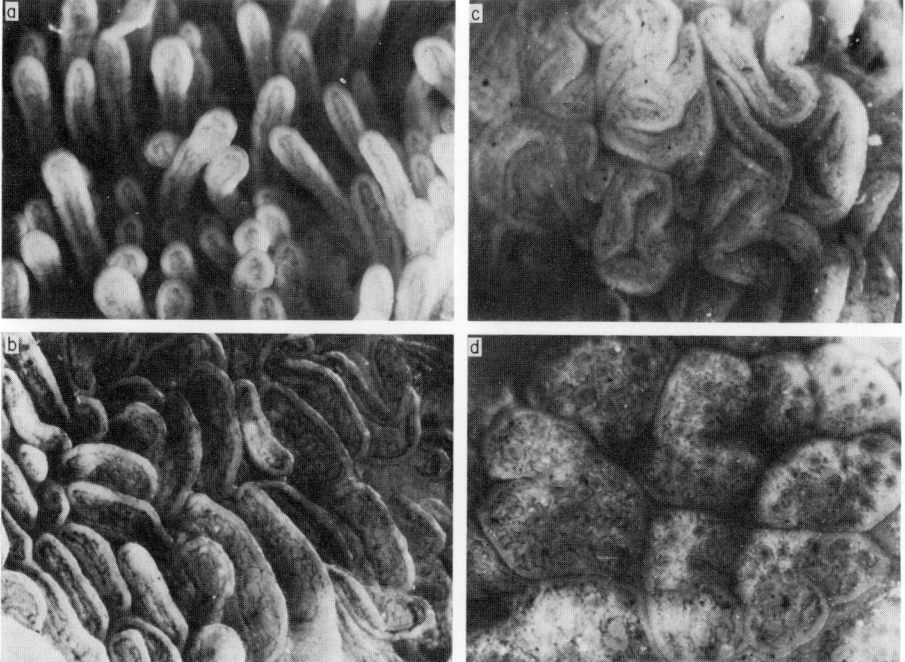

Fig. 1.15. (a) Finger-like villi, Grade 1. (b) Broad leafy villi, Grade 2. (c) Convoluted mucosa, Grade 4. (d) A flat mucosa with mosaic pattern. Grade 5. (× 70) (Courtesy of Dr. J.S. Stewart.)

Dissecting microscopy, however, is best carried out in the laboratory after fixation when the specimen can be handled without fear of damage. The pathology department should provide a photographic record as part of the reporting service. A polaroid camera linked to a dissecting microscope is a convenient tool and the subsequent picture can be attached to the biopsy report.

The biopsy must then be placed in a suitable fixative solution within a few minutes of being taken. The routine fixative for light microscopy is a matter of individual choice, 10% formol-saline being the most widely used. Suitably fixed and photographed, the tissue is processed through to paraffin wax and sectioned perpendicular to the mucosal surface. Haematoxylin and eosin is the standard tissue stain. If the tissue was poorly orientated initially, the technical staff can still produce a satisfactory result by correction at the stage of paraffin embedding. After this, if still unsatisfactory, cutting levels into the biopsy often yields some crypts and villi sufficiently orientated to exclude gross disease. Inspection of 300−600 µm of the central core of the biopsy, either at 50 µm levels or by serial ribbons, is usually satisfactory.

Normal mucosa

The villi are covered by a single layer of columnar absorptive cells (the enterocytes), each with a well-defined brush border (Fig. 1.16). Goblet cells are scattered amongst these enterocytes, the number increasing towards the ileum where the villi become taller. The surface epithelium also contains darkly staining intraepithelial lymphocytes (Ferguson 1977) enmeshed between the enterocytes. Normally these number 6−40/100 enterocytes (Ferguson & Murray 1971). They are a different population from the lymphocytes in the lamina propria and are believed to be of T-cell type (Selby *et al.* 1981).

Two other cell types form part of the epithelial covering of the villus: 'M cells' and 'tuft' cells. The M cell (Owen & Jones 1974) is an epithelial cell present over lymphoid follicles and Peyer's patches. It is void of

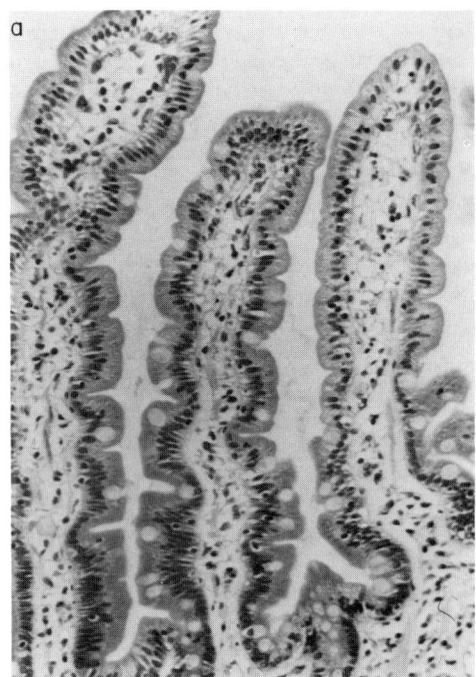

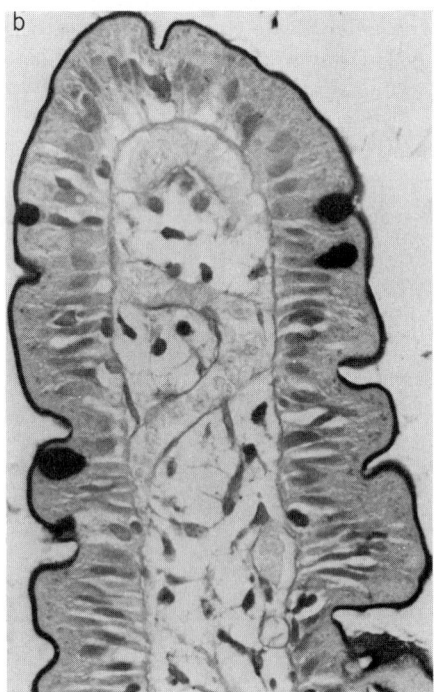

Fig. 1.16. (a) Normal villi covered by a single regular layer of enterocytes (H.E. × 315). (b) The periodic acid−Schiff reagent demonstrates the neat brush border and scattered goblet cells of the villus tip. (P.A.S. × 800).

microvilli but has low surface convolutions. Lymphocytes are present in pockets seemingly within the cells but actually surrounded by cell cytoplasm and produced by invagination of the M-cell surface. Evidence suggests the M cells have a role in protein uptake and are a route for selective antigen absorption, but at the present time the cells have been more easily demonstrated in animal than in human mucosa.

The 'tuft cell' (Nabeyama & Leblond 1974) has a well-developed 'tuft' of microvilli that extends beyond those of the normal enterocyte. The cores of the microvilli penetrate the apical cytoplasm and surround the superficial organelles. In this region many tubular invaginations of the cell surface are present. The role of the 'tuft' cell is still unknown.

At the base of the villi are the crypts of Lieberkühn which extend downwards to the level of the muscularis mucosae. These contain the enteroblasts that mature upwards onto the villous surface. Paneth cells and enterochromafin cells of the APUD system (cf. Chapter 23) are also found within the crypts.

The villous core and the lamina propria around the crypts comprise a delicate framework of connective tissue, blood vessels and lymphatics. Small numbers of plasma cells, lymphocytes and histiocytes are present. Only an occasional neutrophil leucocyte is normally seen and there may be isolated eosinophils. Neutrophils within the crypts or insinuated between the surface enterocytes are abnormal.

Good biopsies should contain muscularis mucosae deep to the mucosa. If any Brunner's glands are seen below this, it usually infers the biopsy capsule was situated in the duodenum but occasionally small numbers of Brunner's glands occur in the upper jejunum. Isolated lymphoid follicles within the mucosa that may produce distortion of the villous pattern are an acceptable part of the normal picture (Fig. 1.17).

The villi are disposed in a regular fashion and vary between 300 μm to 500 μm in height. Crypt depth varies from 110 μm to 230 μm (Lee & Toner 1980). The ratio, villous height : crypt depth, is a useful value in the

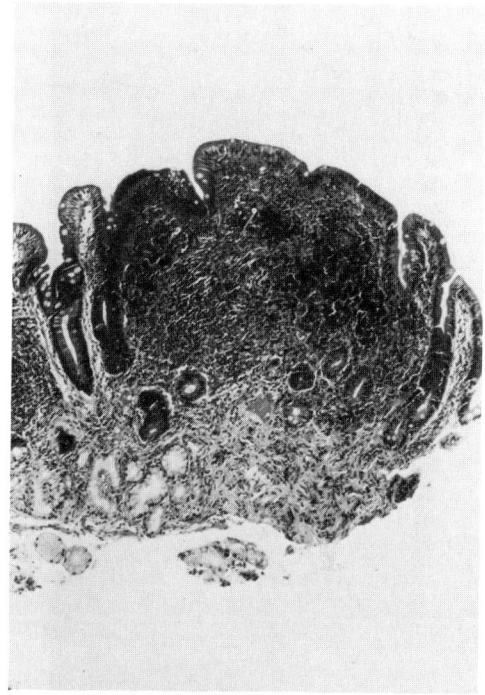

Fig. 1.17. A lymphoid follicle distorting the mucosal architecture (H.E. × 56).

assessment of minor mucosal abnormalities and in monitoring any therapeutic regimen. As a rough guide, a biopsy can be considered adequate for assessment if a row of four villi can be made out.

Assessment of abnormalities

When assessing a biopsy, it is useful to follow a standard format which must include examination of:
1 villous height and overall architecture
2 lumen and surface epithelium
3 crypts
4 cellular constituents of the lamina propria
5 abnormal deposits.

Although this account of how to assess a small intestinal biopsy has been compartmentalized, in practice the pathologist's diagnostic appreciation is usually of the whole picture rather than the sum of the parts.

In almost all mucosal disorders of the small intestine there is some alteration in villous architecture and this is assessed in the

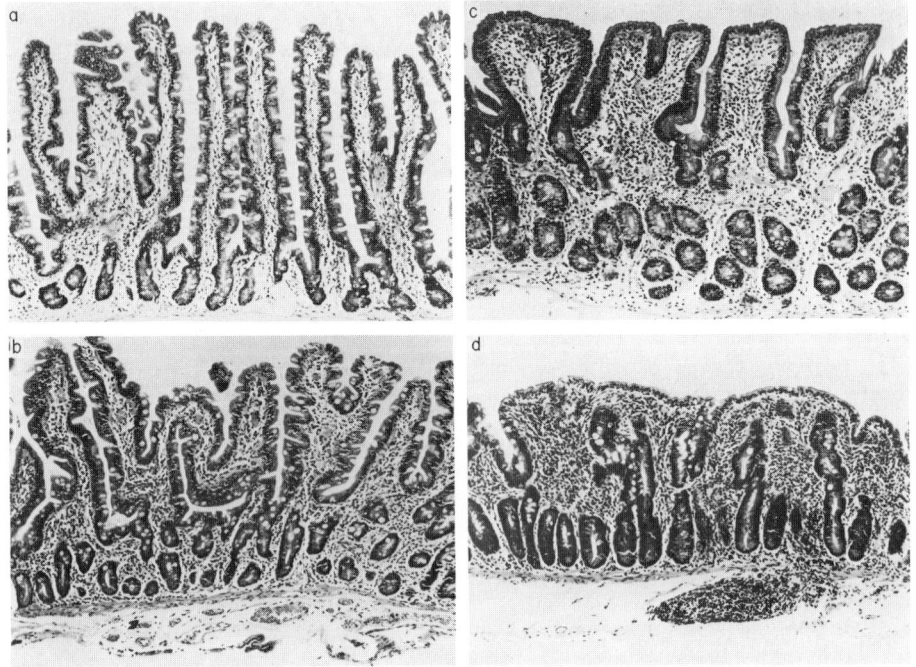

Fig. 1.18. (a) Normal jejunal mucosa corresponding to Fig. 1.15a. (b) Joining leafy villi corresponding to Fig. 1.15b. (c) Moderate partial villous atrophy corresponding to Fig. 1.15c. (d) Subtotal villous atrophy, corresponding to Fig. 1.15d. (H.E. × 100) (Courtesy of Dr. J.S. Stewart)

simplest terms as being mild, moderate or severe (Fig. 1.18). Interpretation must take note of possible artefacts and be tempered with knowledge of the normal range for a particular geographical situation. In tropical climates, for example, the leaf villus predominates and may be accompanied by short ridges. Villus height may be reduced ranging from 150–430 μm. A report of moderate villous atrophy in temperate climates might therefore be regarded as within normal limits in the tropics. Biopsies from children also require special evaluation. Their villi are shorter, the crypts deeper, and inflammatory cells may be increased (Penna et al. 1981).

Tangentially cut villi are a common source of misinterpretation. Significant tangential cutting is recognized by seeing large numbers of crypts in cross section and by appreciating multi-layering of the nuclei of the surface enterocytes. Tangentially cut villi appear broad and blunt leading to a false interpretation of villous atrophy while the absence of the muscularis may also cause the villi to appear artificially broad.

Villi

The assessment begins with whether the villi are of normal height, or show degrees of villous atrophy, which can be mild, moderate or severe. Shiner & Doniach (1960) coined two terms, 'partial villous atrophy' (Fig. 1.18c), which is subclassified mild, moderate or severe, and 'subtotal villous atrophy', indicating a flat biopsy (Fig. 1.18d). This initial architectural assessment is subjective but morphometric analysis provides objective measurements.

Obvious villous atrophy of varying degrees is the main morphological feature in biopsies from patients with coeliac disease, tropical sprue, infectious gastroenteritis, and Kwashiorkor. Accompanying the atrophy is an increase in crypt depth so that, contrary to expectation, the total mucosal thickness increases. Thus in the subtotal villous atrophy of severe untreated coeliac disease the mucosa is not thin but thicker than

Assessment of Small Intestinal Disease

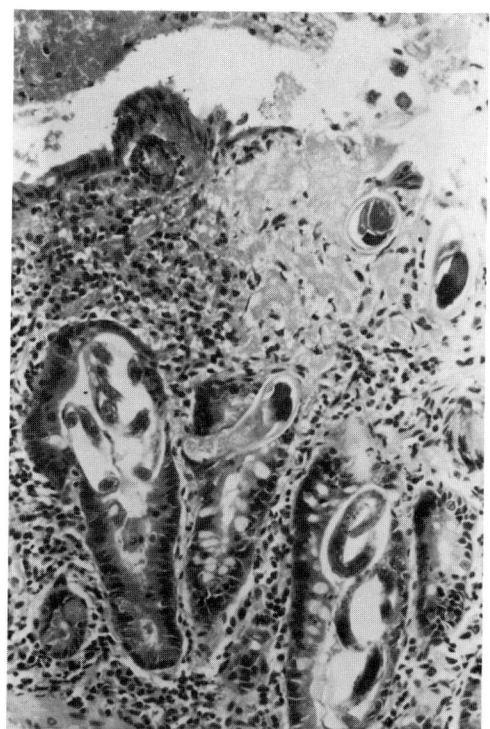

Fig. 1.19. The worms and larvae of *Strongyloides stercoralis* within the crypts (H.E. × 180).

normal. This pattern of villous atrophy is the *hyperplastic form*, in contrast to villous atrophy with hypoplastic crypts, where the crypt depth is diminished and the mucosa is thinned. This pattern, the *hypoplastic form*, is seen in radiation damage, ischaemia, some patients with severe malabsorption unresponsive to treatment with a gluten-free diet and to a mild degree and rarely in vitamin B_{12} and folate deficiency.

Very occasionally a biopsy may exhibit not atrophy of villi but an increase in villus height and crypt depth, the *hypertrophic pattern*. This is seen as an adaptive response in the ileum following extensive small bowel resection (Chapter 6), and in association with glucagonoma (Chapter 23).

Following the assessment of the villus and crypt architecture, the individual constituents of the mucosa can be studied in greater detail and it is easy to overlook examination of the lumen. Giardiasis is the commonest parasite seen, though freshly prepared smears from the mucus covering the biopsy gives a higher detection rate. In tropical climates varieties of worm (Fig. 1.19) may be observed and in immunodeficient patients cryptosporidium and isospora seen on the luminal aspect of the enterocyte can be misinterpreted as stain deposit (Chapter 8).

Lymphocytes

The intraepithelial lymphocytes can be counted per 100 enterocytes (Ferguson & Murray 1971) or per unit length of muscularis mucosa (Skinner & Whitehead 1976). The latter gives the total number per unit length or area of intestine but the former method has the advantage that it can be carried out on nearly any quality of biopsy and it is a simply performed useful clinical guide. However, neither method reflects the absolute pool of lymphocytes in the mucosa. The highest counts are found in untreated coeliac disease and usually diminish in parallel with the return of the normal villous architecture. Abnormal counts may persist in some patients in whom the villi have returned to normal after gluten withdrawal and normal counts may be noted in cases in which, despite treatment, the mucosa remains flat. The count is raised in most cases of tropical sprue, in post-infective malabsorption and many other disorders. In a few patients, unexplained high counts may occur in otherwise normal biopsies. The main value of the intraepithelial lymphocyte count is in monitoring the response of the mucosa to treatment. Marsh (1982) claims that the mitotic index of the epithelial lymphocytes is one of the most specific tests for coeliac disease when considering a flat biopsy.

Enterocytes

An alteration of the regular line of columnar enterocytes to one of low cuboidal cells with loss of their pencil-like brush border and nuclear polarity occurs in coeliac disease (Fig. 1.20). It is nearly always accompanied by increased numbers of lymphocytes and moderate to severe changes in villous architecture. These changes occur in parallel

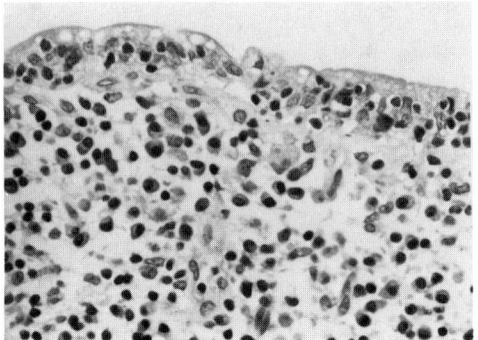

Fig. 1.20. The surface enterocytes in the flat mucosa of coeliac disease. There is loss of nuclear polarity and an increase in intraepithelial lymphocytes (H.E. × 800).

and hence atrophy in the presence of normal enterocytes must raise doubt about a diagnosis of coeliac disease. Rarely, the enterocytes may be macrocytic, a feature restricted to the crypts in conditions such as vitamin B_{12} and folate deficiency, or following myleran therapy. Polymorphs infiltrating the enterocyte layer signify a jejunitis suggesting Crohn's disease or other inflammatory conditions.

Other enterocyte abnormalities include the presence of stainable iron which can be a feature of transfusion siderosis, haemochromatosis or rarer abnormalities in iron transport, while in a-β-lipoproteinaemia the enterocytes are characteristically vacuolated due to the accumulation of fat (cf. Chapter 3). Metaplasia of surface enterocytes can also be observed in specimens. Gastric epithelium is well documented in duodenal biopsies from patients with high acid levels, while pyloric gland metaplasia may occur as a response to chronic inflammation (Price 1980).

Crypts of Lieberkühn

After the villi the crypts are examined. They are elongated in the hyperplastic pattern of mucosal atrophy (Figs. 1.18d) with increased numbers of mitoses. In the hypoplastic pattern they are short and, as already noted, in certain conditions the enteroblasts may exhibit macrocytic changes. The presence of crypt abscesses, like the presence of intraepithelial polymorphs, defines a jejunitis and is in itself non-specific. Focal crypt necrosis is an appearance seen in graft-versus-host disease.

Of the other cellular constituents within the crypts, the numbers of Paneth cells may vary (Sandow & Whitehead 1979). In chronic inflammatory conditions there is often a rise, while in coeliac patients with a poor response to gluten withdrawal, the number may be diminished (Creamer & Pink 1967), though this is disputed (Scott & Brandtzaeg 1981). Abnormalities of Paneth cells at electron microscope level have been described in acrodermatitis enteropathica (Bohane et al. 1977). There is little biopsy data available on variations in the other crypt constituent, the APUD cell (Challacombe & Robertson 1977).

Lamina propria

The lamina propria is next assessed for alterations in the normal cell population or for the presence of an abnormal infiltrate. Relative changes in the normal constituents are non-specific with only a few patterns being diagnostic. Increased numbers of neutrophils and crypt abscesses can be seen in small bowel Crohn's disease while large numbers of eosinophils are seen in parasitic diseases, eosinophilic gastroenteritis and allergic gastroenteropathy of children.

Plasma cell numbers alter to some degree in nearly all small intestinal disorders and become the predominant cell in the lamina propria in coeliac disease. When the increase is insufficient to appear as the primary cause for villous and crypt abnormalities, plasmacytoid lymphoma and α-heavy chain disease must be considered (cf. Chapter 10). An increase in the lymphocyte population of the lamina propria is also part of the non-specific general response to many mucosal 'insults'. Like plasma cells, when they are seen in great excess at the expense of other cell types malignant lymphoma is the likely diagnosis. A confident diagnosis of lymphoma is always difficult, however, from a biopsy alone. The occasional lymphoid follicle may be seen normally but more than two, especially if associated with reduced

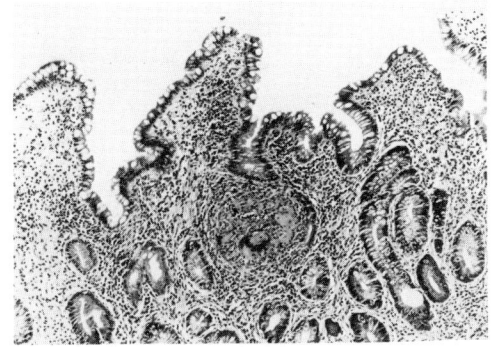

Fig. 1.21. A giant-cell granuloma beneath the surface epithelium from a case of Crohn's disease (H.E. × 157).

numbers of plasma cells, is likely to represent nodular lymphoid hyperplasia and be part of the immunodeficiency syndrome (cf. Chapter 8).

An increase in histiocytes is also likely to be a non-specific mucosal response but certain patterns may be diagnostic. Thus an obvious granuloma in patients from a temperate climate almost certainly indicates Crohn's disease (Fig. 1.21) or, occasionally, tuberculosis. Diffuse infiltration by large periodic acid-Schiff (PAS) reagent positive histiocytes is characteristic of Whipple's disease (cf. Chapter 16), while in a small percentage of coeliac patients, small numbers of highly 'atypical histiocytes' may herald the onset of malignant histiocytosis (Isaacson 1980).

Abnormal infiltrates

Having evaluated the major mucosal compartments, deposits of abnormal materials within the lamina propria should be sought. In collagenous sprue a dense band of collagen appears beneath the surface epithelium, while in Waldenstrom's macroglobulinaemia, prominent hyaline eosinophilic amorphous masses are present in the lamina propria (cf. Chapter 13). Amyloid will give the characteristic red staining with Congo Red and a green birefringence under polarized light. It is easily overlooked unless the diagnosis is suggested by other clinical features.

Morphometry

In routine diagnosis the subjective opinion of the pathologist is adequate but with minor degrees of abnormality or changing degrees of atrophy it is useful to have an objective measurement. Detailed morphometry is time-consuming but there are simple ways of providing values for villus height, crypt depth and intraepithelial lymphocyte numbers. Since many patients with small intestinal disease require a series of biopsies, the measurements form an objective guide to progress and therapeutic response.

The simplest of the methods involves a calibrated micrometer inserted into the eyepiece of the microscope. From this it is easy to measure villus height and crypt depth. A modified linear intercepts technique (Dunnill & Whitehead 1972) will provide an index related to the surface to volume ratio of the mucosa and is suitable for mild degrees of partial villous atrophy. For counting cell types within the mucosa the point counting concept (Aherne & Dunnill 1982) is adequate, though time-consuming. As the most constant structure in a biopsy is the muscularis mucosae, where possible measurements should be expressed per unit of its length (Skinner & Whitehead 1976).

Special techniques

In addition to standard histological stains on paraffin-embedded sections, there is an enlarging battery of immunohistochemical techniques, many incorporating the use of monoclonal antibodies. Most laboratories now carry out simple peroxidase techniques to demonstrate immunoglobulin classes, while more sophisticated procedures such as the identification of lymphocyte subsets is still in the realm of the few.

Transmission electron microscopy

Transmission electron microscopy (TEM) plays little part in routine diagnostic problems but it does have an important role in the understanding of the mechanisms of

20   *Chapter 1*

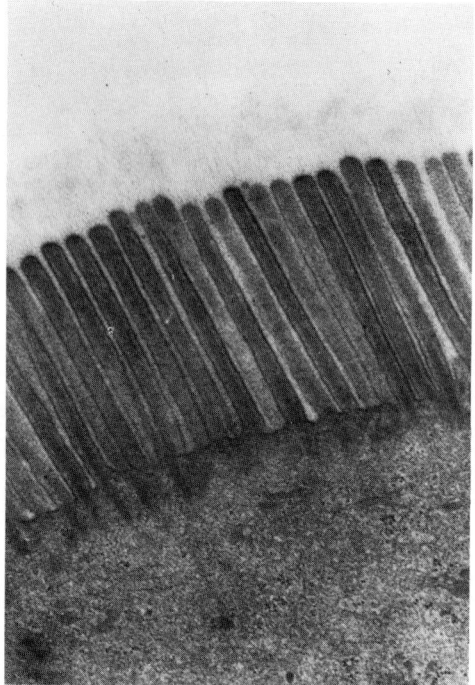

Fig. 1.22. The normal brush border of an enterocyte (E.M. × 56,400). (Courtesy of Dr. A. Phillips.)

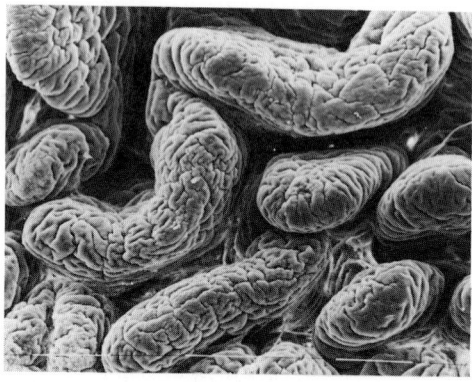

Fig. 1.23. Normal villi seen by scanning electron microscopy (× 280).

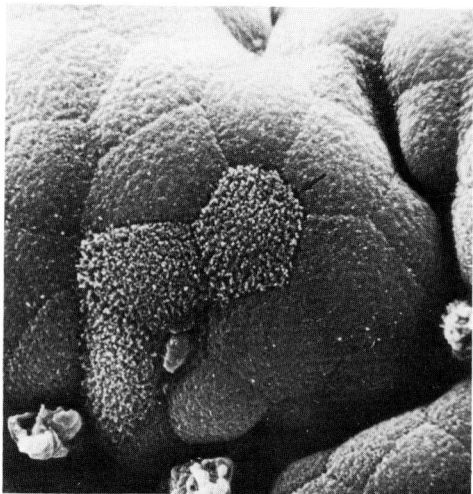

Fig. 1.24. A scanning electron micrograph of the villous surface showing the hexagonal enterocytes. Early extrusion of cells is also seen (arrow) (× 3560). (Courtesy of Dr. A. Phillips.)

disease. For example, in Whipple's disease TEM reveals rod-shaped organisms in the lamina propria (cf. Chapter 16) and in the recovery phase the macrophages are seen to contain their partially degraded cell walls.

Only a 18 mm cube of mucosa is required for electron microscopy and this should be carefully removed from the fresh unfixed biopsy using a new razor blade. It is then placed in special fixative, normally buffered glutaraldehyde, but when EM is anticipated it is preferable to seek advice direct from the laboratory.

By TEM the enterocytes covering the normal villi are seen in close apposition, their lateral walls held together by desmosomes and by an apical junction complex. The most distinctive feature is the luminal striated border of organized rows of microvilli (Fig. 1.22). The villi in turn are covered by a specialized 'fuzzycoat' or glycocalyx comprising mainly sulphated acid-mucopolysaccharides. The villous cores contain actin filaments which link with myosin elements of the terminal web. The system provides motility to the microvillous system.

The remainder of the enterocyte cytoplasm contains the usual complement of organelles and membrane systems. Within the crypts the enterocytes are more primitive; there are fewer microvilli, less well developed organelles and numerous free ribosomes.

Scanning electron microscopy

This technique is not a diagnostic tool but, like TEM, provides another dimension in the appreciation of mucosal abnormalities. The tissue sample does not require trimming as for TEM but the same fixative may be used. Subsequently the technical principle involved is to treat the biopsy so that it can be coated with a conducting metallic layer, usually a gold-containing compound.

With low-power scanning electron microscopy (SEM) the three dimensional pattern of the villous mucosal surface is clear (Fig. 1.23) with the mouths of the crypts apparent between villi. At higher magnifications the goblet cells appear as dimples and the hexagonal pattern of adjacent enterocytes is characteristic (Fig. 1.24), while at the highest powers the microvilli can be seen.

D. INTESTINAL FUNCTION TESTS
M.G. RINSLER AND CHRISTOPHER C. BOOTH

Water and electrolytes 21
Carbohydrates 22
Tests of intestinal permeability 23
Fat 24
Bile salts 25
Protein 26
Water-soluble vitamins 27
Fat-soluble vitamins 28
Iron 29

Tests of intestinal function are complementary to the other diagnostic techniques described elsewhere in this chapter. In the diagnosis of mucosal abnormalities or of gross anatomical lesions of the small intestine, jejunal biopsy and radiological assessment are most useful. Tests of function, however, are particularly helpful in the diagnosis of sugar intolerance, in detecting defects of vitamin B_{12} absorption and in providing indirect evidence of bacterial overgrowth in the small intestine. They may also be used in monitoring the response to treatment of gluten-sensitive enteropathy.

Most absorption tests involve giving a suitable substance to the patient by mouth and sampling from blood, faeces, urine or expired air. Intraluminal aspiration is needed only occasionally. It is used primarily in studies of pancreatic function, but may also be valuable in the microbiological investigation of bacterial overgrowth in the small intestine. Intubation of segments of the small intestine with double or triple-lumen tubes, followed by the infusion of test substances together with a non-absorbable marker is valuable in the study of the physiology and pathology of intestinal absorption (Blankenhorn et al. 1955, Schedl & Clifton 1963, Fordtran et al. 1967, Rambaud et al. 1978). These techniques, however, are rarely necessary in clinical practice. Long term retention of substances such as radiolabelled iron or vitamin B_{12} may be measured using whole-body counting techniques, but the requirements for special and expensive apparatus limit their availability.

Water and electrolytes

Water and electrolytes are absorbed primarily in the jejunum, in close association with special transport mechanisms for bicarbonate, and certain sugars and amino acids. The ileum and colon avidly conserve water, sodium and chloride. In certain pathological situations, the small intestine is stimulated to secrete fluid and ions by certain hormones (VIP and prostaglandin E_2) (Field & Chang 1983) or by microbiological toxins (Sladen 1972).

Formal studies of electrolyte and water balance may be useful in the investigation of ileostomy dysfunction or sometimes when there is severe diarrhoea after small intestinal resection (Griffin et al. 1982). The faecal and urinary losses of sodium, potassium, calcium, magnesium, bicarbonate and chloride can be measured. At the same time, it is worthwhile analysing the stool contents for unabsorbed substances such as sugars. Measurement of stool electrolytes is also helpful in the investigation of diarrhoea due to purgative abuse. Excessive stool magnesium is found in patients who are surreptitiously ingesting magnesium sulphate. In suspected cases of purgative abuse it is also useful and sometimes diagnostic to examine both stool and urine for evidence of ingestion of agents such as senna or phenolphthalein.

The rare condition of congenital chlorridorrhoea (cf. Chapter 3) is diagnosed by measuring faecal electrolyte excretion. Loss of chloride ions exceeds the combined losses of sodium and potassium ions and this leads to a characteristic metabolic alkalosis (Turnberg 1971).

Carbohydrates

Glucose

Glucose is normally absorbed by a sodium-linked active transport process in the brush border membrane of the jejunum. The glucose tolerance test, although often used, is not a good measure of small intestinal function, because the rise in blood glucose may be small in normal individuals (Holdsworth 1969). It may be useful, however, in the assessment of post-gastrectomy dumping. Transient hyperglycaemia after the oral ingestion of 50 g glucose may be followed by hypoglycaemia and this is sometimes associated with weakness, faintness and sweating.

Xylose

Xylose is a pentose monosaccharide absorbed mainly in the jejunum by an energy-dependent mechanism. In man, xylose is ineffectively metabolized so that approximately half of that absorbed from an orally ingested test dose is excreted in the urine. The test is therefore useful in the diagnosis of malabsorption (Benson et al. 1957). After a dose of 25 g (150 mmol), normal adult subjects excrete more than 5 g (30 mmol) in 5 h. Lower values are found in patients with jejunal disease (Sladen & Kumar 1973) and xylose absorption is therefore useful as a screening test in patients with coeliac disease. Accurate urine collections are essential to achieve satisfactory results. Peak plasma concentrations of xylose in normal subjects exceed 2.2 mmol/l and are considerably lower in patients with proximal small intestinal disease. The best results with this test are obtained by measuring xylose in both plasma and urine. In patients with impaired renal function plasma levels alone give a qualitative index of the absorption of xylose, which is particularly useful in the older patient.

^{14}C-D-xylose breath test

Since xylose is metabolized by intestinal bacteria, the demonstration of excessive catabolism may be used as a means of detecting bacterial overgrowth in the small intestine. Xylose is labelled with ^{14}C and the amount of $^{14}CO_2$ excreted in the breath is measured after an oral test dose. With 25 g doses, the test was insufficiently sensitive but using an oral test dose of only 1 g xylose labelled with 10 µCi of ^{14}C, King et al. (1979) claim that the excretion of $^{14}CO_2$ in the breath at 30 and 60 min provides a sensitive screening test for patients with bacterial overgrowth.

Disaccharides

Disaccharides may be present in the diet as lactose and sucrose, or they are derived from the intraluminal digestion of starch and glycogen. Disaccharidases located in the brush border membrane of the enterocyte are responsible for the release of monosaccharides. Tests of absorption may therefore be used for the diagnosis of disaccharidase deficiency.

Lactose

To test lactose absorption, an oral test dose of lactose is given and glucose is measured in capillary blood in the fasting state and at 15, 30, 45, 60, 90 and 120 min after the oral load. A test dose of 50 g gives satisfactory results. In children the dose should be 2 g/kg. A flat glucose curve (rise of blood glucose less than 1.1 mmol/1 (20 mg/100 ml)) usually indicates lactose malabsorption. If at the same time the patient passes a watery stool, the demonstration of lactose in the faecal fluid by thin-layer chromatography provides confirmatory evidence.

Sucrose

A similar test is used for assessing sucrose absorption. Sucrose is given in the same

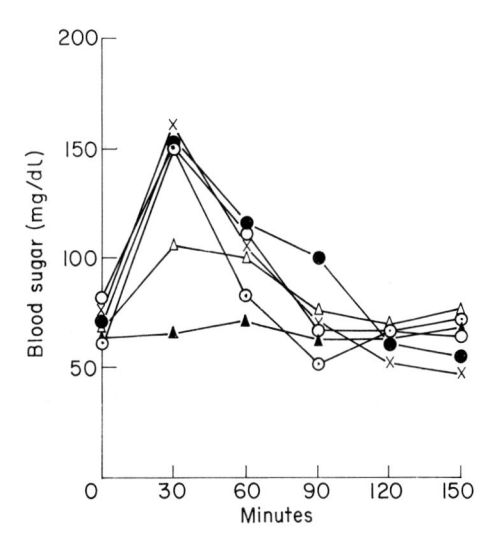

Fig. 1.25. Changes in blood glucose levels after ingestion of 50 g carbohydrate by an adult patient with sucrase−isomaltase deficiency (Neale et al. 1965). ×, 50 g glucose; ⊙, 25 g glucose + fructose; ●, 50 g maltose; ○, 50 g lactose; ▲, 50 g sucrose; △, 50 g starch.

dose as used for the lactose test and glucose measured in capillary blood at half-hourly intervals for 2 h. An example of the result of sucrose and other sugar absorption tests in an adult with the rare condition of sucrase−isomaltase deficiency is shown in Fig. 1.25. There was malabsorption of sucrose and partial malabsorption of starch (as a result of the associated isomaltose deficiency) but normal absorption of lactose and glucose (Neale et al. 1965).

Mucosal disaccharidase assay

The definitive diagnosis of disaccharidase deficiency is made by direct measurement of the enzyme activity in the jejunal mucosa obtained by biopsy. The specimen is collected into 0.9% NaCl and transferred to the laboratory where the capacity of a homogenate of the biopsy to digest the relevant disaccharide is assessed, using the method of Dahlqvist (1964).

Hydrogen breath test

The fermentation of carbohydrate by colonic bacteria generates hydrogen. Under normal circumstances little of an oral test dose of sugar reaches the large intestine and thus there is no increase in breath hydrogen. Increased breath hydrogen may be detected firstly when there is sugar malabsorption (Levitt & Donaldson 1970, Metz et al. 1976) and secondly when there is bacterial overgrowth in the small intestine (King & Toskes 1979).

To detect hypolactasia, 50 g lactose is given by mouth and breath hydrogen is measured in end-expiratory alveolar air from a single breath using a modified Haldane−Priestley tube and mass spectrometry. Measurement of breath hydrogen after oral lactose provides a simple, non-invasive and accurate method of diagnosing hypolactasia (Metz et al. 1975). Hydrogen breath tests, however, are not specific since constipation may lead to some fermentation and an increase in breath hydrogen (Cummings 1983).

Tests of intestinal permeability

The luminal surface membrane of the enterocyte is a complex structure. It behaves as a lipid bilayer, within which are incorporated receptors and transport sites which are essential for the active absorption of the majority of substances in the diet. Lipid-soluble substances, however, may pass by passive diffusion through the lipid phase of the membrane. Water-soluble substances which are not actively transported appear to traverse the intestinal membrane either through pores which permit the entry of solutes up to a limited molecular size or through gaps in the tight junctions that bind the enterocytes together. The intestine is therefore permeable to a variety of solutes, and this permeability has been considered to be inversely proportional to the molecular size of the solute. In normal human intestine, there is a progressive decrease in permeability from proximal to distal small intestine (Fordtran et al. 1965) and colon (Billich & Levitan 1969).

Decreased permeability of the small intestine in coeliac disease was first reported by Fordtran et al. (1967). Using low molecular weight polyethylene glycols, Chadwick et al.

(1977) also showed reduced permeability in coeliac disease and suggested that permeability tests might be useful in diagnosis. Other workers have tested permeability with mono- and disaccharides which the body is unable to metabolize (Menzies et al. 1979). These sugars behave differently from polyethylene glycol (PEG) and indeed from one another. Monosaccharides such as L-rhamnose and mannitol cross normal mucosa quite readily (30–40% of a 5 g dose of mannitol is recovered from control subjects) and transfer is *reduced* in coeliac disease. In contrast, disaccharides such as lactulose and cellobiose pass with difficulty into the circulation (less than 1% of a 5 g dose can be recovered in urine) but transfer is *increased* in coeliac disease. These findings suggest different modes of transfer. PEG is partially lipid-soluble which presumably allows it to follow a transcellular route whereas the water-soluble monosaccharides may use carrier-mediated mechanisms which are not available to the larger disaccharides.

Clinically, comparison of the urinary excretion of a paired monosaccharide/disaccharide provides a sensitive screening test for detecting patients with gluten-sensitive enteropathy. This is expressed as a ratio, for example of lactulose to L-rhamnose (Menzies et al. 1979), or of cellobiose to mannitol (Cobden et al. 1980). Increased permeability using ^{51}Cr-labelled EDTA has also been shown by Bjarnson et al. (1983a) in coeliac disease and in inflammatory bowel disease (Bjarnson et al. 1983b). Although none of these permeability tests are yet in use in the routine laboratory, they may become useful non-invasive methods of screening for small intestinal disease. The ^{51}Cr EDTA-test has the advantage of simplicity and it is less costly.

Fat

The digestion and absorption of dietary fat requires a number of complex steps. Triglyceride present in the diet is first digested by pancreatic lipase, producing monoglycerides and fatty acids, which are then brought into solution in the intestinal contents by combining with bile salts in a physicochemical complex called the micelle. Bile salts are both hydrophilic and hydrophobic and, because of their special qualities, they are able to solubilize monoglycerides and fatty acids by concealing their hydrophobic regions in the interior of the micelle. The exterior of the micelle remains hydrophilic and is therefore water-soluble. The monoglycerides and fatty acids are released from the micelle at the surface membrane of the enterocyte, which they penetrate by virtue of their lipid solubility and they enter the interior of the cell. Here, they are re-synthesized first into triglycerides and they are then encapsulated as chylomicrons, which pass from the cell into the lymphatics and subsequently the general circulation.

Tests of fat absorption therefore measure events in the intestinal lumen (digestion and micelle formation), at or in the mucosa (entry, resynthesis and chylomicron formation) and at the exit into lymphatics and circulation. In general, they do not discriminate between these important steps in fat absorption.

Fat balance

Gross excess of fat in the stool is generally obvious on inspection and may readily be confirmed by staining a wet preparation with an oil-soluble dye and examining it microscopically (Drummey et al. 1961).

Quantitative assessment of fat absorption depends on the measurement of fat in the stool collected over not less than three consecutive 24-h periods. This technique has a number of drawbacks but is, nevertheless, the standard against which other tests of fat absorption are compared (van der Kamer et al. 1949, Frazer 1955). With a standard dietary intake of 100 g of fat a day, the excretion of fat in normal subjects is less than 6 g/24 h. As the faecal output of fat relates to the dietary intake, many subjects who have malabsorption but who eat little fat may not have steatorrhoea (Losowsky et al. 1974). Control of the patient's diet during fat balance is therefore necessary, and the standard diet should preferably precede the collection period for several days. Accurate collection of stools is also essential, for which careful nursing supervision is required. Various systems of marking the beginning and end of the collection period have been employed, such as the use of capsules containing chromic oxide, carmine or polyethylene glycol. They add greatly to the effort required by the procedure and if sufficient care is taken to collect each stool, markers are not essential for general diagnostic purposes.

Other tests of fat absorption depend on the measurement of chylomicrons or triglyceride in plasma following a standard test meal but such tests discriminate poorly between normal and abnormal populations. They may also be unsuitable for investigating diabetic patients or those with hypertriglyceridaemia. Absorption tests using ^{131}I-labelled fats have also been used. In early studies unreliable results were attributed to the use of triolein, and unsatisfactory sample collection. Recent experience, however, has been more favourable (West et al. 1981). For routine purposes, however, the standard fat balance remains the most useful in the investigation of small intestinal disease.

Triolein breath test

The recovery of $^{14}CO_2$ in the expired air after an oral fat load labelled with ^{14}C-labelled triolein or palmitate has provided a simple and reasonably effective test without the disadvantages associated with the collection and analysis of fat in the stools (Newcomer et al. 1979, Kaihara & Wagner 1968). Liquid scintillation counters for measuring the radioactive carbon are now freely available, making the test feasible in many centres. However, attention has been drawn to the many variables which affect the discriminatory power of this procedure. Patients with diabetes mellitus, thyroid disease, or obesity metabolize fatty acids at different rates. The choice of fat carrier and the size of the standard test meal appear to affect the results (Burrows et al. 1974, Strange et al. 1980). More recently ^{13}C-labelled fat has become available; it avoids the use of radioactive material but the test involves the use of a mass spectrometer, and the labelled material is expensive (Watkins et al. 1977).

Bile salts

Bile salts are synthesized by the liver from cholesterol and excreted by the biliary passages and gall bladder into the small intestine where they carry out their important function of micelle formation and the promotion of fat absorption. They are predominantly absorbed in the ileum. Under normal circumstances, for each cycle of the entero-hepatic circulation, less than 5% of the bile salt pool escapes absorption. Tests of bile salt absorption are useful in the diagnosis of bacterial overgrowth in the small intestine and in the demonstration of ileal dysfunction.

Bile salt breath test

Although bile acid metabolism in health and disease may be directly and accurately measured using a wide range of modern biochemical and isotopic techniques (Hofmann 1978), the simple bile acid breath test (Fromm & Hofmann 1971) is currently the most popular technique in clinical practice. An oral dose of cholyl-glycine ^{14}C is given, and the excretion of $^{14}CO_2$ is measured in the breath at varying intervals. With bacterial overgrowth in the small intestine, or malabsorption of bile salts due to ileal resection or disease, there is a greatly increased excretion of $^{14}CO_2$ in the breath when compared to normal individuals (Fromm et al. 1973, Pederson et al. 1973, Hepner 1975).

SeHCAT test

Tauro-23 [^{75}Se] selena-25-homocholic acid (SeHCAT) is the gamma-emitting taurine conjugate of a synthetic tri-hydroxy bile acid which appears to be absorbed, recirculated and excreted at the same rate as natural bile acids. It is resistant to bacterial deconjugation (Boyd et al. 1981).

After being given orally the clearance of SeHCAT can be monitored by external body counting. Early reports suggest that this new method will provide a highly sensitive test for ileal function and may also be useful for measurement of the size of the bile acid pool and for the study of gall bladder function (Merrick *et al.* 1983).

Protein

Proteins, like carbohydrates, require digestion and this takes place not only within the gut lumen but also at the brush border of the enterocyte and to some extent within the intestinal absorbing cell itself. Intraluminal digestion requires pancreatic trypsin which is secreted in response to the ingestion of food and which is derived from the activation of trypsinogen by enterokinase. Pancreatic digestion produces a variety of dipeptides and polypeptides which are further digested by brush border and intracellular peptidases, yielding amino acids which are transported into the portal circulation. There is evidence that a proportion of dietary protein enters the enterocyte as peptide and amino acid-transport systems at the brush border membrane may therefore play only a limited role in the normal absorption of dietary proteins.

Since there are no known defects of brush border peptidase activity, equivalent to disaccharidase deficiency, there are no comparable clinical conditions in which it is necessary to measure protein absorption. Defects of amino acid transport are rare and require special techniques for their elucidation, as described in Chapter 3. Faecal nitrogen is difficult to measure routinely and without a formal nitrogen balance is difficult to interpret. In practice, this procedure is of little value.

In disorders of the small intestine malabsorption of protein rarely causes hypoproteinaemia. It occurs as a result of protein-losing enteropathy and more rarely as a result of excessive catabolism of dietary protein in patients with severe bacterial overgrowth in the small intestine. Tests of protein metabolism which are useful in clinical practice are therefore confined to the assessment of protein-losing enteropathy and to a lesser extent of bacterial breakdown of protein.

Protein-losing enteropathy

^{131}I-labelled serum albumin

Serum proteins labelled with ^{131}I are metabolized in the same way as normal serum proteins. Studies of turnover may therefore be carried out with this material. Unfortunately, ^{131}I-labelled serum proteins are unsatisfactory for the study of protein loss from the gut. The labelled protein passes out into the gut where it is digested and broken down, the released iodide then being reabsorbed and excreted in the urine. It is therefore not possible to detect excess radioactivity in the stool of patients with protein-losing enteropathy using this technique. An ingenious method of circumventing this difficulty was suggested by Jeejeebhoy & Coghill (1961). They gave an ion-exchange resin (Amberlite) orally in an attempt to bind the ^{131}I that entered the gut. Unfortunately, the radioactivity excreted in the faeces was derived from iodide secreted by stomach and salivary glands, as well as from the protein leaked into the intestine.

^{67}Cu-labelled caeruloplasmin

This stable compound is valuable as a research tool for measuring intestinal protein loss (Waldmann *et al.* 1965) but its use in the routine laboratory is precluded by the short half-life of the isotope and by its expense.

^{51}Cr-labelled albumin

Albumin labelled with $^{51}CrCl_3$ *in vitro* or *in vivo* provides the most useful clinical test for protein-losing enteropathy (Waldmann 1961, 1966). Stools are collected for several days after the intravenous injection of ^{51}Cr-labelled albumin or of ^{51}Cr-chloride. The daily faecal excretion of ^{51}Cr is measured and correlated with the plasma radioactivity. Under normal circumstances, less than 1% of the plasma albumin pool is cleared into the gut per day and increased clearance are found in protein-losing enteropathy. The total faecal excretion may be measured for 4 days after the intravenous injection. Normal individuals excrete between 0.1 and 0.7% of the injected radioactivity, whereas up to 40% may be excreted in patients with severe protein-losing enteropathy.

Alpha-1-antitrypsin

The small amount of circulating α-1-antitrypsin which escapes into the lumen of the intestine is excreted in faeces unchanged. Thus the measurement of this protein by sensitive immunoassay provides a non-isotopic method of assessing protein loss from gut which is particularly useful in the study of children (Hill et al. 1981). Results correlate well with those obtained using ^{51}Cr-labelled proteins.

Indicanuria

Indican (indoxyl sulphate) is a metabolic product of certain bacteria within the intestinal lumen which use tryptophan as a substrate. In the normal individual, the amount of indican excreted in urine depends on the dietary intake of protein. Contamination of the upper intestine with bacteria results in the production and subsequent urinary excretion of large amounts of indican. Quantities greater than 400 μmol/l usually indicate bacterial overgrowth. This test is simple to perform, and is particularly useful as a screening test for bacterial overgrowth.

Water-soluble vitamins

It is possible, but rarely necessary, to measure the absorption of a wide range of water-soluble vitamins using biochemical techniques or isotopically-labelled vitamins. In practice, only tests of vitamin B_{12} absorption are used in the investigation of small intestinal disease.

Vitamin B_{12}

Vitamin B_{12} is present in the diet in association with animal protein, being found particularly in muscle, liver, kidney and egg yolk, as well as in milk. Carnivorous creatures and omnivores obtain their requirement of vitamin B_{12} from the diet, whereas in herbivores the vitamin is synthesized by intestinal bacteria from whom it is derived. The capacity to synthesize vitamin B_{12} is one of the major features that distinguishes herbivores from carnivores. Since man has an obligate need for vitamin B_{12} in the diet, strict vegetarians who eat no animal protein run the risk of developing vitamin B_{12} deficiency but this does not usually occur in those who take milk or eggs with a vegetarian diet.

Vitamin B_{12} is a water-soluble vitamin (mol. wt. 1355) which requires the presence of intrinsic factor (IF) secreted by the stomach to ensure its absorption. Two molecules of IF bind with two molecules of vitamin B_{12} and the complex passes down the small intestine to the absorption site which is restricted to the ileum. The B_{12}–IF complex binds to a series of receptors in the ileal brush border membrane where the vitamin B_{12} becomes detached from the complex and passes into the cell. Here further intracellular mechanisms ensure its transport across the ileal enterocyte and into the circulation. Malabsorption of vitamin B_{12} may therefore occur as a result of IF deficiency (as in Addisonian pernicious anaemia), from bacterial binding of B_{12} in the intestinal lumen (as in bacterial overgrowth), if there is a defect in the ileal absorptive cell (as in selective familial vitamin B_{12} malabsorption, or in chronic tropical sprue), as well as when the ileum has been resected.

Tests of absorption should be carried out with an oral test dose of B_{12} alone, then with IF and, if bacterial overgrowth is suspected, after a course of oral broad spectrum antibiotics.

Tests of absorption may be carried out using vitamin B_{12} labelled with ^{57}Co or ^{58}Co. The oral test dose must be within the physiological range of vitamin B_{12} absorption which is between 0.5 and 2 μg. A test dose of 1 μg is most frequently used. The following methods are available for measuring absorption (Pettit 1981):

1 *Faecal excretion method.* The faecal excretion of radioactivity is measured following an oral test dose, absorption being derived from the amount of the radioactivity not recovered in the stool. This method is the most valuable for physiological studies but is rarely used in clinical practice in view of the difficulty and inconvenience of accurate stool collection.

2 *Urinary excretion technique* (Schilling test). Under normal circumstances, little radioactivity is excreted in the urine after an oral test dose of radioactive B_{12} is given. If, however, an injection of 1000 μg of non-radioactive vitamin B_{12} is given intramuscularly 1 or 2 h after the oral dose, approximately a third of the B_{12} absorbed is 'flushed out' into the urine. Urine is therefore collected for 24 h following the oral dose and the radioactivity counted. Since the test relies on urinary excretion of the labelled vitamin, it is unreliable in the presence of renal failure.

Using an oral test dose of 1 μg of labelled B_{12}, control subjects excrete between 11 and 39% of the dose in the urine, whereas patients with pernicious anaemia excrete between 0 and 6.8% if the oral dose is given alone. If given with IF, between 3.1 and 30% is excreted.

3 *Double isotope technique.* Using two different isotopes of cobalt (^{57}Co and ^{58}Co), it is possible to administer two preparations, one of free cobalamin, the other of cobalamin bound to intrinsic factor *in vitro*, in separate capsules at the same time. The loading dose of intramuscular cobalamin is administered 1 h later, as in the conventional Schilling test. By measuring the ratio of the two isotopes in urine collected during the subsequent 24 h, discrimination between failure to produce endogenous intrinsic factor (associated with pernicious anaemia) and failure to absorb cobalamin bound to intrinsic factor (associated with ileal disease) is possible. A recent study has suggested that this simplified test is highly specific and accurate in discriminating between the two types of disease but has a sensitivity of 83% for detecting pernicious anaemia, and yet only 67% for the detection of ileal disease (Domstad *et al.* 1981).

4 *Hepatic uptake method.* Surface counting of the liver 7 days after an oral test dose may be used as a measure of vitamin B_{12} absorption. This method has the disadvantage that it cannot be quantitated accurately.

5 *Plasma radioactivity.* After an oral test dose of radioactive vitamin B_{12} of sufficiently high specific activity, it is possible to measure the changes in radioactivity in the plasma. For the first 3 h there is no rise in plasma radioactivity, this delay representing the time required for B_{12} to pass down the gut to its distal absorption site and to traverse the ileal enterocyte. It then rises to reach a peak at between 8 and 12 h, the period during which blood should be taken to assess plasma radioactivity. As with the hepatic uptake techniques, this test gives only semiquantitative results.

6 *Whole body counting.* The patient is counted in a whole body counter immediately after ingesting the oral dose of radioactive vitamin B_{12}. Seven to 10 days later, when the unabsorbed vitamin B_{12} has been excreted from the body, a further count is carried out, the retained radioactivity representing the proportion of the oral test dose that has been absorbed. This technique provides an accurate and reproducible measurement of vitamin B_{12} absorption and is particularly valuable for research purposes.

Folic acid

Folic acid absorption may be measured either by studying the plasma level or urinary excretion of folic acid after an oral test dose using microbiological techniques or by studying the absorption of isotopically labelled material. Such studies have proved particularly useful in research but are not used in the routine investigation of small intestinal disease.

Fat-soluble vitamins

Although it is possible to label fat-soluble vitamins with isotopes such as ^{3}H and to use these to measure absorption, such studies remain essentially within the realm of the research laboratory. Vitamin A absorption tests have been repeatedly used as an indirect measurement of fat absorption. Such tests, however, are too inaccurate to provide satisfactory data for the assessment of small intestinal function.

Iron

Iron is available to the human in two forms, inorganic iron and haem, which are absorbed by different mechanisms. It is possible to assay the effectiveness of intestinal absorption of both these mechanisms using radioactively labelled preparations but this is not helpful in routine practice. The measurement of plasma iron after a single therapeutic oral dose does not reflect the absorption of iron in normal nutritional circumstances. This test is a measure of either the bioavailability of the pharmaceutical preparation used or patient compliance and is not useful in the investigation of malabsorption.

E. NUTRITIONAL ASSESSMENT
GRAHAM NEALE

Clinical examination 29
Anthropometry and body composition 29
Laboratory and radiological tests............ 32
Prognostic indices 37

Early changes of nutritional deficiency are difficult to detect. Patients often lose weight insidiously or develop deficiencies of specific nutrients. A nutritional disturbance often indicates latent small intestinal disease. Conversely the presence of small intestinal disease should always lead to a search for evidence of nutrient deficiencies. In patients with Crohn's disease, for example, latent deficiencies of many important nutrients such as folic acid, iron, magnesium, zinc and vitamin A are common.

Although malabsorption is a frequent factor in small intestinal disease, it is often reduced nutritional intake rather than defective absorption that leads to nutritional deficiency. The postprandial abdominal pain of Crohn's disease of the small intestine may be of far greater significance in inhibiting appetite than any effect of this disorder on small intestinal function.

Clinical examination

Symptoms and signs of deficiency of specific nutrients usually appear late. Their presence indicates severe and often long-standing deficiency. Many of the clinical pointers are relatively non-specific, for example angular stomatitis or koilonychia, and are thus unreliable. Nevertheless they should not be ignored. The predominant clinical features of nutritional deficiency together with their causes are listed in Table 1.1. Even with such non-specific signs a bedside clinical assessment based on history and examination provides a reproducible and clinically useful technique for evaluating nutritional status (Baker et al. 1982).

Anthropometry and body composition

Anthropometry

Children

Height for age and weight for height are useful primary indicators of nutritional status in children. Reduced height for age is an index of stunting, common with prolonged semi-starvation or with protracted deficiency in nutrient intake (Fig. 1.26), whereas a reduced weight for height indicates wasting often of recent origin. Reference charts include those derived from detailed studies in the UK, Holland, Cuba and the USA. At present charts based on data from the US National Academy of Sciences are probably the best for international use (Waterlow et al. 1977).

Table 1.1. Clinical features of nutritional deficiency.

Organ involved	Symptoms and signs	Cause of deficiency
Integument	Easy bruising	Scurvy (positive Hess test). Vitamin K deficiency
	Dry scaly skin	Usually non-specific. Essential fatty acid deficiency. Zinc deficiency.
	Sparse, depigmented, easily pluckable hair	Long-standing protein calorie malnutrition
	Koilonychia	Iron deficiency (may be congenital)
	Leuconychia	Hypoalbuminaemia
	Angular stomatitis / Naso-labial seborrhoea	Common in the elderly malnourished. Possible relationship to vitamin B status
Gastrointestinal tract	Cheilosis	Occasionally due to vitamin B deficiency
	Aphthous ulcers	Association with iron and folate deficiency and with small intestinal disease
	Atrophic tongue papillae	Association with deficiency of iron, vitamin B, vitamin B_{12}, folic acid
	Parotid swelling	Protein malnutrition; alcoholism
	Dysphagia	Cricopharyngeal web in long-standing iron deficiency
	Hepatomegaly	Fatty infiltration in wasting diseases
Heart	Cardiac failure	Thiamine deficiency
	Extrasystoles	Protein deficiency
Nervous system	Wernicke's encephalopathy/Korsakoff's psychosis	Thiamine deficiency
	Dementia	Nicotinic acid deficiency (pellagra) Vitamin B_{12} deficiency
	Failing vision	Night blindness and xerophthalmia (vitamin A deficiency). Tobacco amplyopia (cyanide toxicity in presence of vitamin B_{12} deficiency)
	Ataxia	Subacute combined degeneration of spinal cord (vitamin B_{12} deficiency)
	Peripheral neuropathy	Vitamin B and B_{12} deficiency
	Tetany	Vitamin D deficiency
Musculo-skeletal	Kyphosis and vertebral fractures	Osteoporosis
	Rickets and osteomalacia	Vitamin D deficiency
	Proximal myopathy	Vitamin D deficiency
	Generalized muscle weakness	Potassium deficiency and generalized undernutrition
Blood	Anaemia	Deficiencies of iron, folic acid and vitamin B_{12}. Rarely vitamin E (in premature infants), pyridoxine (sideroblastic anaemia).
	Bleeding	Hypoprothrombinaemia (vitamin K deficiency) Thrombocytopenia (acute folic acid and more rarely vitamin B_{12} deficiency)

Adults

'Optimal' values for adult weight are usually based on data obtained between 1935 and 1953 by the Metropolitan Life Insurance Company in the USA. It is now recognized, however, that the range of 'healthy weight' is considerably greater than previously thought. Appropriate weights for height based on the criteria of the National Institutes of Health (Fogarty report) as modified by the American 1979 Build Study are given in Table 1.2. The large range of normality limits the clinical usefulness of weight as an index of malnutrition in adults. Patients with disorders of the small intestine may lose substantial weight yet remain

Assessment of Small Intestinal Disease

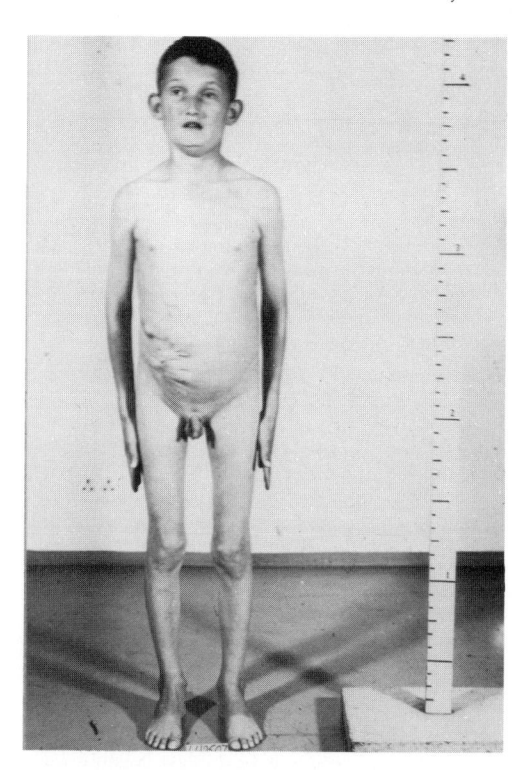

Fig. 1.26. Failure of growth and infantilism in a 19-year-old male with malabsorption due to a stagnant loop syndrome since early life.

Table 1.2. Appropriate body weights in healthy young adults*

Height (cm)	Men Average	Range (kg)	Women Average	Range (kg)
145	—	—	46.0	(37–53)
148	—	—	46.5	(37–54)
150	—	—	47.0	(38–55)
152	—	—	48.5	(39–57)
156	—	—	49.5	(39–58)
158	55.8	(44–64)	50.4	(40–58)
160	57.6	(45–65)	51.3	(41–59)
162	58.6	(46–66)	52.6	(42–61)
164	59.6	(47–67)	54.0	(43–62)
166	60.6	(48–69)	55.4	(44–64)
168	61.7	(49–71)	56.8	(45–65)
170	63.5	(51–73)	58.1	(45–66)
172	65.0	(52–74)	60.0	(46–67)
174	66.5	(53–75)	61.3	(48–69)
176	68.0	(54–77)	62.6	(49–70)
178	69.4	(55–79)	64.0	(51–72)
180	71.0	(58–80)	65.3	(52–74)
182	72.6	(59–82)	—	—
184	74.2	(60–84)	—	—
186	75.8	(62–86)	—	—
188	77.6	(64–88)	—	—
190	79.3	(66–90)	—	—
192	81.0	(68–93)	—	—

*Derived from Build and Blood Pressure Study (1959) and modified in the light of data from the 1979 Build Study (see references). This data applies to slim young adults. The subject is not regarded as overweight unless he exceeds 110 per cent of the upper limit of the quoted range. Obesity begins at 120 per cent.

within 'normal' limits. Thus a history of anorexia and documented loss of weight are far more valuable as nutritional indices.

Body composition

Adipose tissue

In clinical practice body fat is best estimated by measuring skinfold thickness using Harpenden calipers at four sites (triceps, biceps, subscapular, suprailiac) (cf. Tables 1.3 and 1.4), but the method is far from sensitive. Duplicate measurements often vary by as much as 10%. Measurements are likely to be most accurate in healthy young adults close to their ideal body weight; they are least accurate in the elderly, in those with recent weight loss and when there are changes in body hydration. At present there are no reliable percentile values for average skinfold thickness.

Data are available for triceps skinfold thickness (Frisancho 1981) but single measurements are unreliable because of individual differences in the distribution of body fat. There are major differences between the sexes and between ethnic groups. In clinical practice there is usually no difficulty in recognizing the patient with little subcutaneous fat. Recognition of such patients is important because they are prone to hypothermia (Neale et al. 1968). On the other hand it is difficult to assess the progress of patients who are moderately well nourished. At best only relatively large changes (of the order of 4–5 kg) can be detected.

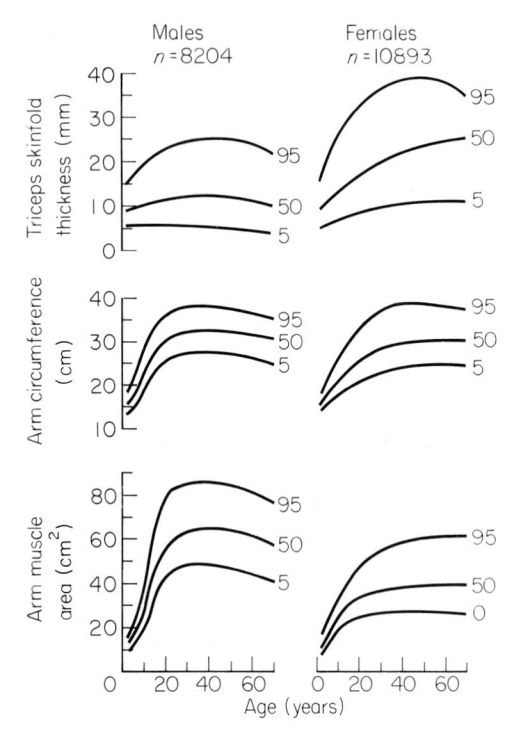

Fig. 1.27. Percentile curves for tricep skinfold thickness, arm circumference and estimated arm muscle area derived from an analysis of data collected from a cross-sectional sample of 19,097 US white subjects during the period 1971–1974 as part of the Health and Nutritional Examination Survey I (Hanes I) of the US (Frisancho 1981).

Table 1.3. Sites for measuring skinfold thickness

Triceps	Over back of left arm at a level corresponding to marked point on left arm halfway between the acromial and olecranon processes.
Biceps	Anterior at marked level with arm resting supinated.
Subscapular	Over wing of L scapula in plane of dermatome.
Suprailiac	1 cm above superior iliac crest in midaxillary line on left in a horizontal plane.

Notes on technique: pull all subcutaneous tissue away gently but firmly from muscle with middle finger and thumb of left hand. Maintain pressure and apply calipers with right hand 1 cm away from left hand. Maintain pressure on skinfold with left hand, release pressure on handle of calipers. Read once needle stops moving or within 3 seconds. Repeat three times and take two closest readings. (Data from Durnin & Womersley, 1974)

Lean body mass

Generalized malnutrition is associated with a loss of body structural protein especially of muscle mass. The relative wasting of fat and body protein will depend on the degree of undernutrition, and the availability of exogenous protein to preserve dynamic structures such as circulating proteins and the activities of tissue enzymes. The degree of physical activity and the amount of metabolic 'stress', for example as a result of trauma or infection, are also important.

Clinical assessment of lean body mass

Muscle circumference of the non-dominant upper arm is the simplest measure of muscle mass (Table 1.3). It is defined as:

(Mid arm circumference $- \pi$ × skinfold thickness).

Alternatively one may calculate upper arm muscle area as.

$$\frac{(\text{Arm circumference} - \pi \times \text{skinfold thickness})^2}{4\pi}$$

Both indices correlate reasonably well with 24-h creatinine excretion (Heymsfield et al., 1982). But as for weight there is a wide range of normality (Fig. 1.27). In patients below the 5th percentile malnutrition is usually obvious to the naked eye except in the unusual patient who has preserved subcutaneous fat, yet has wasted skeletal muscles.

Laboratory and radiological tests

Creatinine–height index (CHI)

The 24-h output of creatinine is a reflection of muscle mass. The CHI is calculated by expressing creatinine as a percentage of the mean normal, corrected for height. In routine practice it is of limited value because of other factors influencing creatinine excretion, including diet, infection, and other disorders, and because of the difficulty in obtaining accurate collections of urine.

Table 1.4. Equivalent fat content (% body weight) derived from the sum of thicknesses of four skin-folds (biceps, triceps, subscapular and suprailiac).

Sum of skinfolds (mm)	Percentage fat							
	Males (age in years)				Females (age in years)			
	17–29	30–39	40–49	50+	17–29	30–39	40–49	50+
20	8	12	12	12.5	14	17	20	21.5
30	13	16	17.5	18.5	19.5	22	24.5	26.5
40	16.5	19	21.5	23	23.5	25.5	28	30
50	19	21.5	24.5	26.5	26.5	28	31	33.5
60	21	23.5	27	29	29	30.5	33	35.5
70	23	25	29.5	31.5	31	32.5	35	37.5
80	25	26.5	31	34	33	34.5	36.5	39.5
90	26	28	33	36	35	36	38.5	41
100	27.5	29	34.5	37.5	36.5	37	39.5	42.5
110	29	30	36	39	38	38.5	41	44
120	30	31	37	40.5	39	39.5	42	45
130	31	32	38	42	40	40.5	43	46
140	32	32.5	39	43	41.5	44	47	
150	33	33.5	40	44	42.5	42.5	45	48
160	33.5	34.5	41	45	43.5	43.5	46	49

Nuclear methods

Several sophisticated methods of measuring lean body mass have been described. These are based on neutron activation analysis for whole body nitrogen, measurements of whole body potassium based on the natural distribution of the radio isotope ^{40}K, and isotopic dilution techniques for total exchangeable potassium and total body water (Shizgal et al. 1979). Lean body mass assessed by anthropometry or by total body potassium correlate reasonably well with total body nitrogen but the coefficient of variation is high. Replenishment of depleted patients leads to a greater rise in total body nitrogen than in lean body mass or total body potassium (Jeejeebhoy, 1981). This may reflect preferential restoration of protein in stores other than those of skeletal muscle. Although it is now possible to measure total body nitrogen with a relatively simple cheap and portable apparatus (Mernagh et al. 1977), the techniques remain primarily of research interest.

Haematology

Haemoglobin, mean corpuscular volume (MCV), mean corpuscular haemoglobin concentration (MCHC), red cell morphology, white cell and platelet counts should be estimated. The recognition of macrocytosis or the presence of Howell–Jolly bodies in the circulating red cells may be the only pointers to a diagnosis of coeliac disease.

Circulating ferritin provides a good index of iron stores but this assay is not yet available routinely. Concentrations of iron and iron-binding capacity (transferrin) are too readily altered by non-nutritional disorders to be of great value in patients with small intestinal disease.

Sternal marrow

Examination of smears of sternal marrow stained for iron provide the most sensitive clinical marker of iron deficiency. The marrow may demonstrate megaloblastic changes indicating either B$_{12}$ or folate deficiency. In the presence of iron deficiency, however, megaloblastic changes may be masked. In these circumstances examination of white cell precursors may reveal giant metamyelocytes.

Folic acid

Circulating folic acid declines rapidly over a few days in the anorectic patient. It is therefore a poor indicator of total body stores, which are best assessed by measurements of red cell folate. Folate deficiency is common in coeliac disease and under appropriate circumstances is an indication for jejunal biopsy.

Acute folate deficiency occasionally occurs in very sick patients, particularly after surgery. In these patients the red cell morphology is normal but leucopenia and thrombocytopenia are common (Beard et al. 1980). There is a rapid response to treatment with folic acid (5 mg three times daily).

Vitamin B_{12}

Serum vitamin B_{12} is a sensitive marker of deficiency. In practice it is estimated either by microbiological means or by radio-immunoassay. The standard reference assay is based on *E. gracilis* but in most laboratories *L. leichmanii* is the preferred organism. Radioimmunoassay is becoming increasingly popular, especially with pure intrinsic factor as the binder. Each laboratory must establish its own normal range. The lower limit is usually about 150 pg/ml. Values between 100–180 pg/ml need careful consideration. Such values need not be associated with any abnormality of B_{12} metabolism, yet on the other hand may indicate early B_{12} deficiency. A low serum vitamin B_{12} by itself, however, is insufficient evidence of B_{12} deficiency. Details of diet, drugs, intestinal function and associated disease must be considered (Chanarin 1979).

Protein status

Many hospital laboratories now offer a routine service for the measurement of a wide range of circulating proteins. Abnormalities are often found in patients with small intestinal disorders but must be interpreted with caution.

Total protein and albumin

Total protein concentration is of little diagnostic value but a low concentration of circulating albumin may indicate malnutrition. In practice hypoalbuminaemia is neither specific nor sensitive. Injury, infection and malignancy may reduce the concentration independent of nutritional status. With disorders of the small intestine protein-losing enteropathy is a common cause of a low serum albumin. It is particularly liable to occur in patients with inflammatory or ulcerative lesions of the small intestine. Hypoalbuminaemia due to malnutrition is unusual in patients with uncomplicated disorders of the small intestine.

Other proteins

Other serum proteins with shorter half-lives than albumin, such as thyroxine-binding pre-albumin and transferrin, have been suggested as more sensitive markers of nutritional status. However, serum concentrations fall rapidly under conditions of stress. Circulating hormones, bacterial toxins and tissue injury may all depress the concentration of these circulating proteins. By contrast, circulating transferrin is increased by iron deficiency.

Amino acids

Absorbed amino acids equilibrate rapidly with extracellular pools. Concentrations in plasma represent the net effect of a number of metabolic pathways associated with the synthesis and degradation of body proteins. Plasma amino acid levels do not therefore give an accurate guide to body protein status and are affected by the type of dietary protein, the metabolic state of the body, the previous nutritional state and the degree of stress (Munro 1970).

Urea and creatinine

In the presence of normal renal function blood urea falls to very low levels if protein intake or absorption is markedly depressed.

The rate of excretion of urea in urine reflects the rate of oxidative metabolism of proteins whether of tissue or dietary origin. In subjects in a stable metabolic state urinary urea may therefore be used as a rough index of protein intake and absorption. It may also be used to assess recovery from malnutrition.

Skeletal structure

Osteoporosis

This is difficult to diagnose in the early stages of its development. Osteoporosis is an acceleration of the ageing process of bone and affects particularly the axial skeleton. X-rays of the spine show under-mineralization and there may be collapse of vertebrae in severe cases. Bone mass may be assessed radiologically using one of several techniques — densitometry, radiogrammetry, photon beam scanning and computerized tomography (Greenfield 1975). These procedures yield interesting epidemiological data but are not used in routine clinical practice. Osteoporosis may be a feature of long-standing malabsorption and occurs most commonly after partial gastrectomy.

Osteomalacia

Biochemical and radiological investigations are the most useful indicators of osteomalacia in clinical practice. Serum calcium, corrected for protein, and phosphate may be reduced and circulating alkaline phosphatase elevated in vitamin D deficiency. These measurements, however, are abnormal only with severe disease and results within the normal range are not uncommon in patients with histologically proven changes of osteomalacia. Circulating levels of 25 hydroxycholecalciferol (25-HCC) provide useful evidence of vitamin D status but do not indicate whether or not the patient has osteomalacia (Schoen et al. 1978, Fraser 1983).

Specific radiological changes such as Looser's zones and signs of secondary hyperparathyroidism are found only in long-standing osteomalacia. More often there is evidence only of demineralization of bone and the distinction from osteoporosis cannot be made with certainty.

Quantitative histology of bone, usually of biopsies from the iliac crest, provides the diagnostic standard. In osteomalacia the osteoid seams are thickened and the percentage calcification front is reduced (Melvin et al. 1970).

Clinicians may have to treat suspected osteomalacia without conclusive evidence of bone pathology. A rise in fasting serum phosphate over a period of 5 days following treatment with 1 mg vitamin D intravenously provides a useful simple marker of response (Whittle et al. 1969). The serum alkaline phosphatase may take several weeks to return to normal.

Body minerals

Sodium

Total body sodium is from 50–60 mEq/kg body weight, and more than one third is tightly held in the skeleton. Powerful homeostatic mechanisms maintain the concentration of circulating sodium within close limits. Patients with disease of the small intestine rarely develop salt depletion except when there are large losses from a high fistula or stoma. In such patients the urinary excretion of sodium may provide useful evidence of sodium status.

Potassium

Total body potassium varies from 40–60 mEq/kg body weight of which 98% is intracellular. Virtually all pools of body potassium can equilibrate within 24 h and thus total body potassium can be estimated fairly readily by isotope dilution techniques. Serum potassium is a moderately sensitive indicator of body potassium, but it may be affected by acid base, hormonal and renal status.

Calcium

Over 99% of total body calcium and approximately 80% of the phosphorus are in bones in a molecular ratio of a little over 2 : 1. The level of circulating calcium is kept remarkably constant by hormonal control.

Circulating calcium levels do not reflect body stores. Low levels occur with vitamin D deficiency, especially in the presence of magnesium deficiency, and to a lesser extent if there is a prolonged reduction of calcium intake (Walker et al. 1954).

Calcium excretion in urine varies widely between normal individuals but tends to be low in patients with severe long-standing malabsorption irrespective of vitamin D status. Measurement of the calcium excretion index or of strontium excretion after an infusion of the appropriate divalent cation is a moderately sensitive index of skeletal avidity for calcium (Joplin et al. 1967).

Phosphorus

Phosphorus is readily absorbed from the small intestine, mainly as free phosphate. At high concentrations transport is mainly passive; at low concentrations it is mediated by vitamin D (Davis et al. 1983). The body content is regulated primarily by urinary excretion and thus phosphate depletion is unusual in disease of the small intestine.

Circulating phosphate rises after meals so that measurements on randomly taken samples of blood are of little clinical value, but fasting values may be helpful in the assessment of osteomalacia (Whittle et al. 1969).

Magnesium

Nearly one half of the body magnesium is extraskeletal. The circulating concentration (55% of which is ionic) is not under direct hormonal control and thus provides a reasonable index of body status. Magnesium deficiency occurs not uncommonly in patients with Crohn's disease or after resection of the small intestine and sometimes in coeliac disease (Booth et al. 1964). There is often hypocalcaemia and hypokalaemia in addition (Shils 1969).

Trace elements

Zinc

Zinc plays a key role in many enzymatic processes and in the synthesis of protein and RNA. Severe deficiency appears to be uncommon in diseases of the small intestine and measurement of circulating zinc, which is bound to α-2-macroglobulin and to albumin, is not a sensitive nor a specific marker of body status. The content of zinc in leucocytes provides a better marker of zinc status in human disease (Keeling et al. 1980) but in most centres only plasma and urine values are available (Main et al. 1982). In a single report (Elmes et al. 1976), zinc deficiency was incriminated in causing severe malabsorption in individuals with coeliac disease initially unresponsive to treatment with a gluten-free diet.

Copper

Copper in the circulation is mostly bound to caerulo-plasmin. Serum values rise in many inflammatory and neoplastic conditions and fall in protein-losing states and in Wilson's disease. The value of measuring serum copper in patients with small intestinal disease is uncertain. Copper deficiency has been described in coeliac disease, tropical sprue and in protein calorie malnutrition but determination of its prevalence awaits better methods of assessment. It has been shown to predispose to anaemia and to scorbutic bone changes in children (Ashkenazi 1973).

Water-soluble vitamins

Assays of water-soluble vitamins (apart from folic acid and vitamin B_{12}) are used rarely in routine clinical practice. Deficiencies of components of vitamin B complex and of vitamin C are readily corrected by appropriate treatment (Drugs & Therapeutic Bulletin 1984) and rarely constitute a problem in management. Vitamin B_6 deficiency occasionally occurs in disease of the small intestine (Dawson et al. 1964) and the plasma concentration of circulating pyridoxal (Rose et al. 1976) may provide a useful screening test.

Fat-soluble vitamins

Vitamin A

The concentration of vitamin A in liver tissue is the most sensitive guide to body status. Plasma retinol values fall only when stores are depleted. At the same time vitamin A deprivation inhibits the release of retinol binding protein (RBP) from the liver and in general there is a good correlation between the concentrations of circulating retinol and RBP. It is worth measuring both variables in the assessment of vitamin A deficiency because of the influence of other factors such as protein malnutrition. Impaired dark adaptation may occur with a plasma retinol or less than 1.4 µmol/l but the the risk of night blindness is high only in those with values below 0.8 µmol/l (Main et al. 1983).

The concentration of circulating carotene is helpful as a marker of dietary deficiency or of intestinal malabsorption but is not of value in assessing vitamin A status.

Vitamin D

Circulating cholecalciferol and its metabolites have provided much useful data regarding the metabolism of vitamin D (Fraser 1983). 25-hydroxy-cholecalciferol in blood is low in patients with small intestinal disease who have histological osteomalacia.

Vitamin E

Vitamin E may be measured as α-tocopherol (Quaife et al. 1949) but is of little clinical value.

Vitamin K

Concentrations of circulating vitamin K are not used in clinical assessment. Prothrombin time is a useful index of deficiency in the absence of liver disease.

Essential fatty acids

The concentrations of ω6 fatty acids in circulating phospholipids fall with deficiency of the essential fatty acids (linoleic and linolenic acids). At the same time ω9 fatty acid (eicosatrienoic acid) becomes easily detectable. The ratio of 20:3 ω9/20:4 ω6 is accepted as the most useful index of essential fatty acid status and a value of greater than 0.4 is diagnostic of deficiency. Minor degrees of depletion occur in several disorders of absorption but the fully developed clinical picture with dermatitis and abnormal platelet function is rare. It has been described most often after massive resection of the small intestine (Press et al. 1974).

Prognostic indices

There has been a recent vogue for constructing prognostic nutritional indices to predict the probability of adverse events after gastrointestinal surgery (Buzby et al. 1980; Mullen et al. 1980; Simms et al. 1982). Most of the measurements used in constructing these indices (such as serum albumin, transferrin, delayed hypersensitivity reactivity) are profoundly affected by non-nutritional factors including age, infection and neoplastic disease. In selecting patients for intensive nutritional rehabilitation these indices remain at best unproven (Simms et al. 1982).

Tests of metabolism and organic function are better than artificially constructed indices in assessing the effects of nutritional deficiency (Solomons & Allan 1983). Most of these tests are not available on a routine basis but they have been used to define the way in which disease of the small intestine may affect nutritional well-being.

References

Aherne W.A. & Dunnill M.S. (1982) *Morphometry*. Edward Arnold Ltd., London.

Alavi A. (1980) Scintigraphic demonstration of acute gastrointestinal bleeding. *Gastrointest. Radiol.* **5**, 205–208.

Anderson G.F., Sfekianakis G., Kind D.R. & Boles E.T. Jr. (1980) Hormonal enhancement of Technetium-99m Pertechnetate uptake in experimental Meckel's diverticulum. *J. Pediatr. Surg.* **15**, 900–905.

Ashkenazi A., Levin S., Djaldetti M., Fishel E. & Benvenisti D. (1973) The syndrome of neonatal copper deficiency. *Pediat. (Springfield)* **52**, 525–531.

Baker J.P., Detsky A.S., Wesson D.E., Wolman S.L., Stewart S., Whitewell J., Langer B. & Jeejeebhoy K.N. (1982) Nutritional assessment: a comparison of clinical judgement and objective measurements. *New Engl. J. Med.* **306**, 969–972.

Baum S. (1983) Arteriography. In *Alimentary Tract Radiology*, 3rd ed. (Ed. by A.R. Margulis & H.J. Burhenne) C.V. Mosby Co., St. Louis. pp. 2132–2183.

Beard M.E., Hatipov C.S. & Hamer J.W. (1980) Acute onset of folic acid deficiency in patients under intensive care. *Crit. Care*, **8**, 500–503.

Benson J.A., Culver P.J., Ragland S., Drummey G.D. & Bougas E. (1957) The D-xylose absorption test in malabsorption syndromes. *New Engl. J. Med.* **256**, 335–339.

Berardi R.S. (1974) Vascular complication of superior mesenteric artery infusion with Pitressin in treatment of bleeding oesophageal varices. *Am. J. Surg.* **127**, 757.

Billich C.O. & Levitan R. (1969) Effects of sodium concentration and osmolality on water and electrolyte absorption from the intact human colon. *J. Clin. Invest.* **48**, 1336–1347.

Bjarnson I., Peters T.J. & Veall N. (1983a) A persistent defect in intestinal permeability in coeliac disease demonstrated by a 51Cr-labelled EDTA absorption test. *Lancet*, **i**, 323–325.

Bjarnson I., O'Morain C., Levi A.J. & Peters T.J. (1983b) Small intestinal permeability in patients with inflammatory bowel disease. *Clin. Sci.* **64**, 61.

Blankenhorn D.H., Hirsch J. & Ahreus E.H. (1955) Transintestinal intubation: technique for measurement of gut length and physiologic sampling at Kurcon loci. *Proc. Soc. Exp. Biol. Med.* **88**, 356–362.

Bohane T.D., Cutz E., Hamilton J.R. & Gall D.G. (1977) Acrodermatitis enteropathica, zinc and the Paneth cell. A case report with family studies. *Gastroenter.* **73**, 587–592.

Bookstein J.J. (1982) Angiographic diagnosis and transcatheter therapy of lower gastrointestinal bleeding. In *Interventional Radiology* (Ed. by R.A. Wilkins & M. Viamonte Jr). Blackwell Scientific Publications, New York.

Booth C.C., MacIntyre I. & Mollin D.L. (1964) Nutritional problems associated with extensive lesions of the distal small intestine in man. *Quart. J. Med.* **33**, 401–420.

Boyd G.S., Merrick M.V., Monks R. & Thomas I.L. (1981) Se-labelled bile acid analogues. New radiopharmaceuticals for investigating the entero-hepatic circulation. *J. Nuclear Med.* **22**, 720–725.

Brandborg L.L., Rubin C.E. & Quinton W.E. (1959) A multipurpose instrument for suction biopsy of the oesophagus, stomach, small bowel and colon. *Gastroenter.* **37**, 1–16.

Burrows P.J., Fleming J.S., Garrett E.S. & Ackery D.M. (1974) Clinical evaluation of the C14 fat absorption test. *Gut*, **15**, 147–150.

Buzby G.P., Mullen J.L., Matthews D.C., Hobbs C.L. & Rosato E.F. (1980) Prognostic nutritional index in gastro-intestinal surgery. *Amer. J. Surg.* **139**, 160–167.

Chadwick V.S., Phillips S.F. & Hofmann A.F. (1977) Measurements of intestinal permeability using low molecular weight polyethylene glycols (PEA 400). *Gastroenterol.* **73**, 247–251.

Challacombe D.N. & Robertson K. (1977) Enterochromaffin cells in the duodenal mucosa of children with coeliac disease. *Gut*, **18**, 373–376.

Chanarin I. (1979) Vitamin B_{12} in serum, liver and cerebro-spinal fluid. In *The Megaloblastic Anaemias*. 2nd ed., Chapter 8, pp. 126–146. Blackwell Scientific Publications, Oxford.

Cobden I., Rothwell J. & Axon A.T.R. (1980) Intestinal permeability and screening tests for coeliac disease. *Gut*, **21**, 512–518.

Coleman R.E., Welch D.M., Baker W.J. et al. (1981) Clinical experience using Indium-111 labelled leucocytes. In *Indium-111 Labelled Neutrophils, Platelets and Lymphocytes* (Ed. by M.L. Thakur & A. Gottschalk), pp. 103–118. Trivirium, New York.

Cooney D.R., Duszynski D.O., Camboa E., Karp M.P. & Jewett T.C. (1982) The abdominal technetium scan (a decade of experience). *J. Pediat. Surg.* **17**, 611–619.

Creamer B. & Pink I.J. (1967) Paneth cell deficiency. *Lancet*, **1**, 304–306.

Crosby W.H. & Kugler H.W. (1957) Intraluminal biopsy of the small intestine. *Amer. J. Digest. Dis.* **2**, 236–241.

Cummings J.H. (1983) Fermentation in the human large intestine: evidence and implications for health. *Lancet*, **i**, 1206–1209.

Dahlqvist P. (1964) Method for assay of intestinal disaccharidases. *Analyt. Biochem.* **7**, 18–25.

Davis G.R., Zerwekh J.E., Parker T.F., Krejs G.J., Pak C.Y.C. & Fordtran J.S. (1983) Absorption of phosphate in the jejunum of patients with chronic renal failure before and after correction of vitamin D deficiency. *Gastroenterol*, **85**, 908–916.

Dawson A.M., Holdsworth C.D. & Pitcher C.S. (1964) Sideroblastic anaemia in adult coeliac disease. *Gut*, **5**, 304–308.

De Lacey G., Benson M., Wilkins R., Spencer J. & Cramer B. (1982) Routine colonic lavage is unnecessary for double contrast barium enema in outpatients. *Br. Med. J.* **284**, 1021–1022.

Domstad P.A., Choy Y.C., Kim E.E. & DeLand F.H. (1981) Reliability of the dual-isotope Schilling test for the diagnosis of pernicious anemia or malabsorption syndrome. *Amer. J. Clin. Pathol.* **75**, 723–726.

Drugs and Therapeutics Bulletin (1984) *Rational use of vitamins.* **22**, 33–36.

Drummey G.D., Benson J.A. & Jones C.M. (1961) Microscopical examination of the stool for steatorrhoea. *New Engl. J. Med.* **264**, 85–87.

Dunnil M.S. & Whitehead R. (1972) A method for the quantitation of small intestinal biopsy specimens. *J. Clin. Path.* **25**, 243–246.

Durnin J.V. & Womersley J. (1974) Total body fat assessed from total body density and its estimation from skin-fold thickness: measurements on 481 men and women aged from 16 to 72 years. *Brit. J. Nutrit.* **33**, 77–97.

Dyet J.F., Pratt A.E. & Flouty G. (1976) The small bowel enema: description and experience of a technique. *B. J. Radiol.* **49**, 1039–1044.

Editorial (1981) Nutritional oedema, albumin and

vanadate. *Lancet,* **i**, 646–647.
Efsing H.O. & Lindroth B. (1980) Small bowel examination after injection of cholecystokinin. *Clin. Radiol.* **31**, 225–226.
Elmes M., Golden M.K. & Love A.H.G. (1976) Unresponsive coeliac disease. *Quart. J. Med.* **45**, 696–697.
Ferguson A. (1977) Intra-epithelial lymphocytes of the small intestine, *Gut*, **18**, 921–937.
Ferguson A. & Murray D. (1971) Quantitation of intraepithelial lymphocytes in human jejunum. *Gut*, **12**, 988–996.
Ferrant A., Dehasque N., Leners N. & Meunier H. (1980) Scintigraphy with In-111 labelled red cells in intermittent gastrointestinal bleeding. *J. Nucl. Med.* **21**, 844–845.
Field M. & Chang E.B. (1983) Pancreatic cholera. *New Engl. J. Med.* **309**, 1513–1515.
Fleckenstein P. & Pedersen G. (1975) The value of the duodenal intubation method (Sellink modification) for the radiological visualization of the small bowel. *Scand. J. Gastroenterol.* **10**, 423–426.
Fordtran J.S., Rector F.C. & Ewton M.F. (1965) Permeability characteristics of the small intestine. *J. Clin. Invest.* **44**, 1935–1944.
Fordtran J.S., Rector F.C. & Locklear T.W. (1967) Water and soluble movement in the small intestine of patients with sprue. *J. Clin. Invest.* **46**, 287–298.
Fraser D. (1983) The physiological economy of vitamin D. *Lancet*, **i**, 969–972.
Frazer A.C. (1955) Steatorrhoea. *Brit. Med. J.* **2**, 805–809.
Fried A.M., Poulos A. & Hatfield D.R. (1981) The effectiveness of the incidental small bowel series. *Radiol.* **140**, 45–46.
Frisancho A.R. (1981) New norms of upper limb fat and muscle areas for assessment of nutritional status. *Amer. J. Clin. Nut.* **34**, 2540–2545.
Fromm H. & Hofmann A.F. (1971) Breath test for altered bile acid metabolism. *Lancet*, **ii**, 621.
Fromm H., Thomas P.J. & Hofmann A.F. (1973) Sensitivity and specificity in tests of distal ileal function: prospective comparison of bile acid and vitamin B_{12} absorption in ileal resection patients. *Gastroenterol.* **64**, 1077–1090.
Furrer A., Grüntzig A., Kugelmeier J. & Goebel N. (1980) Treatment of abdominal angina with percutaneous dilatation of an arteria mesenterica superior stenosis. *Cardiovasc. Intervent. Radiol.* **3**, 43–44.
Goldberg H. I. & Sheft D.J. (1976) Abnormalities in small intestine contour and calibre, a working classification. *Radiol. Clinics North Amer.* **14**, 461–475.
Greenfield G.B. (1975) Loss of bone density. In *Radiology of Bone Diseases*, pp. 13–28. J.B. Lippincott Co., Philadelphia.
Griffin G.E., Fagan E.F., Hodgson H.T. & Chadwick V.S. (1982) Enteral therapy in the management of massive gut resection complicated by chronic fluid and electrolyte depletion. *Dig. Dis. Sci.* **27**, 902–908.
Hattner R.S. (1983) Nuclear medicine of the alimentary tube. In *Alimentary Tract Radiology*, 3rd ed. (Ed. by A.R. Margulis & H.J. Burhenne) C.V. Mosby Co., St. Louis.
Hepner G.W. (1975) Increased sensitivity of the cholylglycine breath test for detecting ileal dysfunction. *Gastroenterol.* **68**, 8–16.
Herlinger H. (1978) A modified technique for the double contrast small bowel enema. *Gastrointest. Radiol.* **3**, 201–207.
Herlinger H. (1983) Double contrast enteroclysis. In *Alimentary Tract Radiology*, 3rd ed. (Ed. by A.R. Margulis & J.H. Burhenne). C.V. Mosby Co., St. Louis.
Herlinger H. & Lintott D.J. (1983) In *Alimentary Tract Radiology* 3rd ed., p. 907. (Ed. by A.R. Margulis & H.J. Burhenne) C.V. Mosby Co., St. Louis.
Heymsfield S.B., McManus C., Stevens V. & Smith J. (1982) Muscle mass: reliable indicator of protein — energy malnutrition severity and outcome. *Amer. J. Clin. Nut.* **35**, 1192–1199.
Hill R.E., Herez A. Corey M.L., Gilday D.L. & Hamilton J.R. (1981) Fecal clearance of alpha-l-antitrypsin — a reliable measure of enteric protein loss in children. *J. Pediat.* **99**, 416–418.
Hoffer P. (1980) Gallium and infection. *J. Nucl. Med.* **21**, 484–488.
Hofmann A.F. (1978) The enterohepatic circulation of bile acids. In *Gastrointestinal Disease* pp. 92–107. (Ed. by M.H. Sleisenger & J.S. Fordtran). W.B. Saunders, Philadelphia.
Holdsworth C.D. (1969) The gut and oral glucose tolerance. *Gut*, **10**, 422–427.
Howarth F.H., Cockel R., Roper B.W. & Hawkins C.F. (1969) The effect of metoclopramide upon gastric motility and its value in barium progress meals. *Clin. Radiol.* **20**, 294–300.
Isaacson P. (1980) Malignant histicoytosis of the intestine: the early histological lesion. *Gut*, **21**, 381–386.
Jeejeebhoy K.M. (1981) Protein nutrition in clinical practice. *Brit. Med. Bull.* **37**, 11–17.
Jeejeebhoy K.N. & Coghill N.F. (1961) The measurement of gastrointestinal protein loss by a new method. *Gut*, **2**, 123–130.
Jeejeebhoy K.N., Chu R.C., Marliss E.B., Greenberg G.R. & Bruce-Robertson A. (1977) Chromium deficiency, glucose intolerance and neuropathy reversed by chromium supplementation in a patient receiving long-term total parenteral nutrition. *Amer. J. Clin. Nutr.* **30**, 531–538.
Joplin G.F., Robinson C.J., Melvin K.E.W., Thompson G.R. & Fraser R. (1967) Results of tracer studies in osteomalacia. In *L'Osteomalacie*, p. 249. Ed. D.J. Hioco, Paris.
Kadir S. & Strauss H.W. (1979) Evaluation of inflammatory bowel disease with 99m-Tc-DTPA. *Radiol.* **130**, 443–446.
Kaihara S., Wagner H.N. (1968) Measurement of

intestinal fat absorption with carbon-14 labelled tracers. *J. Lab. Clin. Med.* **71**, 400–411.

Kamer J.H. van der, ten Bokkel Huinink H. & Weyers H.A. (1949) Rapid method for the determination of fat in feces. *J. Biol. Chem.* **177**, 347–355.

Keeling P.W.N., Jones R.B., Hilton P.J. & Thompson R.P.H. (1980) Reduced leucocyte zinc in liver disease. *Gut*, **21**, 561–564.

King C.E. & Toskes P.P. (1979) Small intestinal bacterial overgrowth. *Gastroenterol.* **76**, 1035–1055.

King C.E., Toskes P.E., Pixey J.C., Lorenz E. & Welkos S. (1979) Detection of small intestinal bacterial overgrowth by means of a ^{14}C-D-Xylose breath test. *Gastroenterol.* **77**, 75–82.

Klidjian A.M., Archer T.J., Foster K.J., & Karran S.J. (1982) Detection of dangerous malnutrition. *J. Parenteral & Enteral. Nutrit.* **6**, 119–121.

Kobayashi S. & Nishiasawa M. (1976) X-ray examination of small intestine: double contrast method by duodenal intubation. *Stomach Intest.* **11**, 157.

Kressel H.Y., Moss A.A., Montgomery C.K., Brito A.C. & Hoffer P. (1978) Radionuclide imaging of bowel infarction complicating small bowel intussusception in dogs. *Invest. Radiol.* **3**, 127–131.

Lee F.D. & Toner P.G. (1980) *Biopsy Pathology of the Small Intestine*. Champman and Hall, London.

Levitt M.D. & Donaldson R.M. (1970) Use of respiratory hydrogen (H_2) excretion to detect carbohydrate malabsorption. *J. Lab. Clin Med.* **90**, 405–411.

Losowsky M.S., Walker B.E. & Kelleher J. (1974) *Malabsorption in Clinical Practice*, Churchill Livingstone, London.

Maglinte D.D., Hall R., Miller R.E., Chernish S.M., Rosenak B., Elmore M. & Burney B.T. (1984) Detection of surgical lesions of the small bowel by enteroclysis. *Amer. J. Surg.* **147**, 225–229.

Main A.N.H., Hall M.J., Russell R.I., Fell G.S., Mills P.R. & Shenkin A. (1982) Clinical experience of zinc supplementation during intravenous nutrition in Crohn's disease: value of serum and urine zinc measurements. *Gut*, **23**, 984–991.

Main A.N.H., Mills P.R., Russell R.I., Bronte-Stewart J., Nelson L.M., McClelland A. & Shenkin A. (1983) Vitamin A deficiency in Crohn's disease. *Gut*, **24**, 1169–1175.

Marsh M.N. (1982) Studies of intestinal lymphoid tissue. IV. The predictive value of raised mitotic indices among jejunal epithelial lymphocytes in the diagnosis of gluten-sensitive enteropathy. J. Clin. *Pathol.* **35**, 517–525.

Marshak R.H. (1980) Enterocylsis (letter) *Gastrointest. Radiol.* **5**, 187.

Martin E.C., Casarella W.J. & Schultz R.W. (1982) Angiographic management of arterial haemorrhage in the upper gastrointestinal tract. In *Interventional Radiology*. (Ed. by R.A. Wilkins & M. Vamonte Jr) Blackwell Scientific Publications, New York.

Melvin K.E.W., Hepner G.W., Bordier P., Neale G. & Joplin G.F. (1970) Calcium metabolism and bone pathology in adult coeliac disease. *Quart. J. Med.* **39**, 83–113.

Menzies I.S., Laker M.F., Pounder R., Bill J., Heyer S., Wheeler P.G. & Creamer B. (1979) Abnormal intestinal permeability to sugars in villous atrophy. *Lancet*, **ii**, 1107–1109.

Mernagh J.R., Harrison J.E. & McNeill K.G. (1977) *In vivo* determination of nitrogen using Pu-Be sources. *Phys. Med. Biol.* **22**, 831–835.

Merrick M.V., Boyd G.S., Eastwood M.A. & Monks R. (1983) SeHCAT — A new radiopharmaceutical for evaluating ileal function and the enterohepatic circulation of bile acids. *Nuclear Medicine and Biology Advances*, pp. 2430–2433. (Ed. by C. Raynaud) Pergamon Press, Oxford.

Metz G., Gassull M., Leeds A. *et al.* (1976) A simple method of measuring breath hydrogen in carbohydrate malabsorption by end expiratory sampling. *Clin. Sci. Mol. Med.* **50**, 237–240.

Metz G., Jenkins D.J.A., Peters T.J., Newman L. & Blendis C.M. (1975) Breath hydrogen as a diagnostic method for hypolactasia. *Lancet*, **i**, 1155–1157.

Miller R.E. (1965) Complete reflux small bowel examination. *Radiol.* **84**, 457–463.

Moossa A.R., Skinner D.B., Stark V. & Hoffer P. (1974) Assessment of bowel viability using 99m Technetium-tagged albumin microspheres. *J. Surg. Res.* **16**, 466–472.

Morton J.L. (1961) Notes on small bowel examination. *Am. J. Roentgenol. Rad. Therapy and Nucl. Med.* **66**, 76–85.

Mullen J.L., Buzby G.P., Waldmann T.G. & Smale B.F. (1980) Reduction of operative morbidity and mortality by combined pre-operative and post-operative nutritional support. *Ann. Surg.* **192**, 604–613.

Munro H.N. (1970) Free amino acid pools and their role in regulation. In *Mammalian Protein Metabolism*, vol. 4, p. 299. (Ed. by H.N. Munro). Academic Press, New York.

Nabeyema A. & Leblond C.P. (1974) 'Caveolated Cells' characterized by deep surface invaginations and abundant filaments in mouse gastrointestinal epithelia. *Am. J. Anat.* **140**, 147–166.

Neale G., Antcliff A.C., Welbourn R.B., Mollin D. & Booth C.C. (1968) Protein malnutrition after partial gastrectomy. *Quart. J. Med.* **36**, 469–494.

Neale G., Clark M. & Levin B. (1965) Intestinal sucrase deficiency presenting as sucrose intolerance. *Brit. med. J.* **11**, 1223–1225.

Newcomer A.D., Hofmann A.F., DiMagno E.P., Thomas P.J. & Carlson G.I. (1979) Triolein breath test: a sensitive and specific test for malabsorption. *Gastroenterol.* **76**, 6–13.

Nice Jr C.M. (1963) Roentgenographic patterns and

motility in small bowel studies. *Radiol.* **80**, 39–45.

Nice Jr C.M. (1974) Controlled roentgen examination of the small bowel. *Minn. Med.* **57**, 281–284.

Nolan D.J. (1979) Rapid duodenal and jejunal intubation. *Clin. Radiol.* **30**, 183–185.

Owen R.L. & Jones A.L. (1974) Epithelial cell specialization within human Peyer's patches: an ultrastructural study of intestinal lymphoid follicles. *Gastroenterol* **66**, 189–203.

Pajewski M., Eshchar J. & Manor A. (1975) Visualization of the small intestine by double contrast. *Clin. Radiol.* **26**, 491–493.

Pederson L., Arnfred T. & Hess Thaysen E. (1973) Rapid screening of increased bile acid deconjugation and bile acid malabsorption by means of the glycine-1-(14C) cholylglycine assay. *Scand. J. Gastroenterol.* **8**, 665–672.

Penna F.J., Hill I.D., Kingston D., Robertson K., Slavin G. & Shiner M., (1981) Jejunal mucosal morphometry in children with and without gut symptoms and in normal adults. *J. Clin. Pathol.* **34**, 386–392.

Perera D.R., Weinstein W.M. & Rubin C.E. (1975) Small Intestinal Biopsy. *Human Pathol.* **6**, 157–217.

Pesquera G.S. (1929) Method for direct visualization of lesions in the small intestine. *Am. J. Roentgenol. Radium Ther. Nucl. Med.* **22**, 254–257.

Petrokuli R.J., Baum S. & Rohrer G.V. (1978) Cimetidine administration resulting in improved pertechnetate imaging of Meckel's diverticulum. *Clin. Nucl. Med.* **3**, 385–388.

Pettit J.E. (1981) Recommended methods for B_{12} absorption. *J. Nucl. Med.*, **22**, 1091–1093.

Press M., Kiruchi H., Shimoyama T. & Thompson G.R. (1974) Diagnosis and treatment of essential fatty acid deficiency in man. *Brit. Med. J.* **2**, 247–250.

Price A.B. (1980) Metaplasia and neoplasia of the gastrointestinal tract. In *Scientific Foundations of Gastroenterology.* (Ed. by W. Sircus & A.N. Smith) William Heinemann Medical Books Ltd., London.

Pringot J. & Bodart P. (1983) Inflammatory diseases. In *Alimentary Tract Radiology*, 3rd ed. (Ed. by A.R. Margulis & H.J. Burhenne) C.V. Mosby & Co., St. Louis, pp. 917–961.

Quaife M.L., Scrimshaw N.S. & Lowry O.H. (1949) Micro method for assay of total tocopherols in blood serum. *J. Biol. Chem.* **180**, 1229–1235.

Rabe F.E., Becker G.J., Besozzi M.J. & Miller R.E. (1981) Efficacy study of the small bowel examination. *Radiol.* **140**, 47–50.

Rambaud J.C., Modigliani R., Edmonds P., Matuchansky C., Vichon N., Besterman H. & Bernier J.J. (1978) Fluid secretions in the duodenum and intestinal handling of water and electrolytes in the Zollinger–Ellison syndrome. *Am. J. digest. Dis.* **23**, 1089–1097.

Read A.E., Gough K.R., Bones J.A. & McCarthy C.F. (1962) An improvement to the Crosby peroral intestinal biopsy capsule. *Lancet* **i**, 894–895.

Rose C.S., Gyjörgy P. & Butler M. (1976) Age differences in vitamin B6 status of 617 men. *Am. J. Clin. Nutr.* **29**, 847–853.

Sanders D.E. & Ho C.S. (1976) The small bowel enema: experience with 150 examinations. *Am. J. Roentgenol.* **127**, 743–751.

Sandow M.J. & Whitehead R. (1979) The Paneth cell. *Gut* **20**, 420–431.

Saverymuttu, S.H., Peters, A.M., Lavender, J.P. & Hodgson, H.J. (1983a) Detection of proteinlosing enteropathy by ^{111}In-Transferrin scanning. *Eur. J. Nucl. Med.* **8**, 40–41.

Saverymuttu, S.H., Peters, A.M., Hodgson, H.J., Chadwick, V.S. & Lavender, J.P. (1983b) ^{111}Indium leucocyte scanning in small bowel Crohn's disease. *Gastrointest. Radiol.* **8**, 157–161.

Schedl H.P. & Clifton J.A. (1963) Solute and water absorption by the human small intestine. *Nature (Lond.)* **199**, 1264–1267.

Schoen M.S., Lindenbaum J., Roginsky M.S. & Holt P.R. (1978) Significance of serum levels of 25-hydroxycholecalciferol in gastrointestinal disease. *Am. J. Dig. Dis.* **23**, 137–142.

Scott H. & Brandtzaeg P. (1981) Enumeration of Paneth cells in coeliac disease: comparison of conventional light microscopy and immunofluorescence staining for lysozyme. *Gut,* **22**, 812–816.

Selby W.S., Janossey G. & Jewell D.P. (1981) Immunohistological characterization of intraepithelial lymphocytes of the human gastrointestinal tract. *Gut,* **22**, 169–176.

Sellink J.L. (1971) *Examination of the Small Intestine by Means of Duodenal Intubation* (Thesis). H.E. Stenfert Kroese, BV, Leiden.

Sellink J.L. (1976) In *Radiological Atlas of Common Disease of the Small Bowel.* H.E. Stenfert Kroese, BV, Leiden.

Sellink J.L. (1983) Single contrast enteroclysis. In *Alimentary Tract Radiology*, 3rd ed. (Ed. by A.R. Margulis & H.J. Buchenne). C.V. Mosby Co., St. Louis. pp. 871–879.

Sfakianakis G.N., Al-Sheikh W., Heal A., Rodman G., Seppa R. & Serafini A. (1982) Comparisons of scintigraphy with In-111 leucocytes and Ga-67 in the diagnosis of acute sepsis. *J. Nucl. Med.* **23**, 618–626.

Shils M.E. (1969) Experimental human magnesium depletion. *Medicine,* **48**, 61–85.

Shiner M. & Doniach I. (1960) Histopathologic studies in steatorrhea. *Gastroenterol.* **38**, 419–440.

Shizgal H.M., Milne C.A. & Spencer A.H. (1979) The effect of nitrogensparing, intravenously administered fluids on post-operative body composition. *Surgery,* **85**, 496–503.

Siegelman S.S., Sprayregm S. & Boley S.J. (1974) Angiographic diagnosis of mesenteric arterial vasoconstriction. *Radiol.* **112**, 533–542.

Skinner J.M. & Whitehead R. (1976) Morphological methods in the study of the gut immune system in man. *J. Clin. Path.* **29**, 564−567.

Sladen G.E. (1972) A review of water and electrolyte transport. In *Transport Across the Intestine* Burland W.L. and Samuel P.B. pp. 14-34. Churchill Livingstone, Edinburgh.

Sladen G.E.G. & Kumar P.J. (1973) Is the xylose test still a worthwhile investigation? *Brit. Med. J.* **3**, 223−226.

Solomons N.W. & Allan L.H. (1983) The functional assessment of nutritional status: principles, practice and potential. *Nut. Rev.* **41**, 33−50.

Soucy, J.P., Eybalin, M.C., Taillefer, R., Levassawe, & Jobin, G. (1983) Lymphoscintigraphic demonstration of intestinal lymphangiectasia. *Clin. Nucl. Med.* **8**, 535−537.

Spencer J.D., Stiel D. & Peters T.J. (1983) Patterns of gastric 99m-Tc-Pertechnetate secretion and their relationship to gastric acid secretion in man (abstract) *Clin. Sci.* **64**, 15P.

Strange R.C., Reid J., Holton D., Jewell N.P. & Percy-Robb I.W. (1980) The glyceryl 14C tripalmitate breath test: a reassessment. *Clin. Chim. Acta.*, **103**, 317−323.

Treves S., Grand R.J. & Eraklis A.J. (1978) Pentagastrin stimulation of Tc-99m uptake by ectopic gastric mucosa in a Meckel's diverticulum. *Radiol.* **128**, 711−712.

Turnberg L.A. (1971) Abnormalities in intestinal electrolyte transport in congenital chloridorrhoea. *Gut*, **12**, 544−551.

Violon D., Steppe R. & Potvliege R. (1981) Improved retrograde ileography with glucagon. *Am. J. Roentgenol.*, **146**, 833−834.

Waldmann T.A. (1961) Gastrointestinal protein loss demonstrated by ^{51}Cr-labelled albumin. *Lancet*, **ii**, 121−123.

Waldmann T.A. (1966) Protein-losing enteropathy. *Gastroenterol.*, **50**, 422−443.

Waldmann T.A., Morell A.G., Wochner R.D. & Sternlieb I. (1965) Quantitation of gastrointestinal protein loss with copper [67]-labelled ceruloplasmin. *J. Clin. Invest.* **44**, 1107.

Walker A.R.P., Arvidsson U.B. & Politzer W.M. (1954) Significance of low serum calcium values in South African Bantu. *South African Med. J.* **28**, 48−51.

Waterlow J.C., Buzina R., Keller W., Lane J.M., Nichaman M.Z. & Tanner J.M. (1977) The presentation and use of height and weight data for comparing the nutritional status of groups of children under the age of 10 years. *Bull. WHO*, **55**, 489−496.

Watkins J.B., Schoeller D.A., Klein P.D., Ott D.G., Newcomer A.D. & Hofmann A.F. (1977) ^{13}C-trioctanoin: a nonradiactive breath test to detect fat malabsorption. *J. Lab. Clin. Med.* **90**, 422−430.

Welch C.A. & Hedberg S. (1973) Gastrointestinal haemorrhage. General consideration of diagnosis and therapy. *Adv. Surg.* **7**, 95.

West P.S., Levin G.E., Griffin G.E. & Maxwell J.D. (1981) Comparisons of simple screening tests for fat malabsorption. *Brit. Med. J.* **1**, 1501−1504.

Whittle H., Neale G., McLaughlin M., Peters T., Blair A., Thalassinos N., Marsh M.N., Wedzicha B. & Thompson G.R. (1969) Intravenous vitamin D in the detection of vitamin D deficiency. *Lancet*, **i**, 747−750.

Williams L.F. & Kim J.P. (1971) Non-occlusive mesenteric ischemia. In *Vascular Disorders of the Intestine*. (Ed. by S.J. Boley, S.S. Schwartz & L.F. Williams). Butterworths, London.

Winzelberg C.G., McKusick K.A., Strauss H.W., Waltman A.C. & Greenfield A.J. (1979) Evaluation of gastrointestinal bleeding by red cells labelled *in vivo* with Technetium-99m. *J. Nucl. Med.* **20**, 1080−1086.

Zarins C.K., Skinner D.B. & James A.E. (1974) Prediction of the viability of revascularised intestine with radioactive microspheres. *Surg. Gynaecol. & Obstetrics.* **138**, 576−580.

Chapter 2
Congenital Anatomical Abnormalities

JOHN WALKER-SMITH AND VANESSA WRIGHT

Embryology of the small intestine 43
Atresia and stenosis 44
Duplication of gastrointestinal tract 46
Small intestinal malrotation with or without volvulus 47
Meckel's diverticulum 49
Congenital short intestine 50
Congenital absence of intestinal muscle 50

Embryology of the small intestine

The primitive gut is a simple tube of endoderm communicating with the extra-embryonic yolk sac by the vitello-intestinal duct. This tube of endoderm is surrounded by mesoderm. Rapid growth in length occurs during early intra-uterine life and this, together with the disproportionate amount of space required by the liver, forces the intestine to herniate into a mesothelial lined sac within the base of the umbilical cord. This herniation commences at about the sixth week of intra-uterine life. The apex of the loop of developing intestine is in continuity with the vitello-intestinal duct which now begins to atrophy and eventually disappears leaving the loop free in the umbilical sac. The cranial limb of the loop then lengthens rapidly to form the small intestine. A small portion of the caudal limb between the attachment of the vitello-intestinal duct and the caecum forms the terminal ileum.

The rotation of the developing gut is shown diagramatically in Fig. 2.1. As the loop lengthens it rotates initially through 90° anti-clockwise around the axis of the superior mesenteric artery, which arises from the aorta and runs through the mesentery of the midgut loop. Thus the cranial part of the loop comes to lie on the right side of the embryo. At about 10 weeks of intra-uterine life the proximal loops of small intestine return to the abdominal cavity which is now more capacious with the liver proportionately occupying a smaller space. The first loop of bowel, destined to form the distal duodenum, lies posteriorly against the abdominal wall and by a further anti-clockwise rotation of the gut comes to be behind the superior mesenteric artery. Gradually the other loops of small intestine are withdrawn from the umbilical sac and eventually the bulbous caecum is also re-

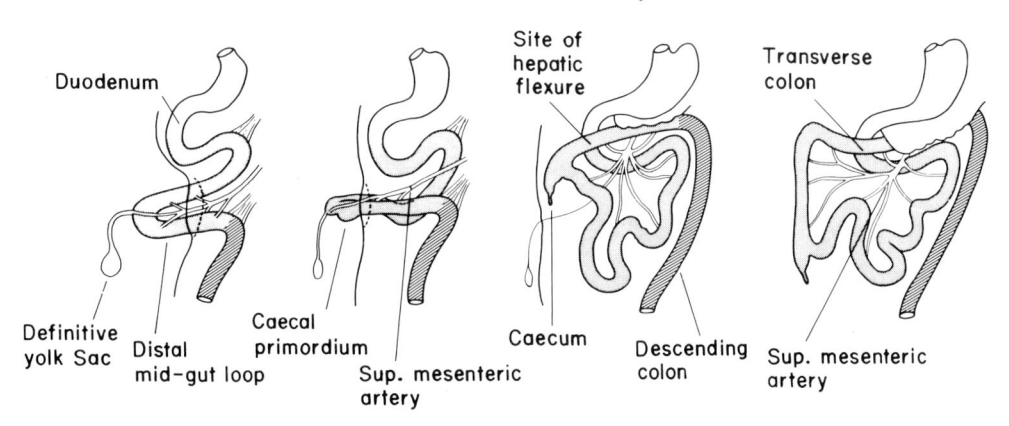

Fig. 2.1. Diagrams of rotation and fixation of the gut, viewed obliquely from the left side. □, Foregut; ▦, midgut; ▨, hindgut.

turned to the peritoneal cavity lying anterior to the other bowel but a further rotation brings the caecum across to the sub-hepatic region. Differential colonic growth then pushes the caecum downwards to the right iliac fossa. Adhesion between apposed surfaces of the primitive mesentery provide gut fixation, the most important being the broad fixation of the small intestinal mesentery from the duodenojejunal flexure, which lies to the left of the first vertebral body, to the ileocaecal junction in the right iliac fossa.

Atresia and stenosis

Aetiology

Tandler suggested in 1902 that duodenal atresia and stenosis are due to a failure of recanalization of the duodenum during the twelfth week of intra-uterine life, duodenal epithelial proliferation having previously produced luminal occlusion. The frequent association of abnormal pancreatic anatomy with these lesions, however, suggests that this theory may be an oversimplification. So far as the jejunum and ileum are concerned, there is good experimental and clinical evidence that vascular accidents occurring during intra-uterine life and after the intestine has developed are responsible for most atresias and stenoses (Barnard 1956, Louw 1959). Occlusion of mesenteric blood vessels, volvulus of a loop or loops of bowel, intussusception, and trapping of bowel in the umbilical sac have all been postulated as possible aetiological factors.

These theories do not explain why other adnormalities outside the gastrointestinal tract occur more often with duodenal than with jejuno-ileal lesions.

Definition

Intrinsic small intestinal obstruction may produce either complete or partial obliteration of the bowel lumen. *Complete obliteration* (atresia) may be due to a mucosal diaphragm occluding the lumen or to a gap between the two ends of the small intestine with or without a connecting band between the ends. There may be an associated V-shaped gap in the mesentery. An *incomplete obstruction* (stenosis) may be due to a narrow segment of intestine or a diaphragm with a small, usually central opening. The latter occurs particularly in the duodenum.

Atresia occurs more commonly than stenosis. In an analysis of forty-two consecutive admissions with small intestinal obstruction to the Royal Alexandra Hospital for Children, Sydney, atresia occurred in thirty children and stenosis in the remaining twelve.

Intrinsic obstruction occurs most commonly in the duodenum. The jejunum and ileum are involved with almost equal frequency. Other abnormalities of the gastrointestinal tract occur in association with intrinsic obstruction (Table 2.1). Duodenal lesions are particularly associated with lesions outside the gastrointestinal tract (Table 2.2), and are a well-known complication of Down's syndrome, occurring in 20–30% of cases.

Table 2.1 Associated abnormalities of the gastrointestinal tract in Atresia & Stenosis (Royal Alexandra Hospital for Children).

	Duodenum	Jejuno-ileum
No. of children	24	18
Malrotation of midgut loop	10	3
Meckel's diverticulum	1	3
Oesophageal atresia	4	—
Imperforate anus	2	—
Volvulus	—	4
Meconium peritonitis	—	2
Meconium ileus	—	2
Perforation	2	—
Annular pancreas	2	—
Atresia of bile ducts	3	—

Table 2.2 Associated abnormalities outside the gastrointestinal tract in Atresia & Stenosis (Royal Alexandra Hospital for Children).

	Duodenum	Jejunum	Ileum
No. of children	24	11	7
Genito-urinary	7	—	—
Musculoskeletal	4	2	—
Down's syndrome	11	—	—
Cardiovascular	6	—	—

Clinical features

Intrinsic obstruction of the small intestine of congenital origin presents most often in the neonatal period. If the obstruction is partial, however, it may first present much later in infancy and childhood, or even in adult life.

Congenital intrinsic duodenal obstruction

When duodenal obstruction is complete, vomiting usually occurs within a few hours of birth and is characteristically bile-stained except when the obstruction is proximal to the ampulla of Vater (10–30% of cases). Vomiting does not occur when there is an accompanying oesophageal atresia, a well-recognized association of this disorder. Meconium may be passed normally and there may be no obvious epigastric distension. In view of the frequent association with other abnormalities outside the gastrointestinal tract, these should be sought for carefully, once the diagnosis has been established. In particular, the infant should be examined carefully for evidence of Down's syndrome. When obstruction is incomplete, the symptoms may be intermittent and the diagnosis is often delayed.

Congenital intrinsic duodenal obstruction may be accompanied by an annular pancreas. This is a congenital disorder in which a ring of pancreatic tissue surrounds the second part of the duodenum and rarely occurs in isolation. It is a sign of failure of duodenal development rather than an obstructing lesion *per se*. In children with duodenal atresia, the appearances at surgery may resemble those of an annular pancreas, since there is inter-position of the pancreas between the two ends of the duodenal atresia. Congenital intrinsic duodenal obstruction is not usually associated with multiple atresias in the remainder of the small intestine.

Jejunal and ileal obstruction

Symptoms of vomiting and abdominal distension usually occur within the first 2 days of life. If meconium is present in the bowel distal to the obstruction, this may be passed but is usually pale and in the form of pellets. In some infants no meconium is passed at all. When obstruction is incomplete the diagnosis may again be long delayed and the condition may present in childhood with intermittent vomiting, abdominal distension and even with features of malabsorption in adult life, the clinical picture resembling coeliac disease. Congenital ileal stricture presenting with vitamin B_{12} deficiency due to a stagnant loop syndrome in adult life has also been described (Chapter 15, p. 265 and Booth & Mollin 1960).

Diagnosis

Plain X-ray of the abdomen is usually diagnostic in infants who present acutely. In duodenal atresia there is the characteristic 'double bubble'. When duodenal obstruction is incomplete there may be small amounts of air in the lower bowel with distension of stomach and proximal duodenum. A barium meal may be necessary in cases of incomplete obstruction and will differentiate a duodenal stenosis from a malrotation producing extrinsic duodenal obstruction.

When there is a complete jejunal or ileal obstruction, there are usually dilated loops of small intestine with fluid levels apparent on plain X-ray of the abdomen and there is no colonic gas. A barium enema may reveal an unused microcolon. When obstruction is incomplete a barium follow-through may be needed to establish the diagnosis. Laparotomy may be necessary in these circumstances.

Management

Delay in diagnosis leads to poor surgical results. Unfortunately such delay sometimes occurs because of the lack of appreciation of the significance of bile-stained vomiting in the first 24 h of life and, therefore, failure to consult surgical advice. Correction of fluid and electrolyte disturbances, if present, should precede surgery. At laparotomy, care should be taken to exclude any accompanying gastrointestinal abnormality. In duodenal obstruction, the operation of choice is duodenoduodenostomy or duodenojejunostomy. Some surgeons use a trans-anastomotic feeding tube during the immediate postoperative period, with a gastrostomy tube draining the stomach. If there are jejunal and ileal lesions, resection is obviously indicated but there should be adequate resection of the proximal dilated gut as gut immediately proximal to an atresia may remain flabby and dilated with ineffective peristalsis postoperatively. This reduces the great discrepancy in size between the two blind ends and so facilitates end-to-end anastomosis, although an oblique-to-end anastomosis is still sometimes necessary. In a high jejunal atresia, where adequate resection of the dilated bowel is impossible, then dilated bowel can be tapered longitudinally to improve motility by reducing the diameter. Despite these manoeuvres, postoperative diarrhoea may occur and this may be due to bacterial overgrowth. There may be disaccharide malabsorption acutely in the postoperative period, or steatorrhoea months or even years later. Sometimes further surgery is necessary to correct this complication by resecting an area of proximally dilated bowel where there is stasis of gut contents above the previous anastomosis.

The shortened intestine provides a further reason for poor intestinal absorption postoperatively. At laparotomy the length of intestine remaining should therefore be measured as accurately as possible and a note made as to whether the intestine is jejunum or ileum and whether the ileocaecal valve remains. Although only a few centimetres of bowel may be removed at laparotomy, the insult which resulted in the atresia may have caused a long length of intestine to reabsorb. Furthermore, multiple atresias requiring resection may leave only a short length of bowel *in situ*. Cystic fibrosis is another occasional cause of failure to thrive following treatment for intestinal atresia. A number of atresias will occur secondary to meconium ileus.

Duplication of gastrointestinal tract

Aetiology

The cause of the developmental aberration producing a cystic or tubular duplication of the intestine remains uncertain. The frequent association with vertebral abnormalities suggests an aetiology in early embryonic life. The notochordal theory postulates that ingrowth of mesoderm between the notochordal plate and the endoderm does not separate these two layers completely and adhesions therefore remain between the notochord and the roof of the developing intestine. These adhesions result in endodermal cells being pulled cranially during rapid meso- and ectodermal growth. Such a column of endoderm might produce a tubular thoracic or thoraco-abdominal duplication or, if only a limited length developed a lumen, a cyst would result. This theory would explain the occasional adhesion of duplications to the vertebral column and abnormalities of vertebral bodies. Another theory postulated is splitting of the notochord with herniation of the yolk sac through the defect with subsequent development of a duplication of the gut. These theories, while attractive, do not completely explain the multiple variations seen with duplications of the gastrointestinal tract.

Definition

Duplications are cystic or tubular structures, the lumen being lined by an epithelium resembling some part of the alimentary tract, supported by smooth muscle. They occur most often within the dorsal mesentery of the gut. They are also sometimes described as enteric cysts, neurenteric cysts and reduplications, but the term duplications seems the most suitable, taking into account their probable embryological origin.

Duplications may occur anywhere along the alimentary tract but they are found most often in relation to the small intestine, particularly the ileum (Bower *et al*. 1978). Cystic duplications occur more commonly than tubular lesions. The tubular duplications usually communicate with the intestine at one end only and run along the mesenteric border of the gut for a variable distance.

Duplications may be found in association with intestinal atresias. Sometimes those in association with the small intestine may be lined by gastric mucosa and peptic ulceration and bleeding may occur.

Clinical features

Duplications present most often in early infancy, less commonly in childhood and only occasionally in adult life.

If large enough, cystic duplications may present as an abdominal mass and, because of their close proximity to the normal bowel obstruction, may result from compression of the lumen by the adjacent cyst. The cyst may also induce a volvulus of the intestine. Small cysts may act as the lead point for an intussusception. Tubular duplications may distend, particularly if the connection with the intestinal lumen is proximal producing a mass or obstruction by compression. Tubular duplication lined by gastric mucosa may induce peptic ulceration in the small bowel mucosa adjacent to its communication with the intestinal lumen and this may present with bleeding or perforation. Occasional cases of duplication present as a mass lesion in the posterior thoracic space with a trans-diaphragmatic extension. These thoracic duplications may be associated with hemivertebrae. A chest X-ray is essential because a significant number of abdominal duplications will be associated with an intrathoracic duplication cyst situated in the posterior mediastinum. The thoracic cyst may be separate from the abdominal duplication or there may be a connection between the thoracic and abdominal components through the diaphragm. The presence of upper thoracic vertebral anomalies makes the diagnosis of a duplication cyst highly likely.

Diagnosis

The clinical diagnosis is often difficult and the diagnosis may sometimes be made only on laparotomy. A technetium scan may sometimes be helpful diagnostically by demonstrating uptake of the isotope by ectopic gastric mucosa.

Management

Surgery is indicated when a duplication produces partial intestinal obstruction, an abdominal mass, severe intestinal haemorrhage, an intussusception or peritonitis as a result of perforation.

Small intestinal malrotation with or without volvulus

Aetiology

Malrotation of the small intestine is due to disordered movement of the intestine around the superior mesenteric artery during the course of embryological development (Fig. 2.2). The complex manoeuvres required to achieve normal gut rotation and fixation may be incomplete or may occur out of

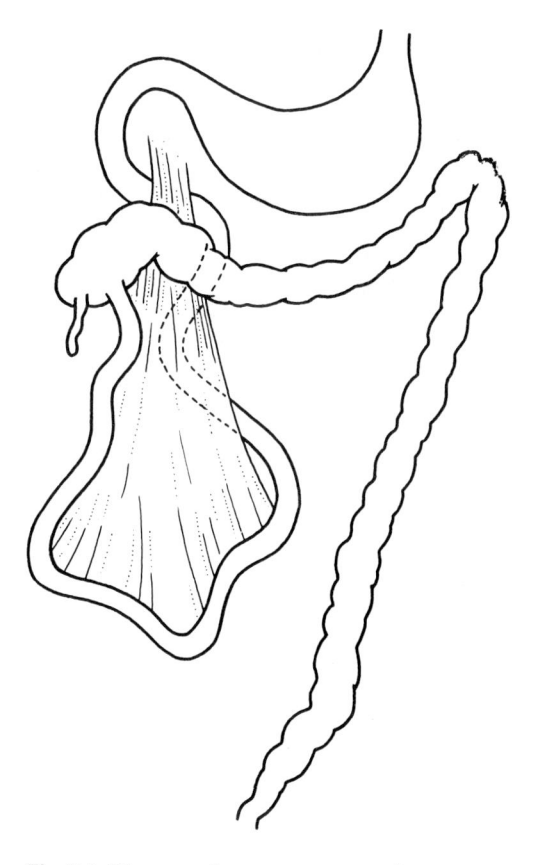

Fig. 2.2. Diagram of commonest type of malrotation viewed from the front.

sequence. An associated abnormality such as a diaphragmatic hernia or abdominal wall defect will result in the bowel developing outside the normal confines of the peritoneal cavity resulting in a high incidence of malrotation and/or malfixation. Figure 2.2 illustrates the anatomical appearance of the intestine usually encountered in a malrotation, producing a duodenal obstruction with or without a volvulus of the midgut.

Two main abnormalities may produce clinical syndromes. First, with gross narrowing of the fixation of the mesentery the midgut may twist sufficiently to cause a volvulus. This may occur acutely, causing complete obstruction, or it may occur intermittently producing bouts of partial or complete obstruction which resolve spontaneously.

Second, there may be partial duodenal obstruction from extrinsic compression of the small intestine by peritoneal bands (Ladd's bands) which extend from the caecum across the duodenum to the subhepatic region.

Stewart *et al.* (1976) in a review of 154 surgically treated patients found 70% had malrotation without other anomalies. The remainder had associated abnormalities, such as partial or complete intrinsic duodenal obstruction, diaphragmatic hernia, exomphalos or gastroschisis.

Clinical features

Malrotation may not produce symptoms or may sometimes be discovered only as an incidental finding on a barium study. The majority of children who develop symptoms related to malrotation do so within the neonatal period, presenting with features of complete or incomplete intestinal obstruction. When there is a volvulus there may also be obstruction to the blood supply of the bowel which, if complete, will lead to extensive gangrene of the small bowel with perforation and peritonitis. The passage of melaena stools may be an early sign of this complication.

Those children with malrotation who present later in childhood may do so with features of intermittent obstruction such as episodes of abdominal pain and the vomiting of bile-stained material, but sometimes they may show features of malabsorption and clinical signs suggestive of coeliac disease. This may be due to intestinal stasis with bacterial overgrowth in the lumen of the small intestine. Such steatorrhoea may be accompanied by protein-losing enteropathy due to obstruction of the mesenteric lymphatics (Burke & Anderson 1966) and sometimes chylous ascites may also be found.

Diagnosis

Malrotation should be considered in the differential diagnosis of small intestinal obstruction in infancy.

Plain X-ray of the abdomen may be useful, typically revealing distension of the stomach with a paucity of distal gas in the intestine (Fig. 2.3). The degree of duodenal obstruction varies and a barium meal and follow-through study may therefore be necessary to reveal the presence of malrotation. The absence of normal duodenal rotation is a constant sign of a malrotation and is more reliable in making the diagnosis than the disposition of the colon as demon-

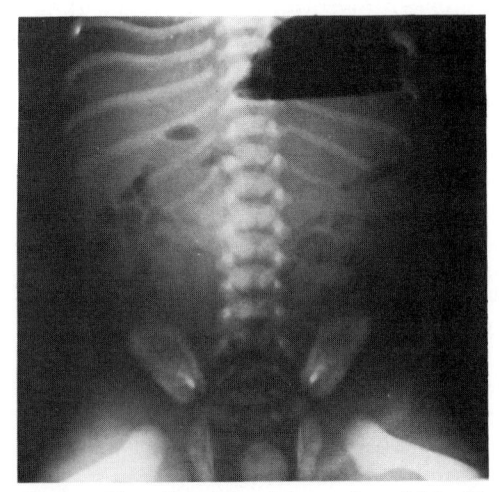

Fig. 2.3. Plain film of the abdomen in a child with duodenal obstruction due to Ladd's bands, together with malrotation. There is gaseous distension of the stomach with a paucity of gas in the intestine.

strated on barium enema. Occasionally repeated barium studies may be necessary to confirm the diagnosis.

Management

Ladd's operation is usually the procedure of choice. In general, this involves the placement of the caecum on the left and the small intestine on the right, having divided any bands and adhesions between the duodenum and large bowel and by dissecting the broadened base of the mesentery as much as possible. Should a volvulus have occurred resulting in intestinal necrosis, bowel resection will be indicated. Fortunately, total necrosis of the entire midgut is rare; ischaemic bowel may recover and 'second look' laparotomies in such cases are useful.

Meckel's diverticulum

This relatively common abnormality results from persistence of the vitello-intestinal duct. Partial atrophy results in a diverticulum on the antimesenteric border of the ileum. This may have a fibrous band at the apex connecting the bowel to the umbilicus or to some other structure within the abdomen. Complete failure of the duct to atrophy produces the patent vitello-intestinal duct with a free communication between the lumen of the ileum and the umbilicus.

Most people who have Meckel's diverticulum are asymptomatic. Out of a series of 250 cases of Meckel's diverticulum reported by Pellerin et al. (1976), 134 were asymptomatic and were only revealed at routine search at laparotomy. Complications may present in a variety of ways. In children these chiefly arise in association with the presence of ectopic gastric mucosa in the diverticulum. Other ectopic tissue, for example pancreatic tissue and colonic mucosa, may be found in some cases. The diverticulum is located in the distal ileum within 100 cm of the ileocaecal valve. It is always antimesenteric in position.

Clinical features

Boys are more often affected than girls. Rectal bleeding is the main symptom. This is usually the passage of bright blood rather than melaena stools.

Typically the stool is at first dark in colour but later bright red. Bleeding may lead to acute shock requiring urgent blood transfusion or it may be chronic. From a practical viewpoint, any child who has a massive painless rectal bleed should be regarded as a case of Meckel's diverticulum until proved otherwise. Most often, bleeding from a Meckel's diverticulum is associated with ulceration of the intestinal mucosa adjacent to the ectopic gastric mucosa in the diverticulum, but this is not always the case as such bleeding on occasions may occur in the absence of ectopic gastric mucosa. Bleeding from the small intestine may also be a feature of Meckel's diverticulum presenting in adult life, as illustrated by the following case report.

> An Iraqi gentleman was referred to Hammersmith Hospital at the age of 28 with five episodes of melaena during the previous 2 years. Radiological studies had suggested the presence of a duodenal ulcer. Subsequent duodenoscopy, however, revealed no evidence of ulceration. A mistaken diagnosis of acute haemorrhage from a pre-existing duodenal ulcer was made. He had four further episodes of melaena during the next 2 years and a repeat barium follow-through examination in Iraq now showed a large pouch arising from the terminal ileum (Fig. 2.4) and the diagnosis of Meckel's diverticulum was suggested. At laparotomy at Hammersmith Hospital, a large Meckel's diverticulum 70 cm proximal to the ileocaecal valve was resected successfully. There was no heterotopic gastric mucosa in the diverticulum but the haemorrhage had occurred from an ulcerated area within a stricture at the midpoint of the diverticulum.

Small intestinal obstruction may also be a mode of presentation. This may result from a volvulus, the Meckel's diverticulum being attached by a band of tissue to the umbilicus

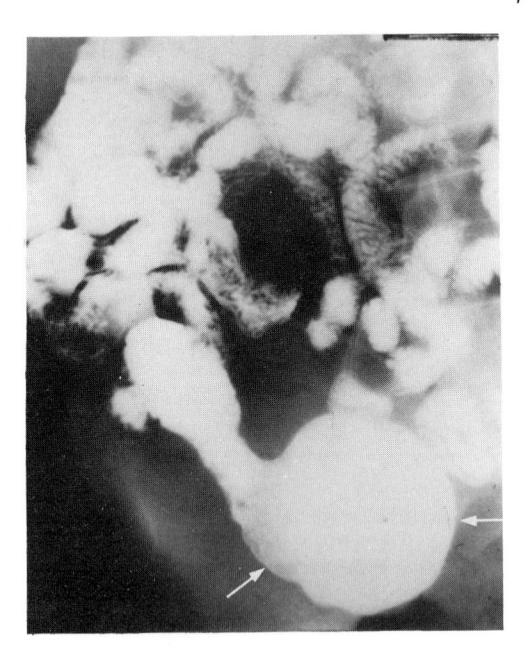

Fig. 2.4. Barium follow-through; the arrows show a large Meckel's diverticulum.

which acts as a fixed point. Intussusception with the diverticulum as the leading part is not uncommon.

Acute Meckel's diverticulitis may produce a clinical picture indistinguishable from acute appendicitis. In the neonatal period passage of meconium or faeces from the umbilicus indicates patency of the vitellointestinal duct. Surgical removal is indicated at an early stage because haemorrhage and intussusception through the umbilicus are common complications.

Diagnosis and management

This depends upon the mode of presentation. When rectal bleeding occurs other causes must be considered. Investigation may include colonoscopy to exclude colonic causes of bleeding and upper gastrointestinal endoscopy to exclude peptic ulceration. Barium follow-through is usually an unrewarding investigation but a small bowel enema may be more successful. A technetium scan is usually the most important investigation. The radionuclide technetium 99m concentrates in the gastric mucosa and may be localized on pictures taken with a gamma camera. The injection of pentagastrin may enhance the appearance. In this way a Meckel's diverticulum with ectopic gastric mucosa or indeed a duplication with such ectopic tissue may be diagnosed. Although the use of this technique should lead to an earlier and more accurate diagnosis of Meckel's diverticulum a negative result in a child with severe bleeding should not deter a surgeon from proceeding with a diagnostic laparotomy, which remains the final diagnostic test. It is, however, often only at laparotomy that the role of a Meckel's diverticulum in the child's intestinal pathology is appreciated (Wilton et al. 1982, Editorial 1983).

Congenital short intestine

A syndrome of congenital short intestine in association with malrotation with clinical features resembling those of massive intestinal resection has been described. Another syndrome of congenital short intestine in association with pyloric hypertrophy and malrotation is also recognized. This latter syndrome is due to an absence or diminution of argyrophil ganglion cells in the small intestinal wall. These cells normally organize peristalsis and ensure that the bolus moves forward at the correct speed. In the absence of such innervation, smooth muscle of the small intestinal wall contracts spontaneously and rhythmically, but segmentation is not co-ordinated, the food does not move forward and there is work hypertrophy of smooth muscle. Both syndromes are rare and often are only diagnosed at laparotomy.

Congenital absence of intestinal muscle

Amuscular segments of small intestine may cause obstruction or perforation in new-born infants. In reported cases there is an abrupt change from normal bowel to a segment with an intact mucosa but little or no muscle. It seems likely that such changes are due to a developmental anomaly rather than to ischaemic damage (Litwin et al 1984). The condition may be recognized at laparotomy and is cured by segmental resection.

References

Barnard C.N. (1956) The genesis of intestinal atresia. *Surgical Forum*, **5**, 393–397.

Booth C.C. & Mollin D.L. (1960) The blind loop syndrome. *Proc. Roy. Soc. Med.* **53**, 658–663.

Bower R.S., Sieber W.K. & Keisewetler W.B. (1978) Alimentary tract duplications in children. *Ann. Surg.* **188**, 669–674.

Burke V. & Anderson C.M. (1966) Sugar intolerance as a cause of protracted diarrhoea following surgery of the gastrointestinal tract in neonates. *Aust. Paed. J.* **2**, 219–227.

Editorial (1983) Meckel's diverticulum: surgical guidelines at last. *Lancet* **2**, 438–439.

Forshall I. (1961) Duplications of intestinal tract. *Postgrad. Med. J.* **37**, 570–589.

Kilby A., Walker-Smith J.A. & Dickson J.S. (1975) Stagnant loop syndrome with evidence of bile salt deconjugation. *Proc. Roy. Soc. Med.* **68**, 417–418.

Litwin A., Avidor I., Schujman E., Grunenbaum M., Wilunsky E., Wolloch Y. & Reisner S.H. (1984) Neonatal intestinal perforation caused by congenital defects of the intestinal musculature. *Amer. J. Clin. Path.* **81**, 77–80.

Louw J.H. (1959) Congenital intestinal atresia and stenosis in the newborn. Observations on pathogenesis and treatment. *Ann. Roy. Coll. Surg. (Eng.)* **25**, 109–115.

Nixon H.H. (1955) Intestinal obstruction in the newborn. *Arch. Dis. Child.* **30**, 13–22.

Pellerin D., Harouch A. & Delmas P. (1976) Meckel's diverticulum: review of 250 cases in children. *Ann. Chir. Inf.* **17**, 157–172.

Rickham P.P., Lister J. & Levine I.M. (1978) *Neonatal Surgery.* 2nd ed. Butterworths, London.

Stewart D.R., Colodny A.L. & Daggetl W.C. (1976) Malrotation of the bowel in infants and children: 15-year review. *Surgery*, **79**, 716–720.

Wilton G. *et al.* (1982) The 'false-negative' Meckel's diverticulum. *Scan. Clin. Nucl. Med.* **7**, 441–443.

Chapter 3
Congenital and Inherited Defects of the Enterocyte

J.T. HARRIES, D.P.R. MULLER AND P.J. MILLA

Carbohydrates 52
Malabsorption of carbohydrate 53
Lipids 55
Malabsorption of lipids 56
Proteins and amino acids 60
Malabsorption of peptides and amino acids . 62
Defects of electrolyte transport 65
Vitamins 68
Minerals 69

Congenital defects of the enterocyte may involve *abnormalities of the brush border membrane* such as alactasia or asucrasia, or *defects of transport* across the enterocyte brush border membrane, as in glucose–galactose malabsorption or in Hartnup disease, where there is malabsorption of the mono-amino monocarboxylic amino acids. There may also be *defects of metabolism within the enterocyte*, as occurs when there is abetalipoproteinaemia which leads to malabsorption of fat due to a failure of the enterocyte to synthesize chylomicrons. Finally, there may be *defects in the exit mechanism* from the cell, as has been suggested in lysinuric protein intolerance.

Carbohydrates

Hydrolysis

The products of the hydrolysis of starch within the gut lumen by salivary and pancreatic α-amylase are maltose, maltotriose and α-limit dextrins. Sucrose and lactose are not digested within the gut lumen but are hydrolysed at the brush border with the products of starch hydrolysis, releasing the monosaccharides glucose, fructose and galactose. Brush border hydrolysis is carried out by the oligosaccharidases lactase, maltase and sucrase–isomaltase which are large glycoproteins with pH optima of approximately 6.0 (Gray 1975). Their maximal activity is in the enterocytes of the proximal jejunum (Newcomer & McGill 1966).

Three species of lactase have been identified — a neutral brush border lactase, a neutral cytoplasmic hetero β-galactosidase and an acid lysosomal β-galactosidase (Asp et al. 1969, Gray & Santiago 1969). Only the brush border enzyme, however, is of importance in the physiology of lactose absorption.

With the exception of trehalase, all the α-glucosidases hydrolyse maltose and can therefore be considered as maltases. Up to 75% of maltase activity can be accounted for by sucrase activity. Sucrase–isomaltase is comprised of two subunits linked by one or more disulphide bonds, with the sucrase and isomaltase subunits having molecular weights of approximately 120,000 and 140,000 daltons respectively. The sucrase–isomaltase complex is anchored to the lipid membrane by a hydrophobic segment of the N-terminal region of the isomaltase subunit (Brunner et al. 1979). The enzyme complex is synthesized as an active protein in the microsomal fraction of the enterocyte and transferred to the brush border membrane where it is cleaved to its sucrase and isomaltase subunits by proteases of pancreatic origin (Frank et al. 1978, Hauri et al. 1979, 1980).

Transport

Following hydrolysis the monosaccharides are translocated across the brush border membrane by carrier-mediated systems, and it is likely that the surface oligosaccharidases are located immediately adjacent to the carriers.

Glucose and galactose

These two hexoses share the same sodium-coupled, energy-dependent electrogenic transport system (Gray 1975). Indirect evidence suggests that the monosaccharides and sodium bind to specific receptor sites on a transmembrane transporting protein and that this is followed by co-transport of sodium and monosaccharide across the membrane into the enterocyte.

It has been suggested (Crane 1965, Kimmich 1973) that the brush border carrier has two binding sites: one for glucose and galactose, and one for the monovalent cations sodium and potassium. Sodium binding increases the carrier's affinity for the monosaccharides whereas potassium has the reverse effect. The intracellular concentration of sodium is kept low as a result of active extrusion of the ion out of the enterocyte into the lateral intercellular spaces, energy being derived from the hydrolysis of ATP by membrane-bound (Na^+-K^+)-ATPase. This allows sodium to diffuse passively down an electrochemical gradient into the enterocyte. Intracellular hexose enters the intercellular spaces and then the portal vein by diffusion down a concentration gradient, almost certainly via a carrier-mediated system.

Fructose

Absorption of fructose appears to be carrier mediated but is independent of energy or sodium (Holdsworth & Dawson 1965, Schultz & Strecker 1970, Gray 1975).

Malabsorption of carbohydrate

Pathogenesis of gastrointestinal symptoms in carbohydrate malabsorption

Symptoms of carbohydrate malabsorption, from whatever cause, are predominantly due to the action of bacteria in the colon. Unabsorbed sugars in the small intestine create an osmotic gradient with bulk movement of fluid and electrolytes from plasma to lumen. The physiological drive provided by glucose and galactose for the absorption of fluid and electrolytes is dissipated. Thus excessive amounts of fluid and sugars enter the large intestine, where bacterial metabolism of sugars generates short-chain organic acids (e.g. acetic, propionic and butyric acids), carbon dioxide and hydrogen. This in turn generates a second osmotic gradient between plasma and lumen with further movement of fluid into the lumen. These events lead to colicky abdominal pain and distension, watery acid stools containing increased amounts of electrolytes and sugars, and perianal excoriation due to increased concentration of H^+ ion. Body losses of fluid and electrolytes, particularly in young infants, may lead to severe dehydration. The need for early diagnosis and treatment cannot be over-emphasized. In adults, however, the colon is usually capable of compensating for the increased load of fluid and organic acids and diarrhoea is therefore less frequent than in children. Many adults with hypolactasia, for example, have no symptoms of diarrhoea.

Lactase deficiency

Congenital

Infants with congenital lactase deficiency present with profuse watery diarrhoea soon after the introduction of milk feeds (Holzel *et al.* 1959). The condition is fatal unless an early diagnosis is established and lactose withdrawn from the diet. A presumptive diagnosis can be made on the basis of a careful clinical history but a definitive diagnosis requires the demonstration of an isolated deficiency or absence of lactase activity in a jejunal biopsy (Levin *et al.* 1970).

Asp & Dahlqvist (1974) studied the activities of the three β-galactosidases present in intestinal mucosa in four children with congenital lactase deficiency. In three of the patients no brush border lactase could be detected and in the fourth there was only a trace. Freiburghaus *et al.* (1976) used polyacrylamide gel electrophoresis of brush border fragments to study lactase in four patients. They found traces of lactase activity with reduced amounts of protein in the lactase position in three patients and lactase completely absent in the fourth; no evidence for an abnormal protein was found. There appears to be a defect in protein regulation with an early 'switch off' of lactase synthesis. The condition is probably inherited as an autosomal recessive.

'Acquired'

From infancy onwards lactose malabsorption is the commonest form of carbohydrate intolerance. In most populations without a tradition of dairying, lactase activity in the brush border of the enterocyte declines in childhood. This may be regarded as physiologically normal and it occurs in most mammalian species. Even in milk-drinking people 3–30% of adults are affected (Bayless et al. 1975, Flatz et al. 1982) and limited studies suggest an autosomal recessive form of inheritance (Neale 1968, Lisker et al. 1975). The biochemical change in the brush border has not been fully elucidated but is presumably caused by regression of the lactase structural gene, an occurrence which is not affected by the prolonged feeding of lactose. The enzyme is, however, more vulnerable to non-specific damage than the other disaccharides and its activity may be drastically reduced in malnutrition (see chapter 18), alcoholism, coeliac disease, tropical sprue, gastroenteritis and other inflammatory disorders of the small intestine.

The extent to which lactase-deficient subjects can tolerate lactose varies considerably (Bayless et al. 1975). The symptoms of abdominal discomfort, cramps, flatulence and diarrhoea after the ingestion of milk are variable although radiological abnormalities may be demonstrated after the ingestion of as little as 5–10 g lactose in barium (Laws & Neale 1966) (Fig. 3.1). The barium column is diluted with fluid, there is intestinal hurry and dilatation of loops of intestine.

Malabsorption of lactose may be diagnosed by oral lactose tolerance tests; by radiology; by measuring $^{14}CO_2$ or hydrogen in the breath and by measuring the excretion of galactose in urine (Ferguson 1981, Arola et al. 1982). These indirect tests are valuable indicators of hypolactasia but only the estimation of lactase activity in a biopsy of jejunal mucosa provides a definitive diagnosis.

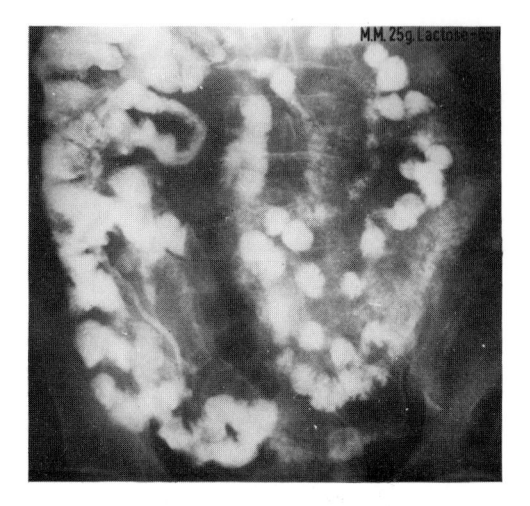

Fig. 3.1. Radiological abnormalities in acquired 'lactase deficiency'. The patient was given 100 ml Micropaque containing 25 g lactose and the radiograph was taken at 65 min. It shows dilution of barium and intestinal hurry.

Many subjects with hypolactasia recognize an intolerance of milk taken orally and may indeed use milk as a means of regulating their bowel habit (Bayless et al. 1975). Sometimes the condition is first recognized during the investigation of a patient complaining of symptoms suggestive of the 'irritable bowel' syndrome. Constitutional hypolactasia leads to symptoms only after the ingestion of milk or foodstuffs containing milk powder or purified lactose. Thus the patient with uncomplicated lactase deficiency requires no more than simple dietetic advice.

Sucrase–isomaltase deficiency

Congenital sucrase–isomaltase deficiency was first described in 1960 by Weijers et al., and although it is generally considered to be a rare condition, it may occur in 0.2% of North Americans (Peterson & Herber 1967) and in as many as 10% of Greenland Eskimos (McNair et al. 1972); the prevalence of the heterozygous state ranges from 9–43%.

Symptoms vary in severity from severe diarrhoea in infancy to intermittent mild symptoms in the older child (Antonowicz et al. 1972, Ament et al. 1973).

The correct diagnosis may be missed for several months or years, symptoms being attributed to conditions such as 'toddler diarrhoea' or 'maternal anxiety'. Occasionally, the condition may only be recognized in adult life. The diagnosis is established by the demonstration of deficient sucrase and isomaltase activities in a morphologically normal jejunal biopsy. Maltase (α-glucosidase) activity is also reduced, because sucrase accounts for a large proportion of the total maltase activity. As with the other congenital disorders of carbohydrate absorption, dietary withdrawal of the offending sugars (predominantly sucrose) results in prompt symptomatic improvement.

The basic molecular defect in sucrase–isomaltase deficiency may be of different types. Eggermont & Hers (1969) demonstrated loss of isomaltase and maltase activities as well as an alteration in their sedimentation characteristics. They suggested that an autosomal recessive gene mutation primarily affected sucrase, with secondary effects on isomaltase and maltase. Conklin et al. (1975) separated the sucrase and isomaltase moieties of the complex and found isomaltase to be labile in the absence of its partner, indicating that the sucrase moiety was deleted or defective and that isomaltase deficiency was a secondary event. Other studies have suggested that the sucrase–isomaltase protein may be structurally altered (Freiburghaus et al. 1977), absent (Gray et al. 1976) or alternatively that there could be a mutation affecting the transfer of the sucrase–isomaltase complex to the brush border region from the endoplasmic reticulum (Schmitz et al. 1980). Whatever the basic defect, sucrase–isomaltase deficiency appears to be inherited in an autosomal recessive fashion.

Trehalase deficiency

Trehalose (α-D-glucopyranoside) is a non-reducing disaccharide which occurs in most lower plants such as mushrooms, some micro-organisms, many insects, and in *Ascaris lumbricoides* and *Artenia salina*. Trehalase deficiency has been well documented in a family who developed symptoms following the ingestion of mushrooms (Madzarovova-Nohejlova 1973). An autosomal dominant type of inheritance was suggested.

Glucose–galactose malabsorption

This condition was first described in 1962 by Lindqvist & Meeuwisse. As with sucrase–isomaltase deficiency, clinical tolerance to the offending carbohydrates improves with age in many patients, despite the fact that the enzyme deficiency and transport defect persist (Ament et al. 1973, Elsas & Lambe 1973, Fairclough et al. 1978).

In vivo and in vitro studies show markedly impaired or absent sodium-coupled mucosal uptake of glucose, and in two studies impaired uptake was present in one or both parents (Meeuwisse & Dahlqvist 1968). Absorption of fructose, xylose, leucine and alanine is intact (Schneider et al. 1966, Phillips & McGill 1973, Wimberley et al. 1974, Hughes & Senior 1975). The finding that amino acid absorption and (Na^+-K^+)-ATPase activity are normal suggests that alterations in the sodium gradient are not basic to the defect in active hexose transport in this condition.

Lipids

Digestion and solubilization

Most dietary lipid is present as triglyceride. The triglyceride is first digested by lipases within the gut lumen to form free fatty acids and monoglyceride. Together with bile salts, the fatty acids and monoglycerides form micelles which are water-soluble. At the brush border of the enterocyte, the lipids are released and enter the enterocyte by passage across the microvillus membrane.

Absorption and handling by the enterocyte

Lipids pass by *passive diffusion* through the lipid phase of the brush border membrane. Since this is a passive process, no congenital defects involving entry of lipid into the enterocyte have been encountered.

Within the enterocyte the fatty acids

are first re-esterified to triglyceride and then packaged into lipoprotein particles (predominantly chylomicrons) for transport in the aqueous environment of the lymphatic system and bloodstream. The synthesis of apoprotein B is essential for the formation of chylomicrons and for the transport of lipid via the lymphatic route. Nascent chylomicrons have been shown to accumulate in the smooth endoplasmic reticulum of the enterocyte (Strauss 1966), and the Golgi apparatus plays an essential role in their secretion. It has recently been demonstrated in both the human (Kane et al. 1980) and rat (Krishnaiah et al. 1980) that there are two species of apoprotein B, one of which is synthesized by the intestine and the other by the liver. Both forms of apoprotein B are absent in classical abetalipoproteinaemia. A single patient with a specific deletion of the hepatic species has also been described (Malloy et al. 1981).

Malabsorption of lipids

Abetalipoproteinaemia (ABL)

The clinical features of ABL were first described by Bassen & Kornzweig in 1950, and total absence of betalipoprotein (low density lipoprotein) from the plasma of affected individuals was later demonstrated independently in three laboratories (Lamy et al. 1960, Mabry et al. 1960, Salt et al. 1960). Approximately fifty patients have been reported in the world's literature (Herbert et al. 1978).

Pathogenesis

In 1971, Gotto et al. showed that apoprotein B (the major apoprotein of betalipoprotein) was undetectable in plasma of patients with ABL. The primary abnormality is not known but the most likely defect is a failure to synthesize apoprotein B. The condition is inherited as an autosomal recessive; affected individuals are therefore homozygous for the condition.

Clinical and biochemical features

The major clinical and biochemical features of abetalipoproteinaemia are listed in Table 3.1. The steatorrhoea and spiky red cells (acanthocytes) are present from birth and the

Table 3.1. Major clinical and biochemical features of abetalipoproteinaemia.

Present from birth
    Absence of apoprotein B
    Absence of low-density lipoprotein
    Absence of very low-density lipoprotein
    Absence of chylomicrons
    Greatly reduced concentrations of serum lipids
    Malabsorption of fat
    Acanthocytes

Typically develop in late childhood or adolescence
    Pigmentary retinopathy
    Ataxic neuropathy

condition commonly presents in early infancy as a result of the fat malabsorption and failure to thrive. Other clinical features such as neuropathy and retinopathy tend to develop around the age of 10 years. The absence of low density lipoproteins, very low density lipoproteins and chylomicrons from the serum of these patients reflects the necessity of apoprotein B for their formation and results in the markedly reduced concentrations of the serum lipids. Heterozygotes for the condition are symptom-free and their serum lipids and lipoproteins are normal.

The gastrointestinal symptoms are present from birth and are characterized by poor appetite, vomiting, failure to thrive and large loose stools. These symptoms have led to the correct diagnosis by the age of four weeks (Lloyd 1968). Faecal fat determinations have shown that 50–80% of dietary fat is absorbed. The activities of pancreatic amylase, lipase, and trypsin, and the concentrations of bile salts in duodenal juice are normal (Salt et al. 1960).

Studies on intestinal mucosa obtained by peroral biopsy have localized the defect within the enterocyte. The biopsy has a characteristic 'white sea-anemone' appearance under the dissecting microscope. Under light microscopy the villus architecture is normal but the cells are distended and vacuolated. Histochemical techniques show the vacuolation to be due to lipid accumulation within the mucosal cells which is particularly evident at the villus tip (Fig. 3.2). Studies using both light and electron microscopy have failed to demonstrate the presence of lipid droplets in the intercellular spaces and lacteals of the intestinal mucosa

(Dobbins 1966), or accumulation of lipid droplets in the Golgi apparatus of patients with ABL. The lipid droplets which are visible lack the characteristic ring of increased density around their surface. It would therefore appear that the triglyceride present in the enterocyte in ABL is not surrounded by the typical specific protein coat. The lipid droplets are not transported through the endoplasmic reticulum to the Golgi apparatus, and are not 'packaged' and secreted into the lymphatics in the normal way. These observations, together with the lack of chylomicrons in the serum and the failure of serum triglyceride concentrations to rise after a fat meal, provide evidence that apoprotein B is essential for the synthesis of chylomicrons and the efficient transport of fat by the enterocyte. Despite the inability to form chylomicrons, fat malabsorption is relatively mild, which implies the existence of an alternative absorptive pathway. Direct entry into the portal vein of unesterified long chain fatty acids bound to albumin has been shown to occur to a limited extent in normal animals and is apparently increased under conditions where protein synthesis and chylomicron formation are inhibited (Kayden & Medick 1969). Barnard et al. (1970) also reported that after a meal of corn oil was given to one child with ABL, there was no detectable increase in the plasma triglyceride concentration. Evidence of fat absorption was, however, provided by an increase in the proportion of linoleic acid (the principal fatty acid of corn oil) in the free fatty acid and cholesterol–ester fractions of the plasma. A limited but significant absorption of vitamin E from large oral loads is also possible.

It is generally agreed that symptoms related to steatorrhoea improve with age in patients with ABL. This may reflect acquired adaptive mechanisms but is more likely to be related to unconscious dietary changes. Attention to diet from a young age may allow normal growth (Muller et al. 1977).

Diagnosis

The diagnosis should be suspected in all patients with unexplained malabsorption,

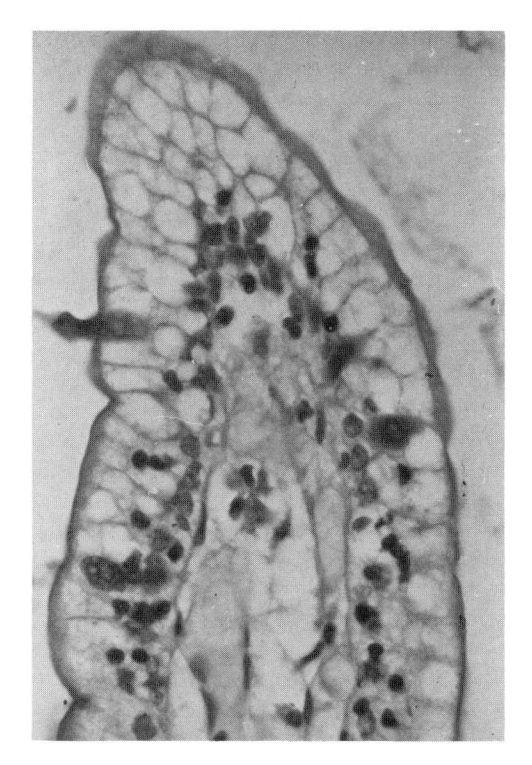

Fig. 3.2. Jejunal biopsy showing villus tip from a patient with abetalipoproteinaemia stained with PAS. The cytoplasm of the epithelial cells appears foamy and vacuolated due to accumulation of unstained lipid which also displaces the nuclei to the basal region of the cells (× 650).

particularly if the symptoms date from birth, and in older children and young adults who have atypical retinitis pigmentosa or an ataxic neuropathy similar to that of Friedreich's ataxia. The finding of acanthocytes in a fresh wet undiluted blood film, together with abnormally reduced serum cholesterol and triglyceride concentrations is virtually diagnostic. The absence of apoprotein B-containing lipoproteins can then be confirmed by immunochemical, ultracentrifugal and electrophoretic techniques. The appearance of the jejunal mucosa, both under the dissecting and electron microscope, although not pathognomonic, is highly characteristic of the condition (Fig. 3.2).

Treatment

Prolonged deficiency of a fat-soluble compound normally carried by the lipoproteins has been suggested as an explanation for the neurological and retinal lesions. Vitamin E, which normally depends on chylomicrons for its absorption and on the low density lipoproteins for its transport, is such a substance and is undetectable from birth in serum of patients with ABL (Kayden et al. 1965, Muller et al. 1974). For these reasons we have treated children with ABL with very large oral doses of vitamin E (approximately 100 mg/kg per day). Eight patients have been followed for periods of 11–16½ years. Vitamin E is detectable in the serum of all these patients and *in vitro* red cell haemolysis, an indicator of tissue concentrations of the vitamin, is normal (Muller et al. 1974). The long-term effects are summarized in Table 3.2 (Muller et al. 1977, Muller & Lloyd 1982).

> The five youngest patients (aged 12–16 years) were all treated with vitamin E supplements from early infancy, attended normal school and showed no clinical abnormalities; motor nerve conduction studies and electrodiagnostic tests of retinal function remain normal. The three oldest patients already showed some neurological dysfunction before supplementation with vitamin E in childhood. The condition of two of them has remained essentially unchanged. One is now 19 years old, works in a car body repair workshop and attends a college of further education. The other patient who was first reported by Salt et al. in 1960 is now aged 25 years and is a secondary school teacher with a university degree. The third patient is now almost 27 years old. He was diagnosed at the age of 7 years and first received vitamin E at the age of 10, by which time he already had marked ataxia, absent tendon reflexes, delayed motor nerve conduction velocities, a pigmentary retinopathy and abnormal retinal function. Within 2 years of starting vitamin E his gait, motor nerve conduction velocities, the electroretinogram and electro-oculogram had improved although his tendon reflexes remained absent. Over the following 14½ years there has been further improvement in his gait and his motor nerve conduction velocities and retinal function tests have returned to normal. He is employed making furniture in a sheltered workshop and is able to drive a car. Other investigators have also reported similar beneficial effects of large oral doses of vitamin E in ABL (Azizi et al. 1978, Herbert et al. 1978, Miller et al. 1980).

These long-term studies in patients with ABL indicate that vitamin E is important for normal neurological function (Muller et al. 1983). This has recently been confirmed by two other lines of evidence. Firstly, patients with other chronic disorders of fat absorption and a severe deficiency of vitamin E have been reported who have similar neurological features to those found in ABL. Some of these patients have also responded to vitamin E supplementation. Secondly, the neuropathological changes observed in vitamin-E-deficient states in man, including ABL, are similar to those found in the vitamin-E-deficient rat and monkey.

A deficiency of vitamin A could also play a role in the development of the retinal lesions. Gouras et al. (1971) treated two patients in their twenties with large doses of vitamin A and reported a partial or complete reversal of abnormalities of dark adaptation and of the electroretinogram. Less dramatic improvement has been seen in two younger children receiving similar treatment (Sperling et al. 1972). However, one child with ABL developed a retinopathy despite normal serum levels of vitamin A for 3 years (Wolff et al. 1964).

A restriction of dietary fat and supplements of the fat-soluble vitamins is the currently recommended treatment for ABL (Lloyd & Muller 1972). Normally, 15,000–20,000 iu/day of vitamin A is required to maintain normal plasma levels and sufficient vitamin K is given to maintain a normal clotting time. Massive doses of vitamin E (100 mg/kg per day) are recommended to maintain an adequate vitamin E status.

Table 3.2. Effect of long term treatment in abetalipoproteinaemia.

Case[*]	Age (year. month) At D	Vit. E	Current	Neurological status[†] Clinical D	1	2	Nerve conduction D	1	2	Ophthalmoscopy D	1	2	Visual function D	1	2
1	0.1	0.2	12.8	N	N	N	—	N	N	N	N	N	—	—	N
2	0.3	0.3	15.9	N	N	N	N	—	—	N	N	N	—	—	—
3	0.5	0.5	13.5	N	N	N	—	N	—	N	N	N	—	—	—
4	0.11	0.11	11.10	N	N	N	N	N	N	N	N	N	—	N	N
5	1.1	1.4	14.3	Hypotonic; No KJ, AJ	N	N	—	—	N	N	N	N	—	—	N
6	1.7	3.5	19.0	No KJ, AJ	No KJ, AJ, reduced vibration	No KJ, AJ, reduced vibration & proprioception	N	N motor reduced sensory	N[†]	N	N	N	N	N	N
7	1.5	8.9	24.11	No KJ, AJ	No KJ, AJ	No KJ, AJ	—	N	N[s]	'N	Slight PR	Unchanged PR	—	N	N
8	7.3	10.3	26.8	Ataxia; areflexia; pes cavus	Less ataxic; areflexia; pes cavus	Slightly ataxic; areflexia; pes cavus	Reduced motor	N	N	PR	Unchanged PR	Unchanged PR	Abnormal EOG, ERG	N	N

[*]Case numbers are the same as in the previous reports.
[†]D = at diagnosis, 1 = at follow-up in 1975, 2 = at follow-up in 1981; N = normal; KJ = knee jerks AJ = ankel jerks; PR = pigmentary retinopathy; EOG = electro-oculogram; ERG = electroretinogram.
[‡]Except for reduced sural and radial action potentials.
[§]Except for reduced sural action potential.

Familial hypobetalipoproteinaemia

This condition (Herbert et al. 1978) is thought to be a genetic disorder distinct from classical ABL. It appears to be transmitted as an autosomal dominant trait and both heterozygotes and homozygotes for the condition have been described.

Heterozygous condition

Fredrickson et al. (1972) proposed three diagnostic criteria for the heterozygous condition:
1 Abnormally low concentrations of low density lipoprotein, which are nonetheless present and identifiable immunochemically, together with normal concentrations of very low density and high density lipoproteins.
2 No secondary cause of the hypobetalipoproteinaemia.
3 Similar lipoprotein and lipid findings in a first degree relative.
The majority of the affected individuals from the seventeen families reported with heterozygous hypobetalipoproteinaemia have been fit and healthy without any features of ABL. Patients have, however, been reported with some of the features of classical ABL, including acanthocytosis, steatorrhoea, the characteristic accumulation of lipid in the mucosa, retinopathy and neuropathy (Herbert et al. 1978, Scott et al. 1979). Heterozygous individuals have been shown to have greatly reduced concentrations of apoprotein B but the concentrations of the other apoproteins fell within the normal range (Alaupovic, Personal communication). Studies in five patients have suggested that the reduced low density lipoprotein concentrations result from reduced synthesis rather than increased catabolism of low density lipoproteins (Levy et al. 1970, Sigurdsson et al. 1977).

Homozygous condition

Only four patients with the homozygous form of the condition have been reported. They are clinically and chemically indistinguishable from subjects with classical ABL but the first degree relatives, who are heterozygotes, have a reduced serum cholesterol and low density lipoprotein concentration.

Bile salt malabsorption

Bile salts are nature's detergents. Above a certain concentration, known as the critical micellar concentration, they aggregate to form micelles which are able to solubilize the products of lipolysis, monoglyceride and free fatty acids and carry them to the brush border membrane of the enterocyte (Carey & Small 1972). In health, the bile salts are conserved by a highly efficient enterohepatic circulation (Heaton 1972, Hofmann 1977), and are absorbed principally by an active carrier-mediated sodium-dependent transport system in the terminal ileum (Fig. 6.3 in Chapter 6).

A primary malabsorption of bile acids has been described by Heubi et al. (1982) in two boys with persistent severe diarrhoea from birth who failed to thrive, and who had malabsorption of fat. There was evidence of bile acid malabsorption. Faecal excretion of orally administered labelled cholic acid was increased; luminal, serum and urinary concentrations of the bile acids and pool size were decreased and the fractional turnover rate increased; the serum concentrations of cholylglycine following stimulation of the gall bladder by a liquid test meal were greatly reduced and impaired ileal uptake of bile acid was documented following the *in vitro* incubation of terminal ileal biopsies with radiolabelled taurocholate.

A similar defect in bile acid absorption has also been reported in cystic fibrosis by Fondacaro et al. (1981).

Proteins and amino acids

Digestion and absorption

Proteins are digested by pancreatic enzymes within the gut lumen to small peptides up to two to six amino acid residues in length (Gray & Cooper 1971), and amino acids. The principal enzyme responsible for protein digestion is trypsin, which is not secreted by the pancreas in its active form, but as a precursor, trypsinogen. The activation of trypsinogen requires an enteropeptidase, *enterokinase*, which is present in the brush border membrane of the enterocyte of the proximal small intestine. Enterokinase is easily removed from the surface of the brush border by the action of bile and proteolytic enzymes and increased luminal enterokinase concentrations have been observed after injection of cholecystokinin and secretin. This suggests that enterokinase is released from the brush border by normal physiological events that occur after the ingestion of food, and that the activation of trypsin from trypsinogen follows.

Peptide absorption

Two schemes of enterocyte handling of di- and tripeptides have been proposed. The first suggests that all peptides are hydrolysed by brush border peptidases, and that the liberated amino acids are then absorbed by specific amino acid translocation mechanisms. The second scheme proposes that the peptides are translocated intact and hydrolysed by intracellular cytoplasmic peptidases. Neither proposal wholly explains all the experimental data and a more satisfactory scheme combines both (Silk 1974, Matthews 1975, Matthews & Adibi 1976). Thus di- and tripeptides with a high affinity for brush border peptidases are largely handled by the first scheme — brush border hydrolysis and to a lesser extent by intact translocation — whereas those with a low affinity for brush border peptidases are transported intact.

The translocation mechanisms utilized by unhydrolysed peptides are different and separate from those used by free amino acids. In the experimental animal the addition of large amounts of free amino acids to peptide solutions does not inhibit absorption of di- and tripeptides (Rubino *et al.* 1971, Chung *et al.* 1979) and in inherited disorders of amino acid transport, such as cystinuria, normal absorption of dipeptides occurs despite the transport defect of the affected free amino acids (Hellier *et al.* 1972, Leonard *et al.* 1976).

Amino acid transport

There are four major group-specific active transport systems at the apical membrane of the enterocyte:
1 Monoamino—monocarboxylic (neutral) amino acids.
2 Dibasic amino acids + cystine.
3 Dicarboxylic (acidic) amino acids.
4 Imino acids + glycine.

Studies of amino acid transport in the inherited conditions Hartnup disease and cystinuria have firmly established the existence of specific transport systems for amino acids in Groups 1 and 2. Studies in iminoglycinuria have also suggested that there is a group-specific system for glycine and the imino acids, proline and hydroxyproline.

Intracellular events and exit

It has been generally assumed that unhydrolysed peptides translocated across the apical membrane are rapidly hydrolysed to their constituent amino acids by high specific activity cytoplasmic peptidases before crossing the basolateral membrane. Evidence for this is indirect. Unhydrolysed peptides are not found in portal blood nor on the serosal side of *in vitro* preparations, except for those peptides which have a particularly low affinity for the cytoplasmic peptidases such as those containing carnosine, hydroxyproline or sarcosine (Perry *et al.* 1967, Prockop *et al.* 1962). These may appear in the urine intact after oral ingestion.

There is little information regarding exit of amino acids from the cell but the evidence points to facilitated diffusion (Danisi *et al.* 1976, Mircheff *et al.* 1980). The recent description of a defect in lysine transport at the basolateral membrane of the enterocyte in lysinuric protein intolerance (Desjeux *et al.* 1980) suggests that special exit mechanisms are present, that they are group-specific, and that the basolateral translocation mechanisms are under different genetic control from those involved at the apical membrane.

Malabsorption of peptides and amino acids

Enterokinase deficiency

Deficiency of enterokinase is rare. The clinical symptoms are indistinguishable from those of pancreatic insufficiency affecting only proteolytic enzymes (Hadorn et al. 1969, Hadorn 1972). The first symptoms may not appear immediately after birth and frequently develop only after weaning, suggesting that digestion of breast milk protein is less dependent on the presence of active trypsin than dietary protein ingested after weaning.

Clinically hypoproteinaemia and oedema may occur. The diagnosis is established by a zymogen activation test. Exogenous enterokinase added to the duodenal contents of the patient will activate trypsinogen and other zymogens (Hadorn 1972).

Defects of amino acid transport

The majority of defects of amino acid transport are of theoretical rather than practical importance, since the normal absorption of amino acids as peptides ensures that nutritional deficiencies are unusual. In cystinuria, for example, although the renal tubular defect is of major clinical significance because of renal stone formation, the intestinal defect is important only to physiologists interested in transport mechanisms. Studies of intestinal function in patients with amino acid transport defects have helped elucidate the pathways of absorption of both free amino acids and peptides.

Hartnup disease

In this condition there is a congenital defect of transport of the monoamino–monocarboxylic amino acids in the proximal renal tubule (Baron et al. 1956) and the small intestine (Milne 1964). In spite of this transport defect involving many essential amino acids, the absorption of small peptides of two to three residues is unaffected (Asatoor et al. 1970, Leonard et al. 1976).

Patients usually remain well but pellagra may occur because of the abnormally small proportion of dietary tryptophan available for the synthesis of nicotinamide. Unabsorbed free tryptophan is metabolized by intestinal bacteria to produce indoles, some of which may be potent inhibitors of the kynurenine–nicotinamide pathway, thereby further decreasing the production of nicotinamide (Milne et al. 1960). As tryptophan can be absorbed in the form of di- and tripeptides, it is perhaps surprising that clinical symptoms occur at all. Clinical attacks are associated with an inadequate or irregular diet, and this may well result in insufficient absorption of peptide-bound tryptophan. If conversion of tryptophan to nicotinamide is restricted by metabolites, then symptoms may occur. Bacterial metabolism of the other neutral amino acids does not seem to cause clinical symptoms.

Clinical manifestations

The onset is in early childhood with a pellagra-like rash, mental retardation, with a dementing psychiatric disturbance similar to that seen in pellagra. Less often, there is a reversible cerebellar ataxia. These clinical manifestations are intermittent and variable, the skin rash being the primary cause of referral to hospital. With increasing age, attacks are less common, presumably because of the decreased requirements for nicotinamide. The biochemical lesion, however, persists.

Laboratory findings and diagnosis

The key finding is malabsorption of the neutral amino acids by both gut and renal tubule. Peripheral blood neutral amino acid levels fail to rise after an oral load of amino acids and bacterial degradation products appear in the stool and urine.

There is no specific treatment for the condition other than supplements of nicotinamide (25–50 mg/day). Monoamine oxidase inhibitors are contra-indicated. The ultimate prognosis is good, with amelioration of the condition in adult life.

Cystinuria

Cystinuria is a disorder of dibasic amino acid transport affecting the epithelial cells of both the small intestine and the renal tubule. The disorder is inherited in a complex autosomal recessive manner as a result of allelic mutations. The condition is characterized by the formation of urinary tract stones, with the potential for obstruction, infection and ultimately renal failure.

Pathogenesis

Originally, the condition appeared to be only of tubular epithelial cells (Dent & Rose 1951), but after tests of intestinal absorption with cystine and the dibasic amino acids, Milne et al. (1961) suggested the presence of a similar defect in the intestine. In vitro uptake studies in jejunal biopsies demonstrated a defect in the active carrier-mediated uptake of dibasic amino acids and cystine in homozygous cystinuria (McCarthy et al. 1964, Thier et al. 1965). On the basis of these and other in vitro studies, three types of homozygous cystinuria were described (Rosenberg et al. 1966): Type I — no active accumulation of cystine or dibasic aminoacids; Type II — active accumulation of cystine, but not of dibasic amino acids; Type III — reduced accumulation of cystine and dibasic amino acids. In a study of intestinal and renal transport Morin et al. (1971) confirmed the presence of Types I and II but not of Type III cystinuria.

Clinical manifestations

The incidence of cystinuria world wide is approximately 1 in 7000 live births (Levy 1973), but in England it may be as high as 1 in 2000 (Woolf 1967) and in the USA 1 in 15,000 (Levy 1973). The disorder occurs equally in both sexes though males tend to be more severely affected. Clinical expression of the disease may occur as early as the first years of life and in one large series (Dahlberg et al. 1977) nearly a quarter of the patients presented under the age of 14 years with a median age of 19 years. The most common presenting features are those of nephrolithiasis. Cystine stones occur as staghorn or recurrent multiple stones and frequently necessitate surgery. Cystinuria has been noted in association with many other conditions and mental retardation has been linked but this only occurred in 1 out of 89 of the cases reported by Dahlberg et al. (1977).

Growth of patients is normal (Dahlberg et al. 1977) because, as in Hartnup disease, the affected amino acids are absorbed normally when presented as dipeptides (Hellier et al. 1972, Silk et al. 1975).

Laboratory findings and diagnosis

The diagnosis is made by estimating the daily urinary excretion of cystine, lysine, arginine and ornithine (>18, 130, 16 and 22 mg/g creatinine respectively in the adult) or by chemical analysis of a cystine stone. The cyanide nitroprusside test has been widely used as a screening procedure and is positive in the presence of about 100 mg/g creatinine. It may not, therefore, separate some heterozygotes.

Treatment

Alkalinizing the urine is an effective means of keeping cystine in solution. A standard treatment programme includes a high oral fluid intake and alkalinization of the urine to a pH >7.5. D-penicillamine may be given because it complexes with cystine to produce a relatively soluble compound which is easily excreted without further stone formation. Toxic side-effects, especially fever, rash, arthralgia and lymphadenopathy, occur in up to 25% of patients treated with D-penicillamine. Occasional more serious side-effects occur, including nephrosis, agranulocytosis, and both lupus erythematosus-like and Goodpasture-like syndromes. These side-effects nearly always necessitate withdrawal of the drug. D-penicillamine also inhibits pyridoxal-5-phosphate and prophylactic administration of pyridoxine (100 mg/daily) will prevent pyridoxine deficiency. To minimize side-effects the drug should be withdrawn when stones have dissolved and the patient maintained on a large fluid intake plus alkalis.

Lysinuric protein intolerance

This condition, unlike Hartnup disease and cystinuria, presents with severe symptoms including marked failure to thrive, diarrhoea, vomiting, protein intolerance, hepatosplenomegaly, and often mental retardation (Perheentupa & Visakorpi 1965). Lysinuric protein intolerance (LPI) is a defect of dibasic amino acid transport which is inherited as an autosomal recessive trait. The transport defect has been demonstrated in small intestine (Desjeux et al. 1980), liver (Simell 1975) and proximal renal tubules (Simell et al. 1975).

Pathogenesis

Oral load studies in LPI homozygotes have shown impaired intestinal absorption for lysine, ornithine and arginine with normal absorption for citrulline. However, unlike the situation in cystinuria and Hartnup disease, no significant absorption of dipeptide-bound lysine occurs in LPI (Rajantie et al. 1980a, b). These findings suggested that the defect for lysine transport may be present at the basolateral border of the enterocyte. This suggestion was confirmed by an *in vitro* study of initial uptake, cellular accumulation and steady state transepithelial fluxes, in jejunal mucosa obtained by peroral biopsy in patients with LPI (Desjeux et al. 1980). This demonstration of a genetically determined basolateral membrane defect clearly shows the presence of special systems for amino acid transport across the basolateral membrane of the enterocyte and suggests that this is under different genetic control than that for translocation across the apical membrane.

Clinical manifestations

In infancy diarrhoea and vomiting occur with weaning to cow's-milk-containing formulae. This is associated with failure to thrive. After the first year of life, protein aversion is common and symptoms ameliorate as protein intake decreases. If a high protein intake is maintained, hyperammonaemia, hepatosplenomegaly and sometimes coma develop. Growth is retarded and in four of twenty patients mental retardation occurred (Simell et al. 1975).

Laboratory findings and diagnosis

The pathognomonic features are increased faecal and urinary excretion of the dibasic amino acids and hyperammonaemia after a protein load. An intravenous alanine load (6.6 mmol/kg body weight) in 5% w/v aqueous solution produces hyperammonaemia which is prevented if ornithine (1.1 mmol/kg body weight) is infused at the same time; thus provision of a urea cycle intermediate allows the alanine to be metabolized. Liver function is mildly deranged and may be associated with portal hypertension.

Treatment

The corner-stone of treatment is a low protein diet (1.5 g/kg body weight). Early attempts at preventing hyperammonaemia with arginine or ornithine supplements were not entirely successful, no doubt due to poor intestinal absorption (Simell et al. 1975) and diarrhoea occurs if more than 22.0 g arginine is given as a single dose. However, the use of a urea cycle intermediate appears to allow sufficient protein to be taken for catch-up growth.

Blue diaper syndrome

The blue diaper syndrome occurs with the isolated malabsorption of tryptophan. It is associated with increased calcium absorption. This rare condition is inherited as an autosomal recessive trait and presents in the neonatal period with failure to thrive, recurrent pyrexia, irritability, constipation and a blue discoloration of the nappies (Drummond et al. 1964). The stools contain large quantities of indoles, tryptophan, tryptamine and indolic acid. The blue discoloration results from the presence of indigotin (indigo blue), an oxidation product of urinary indican. Malabsorption of tryptophan has been suggested by the findings of low plasma tryptophan levels during oral loading tests. Hypercalcaemia and nephrocalcinosis are presumed to be due to increased Ca^{++} absorption. There is no evidence that this disorder affects renal tubules, and urinary excretion of amino acids is normal.

Oast-house syndrome (methionine malabsorption)

This extremely rare condition, so called because of the patient's odour, presents with convulsions, diarrhoea and severe mental retardation (Hooft et al. 1964). An isolated defect of methionine transport in both intestine and kidney has been demonstrated. In the patient described by Hooft et al. (1964), α-hydroxybutyric acid (a bacterial breakdown product of methionine) was found in both urine and faeces following oral loads of methionine, and was responsible for the characteristic odour. On treating the patient with a methionine-free diet, the symptoms improved.

Iminoglycinuria

This has been reported both in healthy individuals (Scriver & Wilson 1967, Whelan & Scriver 1968) and in a child with convulsions (Joseph et al. 1958). There is little information regarding intestinal involvement but one report described normal glycine and decreased proline absorption after oral load tests (Goodman et al. 1967) and another showed increased faecal excretion of both proline and glycine after oral loading (Morikawa et al. 1966). In the latter case when either proline, hydroxyproline or glycine were given orally the faecal excretion of the other two amino acids increased. This data supports the presence of a group-specific transport system for imino acids and glycine and indicates that it is defective in this condition.

Lowe's syndrome

This condition, inherited as a sex-linked trait, is characterized by mental retardation, cataracts, renal tubular acidosis with aminoaciduria. Defective absorption of lysine and arginine has been demonstrated.

Defects of electrolyte transport

Congenital chloridorrhoea is the only defect of intestinal electrolyte transport which has so far been clearly described. Infants with protracted lethal diarrhoea (often occurring in families) may be examples of as yet undefined defects of electrolyte transport (Fordtran 1967, Davidson 1978, Candy et al. 1981).

Congenital chloridorrhoea (CCD)

Darrow (1945) and Gamble et al. (1945) simultaneously described an unusual form of severe watery diarrhoea with hypokalaemia, hypochloraemia and metabolic alkalosis. A unique and striking feature was the high concentration of Cl^- in the stools, often as high as 150 mmol/l and always exceeding the sum of the concentrations of Na^+ and K^+.

Forty-four cases have been reported, half of which come from Finland (Holmberg et al. 1977a), and in particular from the north and eastern parts where there is a high incidence of rare recessive genes (Norio et al. 1973). The condition is inherited as an autosomal recessive trait.

Pathogenesis

Investigation of patients with CCD using *in vivo* perfusion techniques (Turnberg 1971, Bieberdorf et al. 1972, Rask-Madsen et al. 1976) have shown that the principal defect is of active Cl^-/HCO_3^- transport and that the defect is restricted to the ileum and colon. Secretion of Cl^- by the stomach and renal Cl^- transport are normal (Pearson et al. 1973). Studies of jejunal transport show normal absorption of glucose, sodium, water and bicarbonate (Turnberg 1971, Pearson et al. 1973, Rask-Madsen et al. 1976). Na^+ and Cl^- are secreted into the lumen of the intestine. Cl^- enters at a faster rate than Na^+ and the ionic balance is maintained by the absorption of HCO_3^-. This leads to a fall in luminal pH (Turnberg 1971). Rask-Madsen et al. (1976) have made similar observations. In

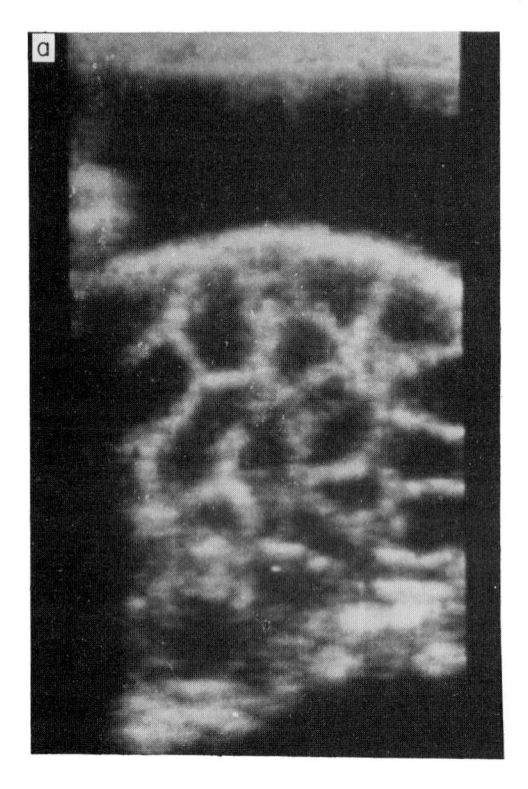

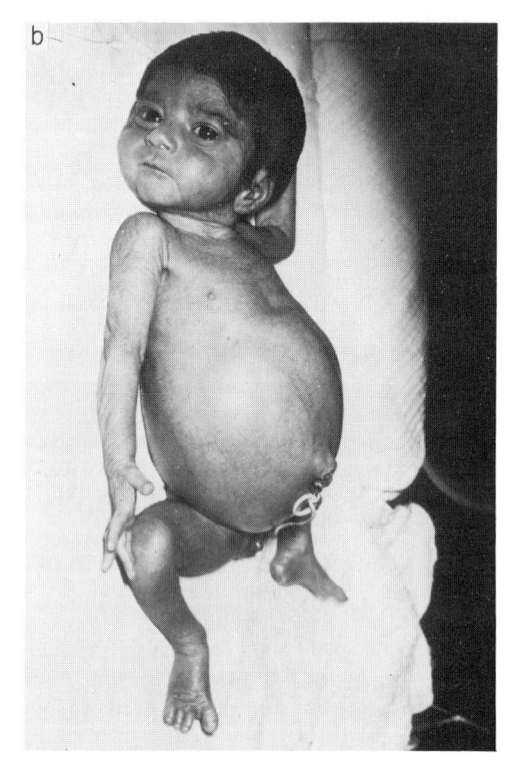

Fig. 3.3. (a) Abdominal ultrasound of fetal abdomen in congenital chloridorrhea showing dilated fluid filled loops of gut. (b) A neonate with congenital chloridorrhea with grossly distended abdomen.

a study of the colon of three patients with CCD and their healthy siblings, Holmberg et al. (1975) showed that Na^+ transport was intact but absorption was dependent on the luminal presence of HCO_3^-.

Clinical manifestations

The condition is present in fetal life and so far has always been associated with maternal hydramnios (Holmberg et al. 1977a). Figure 3.3a shows the affected fetal abdomen on abdominal ultrasound of the maternal uterus.

The infants are all born prematurely. Growth is appropriate for the period of gestation, and the abdomen is often distended at birth (Fig. 3.3b). Although diarrhoea and an absence of meconium is often recognized on the first day of life, it may go unnoticed, as fluid on the napkin is usually thought to be urine.

The abdominal distension is associated with a paralytic ileus which may last several weeks, and which is unrelated to K^+ depletion. Excitatory adrenergic stimulation of smooth muscle cells is dependent on a change in Cl^- membrane conductance. Thus Cl^- depletion is the probable cause of the ileus (Szurszewski & Bulbring 1973).

The majority of affected infants become hyponatraemic and hypochloraemic in the first week of life, but not hypokalaemic or alkalotic. This may be due to the degree of functional development of the ileum and colon in early life.

In the neonatal period acidosis is the rule rather than alkalosis and the original name of the disease 'congenital alkalosis with diarrhoea' is a misnomer. During this period jaundice is common, aggravated by a combination of acidosis, dehydration and prematurity. If adequate electrolyte replacement is not instituted severe alkalosis develops. In the eighteen families studied by Holmberg et al. (1977a) there had been seven previous deaths in infancy almost certainly due to CCD and one death of a known patient due to inadequate intravenous replacement therapy.

Infants who present later invariably have a history of diarrhoea or the passage of unformed stools since birth with moderate to severe growth retardation. At this stage there is alkalosis, hypochloraemia, hypokalaemia and hyponatraemia. Later sodium levels return to normal because of secondary hypoaldosteronism. If inadequate replacement therapy is prolonged, osteoporosis may develop as a result of excessive urinary phosphate loss.

Laboratory findings and diagnosis

The diagnosis may be suspected *in utero* by the presence of maternal hydramnios. Ultrasound of the fetal abdomen shows the characteristic picture of intra-uterine diarrhoea (Fig. 3.3a). Examination of amniotic fluid is not helpful, however, because electrolyte concentrations are normal.

The Cl^- concentration of the stool is always more than 90 mmol/l and after the first few months of life the stool electrolyte excretion assumes its unique and striking pattern in which the Cl^- concentration always exceeds the sum of Na^+ and K^+ concentrations. This finding confirms the diagnosis. Urine from these patients contains little or no chloride (Holmberg *et al.* 1977a).

Treatment

Initially electrolytes are infused intravenously but by 1 month it is usually possible to maintain normality by oral supplements. Many of the early patients were treated with KCl supplements only; although this corrected the hypokalaemia and hypochloraemia, normal plasma Na^+ concentrations were only achieved by marked and persistent hypoaldosteronism. This causes juxtaglomerular hyperplasia with increased secretion of Angiotensin II which results in vascular changes and hyperaldosteronism, which causes hypokalaemic alkalosis, predisposing to nephrocalcinosis. Although these patients were clinically well, hyalinized glomeruli, juxtaglomerular hyperplasia, calcium deposits and hypertensive vascular changes were found on examining renal biopsies (Pasternack *et al.* 1967). Similar vascular changes were also present in muscle (Pasternack & Perheentupa 1966). As excess K^+ and low Na^+ are known to stimulate aldosterone production, and children with congenital chloridorrhoea lose Na^+ in their stools, Holmberg *et al.* (1977b) have recommended that oral replacement solutions should contain both NaCl and KCl in the smallest dose that would maintain urinary chloride excretion (0.7% NaCl and 0.3% KCl for infants, and 1.8% NaCl and 1.9% KCl for 3-year-olds.) Using this regimen, the previously described renal and arteriolar changes have not occurred, acute episodes of dehydration have been less frequent and less severe, and growth has been normal. Mental retardation, which occurred in some patients treated solely with potassium, has not developed in those treated with full replacement therapy (Holmberg *et al.* 1977a).

Lethal familial protracted diarrhoea

Recently a group of infants have been described who present in the first few days of life with severe watery diarrhoea, which persists despite withdrawal of all feeds (Davidson *et al.* 1978, Candy *et al.* 1981). Siblings of the affected infants had suffered from similar illnesses and the familial pattern suggests an autosomal recessive mode of inheritance. Despite exhaustive investigations, no known disease entities have been detected. The mortality rate, even with prolonged intravenous feeding and the use of a wide variety of pharmacological agents, is more than 80%.

Pathogenesis

In the cases described by Davidson *et al.* (1978) the jejunum was uniformly affected by a crypt hypoplastic villous atrophy with no inflammatory cell infiltrate in the lamina propria, whereas in those described by Candy *et al.* (1981) jejunal mucosal appearance ranged from normal through partial villous atrophy and crypt hyperplastic villous atrophy to crypt hypoplastic villous atrophy. Steady state perfusion studies of the jejunum in both groups of patients showed the presence of a secretory state with respect to Na^+ and water, and marked impairment of Na^+ coupled solute transport. In the infants studied by Candy et al. (1981) there was marked reduction of $Na^+-K^+-ATPase$ but normal adenylate cyclase activity. The evidence suggests that in this group of infants the diarrhoea results from small intestinal secretion overwhelming the reabsorptive capacity of the colon.

Clinical manifestations

The affected infants present either at birth or within the neonatal period with severe watery diarrhoea and failure to thrive. In twenty-one of twenty-four cases, protracted diarrhoea persisted until death, resulting in a mortality rate of 87.5% (Candy et al. 1981). Withdrawal of feeds makes little difference to the stool output which is cholera-like and in an extreme case the 24-h stool volume was nearly 7 litres in a girl 22 months old weighing 8.2 kg.

Gastrointestinal-related and extra-gastrointestinal anomalies are common. Extragastrointestinal anomalies have included craniosynostosis, absence of the organ of Corti, bifid phalanges, renal dysplasia and absence of the corpus callosum. Other gastrointestinal-related problems have been reported, for example hiatus hernia and inguinal hernia, Meckel's diverticulum, universal mesentery and intra-abdominal adhesions and calcification.

Laboratory findings and diagnosis

A severe secretory diarrhoea with plasma-like stool electrolyte concentrations is the only constant finding in this condition. Numerous investigations including pancreatic function tests, small intestinal perfusion studies, trace metal and gastrointestinal polypeptide hormone assays, barium studies, sweat electrolytes and rectal biopsies have all failed to reveal a primary abnormality. Immunological studies have frequently been abnormal and, although results are difficult to interpret in malnourished infants, a primary defect is suspected in at least some cases (Candy et al. 1981).

Treatment

Dietary exclusion of disaccharides, monosaccharides, cow's milk, soya protein or gluten have had no effect on the diarrhoea. In nearly all cases life has been sustained only by intravenous feeding. A wide variety of drugs such as oral broad-spectrum antibiotics, disodium cromoglycate, prostaglandin synthetase inhibitors, beta blockers, H_1 and H_2 histamine blockers, cholestyramine, chlorpromazine and non-specific antidiarrhoeal agents have failed to reduce the diarrhoea. In a few cases adrenocorticoids have been effective but usually only in high dosage (Prednisolone 1−2 mg/kg per day) which has invariably led to severe cushingoid side-effects. More recently the opiate analogue loperamide has been used in this condition and in some instances has been life-saving (Sandhu et al. 1983).

Vitamins

Congenital and selective vitamin B_{12} malabsorption (Imerslund−Gräsbeck syndrome)

In 1960, Imerslund and Gräsbeck et al. independently described an autosomal recessive disorder with megaloblastic anaemia associated with proteinuria; to date more than 100 such cases have been described. The age of presentation has varied from 2−15 years of age. The clinical features are pallor, weakness, irritability and loss of appetite, often associated with vomiting, pyrexia, glossitis and constipation. There may also be evidence of diminished vibration sense, extensor plantar responses and mental retardation. Older children often present with the signs and symptoms of anaemia. Approximately 90% of reported cases have proteinuria which persists after treatment in the absence of any other abnormalities of renal function.

Malabsorption of vitamin B_{12} occurs in

these patients and is not improved by the addition of gastric intrinsic factor (GIF). Gastric and intestinal function are normal in all other respects and serum concentrations of transcobalamin II are also normal. Mackenzie et al. (1972) described uptake studies of free B_{12} and the B_{12}–GIF complex using ileal biopsy homogenates from a patient with congenital B_{12} malabsorption and from controls. The results were similar for the patient and controls, with GIF causing a marked stimulation of B_{12} uptake. It was therefore concluded that the receptor was present and functioned normally in this condition, and that the defect was at some point beyond the attachment of the B_{12}–GIF complex to the receptor but before the vitamin was bound to transcobalamin II.

The condition is treated by monthly injections of 250 µg hydroxocobalamin which must be continued for life.

Deficiency of transcobalamin II

A deficiency of transcobalamin II is a very rare condition with less than ten patients having been reported (Hakami et al. 1971, Hitzig et al. 1974, Chanarin 1982). Patients have generally presented during the first few weeks of life with failure to thrive. The blood shows severe anaemia, leucopenia and thrombocytopenia, and the marrow severe megaloblastic haemopoiesis. The diagnosis is dependent on the demonstration of an absence of transcobalamin II. Serum concentrations of vitamin B_{12} are normal. This apparent anomaly results from sequestration of the vitamin in the bloodstream because in the absence of transcobalamin II it is unavailable for tissue uptake.

Vitamin B_{12} is malabsorbed in this condition; studies in two children using whole body counting after an oral load of radiolabelled B_{12} showed virtually zero absorption (Chanarin 1982). This indicates that transcobalamin II is necessary for the transport of vitamin B_{12} away from the enterocyte and that this carrier protein is normally synthesized by the enterocyte. Direct evidence for the intestinal synthesis of transcobalamin II is not available, although Chanarin et al. (1978) have provided indirect evidence for this hypothesis by following plasma binding of newly absorbed radiolabelled B_{12} after the saturation of available binding sites by an intramuscular injection of the unlabelled vitamin.

Congenital folate malabsorption

Congenital folate malabsorption is a rare condition (Luhby et al. 1961, Lanzkowsky et al. 1969, Santiago-Borrero et al. 1973) in which patients develop a megaloblastic anaemia and other manifestations of folate deficiency (Chanarin 1982) as a result of a specific defect in folate absorption. All other parameters of intestinal function are normal.

Minerals

Acrodermatitis enteropathica

Acrodermatitis enteropathica (AE) is due to defective intestinal absorption of zinc. It is inherited in an autosomal recessive fashion. The clinical features were first described by Brandt in 1936 and the entity was later given its name by Danbolt & Closs (1942). In 1973, Moynahan & Barnes showed that the manifestations of AE were a direct consequence of zinc deficiency, and that the administration of zinc supplements led to rapid and complete recovery.

Pathogenesis

Zinc absorption has been shown to be abnormal by measuring the body retention of ^{65}Zn (Lombeck et al. 1975) and by balance studies (Aggett et al. 1978) showing a net intestinal secretion of zinc in patients with AE not receiving Zn supplements. Atherton et al. (1979) demonstrated a marked defect in the uptake of zinc by jejunal biopsies obtained from patients with AE irrespective of their Zn status.

Clinical manifestations

The classical clinical manifestations of AE are dramatic and include skin rashes, diarrhoea, failure to thrive, infections, alopecia, nail dystrophy, psychological and behaviour problems, stomatitis, glossitis, blepharitis, conjunctivitis and photophobia.

The skin lesions are distributed at acral and mucocutaneous regions of the body and are vesicular eczemtoid and/or pustular. In the acute stage the rash may become generalized and very disfiguring and hyperkeratotic skin plaques occur (Fig. 3.4). Alopecia may be complete and the skin is often infected with candida and staphylococci. Typically the lesions develop following the transition from breast to formula feeding and may resolve if breast milk is reintroduced. It has been suggested that the ligands present in breast milk facilitate zinc absorption.

Diarrhoea is common and may be severe. There is failure to thrive and often profound lethargy and irritability. The condition was frequently fatal in childhood until the fortuitous discovery that the antifungal agent 5,7-di-iodo-8-hydroxyquinoline (Diodoquin) could induce a complete clinical remission (Dillaha et al. 1953, Aggett et al. 1978). Diodoquin acts as an ionophore in enhancing zinc absorption (Aggett et al. 1979).

There are reports of three women who survived to adulthood without zinc therapy, and two of these had children with fatal congenital malformations similar to those seen in the offspring of zinc-deficient rats. This suggests that zinc deficiency may be teratogenic in the human (Hambidge et al. 1975). Subsequently plasma zinc concentrations were carefully monitored during two pregnancies in a patient with AE treated with oral zinc supplements (Brenton et al. 1981). The offspring had no congenital abnormalities and developed normally.

Laboratory findings and diagnosis

Zinc is essential for the optimal activity of a large number of enzymes which participate in a wide variety of metabolic processes throughout the body (Riordan & Vallee 1976). Deficiency of this divalent cation causes impairment of both cellular and humoral mediated immunity (Good et al. 1980, Gross & Newberne 1980).

The diagnosis of AE is made on clinical grounds, documentation of zinc deficiency and the prompt and dramatic resolution following zinc supplementation (Fig. 3.5). The primary defect in AE is permanent, and therefore the diagnosis can be made with

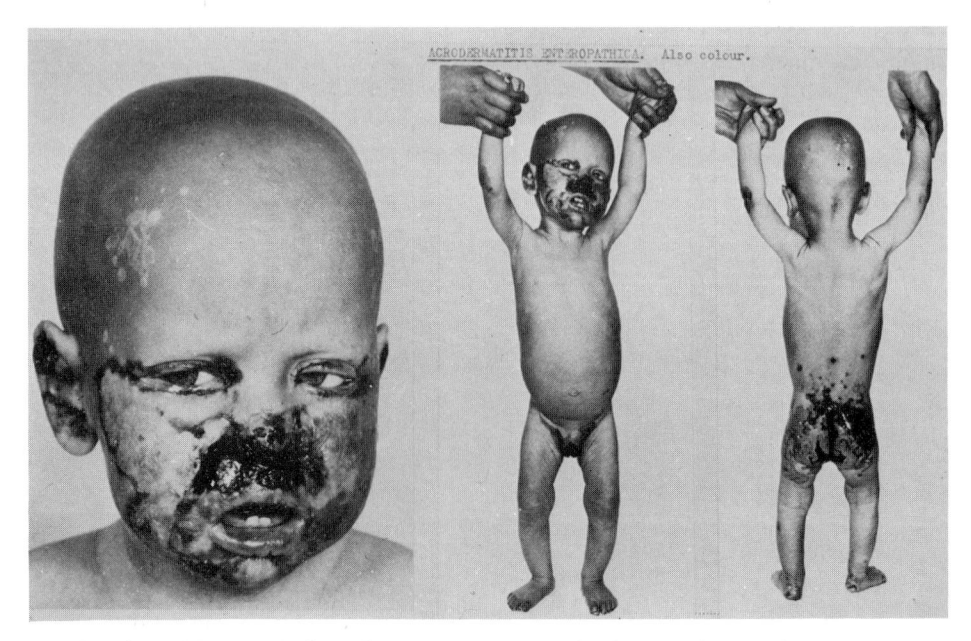

Fig. 3.4. Acrodermatitis enteropathica, demonstrating severe skin lesions, alopecia, failure to thrive and depression; age 16 months.

certainty by discontinuing zinc therapy following a prolonged remission, and inducing a relapse. Measurements of serum and plasma zinc concentrations are the most useful techniques for assessing total body zinc status.

Treatment

Oral zinc supplementation has now superceded diodoquin as the treatment of choice in AE, and should be continued on an indefinite basis (Fig. 3.5). It is crucial to carefully monitor body zinc status during growth and pregnancy, and to adjust the dose of zinc as necessary.

Idiopathic primary haemochromatosis

Idiopathic primary haemochromatosis (IPH) was first proposed as an inborn error of iron metabolism by Sheldon (1935). All the features result from a progressive increase in body iron stores and accumulation of iron in a variety of organs which results in structural and functional abnormalities.

Pathogenesis

An excessive absorption of iron from the small intestine may be the primary abnormality in IPH. Normally the small intestine controls total iron balance by a homeostatic mechanism which adjusts absorption to meet body requirements (McCance & Widdowson 1937).

Recent studies of the uptake and kinetics of iron transport in human duodenal biopsies have provided evidence for specific iron protein binding sites on the mucosa, and have suggested that uptake is by an active process displaying saturation kinetics. In patients with IPH there is an apparent increase in iron uptake due to a reduction in the affinity constant (K_t). It was independent of iron stores since values in patients with iron overload were no different from controls (Cox & Peters 1978, 1980). These studies suggest that the basic defect in IPH is increased intestinal absorption of iron due to high affinity enterocyte receptors whose activity is not modulated by mucosal iron

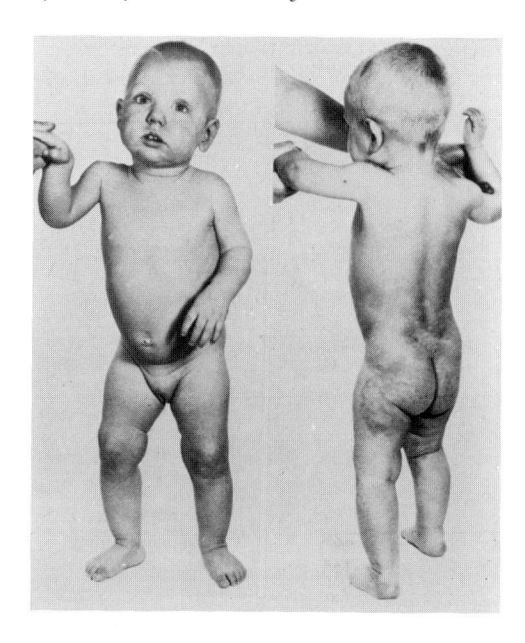

Fig. 3.5. Patient shown in Fig. 3.4, 2 months after starting oral zinc therapy.

transport or total body iron stores.

Primary hypomagnesaemia

Primary hypomagnesaemia is a genetically determined disorder which is probably inherited in an autosomal recessive fashion. The condition presents in early infancy with convulsions and/or tetany, and the biochemical hallmarks are hypomagnesaemia and hypocalcaemia.

Pathogenesis

Balance studies (Paunier et al. 1968) and steady state perfusion studies of the small gut (Milla et al. 1979) have now clearly demonstrated that the magnesium deficiency is related to a primary defect in magnesium transport. Milla et al. (1979) showed that net loss of magnesium into the lumen occurred when low concentrations (1 and 2mM) of magnesium were perfused compared with control subjects. At high concentrations (10mM) net absorption similar to that observed in controls occurred. Kinetic studies suggested that the primary abnormality in this condition is a defect in a carrier-mediated transport system which saturates at a low intraluminal concentration. Normal absorption of magnesium from higher intraluminal concentrations occurs by simple passive diffusion, and allows hypomagnesaemia to be corrected with large oral doses.

Clinical manifestations, diagnosis and treatment

Patients present at the age of a few weeks with generalized convulsions and tetany, but in some cases, the clinical onset is delayed until later in infancy. Hypotonia may be marked and the convulsions fail to respond to conventional anticonvulsant drugs. Hypoproteinaemia and peripheral oedema secondary to a protein-losing enteropathy, which improved with magnesium therapy, have been reported in one patient (Milla et al. 1979).

The diagnosis is established by the demonstration of otherwise inexplicable severe hypomagnesaemia and hypocalcaemia responding promptly to treatment with magnesium which is required permanently.

Magnesium (1–2 mmol/kg per day) given orally as one of the soluble salts usually has a rapid effect in controlling convulsions and tetany, as well as correcting plasma magnesium and calcium levels; higher doses may be necessary in some cases and may cause diarrhoea. Conventional anticonvulsant therapy and calcium supplements may be required during the early stages of treatment.

Familial hypophosphataemic rickets

Familial hypophosphataemic rickets (vitamin-D-resistant hypophosphataemic rickets) is usually inherited in an X-linked fashion, but occasionally transmission may be autosomal dominant (Harrison & Harrison 1979).

Pathogenesis

The major abnormality is a defect in the renal tubular reabsorption of phosphate (Rasmussen & Anast 1978), but intestinal absorption of phosphate and calcium is also impaired.

Clinical manifestations, diagnosis and treatment

Initially growth is normal. Later it is impaired with the clinical signs of rickets often not noticed until the patient is 1–3 years old or more.

The association of hypophosphataemia, a raised alkaline phosphatase, and radiological evidence of rickets or osteomalacia, suggests the diagnosis.

Calcitriol (1,24-dihydroxy-D_3) together with phosphate supplements is the treatment of choice (Glorieux et al. 1980).

References

Aggett P.J., Atherton D.J., Delves H.T., Thorn J.M., Bangham A., Clayton B.E. & Harries J.T. (1978) Studies in acrodermatitis enteropathica. In *3rd International Symposium on Trace Element Metabolism in Man and Animals*, pp. 418–422. (Ed. by M. Kirchgessner). Freising-Weihenstephan.

Aggett P.J., Delves H.T., Harries J.T. & Bangham A.D. (1979) The possible role of diodoquin as a zinc ionophore in the treatment of acrodermatitis enteropathica. *Biochem. Biophys. Res. Comm.* **87**, 513.

Ament M.E., Perera D.R. & Esther L.J. (1973) Sucrase-isomaltase deficiency — a frequently misdiagnosed disease. *J. Paediat.* **83**, 721–727.

Antonowicz L., Lloyd-Still J.D., Khaw K.T. & Shwachman H. (1972) Congenital sucrase-isomaltase deficiency. Observations over a period of six years. *Pediat.* **49**, 847–853.

Arola H., Jokela H., Koivula T. & Isokoski M. (1982) Simple urinary test for lactose malabsorption. *Lancet*, **ii**, 524–525.

Asatoor A.M., Clegg B., Edwards K.D.G., Lant A.F., Matthews D.M., Milne M.D., Navab F. & Richard A.J. (1970) Intestinal absorption of two dipeptides in Hartnup disease. *Gut*, **11**, 380–387.

Asp N.-G. & Dahlqvist A. (1974) Intestinal β-galactosidases in adult low lactase activity and in congenital lactase deficiency. *Enzymes*, **18**, 84–102.

Asp N.-G., Dahlqvist A. & Koldovsky O. (1969) Human small intestinal β-galactosidase. Separation and characterization of one lactase and one hetero β-galactosidase. *Biochem. J.* **114**, 351–359.

Atherton D.J., Muller D.P.R., Aggett P.J. & Harries J.T. (1979) A defect in zinc uptake by jejunal biopsies in acrodermatitis enteropathica. *Clin. Sci.* **56**, 505–507.

Azizi E., Aaidman J.L., Eshchar J. & Szeinberg A. (1978) Abetalipoproteinaemia treated with parenteral and oral vitamin A and E with medium chain triglycerides. *Acta Paediat.*

Scand. 67, 797−801.

Barnard G., Fosbrooke A.S. & Lloyd J.K. (1970) Neutral lipids of plasma and adipose tissue in abetalipoproteinaemia. Clin. Chim. Acta 28, 417−422.

Baron D.N., Dent C.E., Harris H., Hart E.W. & Jepson J.B. (1956) Hereditary pellagra-like skin rash with temporary cerebellar ataxia, constant renal amino aciduria and other bizarre biochemical features. Lancet, ii, 421−428.

Bassen F.A. & Kornzweig A.L. (1950) Malformation of the erythrocytes in a case of atypical retinitis pigmentosa. Blood, 5, 381−387.

Bayless T.M., Rothfield B., Massa C., Wise L., Paige D. & Bedine M.S. (1975) Lactose and milk intolerance: clinical implications. New Engl. J. Med. 292, 1156−1159.

Bieberdorf F.A., Gorden P. & Fordtran J.S. (1972) Pathogenesis of congenital alkalosis with diarrhoea. J. Clin. Invest. 51, 1958−1968.

Brandt T. (1936) Dermatitis in children with disturbances of the general condition and absorption of food elements. Acta Dermatol. Venereol. 17, 513−546.

Brenton D.P., Jackson M.J. & Young A. (1981) Two pregnancies in a patient with acrodermatitis enteropathica treated with zinc sulphate. Lancet, ii, 500−502.

Brunner J., Hauser H, Braun H, Wilson K.J., Wacker H., O'Neill B. & Semenza G. (1979) The mode of association of the enzyme complex sucrase-isomaltase with the intestinal brush border membrane. J. Biol. Chem. 250, 7802−7809.

Candy D.C.A., Larcher V.F., Cameron D.J.S., Norman A.P., Tripp J.H., Milla P.J., Pincott J.R. & Harries J.T. (1981) Lethal familial protracted diarrhoea. Arch. Dis. Child. 56, 15−23.

Carey M.C. & Small D.M. (1972) Micelle formation by bile salts. Physical−chemical and thermodynamic considerations. Arch. Intern. Med. 130, 506−527.

Chanarin I. (1982) Disorders of vitamin absorption. Clin. Gastroenterol. 11, 73−85.

Chanarin I., Muir M., Hughes A.V. & Hoffbrand A. (1978) Evidence for an intestinal origin of transcobalamin II during vitamin B_{12} absorption. Brit. Med. J., 1, 1453−1455.

Chung Y.C., Silk D.B.A. & Kim Y.S. (1979) Intestinal transport of a tetrapeptide, L-leucylgiycylglycylglycine, in rat intestine in vivo. Clin. Sci. 57, 1−11.

Conklin K.A., Yamashiro L.M. & Gray G.M. (1975) Human intestinal sucrase−isomaltase. Identification of free sucrase and isomaltase and cleavage of the hybrid into active distinct subunits. J. Biol. Chem. 250, 5735−5741.

Cox T.M. & Peters T.J. (1980) In vitro studies of duodenal iron uptake in patients with primary and secondary iron storage disease. Quart. J. Med. 49, 249−257.

Cox T.M. & Peters T.J. (1978) Uptake of iron by duodenal biopsy specimens from patients with iron-deficiency anaemia and primary haemochromatosis. Lancet, i, 123−124.

Crane R.K. (1965) Na^+-dependent transport in the intestine and other animal tissues. Fed. Proc. 24, 1000−1006.

Dahlberg P.J., Van den Berg C.J., Kurtz S.B., Wilson D.M. & Smith L.H. (1977) Clinical features and management of cystinuria. Mayo Clin. Proc. 52, 533−542.

Danbolt N. & Closs K. (1942) Acrodermatitis enteropathica. Acta Dermatal. Venereol. 23, 127−169.

Danisi G., Tai Y.H. & Curran P.F. (1976) Mucosal and serosal fluxes of alanine in rabbit ileum. Biochem. Biophys. 455, 200−213.

Darrow D.C. (1945) Congenital alkalosis with diarrhoea. J. Paediat. 26, 519−532.

Davidson G.P., Cutz E., Hamilton J.R. & Gall D.G. (1978) Familial enteropathy: a syndrome of protracted diarrhoea from birth, failure to thrive and hypoplastic villous atrophy. Gastroenterol. 75, 783−790.

Dent C.E. & Rose G.A. (1951) Amino acid metabolism in cystinuria. Quart. J. Med. 20, 205−219.

Desjeux J.F., Ragantie J., Simell O., Dumontier A.M. & Perheentupa J. (1980) Lysine fluxes across the jejunal epithelium in lysinuric protein intolerance. J. Clin. Invest. 65, 1382−1387.

Dillaha C.J., Lorinez A.L. & Aavik O.R. (1953) Acrodermatitis enteropathica: A review of the literature and report of a case successfully treated with diodoquin. J. Amer. Med. Assoc. 152, 509−512.

Dobbins W.O. III (1966) An ultrastructural study of the intestinal mucosa in congenital β-lipoprotein deficiency with particular emphasis upon the intestinal absorptive cell. Gastroenterol. 50, 195−210.

Drummond K.N., Michael A.F., Ulstrom R.A. & Gould R.A. (1964) The blue diaper syndrome: familial hypercalcaemia in nephrocalcinosis and indicanuria. Amer. J. Med. 37, 928−948.

Eggermont E. & Hers H.G. (1969) The sedimentation properties of the intestinal α-glucosidases of normal human subjects and of patients with sucrose intolerance. Europ. J. Biochem. 9, 488−496.

Elsas L.J. & Lambe D.W. (1973) Familial glucose-galactose malabsorption. Remission of glucose intolerance. J. Paedia. 83, 226−232.

Fairclough P.D., Clark M.L., Dawson A.M., Silk B.D.A., Milla P. & Harries J.T. (1978) Absorption of glucose and maltose in congenital glucose-galactose malabsorption. Pediat. Res. 12, 1112−1114.

Ferguson A. (1981) Diagnosis and treatment of lactose intolerance. Brit. Med. J. 283, 1423−1424.

Flatz G., Howell J.N., Doench J. & Flatz S.D. (1982) Distribution of physiological adult lactase phenotypes, lactose absorber and malabsorber, in Germany. Hum. Genet. 62, 152−157.

Fondacaro J.D. & Wolcott R.H. (1981) Effect of dietary nutrients on intestinal taurocholic acid absorption. Proc. Soc. Exp. Biol. Med. 168, 276−281.

Fordtran J.S. (1967) Speculations on the pathogenesis of diarrhoea. *Fed. Proc.* **26**, 1405–1414.

Frank G., Brunner J., Hauser H., Wacker H., Semenza G. & Zuber H. (1978) The hydrophobic anchor of small intestinal sucrase–isomaltase. *FEBS Lett.*, **96**, 183–187.

Fredrickson D.S., Gott A.M. & Levy R.I. (1972) Familial lipoprotein deficiency. In *The Metabolic Basis of Inherited Disease*, 3rd Ed. (Ed. by J.B. Stanbury, J.B. Wyngaarden & D.S. Fredrickson). McGraw-Hill, New York.

Freiburghaus A.U., Schmitz J., Schindler M., Rotthauwe H.W., Kuitunen P., Launiala K. & Hadron B. (1976) Protein patterns of brush border fragments in congenital lactose malabsorption and in specific hypolactasia of the adult. *New Engl. J. Med.* **294**, 1030–1032.

Freiburghaus A.U., Dubs R., Hadorn B., Gaze H., Hauri H.P. & Gitzelmann R. (1977) The brush border membrane in hereditary sucrase–isomaltase deficiency: abnormal protein pattern and presence of immunoreactive enzyme. *Eur. J. Clin. Invest.* **7**, 455–459.

Gamble J.L., Gahey K.R., Appleton J. & MacLachlan E. (1945) Congenital alkalosis with diarrhoea. *J. Paediat.* **26**, 509–518.

Glorieux F.H., Marie P.J., Pettifor J.M. & Delvin E.E. (1980) Bone response to phosphate salts, ergocalciferol and calcitriol in hypophosphatemic vitamin D-resistant rickets. *New Engl. J. Med.* **303**, 1023–1031.

Good R.A., West A. & Fernandes G. (1980) Nutritional modulation of immune responses. *Fed. Proc.* **39**, 3098–3104.

Goodman S.I., McIntyre C.A. & O'Brien D. (1967) Impaired intestinal transport of proline in a patient with familial amino aciduria. *J. Paediat.* **71**, 246–249.

Gotto A.M., Levy R.L., John K. & Fredrickson D.S. (1971) On the nature of the protein defect in abetalipoproteinaemia. *New Engl. J. Med.* **284**, 813–818.

Gouras P., Carr R.E. & Gunkel R.D. (1971) Retinitis pigmentosa in abetalipoproteinaemia: effects of vitamin A. *Invest. Ophthalmol.* **10**, 784–793.

Grasbeck R., Gordin R., Kantero I. & Kuhlback B. (1960) Selective vitamin B_{12} malabsorption and proteinuria in young people. A syndrome. *Acta Med. Scand.* **167**, 289–296.

Gray G.M. (1975) Carbohydrate digestion and absorption. Role of the small intestine. *New Engl. J. Med.* **292**, 1225–1230.

Gray G.M., Conklin K.A. & Townley R.R.W. (1976) Sucrase–isomaltase deficiency. Absence of an inactive enzyme variant. *New Engl. J. Med.* **294**, 750–753.

Gray G.M. & Cooper H.L. (1971) Protein digestion and absorption. *Gastroenterol.* **61**, 535–544.

Gray G.M. & Santiago N.A. (1969) Intestinal β-galactosidase. I. Separation and characterization of three enzymes in normal human intestine. *J. Clin. Invest.* **48**, 716–728.

Gross R.L. & Newberne P.M. (1980) Role of nutrition in immunologic function. *Physiol. Rev.* **60**, 188–299.

Hadorn B. (1972) Disease of the pancreas in children. *Clin. Gastroenterol.* **1**, 125–145.

Hadorn B., Tarlow M.J., Lloyd J.K. & Wolff O.H. (1969) Intestinal enterokinase deficiency. *Lancet*, **i**, 812–813.

Hakami N., Neiman P.E., Canellos G.P. & Lazerson J. (1971) Neonatal megaloblastic anemia due to inherited transcobalamin II deficiency in two siblings. *New Engl. J. Med.* **285**, 1163–1170.

Hambidge K.M. Neldner K.H. & Walravens P.A. (1975) Zinc, acrodermatitis enteropathica and congenital malformations. *Lancet*, **i**, 577.

Harrison H.E. & Harrison H.C. (1979) Disorders of calcium and phosphate metabolism in childhood and adolescence. In *Major Problems in Clinical Pediatrics*, p. 219. W.B. Saunders, Philadelphia.

Hauri H.P. Quaroni A. & Isselbacher K.J. (1979) Biogenesis of intestinal plasma membrane: post-translational route and cleavage of sucrase–isomaltase. *Proc. Nat. Acad. Sci. USA* **76**, 5183–5186.

Hauri H.P., Quaroni A. & Isselbacher K.J. (1980) Monoclonal antibodies to sucrase–isomaltase: probes for the study of postnatal development and biogenesis of the intestinal microvillus membrane. *Proc. Nat. Acad. Sci. USA* **77**, 6629–6633.

Heaton K.W. (1972) The enterohepatic circulation. In *Bile Salts in Health and Disease*, pp. 58–81. Churchill Livingstone, Edinburgh.

Hellier M.D., Holdsworth C.D., Perrett D. & Thirumalai C. (1972) Intestinal dipeptide transport in normal and cystinuric subjects. *Clin. Sci.* **43**, 659–668.

Herbert P.N. Gotto A.M. & Fredrickson D.S. (1978) Familial lipoprotein deficiency. In *The Metabolic Basis of Inherited Disease*, 4th Ed. pp. 544–588. (Ed. by J.B. Stanbury, J.B. Wyngaarden & D.S. Fredrickson). McGraw-Hill, New York.

Heubi J.E., Balistreri W.F., Fondacaro J.D., Partin J.C. & Schubert W.K. (1982) Primary bile acid malabsorption: defective *in vitro* ileal active bile acid transport. *Gastroenterol.* **83**, 804–811.

Hitzig W.H., Dohmann U., Pluss H.J. & Vischer D. (1974) Hereditary transcobalamin II deficiency: clinical findings in a new family. *J. Paediat.* **85**, 622–628.

Hofmann A.F. (1977) The enterohepatic circulation of bile acids in man. In *Clinics in Gastroenterology*, vol. 6, no. 1, pp. 3–24. (Ed. by G. Paumgartner). W.B. Saunders, London.

Holdsworth C.D. & Dawson A.M. (1965) Absorption of fructose in man. *Proc. Soc. Exp. Biol. Med.* **118**, 142–145.

Holmberg C., Perheentupa J. & Launiala K. (1975) Colonic electrolyte transport in health and in congenital chloride diarrhoea. *J. Clin. Invest.* **56**, 302–310.

Holmberg C., Perheentupa J., Launiala K. & Hallman N. (1977a) Congenital chloride diarrhoea. *Arch. Dis. Child.* **52**, 255–267.

Holmberg C., Perheentupa J. & Pasternack A. (1976b) The renal lesion in congenital chloride diarrhoea. *J. Paediat.* **91**, 738–743.

Holzel A., Schwarz V. & Sutcliffe K.W. (1959) Defective lactose absorption causing malnutrition in infancy. *Lancet*, **i**, 1126–1128.

Hooft C.J., Timmermans J., Snoeck J., Antener I. & Van den Hende C. (1964) Methionine malabsorption in a mentally defective child. *Lancet*, **ii**, 20–21.

Hughes W.S. & Senior J.R. (1975) The glucose-galactose malabsorption syndrome in a 23-year-old woman. *Gastroenterol.* **68**, 142–145.

Imerslund O. (1960) Idiopathic chronic megaloblastic anemia in children. *Acta Pediat. (Stockholm)*, **49** (Suppl 119).

Joseph R., Ribierre M., Job J.C. & Girault M. (1958) Maladie familiale associent des convulsions à début très précoce, une hyperalbuminorachie et une hyperaminoacidurie. *Arch. Franc. de Pédiat.* **15**, 374–387.

Kane J.P., Hardman D.A. & Paulus H.E. (1980) Heterogeneity of apolipoprotein B: isolation of a new species from human chylomicrons. *Proc. Nat. Aca. Sci. USA*, **77**, 2465–2469.

Kayden H.J. & Medick M. (1969) The absorption and metabolism of short and long chain fatty acids in puromycin-treated rats. *Biochim. Biophys. Acta*, **176**, 37–43.

Kayden H.J., Silber R. & Rossmann C.E. (1965) The role of vitamin E deficiency in the abnormal autohemolysis of acanthocytosis. *Trans. Assoc. Amer. Physic.* **78**, 334–342.

Kimmich G.A. (1973) Coupling between Na^+ and sugar transport in small intestine. *Biochim. Biophys. Acta* **300**, 31–78.

Krishnaiah K.V., Walker L.E., Borensztajn J., Schonfeld G. & Getz G.S. (1980) Apolipoprotein B varient derived from rat intestine. *Proceed. Nat. Acad. Sci. USA* **77**, 3806–3810.

Lamy M.J., Frezal J., Polonovski J. & Rey J. (1960) L'absence congenitale de betalipoproteins. *Comp. Rend. Séanc. Soc. Biolog. (Paris)* **154**, 1974–1978.

Lanzkowsky P., Erlandson M.E. & Bezan A.I. (1969) Isolated defect of folic acid absorption associated with mental retardation and cerebral calcification. *Blood*, **34**, 452–465.

Laws J.W. & Neale G. (1966) Radiological diagnosis of disaccharidase deficiency. *Lancet*, **ii**, 139–143.

Leonard J.V., Marrs T.C., Addison J.M., Burston D., Clegg K.M., Lloyd J.K., Matthews D.M. & Seakins J.W. (1976) Intestinal absorption of amino acids and peptides in Hartnup disorder. *Pediat. Res.* **10**, 246–249.

Levin B., Abraham J.M., Burgess E.A. & Wallis P.G. (1970) Congenital lactose malabsorption. *Arch. Dis. Child.* **45**, 173–177.

Levy H.L. (1973) Genetic screening. In *Progress in Human Genetics*, vol. 4, pp. 1–15. (Ed. by H. Herns & K. Hirschorn). Plenum Press, New York.

Levy R.I., Langer T., Gotto A.M. & Fredrickson D.S. (1970) Familial hypobetalipoproteinaemia, a defect in lipoprotein synthesis. *Clin. Res.* **18**, 539A.

Lindqvist B. & Meeuwisse G.W. (1962) Chronic diarrhoea caused by monosaccharide malabsorption. *Acta Paediat.* **51**, 674–685.

Lisker R., Gonzalez B. & Daltabuct M. (1975) Recessive inheritance of the adult types of intestinal lactase deficiency. *Amer. J. Human Genetics* **27**, 662–664.

Lloyd J.K. (1968) Disorders of the serum lipoproteins. I. Lipoprotein deficiency states. *Arch. Dis. Child.* **43**, 393–403.

Lloyd J.K. & Muller D.P.R. (1972) Management of abetalipoproteinaemia in childhood. In *Protides of the Biological Fluids*, p. 331. (Ed. by H. Peeters). Pergamon Press, Oxford.

Lombeck I., Schnippering H.G., Ritzl F., Feinendegen L.E. & Bremer H.J. (1975) Absorption of zinc in acrodermatitis enteropathica. *Lancet*, **i**, 855.

Luhby A.L., Eagle F.J., Roth E. & Cooperman J.M. (1961) Relapsing megaloblastic anemia in an infant due to a specific defect in gastrointestinal absorption of folic acid. *Amer. J. Dis. Child.* **102**, 482–483.

Mabry C.C., Di George A.M. & Auerbach V.H. (1960) Studies concerning the defect in a patient with acanthocytosis. *Clin. Res.* **8**, 371A.

Mackenzie I.L., Donaldson R.M. Jr, Trier J.S. & Mathan V.I. (1972) Ileal mucosa in familial selective vitamin B_{12} malabsorption. *New Engl. J. Med.* **286**, 1021–1025.

Madzarovova-Nohejlova J. (1973) Trehalase deficiency in a family. *Gastroenterol.* **65**, 130–133.

Malloy M.J., Kane J.P., Hardman D.A., Hamilton R.L. & Dalal K.B. (1981) Normotriglyceridemic abetalipoproteinaemia. Absence of the B-100 apolipoprotein. *J. Clin. Invest.* **67**, 1441–1450.

Matthews D.M. (1975) Intestinal absorption of peptides. *Physiol. Rev.* **55**, 537–608.

Matthews D.M. & Adibi S.A. (1976) Peptide absorption. *Gastroenterol.* **71**, 151–161.

McCance R.A. & Widdowson E.M. (1937) Absorption and excretion of iron. *Lancet*, **233**, 680–684.

McCarthy C.F., Borland J.L., Lynch H.J., Owen E.E. & Tyor M.P. (1964) Deficient uptake of basic amino acids and cystine by intestinal mucosa of patients with cystinuria. *J. Clin. Invest.* **43**, 1518–1524.

McNair A., Gudmand-Hoyer E., Jarman S. & Orrild L. (1972) Sucrose malabsorption in Greenland. *Brit. Med. J.* **ii**, 19–21.

Meeuwisse G.W. & Dahlqvist A. (1968) Glucose-galactose malabsorption: a study with biopsy of the small intestinal mucosa. *Acta Paediat. Scand.* **57**, 273–280.

Milla P.J., Aggett P.J., Wolff O.H. & Harries J.T. (1979) Studies in primary hypomagnesaemia:

evidence for defective carrier-mediated small intestinal transport of magnesium. *Gut*, **20**, 1029–1033.

Miller R.G., Davis C.J.F., Illingworth D.R. & Bradley W. (1980) The neuropathy of abetalipoproteinemia. *Neurol.* **30**, 1286–1291.

Milne M.D. (1964) Disorders of amino acid transport. *Brit. Med. J.* **i**, 327.

Milne M.D. Asatoor A.M., Edwards K.D.G. & Loughridge L.W. (1961) The intestinal absorption defect in cystinuria. *Gut*, **2**, 232–337.

Milbe M.D., Crawford M.A., Girao C.B. & Loughridge L.W. (1960) The metabolic disorder in Hartnup disease. *Quart. J. Med.* **29**, 407–421.

Mircheff A.K., van Os C.H. & Wright E.M. (1980) Pathways for alanine transport in intestinal baso-lateral membrane vesicles. *J. Membr. Biol.* **52**, 83–92.

Morikawa T, Tada K., Ando T., Yoshida T., Yokoyama Y. & Arakawa T. (1966) Prolinuria: deficient intestinal absorption of amino acids and proline. *J. Exp. Med.* **90**, 105–116.

Morin C.L., Thompson M.W., Jackson S.H. & Sassokorlsak A. (1971) Biochemical and genetic studies in cystinuria: Observations on double heterozygotes of genotype I/II. *J. Clin. Invest.* **50**, 1961–1976.

Moynahan E.J. & Barnes P.M. (1973) Zinc deficiency and a synthetic diet for lactose intolerance. *Lancet*, **i**, 676.

Muller D.P.R., Harries J.T. & Lloyd J.K. (1974) The relative importance of the factors involved in the absorption of vitamin E in children. *Gut*, **15**, 966–971.

Muller D.P.R., Lloyd J.K. & Bird A.C. (1977) Long-term management of abetalipoproteinaemia. Possible role for vitamin E. *Arch. Dis. Child.* **52**, 209–214.

Muller D.P.R. & Lloyd J.K. (1982) Effect of large oral doses of vitamin E on the neurological sequelae of patients with abetalipoproteinaemia. *Ann. New York Acad. Sci.* **393**, 133–144.

Muller D.P.R., Lloyd J.K. & Wolff O.H. (1983) Vitamin E and neurological function. *Lancet*, **i**, 225–228.

Neale G. (1968) The diagnosis, incidence and significance of disaccharidase deficiency in adults. *Proc. Roy. Soc. Med.* **61**, 1099–1102.

Newcomer A.D. & McGill D.B. (1966) Distribution of disaccharidase activity in the small bowel of normal and lactase deficient subjects. *Gastroenterol.* **51**, 481–488.

Norio R., Nevanlinna H.R. & Perheentupa J. (1973) Hereditary disease in Finland, rare flora in rare soil. *Ann. Clin. Res.* **5**, 109–141.

Pasternack A. & Perheentupa J. (1966) Hypertensive angiopathy in familial chloride diarrhoea. *Lancet*, **ii**, 1047–1049.

Pasternack A., Perheentupa J., Launiala K. & Hallman N. (1967) Kidney biopsy findings in familial chloride diarrhoea. *Acta Endocrinol.* **55**, 1–9.

Paunier L., Radde I.C., Kooh S.W. & Fraser D. (1968) Primary hypomagnesemia with secondary hypocalcemia in an infant. *Pediat.* **41**, 285–402.

Pearson A.J., Sladen G.E., Edmonds C.J., Tavill A.S., Wills M.R. & McIntyre N. (1973) The pathophysiology of congenital chloridorrhoea. *Quart. J. Med.* **42**, 453–466.

Perheentupa J. & Visakorpi J. (1965) Protein intolerance with deficiency transport of basic amino acids; another inborn error of metabolism. *Lancet*, **ii**, 813–816.

Perry T.L., Hansen S., Tischler B., Butning R. & Berry K. (1967) Carnosinaemia: a new metabolic disorder associated with neurologic disease and mental defect. *New Engl. J. Med.* **277**, 1219–1227.

Peterson M.L. & Herber R. (1967) Intestinal sucrase deficiency. *Trans. Assoc. Amer. Physic.* **80**, 275–283.

Phillips S.F. & McGill D.B. (1973) Glucose–galactose malabsorption in an adult: perfusion studies of sugar, electrolyte and water transport. *Amer., J. Digest. Dis.* **18**, 1017–1024.

Prockop D.J., Keiser H.R. & Sjoerdsma A. (1962) Gastrointestinal absorption and renal excretion of hydroxyproline peptides. *Lancet*, **ii**, 527–528.

Rajantie J., Simell O. & Perheentupa J. (1980a) Intestinal absorption in lysinuric protein intolerance: impaired for diamino acids, normal for cirtulline. *Gut*, **21**, 519–524.

Rajantie J., Simell O. & Perheentupa J. (1980b) Basolateral membrane transport defect for lysine in lysinuric protein intolerance. *Lancet*, **i**, 1219–1221.

Rask-Madsen J., Kamper J., Oddsson E. & Krog E. (1976) Congenital chloridorrhoea, a question of reversed brush border processes and varying junctional tightness. *Scand. J. Gastroenterol.* **2**, 377–383.

Rasmussen H. & Anast C. (1978) Familial hypophosphatemic (vitamin D-resistant) rickets and vitamin D-dependent rickets. In *The Metabolic Basis of Inherited Disease*, 4th ed., pp. 1537–1562. (Ed. by J.B. Stanburg, J.B. Wyngaarden & D.S. Fredrickson). McGraw-Hill, New York.

Riordan J.F. & Vallee B.L. (1976) Zinc and metalloproteins. Structure and function of zinc metalloenzymes in trace elements. In *Human Health and Disease*, vol. 1, pp. 227–256. (Ed. by A.S. Prasad). Academic Press, New York.

Rosenberg L.E., Downing J., Durant J.L. & Segal S. (1966) Cystinuria: biochemical evidence for three genetically distinct diseases. *J. Clin. Invest.* **45**, 365–371.

Rubino A., Field M. & Shwachman H. (1971) Intestinal transport of amino acid residues of dipeptides. I. Influx of the glycine residue of glycyl-L-proline across mucosal border. *J. Biol. Chem.* **246**, 3342–3548.

Salt H.B., Wolff O.H., Lloyd J.K., Fosbrooke A.S., Cameron A.H. & Hubble D.V. (1960) On having no betalipoprotein — a syndrome comprising abetalipoproteinaemia, acanthocytosis and steatorrhoea. *Lancet*, **ii**, 325–329.

Sandhu B.K., Tripp J.H., Milla P.J. & Harries J.T. (1983) Loperamide in severe protracted diarrhoea. *Arch. Dis. Child.* **58**, 39–43.

Santiago-Borrero P.J., Santini R. Jr, Perez-Santiago E., Maldonado N., Millan S. & Coll-Camalez G. (1973) Congenital isolated defect of folic acid absorption. *J. Paediat.* **82**, 450–455.

Schmitz J., Bresson J.L., Triadou N., Bataille J. & Rey J. (1980) Analyse en eléctrophorèse sur gel de ployacrylamide des protéines de la membrane microvillositaire et d'une fraction cytoplasmatique dans 8 cas d'intolérance congénitale au saccharose. *Gastroenterol. Clin. et Biolog.* **4**, 251–256.

Schneider A.J., Kinter W.B. & Stirling C.E. (1966) Glucose-galactose malabsorption. *New Engl. J. Med.* **274**, 305–312.

Schultz S.G. & Strecker C.K. (1970) Fructose influx across the brush border of rabbit ileum. *Biochem. Biophys. Acta*, **211**, 586–588.

Scott B.B., Miller J.P. & Losowsky M.S. (1979) Hypobetalipoproteinaemia — a variant of the Bassen-Kornzweig syndrome. *Gut*, **20**, 163–168.

Scriver S.R. & Wilson O.H. (1967) Amino acid transport: evidence for genetic control of two types in human kidney. *Science*, **155**, 1428–1430.

Sheldon J.H. (1965) *Haemochromatosis*. Oxford University Press, London.

Sigurdsson G., Nicoll A. & Lewis B. (1977) Turnover of apolipoprotein-B in two subjects with familial hypobetalipoproteinaemia. *Metabolism*, **26**, 25–31.

Silk D.B.A. (1974) Peptide absorption in man. *Gut*, **15**, 494–501.

Silk D.B.A., Perrett D. & Clark M.L. (1975) Jejunal and ileal absorption of dibasic amino-acids and an arginine-containing dipeptide in cystinuria. *Gastroenterol.* **68**, 1426–1432.

Simell O. (1975) Diamino acid transport into granulocytes and liver slices of patients with lysinuric protein intolerance. *Pediat. Res.* **9**, 504–508.

Simell O., Perheentupa J., Rapola J., Visakorpi J.K. & Eskelin L.E. (1975) Lysinuric protein intolerance. *Amer. J. Med.* **59**, 229–240.

Sperling M.A., Hiles D.A. & Kennerdell J.S. (1972) Electroretinographic responses following vitamin A therapy in abetalipoproteinaemia. *Amer. J. Ophthalmol.* **73**, 342–351.

Strauss E.W. (1966) Morphological aspects of triglyceride absorption. In *Handbook of Physiology*, section 6, vol. 3, pp. 1377–1406. (Ed. by C.F. Code). American Physiological Society, Washington D.C.

Szurszewski J. & Bulbring E. (1973) The stimulant action of acetylcholine and catecholamine on the uterus. *Phil. Trans. Roy. Soc., Lond. Series B*, **265**, 149–156.

Thier S.O., Segal S, Fox M. Blair A. & Rosenberg L.E. (1965) Cystinuria: defective intestinal transport of dibasic amino acids and cystine. *J. Clin. Invest.* **44**, 442–448.

Turnberg L.A. (1971) Abnormalities in intestinal electrolyte transport in congenital chloridorrhoea. *Gut*, **12**, 544–551.

Weijers H.A., Van de Kamer J.H., Mossel D.A.A. & Dicke W.K. (1960) Diarrhoea caused by deficiency of sugar splitting enzymes *Lancet*, **ii**, 296–297.

Whelan D.T. & Scriver C.R. (1968) Cystathioninuria and renal iminoglycinuria in a pedigree. *New Engl. J. Med.* **278**, 924–927.

Wimberley P.D., Harries J.T. & Burgess E.A. (1974) Congenital glucose–galacrose malabsorption. *Proc. Roy. Soc. Med.* **67**, 755–756.

Wolff O.H., Lloyd J.K. & Tonks E.L. (1964) Abetalipoproteinaemia with special reference to the visual defect. *Exp. Eye Res.* **3**, 439–442.

Woolf L.I. (1967) Large scale screening for metabolic disease in the newborn in Great Britain. In *Phenylketonuria and Allied Metabolic Disorders*, pp. 50–59. (Ed. by J.A. Anderson & K.F. Swaiman). U.S. Department of Health, Education and Welfare, Washington DC.

Chapter 4
Motility and its Disorders

D. G. THOMPSON AND D. L. WINGATE

Introduction 78
The normal pattern of small intestinal motility 78
Control of small intestinal motility 80
Normal motility in clinical practice 83
Disorders of intestinal motility 83
Clinical syndromes with disordered small intestinal motility 84
Treatment of motility disorders 89

'The gastroenterologist should always keep in mind two facts . . . One, that the important organ of digestion is the small bowel, and the other, that most of the symptoms of indigestion appear to arise in disturbances in the motor functions of the digestive tract'.
Walter C. Alvarez (1948)

Introduction

Despite the length of time for which a relationship between abnormal small intestinal motility and gastrointestinal symptoms has been assumed to exist, knowledge derived from systematic scientific observation remains scarce and our understanding of the physiology and pathophysiology of human intestinal motility is far from complete. An appreciation of the underlying mechanisms is only now beginning to be realized, and to date, the practical applications of this knowledge have barely influenced the practice of clinical medicine.

This chapter summarizes the present state of knowledge of human small intestinal motility, demonstrates the relationship of this knowledge to disease states and indicates areas where future study might advance both clinical science and clinical practice.

The normal pattern of small intestinal motility

The normal pattern of small intestinal motility is more easily understood when its physiological role is considered. Essentially, the small intestine is in one of two conditions; it is either receiving chyme from the stomach after feeding, or it is in the fasted state with the lumen void of nutrient. It is still not widely appreciated that the pattern of motor activity which prevails is, in health, entirely dependent upon which of these two conditions applies. That this is the case seems less surprising when the task demanded of the bowel is considered.

After the ingestion of food, small bowel motility is required to ensure transit of its contents through the intestine at a rate which is appropriate for optimal mixing with intestinal secretions for digestion and for optimal contact with the mucosal surface for absorption. Since there is considerable variation in the physical and chemical nature of meals, it seems probable that the postprandial motility pattern, even if stereotyped, is susceptible to modulation according to the content of the meal, and that receptors linked to the motor control system exist for this purpose.

Between meals, however, the motor activity of the small intestine functions to ensure that its lumen remains empty by means of intermittent propulsive episodes, which migrate caudally throughout its length and which expel non-digested residue. In man, such propulsive episodes may also serve to repel the oral migration of the colonic bacterial flora and prevent small intestinal bacterial overgrowth.

The fasted pattern

The fasted pattern of mammalian small intes-

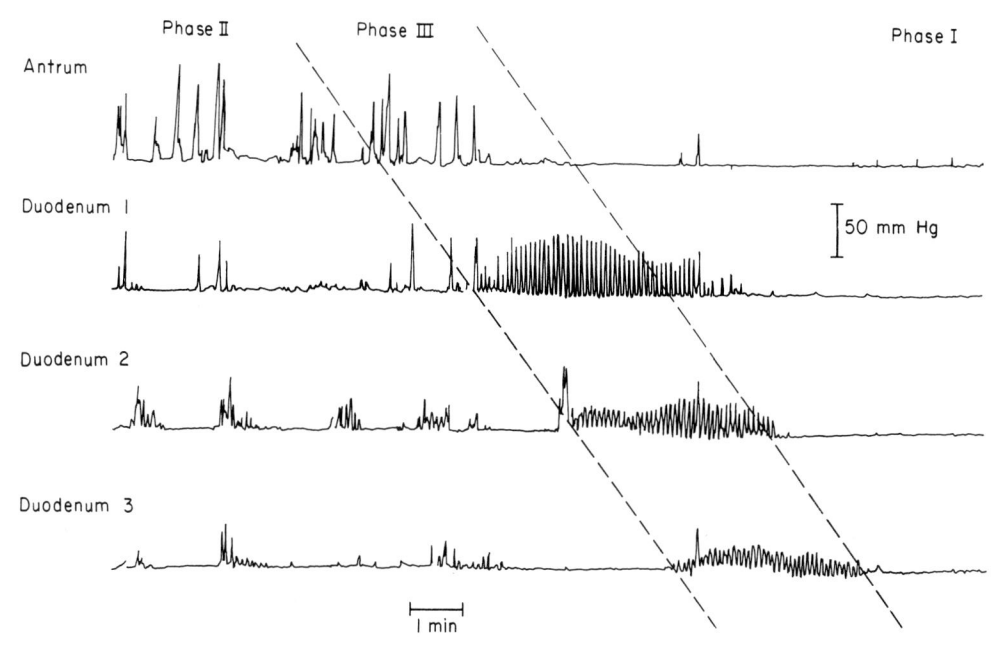

Fig. 4.1. Recording of human antral and duodenal fasting motor activity obtained using an ingested multi-lumen tube with four channels 10 cm apart. A period of irregular motor activity (Phase II) can be seen to terminate in regular contractions (Phase III) at a rate of approximately three per minute in the antrum and eleven per minute in the duodenum. The Phase III pattern migrates aborally through the duodenum and is replaced by a period of quiescence (Phase I).

tinal activity has been studied for nearly a century since the pioneering work of Boldyreff (1905), but only in recent years, since the studies of Szurszewski (1969) and Code & Marlett (1975) has it been clearly defined. The pattern in man is essentially similar to that of most other mammalian species, with a triphasic cycle (Fig. 4.1). Periods of motor quiescence (Phase I) alternate with irregular activity (Phase II) which then terminates with a shorter period of regular contractile activity (Phase III) at a frequency of twelve to fourteen contractions per minute. Each phase of the cycle may progress slowly down from duodenum to ileum, although some cycles may begin distal to the duodenum, while others may fail to progress for the complete length of the small bowel. The pattern is thus one of recurring cyclical or *periodic* activity and has been termed the *migrating myoelectric*, or *migrating motor, complex*, for which the abbreviation *MMC* is a useful common denominator.

Because it 'sweeps' slowly down the small intestine, the regular Phase III activity has been likened to a broom and described by Code and other workers as 'the intestinal housekeeper' of the small intestine. It has been assumed that this pattern is necessary for maintaining an empty gut and preventing bacterial overgrowth. Indeed, it has been claimed that small intestinal bacterial overgrowth is a consequence of impaired Phase III activity in some patients (Vantrappen et al. 1977). In view of the cyclical changes in secretion which are now recognized to accompany the motility phases (Vantrappen et al. 1979, Keane et al. 1980), the Phase III pattern is probably better compared with the 'mop and bucket' of the housekeeper, washing as well as sweeping the fasted gut. Although an attractive concept, it seems likely, however, that most caudal transit of intestinal debris occurs during Phase II and not Phase III, simply because the duration of Phase II is much longer than Phase III, even though its propulsive efficiency may be less.

The fed pattern

Feeding disrupts the fasting pattern, replacing it by a period of irregular contractile activity throughout the small intestine, the duration of which is dependent upon the nutrient load and upon the rate of gastric emptying. When gastric emptying ceases, the fasting pattern resumes, although the exact time relationship of these events has not been determined. In most developed countries, three meals a day are consumed, spaced at intervals of 5–6 h. Under these circumstances, the commonest pattern of motor activity in the small intestine will be the fed pattern, with the fasting pattern restricted largely to the night, although occasionally, fasted activity is recognizable between meals (Thompson et al. 1981).

One of the major problems in human intestinal motility is a full understanding of the fed pattern; thus far it has defied adequate analysis. It seems probable that the description of irregular contractile activity embraces a number of different patterns which have different mechanical consequences in terms of both mixing and transit, but identification and interpretation of these variations requires further study. To give one example; it has been shown that in normal volunteers, enteral administration of an easily absorbed feeding solution produces a different pattern of motility from that induced by an elemental feeding solution which is known to induce fluid secretion and, hence, diarrhoea (Wilson & Goode 1981), but which is cause, and which is effect, is unknown.

Retroperistalsis

It is often believed that the propagation of intestinal contractions is unidirectional, oral to caudal. While this seems largely true, caudal to oral retroperistalsis does undoubtedly occur (Alvarez 1925). Such activity furthermore seems to be an integral part of the emetic mechanism and immediately precedes vomiting in most, if not all, mammalian species.

At present the mechanism inducing retroperistalsis defies adequate explanation. If the normal propagation of contractions is consequent upon aboral polarity of the slow wave, then retroperistalsis would logically be expected to result from a reversal of this polarity.

Control of small intestinal motility

The efficient transit of nutrients through many centimetres of intestine requires a sophisticated control system. This control is exerted upon the small intestinal smooth muscle at a number of levels which summate to produce the required effect. The operation of this control remains arguably the major unsolved problem in gastrointestinal physiology today. It is clear that the rational treatment of small intestinal motility disorders must depend upon understanding the control mechanisms both in health and in disease. Furthermore, this knowledge may provide the key to the unlocking of other more complex neuronal systems in the central nervous system.

Intestinal smooth muscle

To understand the control of small intestinal motility, we must start with the muscle itself, which is arranged in two distinct layers, an inner circular and an outer longitudinal layer. While each smooth muscle cell is a discrete unit, it is closely attached to its neighbour by tight junctions (Burnstock 1970). These close approximations of adjacent cell membranes allow low resistance electrical connections, producing a functional, if not structural, syncitium.

Intestinal smooth muscle cells show a rhythmic variation in transmembrane potential difference. This activity is a basic function of intestinal smooth muscle, being recordable throughout its life, even during complete motor quiescence (Duthie 1974). While the exact mechanism for the fluctuation in membrane potential remains imperfectly understood, it seems to result from rhythmic changes in the sodium pump of the cell membrane (Connor et al 1974). The syncitial organization of the muscle mass ensures that cells which are close to each other depolarize their membranes synchronously, producing a rhythmic fluctuation in voltage at the surface of the muscle mass, which may be detected by a large volume surface electrode. This fluctuation is conveniently termed the *electrical slow wave*, and the rhythmic succession of slow waves has been called the *basic electrical rhythm (BER)*. It is important to understand that the slow wave is an electrical and not a mechanical event, but the rhythmic electrical changes determine the timing of contractions.

The frequency of the slow wave varies with position in the small intestine. In the duodenum and upper jejunum the frequency of the slow wave is approximately eleven per min while, in the ileum, it is slower at approximately eight per min. In the dog and almost certainly in man, the slow waves can be shown to migrate caudally down the small intestine from a duodenal pacemaker (Hermon-Taylor & Code 1971) with regions of higher intrinsic slow wave frequency tending to capture more caudal regions and drive them at a faster rate (Christensen *et al.* 1966).

The frequency of the slow wave at a given site in the small intestine is normally altered very little by external influences, such as autonomic nervous activity. Frequency of the slow wave does, however, vary with the basal metabolic rate, increasing with thyrotoxicosis or fever (Christensen *et al.* 1966).

Electrical recording of small intestinal slow wave activity often shows the presence of faster, shorter duration electrical deflections superimposed upon slow waves at the point in the slow wave cycle which corresponds to maximal depolarization of the underlying muscle cells. These are known conventionally as *spike potentials* and are associated with the initiation of contractile activity (Daniel & Chapman 1963). Some authors refer to them as action potentials, but an action potential refers to changes in the membrane potential of a single cell; spike potentials represent the summated action potentials occurring within the vicinity of a surface electrode.

Thus, contractions in the small intestine are synchronized with the underlying slow wave, the frequency and propagation of contractions at any point in the small intestine being linked by the slow wave at that point. The slow wave determines the timing of each contraction, and the number of slow waves per minute represents the maximum number of contractions which can (but may not) occur during that time. Whether or not contraction will occur during the passage of a slow wave at a given site thus depends, not upon the muscle itself, but upon the control system.

Intrinsic nervous control

The control of the action potential remains uncertain. Neural input from the myenteric plexus, however, is of major importance. Furthermore, it seems likely that myenteric neural control of smooth muscle is predominantly inhibitory, since tetrodotoxin, a non-specific neurotoxin with little or no effect upon smooth muscle function, induces a florid action potential discharge and small intestinal contraction at the underlying slow wave frequency (Biber & Fara 1973). Thus, muscle contraction in the intact small intestine seems to occur as a result of an inhibition of the underlying background inhibitory neural input.

The myenteric plexus

That the immediate level of control of the smooth muscle is by neural input from the myenteric plexus can be shown by the anatomical network of neurones which link the plexus to the muscle mass. The conventional view of the myenteric plexus is that it is simply a relay station which co-ordinates the movements of the muscle and conveys instructions from higher centres. However, recent work has shown that it is probably the main level of control of small intestinal motor activity, and that it contains 'programmes' for integrated and purposive movements. Furthermore, it responds to neural input, both from the local receptors, and from higher centres, by selecting the appropriate programme. That the circuitry required to organize intestinal contractions is located within the myenteric plexus is further shown by observation of MMC-like motor activity in isolated autotransplanted small intestine (Sarr & Kelly 1981). When the small intestine is transected in several places and then reanastomosed in continuity, each segment exhibits autonomous and independent MMC-like activity for a period of weeks; at the end of that time, as the myenteric plexus regenerates across the anastomoses (whereas fibrous tissue permanently separates the muscle layers), the MMC activity again becomes co-ordinated and synchronized.

Knowledge of myenteric nervous organization is increasing. In addition to the traditional adrenergic and cholinergic branches of the autonomic nervous system, a third branch, the so-called 'non-adrenergic, non-cholinergic' system is now recognized. The small intestinal cholinergic nerve activity is predominantly excitatory while adrenergic nervous stimulation is inhibitory; the inhibitory input is probably applied to the intrinsic nerve plexuses rather than directly to the muscle cells (Furness & Costa 1974). Inhibitory control is also exerted upon the small intestine by the non-adrenergic, non-cholinergic nerves. The neurotransmitter for this system is uncertain; a number of candidate substances have been proposed of which ATP (Burnstock 1972), VIP (Furness et al. 1981) and serotonin (Gershon & Erde 1981) are presently most popular.

Gut peptides

In addition to the more traditional concept of neural control, additional local control systems operating through the local release of peptides have been proposed, the so-called paracrine system. A multitude of peptides capable of influencing small intestinal motility in experimental circumstances have now been described, but their role in the physiology of human small intestinal motility remains far from clear. Theoretically, gut peptides may act in three ways; as humoral agents (endocrine), as locally active agents (paracrine), and as neurotransmitters or neuromodulators (neurocrine). Experiments to distinguish between these effects are difficult to design and perform, and much of what is known is inferred indirectly from immunoassay of plasma and tissue peptides, and from histochemical study of their distribution (cf Chapter 23).

Motilin

Motilin has been stongly implicated as the controller of small intestinal motility, based on observations that cyclical variations in plasma levels usually coincide with the incidence of fasting Phase III activity in the stomach and duodenum (Peeters et al. 1980). Exogenous motilin also seems to have the potential to initiate Phase III activity in fasting man (Vantrappen et al. 1979). On the other hand, it seems that motilin requires a receptive intestine induced by neural activity; cholinergic blockade seems to block the effect of exogenous motilin (Green et al. 1976), whereas the gastrointestinal response to exogenous motilin is dependent upon the phase of activity of infusion (Itoh et al. 1977). In the early experiments with motilin it was assumed that the peptide affected both the foregut (stomach and duodenum), and the midgut (jejunum and ileum), but it now seems probable that motilin does not directly affect the midgut. Furthermore, while it is true that MMC-like activity initiated in the duodenum by motilin will be propagated along the small bowel through the intrinsic nerve network, experiments in dogs with Thiry–Vella lengths of small intestine, disconnected from the proximal bowel, show a failure of the loop to respond to motilin (Pinnington & Wingate 1981).

Somatostatin

Exogenous somatostatin has a potent effect on the motor activity of the small bowel; exogenous somatostatin will covert the fed pattern into a fasting pattern (Konturek 1977). From this it is tempting to assume that somatostatin plays a physiological role, but given the ability of exogenous somatostatin to block many endogenous peptides, the effect may not be physiological.

Gastrin and CCK

In the intact gut, both gastrin and CCK will interrupt the fasting pattern, at least in the proximal gut (Wingate et al. 1978). This has led to suggestions that gastrin release converts the fasted to the fed pattern, but in the small intestine, it seems more likely that the effect is mediated through the extrinsic nerves. Apart from anything else, the postprandial plasma rise in gastrin is much more brief than the duration of the fasting pattern (Wingate et al. 1979), although it is conceivable that gastrin release triggers another mechanism which has a more sustained action.

Opioids

Opioid peptides, such as enkephalin, given systemically, have profound effects on small bowel motility, abolishing irregular contractile activity (Konturek et al. 1980) and inducing powerful MMC-like propagated bursts. Whether or not opioids play a physiological or pathological part in the control of motility remains obscure.

Extrinsic nervous control

While present evidence seems to indicate that initiation and propagation of the fasting cyclical pattern is intrinsic to the small intestine, it seems likely that the control of the feeding response is dependent upon extra-intestinal influences. For example, feeding fails to inhibit the occurrence of migratory Phase-III-like activity in autotransplanted segments of small intestine (Sarr & Kelly 1981) which are isolated from external neural innervation. Also stimulation of brainstem vagal nuclei can inhibit established fed activity (Thompson et al. 1982) as does acute vagal blockade in animals (Diamant et al. 1980).

The normal control of intestinal motility is, thankfully, independent of conscious thought. Higher neural centres, however, do seem to influence small intestinal motility under normal conditions. For example, the fasting pattern is altered during sleep with a reduction in the quantity of Phase II activity (Ritchie et al. 1980). It has also been claimed that the onset of Phase III activity correlates with rapid eye movement (REM) sleep, thus implying that the two phenomena are inter-related (Finch et al. 1980). On the other hand, abolition of REM sleep by drugs does not abolish Phase III activity which suggests that it is not directly causally related (Evans et al. 1982).

Normal motility in clinical practice

How is knowledge of normal small intestinal motility relevant to clinical practice? There are a number of important practical points for the clinician to remember. First, the recurrent cyclical pattern of both motility and secretion means that the concept of a 'steady-state' in the small intestine during fasting is no longer acceptable and that 'bowel rest' can never be completely achieved by starvation alone.

Fasting Phase III activity in the upper small intestine is also relevant because its presence may be recognized by normal fasting subjects as a transient vague 'sinking' nauseating feeling.

Finally, the variability of intestinal transit during the different phases of fasting motor activity could influence the bioavailability of drugs ingested during the different phases. Slow release and enteric-coated drugs might be rapidly propelled through the small intestine without complete absorption if ingested just before Phase III of the migrating complex. While this hypothesis remains to be fully tested, it has been shown that digoxin blood levels following the ingestion of enteric-coated preparations are influenced by other drugs which speed enteric transit (Manninen et al. 1973).

Disorders of intestinal motility

Since the first observation of the normal triphasic human fasting pattern, many studies have been performed upon patients with abdominal symptoms in an attempt to demonstrate abnormalities associated with particular diseases. To date, published reports of recognizable and consistent abnormalities in disease are few. One major problem which has confronted researchers in this field has been the wide range of the normal pattern (Thompson et al. 1980) which has necessitated prolonged studies of at least

24 h. Further problems have been the correlation of any alleged abnormality with the manifestation of the disease process, and the uncertainty in most instances, whether the observed abnormality is the cause of or the result of the underlying disease. Furthermore, the fasted pattern may not be the most appropriate phase to study in many disorders; it is studied principally because a reproducible pattern can be seen, in contrast to the fed state where no obvious normal pattern has been recognized. Even studies of the fasted pattern have been largely restricted to observations of periodicity of Phase III activity since this phase is most easily identified and measured.

Theoretical mechanisms of disordered motility

Disorders of small intestinal motility could theoretically result from dysfunction of smooth muscle of the intrinsic control system, or of extrinsic control.

Smooth muscle

Damage to the intestinal smooth muscle would be expected to reduce the intraluminal pressure generated in the small intestine and to delay transit. Pressure recordings would show a normal incidence and pattern of contractions, but a reduction in amplitude. Impaired transit would allow accumulation of nutrient residue and result in bacterial colonization and malabsorption. It is likely that the disordered intestinal transit seen in scleroderma, and in some cases of chronic idiopathic pseudo-obstruction (discussed below), are predominantly the result of smooth muscle damage.

Intrinsic nervous system

Damage to the myenteric plexus would be expected to disrupt the normally observed patterns of contractile activity both during fasting and after food. Complete denervation might be expected to release the intestinal smooth muscle from its customary inhibition and to result in a hyperkinetic gut. However, it would be unwise to expect consistent patterns of abnormality when destruction of the intrinsic plexuses is incomplete; the intrinsic nerve plexuses include at least three (and probably many more) separate nerve networks with specialized functions which are both agonist and antagonist.

Pathological processes may damage the myenteric plexus and diseases such as diabetes, ischaemia, Chagas' disease and toxigenic intestinal pathogens probably cause motility disorders via damage at this level.

The extrinsic nervous control

Abnormalities of the control mechanisms sited outside the gut could disrupt the normal pattern, the disruption varying with the level of extrinsic nervous involvement. For example, disruption of afferents from the gut could disturb the recognition of food, whereas disruption of efferent pathways to the gut via vagal and sympathetic channels would disrupt the normal pathways by which higher nervous control is exerted.

The central nervous system might also disturb the normal small intestine by effects mediated through the autonomic nervous system.

In general, parasympathetic influences upon the small intestine stimulate motor activity whereas sympathetic stimulation suppresses it. Increased sympathetic nervous activity is a well-recognized accompaniment of stress which has been shown to disturb fasting small intestinal motility. Could stress then, be a factor in clinical disorders of intestinal function?. The answer is uncertain. Although reports of abnormal small intestinal motility patterns in patients with functional bowel disorders do exist (Horowitz & Farrar 1962, Thompson *et al.* 1979), it still remains to be determined whether such changes are the cause of the clinical problem and not a consequence of it.

Clinical syndromes with disordered small intestinal motility

Abnormal fasting motility

Fasting small intestinal motor activity is an

efficient mechanism for evacuating both solid and liquid material from the small intestine. Failure of the normal pattern of motility or failure to achieve adequate pressure gradients might, therefore, result in the accumulation of food residue in the small intestine and in bacterial overgrowth.

There are few systematic studies of motility in patients with overgrowth in the absence of structural abnormalities of the small intestine. One group has asserted that the absence of observable Phase III motor activity may be related to small intestinal bacterial overgrowth (Vantrappen et al. 1977). Whilst attractive, the concept seems unlikely to be the sole cause of overgrowth in such patients unless Phase II activity is also abnormal, since significant aboral intestinal transit also occurs during this phase. It is also probably necessary to postulate an accompanying abnormality of postprandial transit in view of the predominance of this activity, the fasting pattern in most Western adults being restricted to less than half of each 24 h.

Intestinal pseudo-obstruction

In this syndrome, small intestinal transit is abnormally slow and secondary bacterial overgrowth occurs. Recurrent intestinal obstruction without mechanical blockage of the small intestinal lumen is the predominant feature. It is usually found secondary to a number of systemic diseases but also occurs as a primary phenomenon. The abnormality of transit characterizing this syndrome could result from either smooth muscle and/or neurological dysfunction.

Thus, three main types of the syndrome can be postulated, i.e. normal muscle with abnormal neural control; normal neural control with abnormal muscle; impaired neural control with abnormal muscle.

Evidence is now accumulating to support the three types of the syndrome. In some cases (Schuffler et al. 1978), myenteric plexus neurones have been found to be abnormal or absent in the presence of normal smooth muscle. This would be expected to result in delayed transit by disordered propulsion and to show abnormalities of both fasted and fed patterns of motor activity. Such abnormalities have, in fact, been shown in those few cases studied by intestinal manometry. In other reports, a myopathy has been found to be the primary disorder (Schuffler et al. 1977).

The clinical presentation of the three types is very similar. Recurrent upper abdominal pain after food in association with bloating, nausea and vomiting are the most common features indicating combined gastric and small intestinal disease.

Change in bowel habit with constipation and dysphagia also occurs but less frequently. In some patients, urinary retention coincides indicating the presence of extra-intestinal involvement.

Commonly, patients undergo surgery at initial presentation because acute intestinal obstruction is diagnosed. Abdominal X-rays often show dilated loops of small bowel and fluid levels making surgical intervention virtually impossible to avoid without prior knowledge of the disorder in the patient. In some cases, it is possible to obtain a family history of similar symptoms and asymptomatic relatives, sometimes with quite marked radiological abnormalities, are also found. This type of enquiry (and indeed a differential diagnosis which includes pseudo-obstruction) is often only made after surgery has failed to reveal mechanical obstruction.

Radiological features include oesophageal dilatation with absent peristalsis, gastric dilatation and delayed emptying. Megaduodenum is a common feature, together with segmental dilatation of the jejunum and ileum. Barium enema examination often shows colonic dilatation with faecal concretions and impaction.

Small intestinal bacterial overgrowth is an expected result of the impaired intestinal transit. Manometric and myoelectric studies have been performed on selected patients with variable results. Management of the condition is generally unsuccessful. Surgery is often advised in an attempt to bypass an allegedly abnormal segment but almost always fails to ensure permanent relief of symptoms because of the widespread involvement of the gut. Multiple laparotomies also make future management difficult since the possibility of mechanical obstruction due to adhesions then requires exclusion every time symptoms worsen.

Pharmacological intervention has been similarly futile. While cholinergic drugs are capable of inducing mechanical activity, they cannot produce the appropriate patterns of organized activity required for optimum transit, and they are ineffective when the intrinsic nerve plexuses, which contain the 'programmes' for organized motility, are damaged. Management, therefore, is directed principally towards reducing the secondary manifestations of of the disease. Small intestinal bacterial overgrowth can be reduced by appropriate antibiotic therapy, but in severe cases, parenteral nutrition may offer the only way of providing adequate long-term care.

Systemic sclerosis

Patients with systemic sclerosis commonly suffer from gastrointestinal involvement. Although the clinical manifestations are predominantly oesophageal or colonic, the small intestine is usually also affected (Bluestone et al. 1969). Atrophy of the small intestinal smooth muscle is accompanied by collagen deposition and there is disruption of contact between adjacent smooth muscle cells (Greenberger et al. 1968) which disturbs the normally co-ordinated pattern of muscle activity, with consequent impairment of intraluminal propulsion. Although reduced in number, the smooth muscle cells appear morphologically normal (Schuffler & Beegle 1979). Small intestinal damage is commonly subclinical (Bluestone et al. 1969) and usually discovered incidentally as symptomless small intestinal distension during radiological examination. Occasionally, however, a full-blown pseudo-obstruction syndrome results identical in its manifestations to that described above.

Fasting small intestinal motor activity has been recently examined in patients with systemic sclerosis, both with and without clinical evidence of small intestinal disease (Rees et al. 1982). A normal triphasic cyclical pattern was recordable from the asymptomatic patients, but in those with evidence of small intestinal involvement, the pattern was abnormal, with disrupted cycles and reduction in motor activity. Plasma motility is increased in all phases of the MMC in both symptomatic and asymptomatic patients. Whether this elevation represents a true increase in motilin release or is a consequence of impaired clearance from the circulation, perhaps the result of coincident renal impairment remains to be determined.

Therapy, like that for pseudo-obstruction in general, remains symptomatic and usually does not influence the course of the disease. Oral broad spectrum antibiotics may be helpful if there is significant bacterial overgrowth.

Episodic functional abdominal pain

Many patients with gastrointestinal symptoms have no demonstrable structural abnormality. Their episodic abdominal pain is usually ascribed to a disorder of gut function. Because their predominant symptoms are usually defaecatory, such patients are conventionally termed 'irritable colon', or 'irritable bowel'. Most patients, however, have widespread gut symptoms and probably show dysfunction of the entire gastrointestinal tract.

It is natural, therefore, to suspect that such patients should show an abnormal pattern of small intestinal motility. Several case reports of an abnormal fasting pattern have now been published (Horowitz & Farrar 1962, Thompson et al. 1979), but many more unpublished studies of similar patients have failed to show a difference from the normal pattern. In part, this probably reflects the difficulties in demonstrating any significant deviation from the wide range of patterns found in healthy people, together with the still primitive methods of data analysis.

It must also be remembered that episodic symptoms may result from episodic abnormalities in motor pattern, and it is perhaps not surprising that studies of patients, when free of symptoms, show no abnormality. To study patients at a time when they have symptoms probably requires ambulatory monitoring. Postprandial motor patterns may be particularly important because

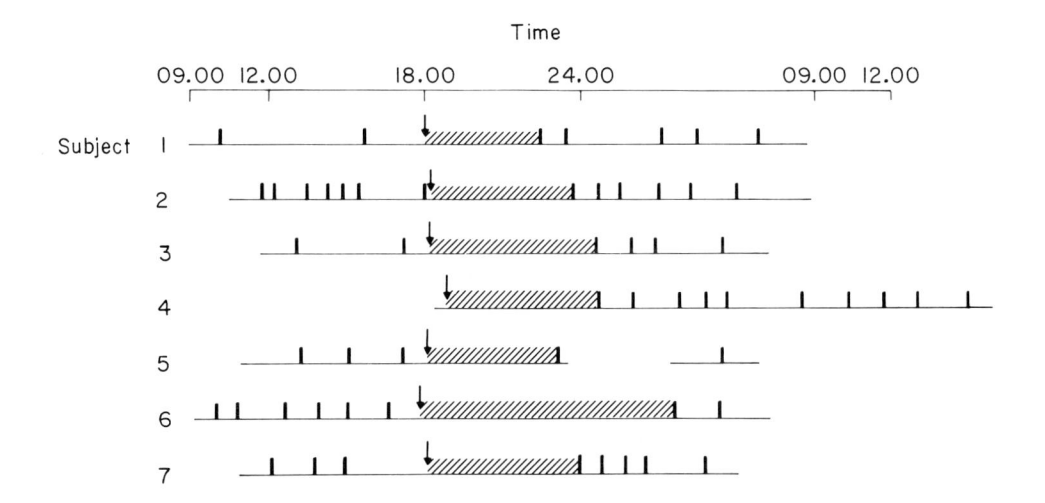

Fig. 4.2. Diagrammatic representation of small intestinal motility at the duodeno-jejunal junction in seven non-operated patients with duodenal ulcer disease. The horizontal lines indicate that duration of study in each patient. Vertical blocks represent periods of Phase III activity. Arrows indicate time of ingestion of a standard mixed meal. Hatched regions represent duration of interruption of fasting activity until the next observed Phase III period indicates the fasted state (Thompson et al. 1982).

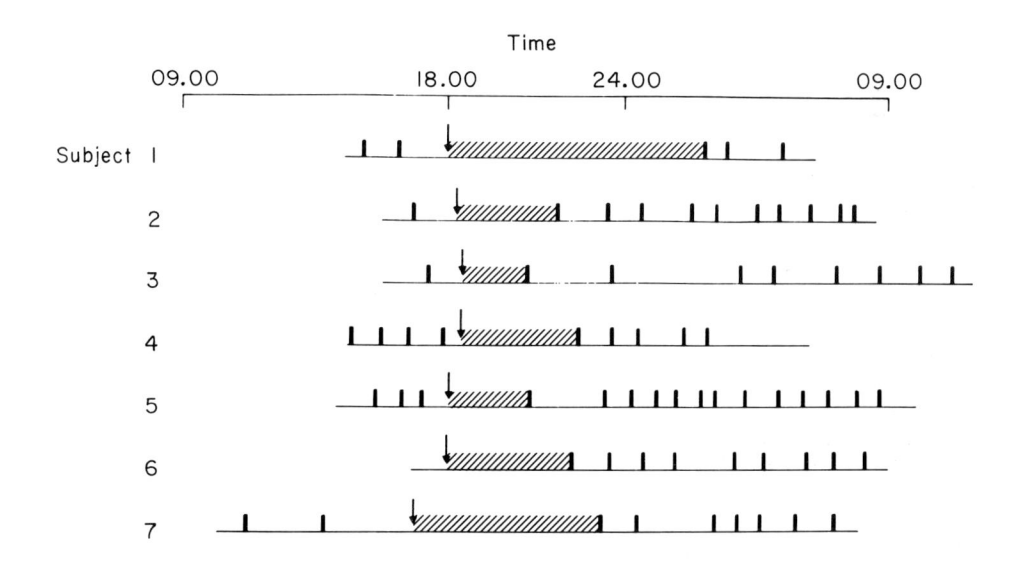

Fig. 4.3. Diagrammatic representation of small intestinal motility in seven patients following truncal vagotomy for duodenal ulceration. (Symbols as in Fig. 4.2). There is a reduction in the duration of Phase III inhibition for this group, compared to the duodenal ulcer patients (Thompson et al. 1982).

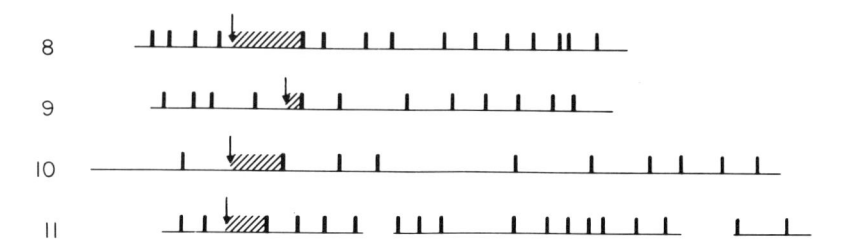

Fig. 4.4. Small intestinal motility in four patients with persistent post-vagotomy diarrhoea (symbols as in Fig. 4.2). A further reduction in duration of Phase III inhibition is present in this group.

symptoms are often related to meals.

Duodenal ulcer and truncal vagotomy

It has been claimed that the pain of duodenal ulcer bears a temporal relationship to the occurrence of 'hunger contractions' in the duodenum. It is not certain, however, that the symptoms are related to the motility since an increased acid load to the duodenal cap also occurs with the cyclical changes in fasting gastric secretion (Hoelzel 1925). Studies of fasting small intestinal motor activity in duodenal ulcer are indistinguishable from normal (Fig. 4.2) suggesting that disordered fasting motility has no major role in its aetiology.

In contrast to unoperated ulcer patients, patients following truncal vagotomy do show abnormalities of small intestinal motility (Thompson et al. 1982) with an earlier return of recognizable Phase III activity after a standard meal (Fig. 4.3). This premature return of Phase III activity is even more marked in patients suffering from persistent post-vagotomy diarrhoea (Fig. 4.4) making it tempting to relate the two phenomena. It remains to be determined, however, whether the premature Phase III is merely an innocent by-stander in the process, the result of rapid gastric emptying and premature return of the 'fasting state' or whether it is the culprit, and by occurring prematurely in the upper gut, is responsible for early emptying of the small intestine and diarrhoea.

Small intestinal ischaemia

In experimental animals hypoxia of the small intestine disrupts myoelectric activity and results in a chronically disordered pattern (Szurszewski & Steggerda 1968). While similar human studies have not been reported, it seems possible that some of the symptoms of chronic intestinal ischaemia may result from motor dysfunction secondary to neuronal damage.

Small intestinal infection

A number of infective agents, including *Vibrio cholerae* (Mathias et al. 1976) and invasive organisms (Burns et al. 1980), are capable of markedly altering intestinal motility in experimental animals, producing bursts of irregular, caudally migrating, myoelectric activity. Some of the diarrhoea resulting from similar infections in man could result from similarly induced dysfunction of the myenteric ganglia leading to inappropriately rapid transit. Recent studies (Sinar et al. 1982) have shown that one of the sub-units of cholera toxin disrupts myoelectric activity in an experimental animal model without inducing concomitant fluid secretion, suggesting that the disordered motility in diarrhoea may be a primary effect of the pathogen rather than merely secondary to fluid distension of the bowel. These observations also point to a possible explanation for the clinically observed development of functional bowel disease after acute gastrointestinal infection.

Chagas' disease also disrupts intestinal motility, with development of a pseudo-obstruction syndrome consequent upon damage to smooth muscle and the myenteric plexus.

Secondary autonomic neuropathy

Autonomic neuropathy affecting the intrinsic innervation of the gut may be a consequence of metabolic disorders, of which the best recognized is diabetes mellitus. However, it should be remembered that nerve destruction in the small bowel in this condition is usually assumed rather than proven. It has recently been reported (Gorchein et al. 1982) that a pseudo-obstruction syndrome may be associated with acute intermittent porphyria, presumably due to autonomic neuropathy; again neuropathy is an assumption rather than a fact.

Ileus

Motor paralysis of the small intestine (paralytic ileus) is a well-recognized phenomenon following surgery, when it is usually only a transitory state. The cause of ileus is not known, although it appears to be associated with manipulation of the viscera during surgery. It has often been suggested that it is due to adrenergic stimulation, leading to a neural inhibition, but this explanation does not answer the question why the inhibition should be so prolonged in relation to the duration of the stimulus, nor why the condition should be so refractory to adrenergic blocking agents. Because the condition is both clinically obvious and generally self-limiting, it has been studied but little in man; it may well be that further studies would be both useful and important.

Incomplete obstruction

Incomplete obstruction of the bowel leads to disruption of the normal fasted pattern of motility proximal to the site of obstruction. It has been shown that in cases of Crohn's disease with partial obstruction, there is replacement of the normal periodic fasting activity with bursts of contractions recurring at intervals of only a few minutes (Summers et al. 1981); it is possible that intestinal manometry may prove to be a diagnostic test when recurrent pain in inflammatory bowel disease leads to the suspicion of subacute obstruction.

Treatment of motility disorders

The therapy of patients with a recognized motility disturbance of the small intestine is even more difficult than is the study of the disease. Where there is structural damage to the neural control, no drug can be expected to be successful. Where the disorder is thought to be secondary to another disease, for example intestinal infection, the rational therapy is of the primary disease and not of the secondary manifestation.

Until an understanding of the disease process itself is obtained, drugs can provide only marginal relief. Meanwhile, some types of drugs are alleged or assumed to be beneficial, although placebo effects must be common.

Dopamine antagonists

Dopamine antagonists, such as metoclopramide, and more recently, domperidone, are often alleged to 'improve motility'. While there are some patients with motility disorders in whom these drugs are beneficial, these are usually patients in whom gastric emptying is impaired. There is no evidence that dopamine antagonists are therapeutically useful in disorders of small intestinal motility, just as there is no evidence that excessive dopamine, or dopaminergic activity, is aetiologically important in such disorders.

Opiates

Although opiates have been traditional remedies for gastrointestinal disorders for centuries, there is no evidence that they have any specific beneficial effect on particular forms of disordered small bowel motility. However, it is fair to say that the evidence is lacking because it has not been sought and the history of pharmacology teaches us that many effective synthetic chemical agents bear a close resemblance in their action to long established 'folk medicine'. Again,

Antispasmodics and cholinergics

These have not been found to be useful in the treatment of small bowel motility disorders but again experimental studies are lacking.

Backward pacing

In experimental animals, the possibility of reducing transit through the small intestine has been explored by the use of reverse pacing (Collin et al. 1979).

The electrical slow wave frequency of the lower small intestinal smooth muscle can be increased by directly applied electrodes which results in a reversal of the normal aboral progression of the slow wave. It has been claimed that by such means, transit may be reduced, presumably by inducing reversal of contractions. This technique would have important application in the treatment of patients following major intestinal resection and in other circumstances where rapid transit through the small intestine is a problem.

Recently, however, doubt has been cast upon the likely value of this technique by the demonstration that Phase III activity continues normally in paced animals (Monson et al. 1982) indicating that myoelectric activity seems to remain aborally polarized despite slow wave reversal.

References

Alvarez W.C. (1948) *An Introduction to Gastroenterology*. W.M. Heinemann, London.
Alvarez W.C. (1925) Reverse peristalsis in the bowel; a precusor of vomiting. *J. Amer. Med. Assoc.* **85**, 1051–1054.
Biber B. & Fara J. (1973) Intestinal motility increased by tetrodotoxin lidocaine and procaine. *Experientia*, **29**, 551–552.
Bluestone R., Macmahon M. & Dawson J. (1969) Systemic sclerosis and small bowel involvement. *Gut*, **10**, 185–193.
Boldyreff W.N. (1905) Le travail periodique de l'appareil digestif en dehors de la digestion. *Arch. Des. Sci. Biol.* **11**, 1–157.
Burns T.W., Mathias J.R., Martin J.L., Carlson G.M. & Sheilds R.P. (1980) Alteration of myoelectric activity of small intestine by invasive Escherichia coli. *Amer. J. Physiol.* **238**, G57–G62.
Burnstock G. (1970) Structure of smooth muscle and its innervation. In *Smooth Muscle*. (Ed. by E. Bulbring, A.F. Brading, A.W. Jones & T. Tomita). Edward Arnold, London.
Burnstock G.W. (1972) Purinergic neurons. *Pharmacol. Rev.* **34**, 509–581.
Christensen J., Schedl H.P. & Clifton J.A. (1966) The small intestine basic electrical rhythm (slow wave) frequency gradient in normal men and in patients with a variety of diseases. *Gastroenterol.* **50**, 309–315.
Code C.F. & Marlett J.A. (1975) The interdigestive myoelectric complex of the stomach and small bowel of dogs. *J. Physiol.* **246**, 298–309.
Collin J., Kelly K.A. & Phillips S.F. (1979) Absorption from the jejunum is increased by forward and backward pacing. *Brit. J. Surg.* **66**, 489–492.
Connor J.A., Prosser C.L. & Weems W.A. (1974) A study of pacemaker activity in intestinal smooth muscle. *J. Physiol.* **240**, 671–701.
Daniel E. & Chapman K.M. (1963) Electrical activity of the gastrointestinal tract as an indication of mechanical activity. *Amer. J. Dig. Dis.* **8**, 54–102.
Diamant N.E., Hall K., Mui H. & El-Sharkawy T.Y. (1980) Vagal control of the feeding motor pattern in the lower oesophageal sphincter, stomach and upper small intestine of dog. *Proc. 7th Int. Symp. on G.I. Motility*. Raven Press, New York.
Duthie H. (1974) Electrical activity of gastroinstestinal smooth muscle. *Gut*, **15**, 669–681.
Evans D.F., Foster G.E. & Hardcastle J.D. (1982) The effect of pentobarbitone sedation on jejunal migrating motor complex. *Gastroenterol.* **82**, 1051 (abst.).
Finch P., Ingram D., Henstridge J. Catchpole B. (1980) The relationship of sleep stage to the migrating gastrointestinal complex in man. *Proc. 7th Int. Symposium G.I. Motility*, pp. 261–265. Raven Press.
Furness J.B. & Costa M. (1974) The adrenergic innervation of the gastrointestinal tract. *Ergebn. Physiol.* **69**, 1–40.
Furness J.B., Costa M. & Walsh J.H. (1981) Evidence for and significance of the projection of VIP neurons from the myenteric plexus to the taenia coli in the guinea pig. *Gastroenterol.* **80**, 1557–1561.
Gershon M.D. & Erde S.M. (1981) The nervous system of the gut. *Gastroenterol.* **80**, 1571–1594.
Gorchein A., Valori R.M., Wingate D.L. & Bloom S.R. (1982) Abnormal proximal gut motility in acute intermittent porphyria: a neuropathic model. *Gastroenterol.* **82**; 1070.
Green W.E.R., Ruppin H. & Wingate D.L. (1976) Effects of 13-Nle-Motilin in the electrical and mechanical activity of the isolated perfused canine stomach and duodenum. *Gut*, **17**, 362–370.

Greenberger N.J., Dobbins W.O., Ruppert R.D. & Jesseph J.E. (1968) Intestinal atony in progressive systemic sclerosis. *Amer. J. Med.* **45**, 301–308.

Hermon-Taylor J. & Code C.F. (1971) Localization of the duodenal pacemaker and its role in the organization of duodenal myoelectric activity. *Gut*, **12**; 40–47.

Hoelzel J. (1925) The relation between the secretory and motor activity in its role in the fasting stomach (Man). *Amer. J. Physiol.* **73**, 463–469.

Horowitz L. & Farrar J.T. (1962) Intraluminal small intestinal pressures in normal patients and in patients with functional gastrointestinal disorders. *Gastroenterol.* **42**, 455–464.

Itoh Z., Takeuchi S., Aizawa I. & Takayanagi R. (1977) Effect of synthetic motilin on gastric motor activity in conscious dogs. *Amer. J. Dig. Dis.* **22**, 813–819.

Keane F.B., DiMagno E.P. & Malagelade J-R. (1980) Role of the migrating motor complex and its secretory counterpart on duodenogastric reflux in man. *Gastroenterol.* **78**, 1192 (abst.).

Konturek S.J. (1977) Somatostatin and gastrointestinal secretion and motility. In *Gastrointestinal Hormones and Pathology of the Digestive System*. (Ed. by M. Grossman, V. Speranze, N. Basso & E. Lezoche), pp. 227–234. Plenum Press, New York.

Konturek S.J., Thor P., Krol R., Dembinski A. & Schally A.V. (1980) Influence of methionine-enkephalin and morphine on myoelectric activity of small bowel. *Amer. J. Physiol.* **238**, G384–G389.

Manninen V., Apajalahti A., Melin J. & Karesoja M. (1973) Altered absorption of digoxin in patients given propantheline and metoclopramide. *Lancet*, **i**; 398–399.

Mathias J.R., Carlson G.M., DiMarino A.J., Bertiger G., Morton H.E. & Cohen S. (1976) Intestinal myoelectric activity in response to live Vibrio cholera enterotoxin. *J. Clin. Invest.* **58**, 91–96.

Monson J., Keane F.B., Byrne P.J. & Hennessy T.P.J. (1982) Effect of retrograde pacing on the jejunal interdigestive migrating motor complex. *Gut*, A443.

Peeters T.L., Vantrappen G. & Janssens J. (1980) Fasting plasma motilin levels are related to the interdigestive motility complex. *Gastroenterol.* **79**, 716–719.

Pinnington J. & Wingate D.L. (1981) Motilin and the canine migrating myoelectric complex (MMC) a reassessment. *J. Physiol.* **319**, 49–50.

Ress W.D.W., Leigh R.J., Chistofides N.D., Bloom S.R. & Turnberg L.A. (1982) Interdigestive motor activity in patients with systemic sclerosis. *Gastroenterol.* **83**; 575–580.

Ritchie H.D., Thompson D.G. & Wingate D.L. (1980) Diurnal variation in human jejunal fasting motor activity. *J. Physiol.* **304**, 54.

Sarr M.G. & Kelly K.A. (1981) Myoelectric activity of the autotransplanted canine jejunoileum. *Gastroenterol.* **81**, 303–310.

Schuffler M.D. Lowe M.C. & Bill A.H. (1977) Studies of idiopathic intestinal pseudo-obstruction. Hereditary hollow visceral myopathy. Clinical and Pathological studies. *Gastroenterol.* **73**, 327–338.

Schuffler M.D. & Beegle R.G. (1979) Progressive systemic sclerosis of the gastrointestinal tract and hereditary hollow visceral myopathy. Two distinguishable disorders of intestinal smooth muscle. *Gastroenterol.* **77**, 664–671.

Schuffler M.D., Birol T.D., Sumi S.M. & Cook A. (1978) Familial neuronal disease presenting as intestinal pseudo-obstruction. *Gastroenterol.* **75**, 889–898.

Sinar D.R., Charles L.G. & Burns T.W. (1982) Migrating action-potential complex is produced by B subunit of cholera enterotoxin. *Amer. J. Physiol.* **242**, G47–G51.

Summers R.W., Anuras S. & Green J. (1981) Jejunal motility patterns in normal subjects and symptomatic patients with partial mechanical obstruction or pseudo-obstruction. *Z.F. Gastroenterol.* **19**, 413 (abst.).

Szurszewski J.H. (1969) A migrating electric complex of the canine small intestine. *Amer. J. Physiol.* **217**, 1757–1763.

Szurszewki J. & Steggerda F.R. (1968) The effect of hypoxia on the electrical slow wave of the canine small intestine. *Amer. J. Dig. Dis.* **13**, 168–177.

Thompson D.G., Archer L., Green W.J. & Wingate D.L. (1981) Fasting motor activity occurs during a day of normal meals in healthy subjects. *Gut*, **22**, 489–492.

Thompson D.G., Laidlow J.M. & Wingate D.L. (1979) Abnormal small bowel motility demonstrated by radiotelemetry in a patient with irritable colon. *Lancet*, **ii**, 1321–1323.

Thompson D.G., Richelson E. & Malagelada J-R. (1982) Perturbation of gastric emptying and duodenal motility via the central nervous system. *Gastroenterol.* **83**, 1200–1206.

Thompson D.G., Ritchie H.D. & Wingate D.L. (1982) Patterns of small intestinal motility in duodenal ulcer patients before and after vagotomy. *Gut*, **23**, 517–523.

Thompson D.G., Wingate D.L., Archer L., Benson M.J., Green W.J. & Hardy R.J. (1980) Normal patterns of human upper small bowel motor activity recorded by prolonged radiotelemetry. *Gut*, **21**, 500–506.

Vantrappen G., Janssens J., Peeters T.L., Bloom S.r., Christofides N.D. & Hellemans J. (1979) Motilin and the interdigestive migrating motor complex in man. *Dig. Dis. Sci.*, **24**, 497–500.

Vantrappen G., Janssens J., Hellemans J. & Ghoos Y. (1977) The interdigestive motor complex of normal subjects and patients with bacterial over-growth of the small intestine. *J. Clin. Invest.* **59**, 1158–1166.

Vantrappen G.R., Peeters T.L. & Janssens J. (1979) The secretory component of the interdigestive migrating motor complex in man. *Scand. J. Gastroenterol.* **14**, 663–667.

Wilson I.A.I. & Goode A.W. (1981) The effect of enteral infusion of elemental amino acid and whole protein hydrolysate on small bowel motility in man. *J. Par. Ent. Nutrit.* **5**, 560.

Wingate D.L., Pearce E.A., Hutton M., Dand A., Thompson H.H. & Wunsch E. (1978) Quantitative comparison of the effects of cholecystokinin, secretin and pentagastrin on gastrointestinal myoelectric activity in the conscious dog. *Gut*, **19**, 593-601.

Wingate D.L., Pearce E.A., Ling A., Boucher B.J., Thompson H.H. & Hutton M.R. (1979) Quantitative effect of oral feeding on gastrointestinal myoelectric activity in the conscious dog. *Dig. Dis. Sci.* **24**, 417–423.

Chapter 5
Effects of Gastric Operations

J. ALEXANDER-WILLIAMS AND I.A. DONOVAN

Introduction 93
Effects on intestinal motility 93
Intestinal morphology 94
Bacteria and parasites 95
Digestion and absorption 95
Nutritional deficiency 97

Introduction

In recent years, there has been a considerable decline in the frequency with which partial gastrectomy is carried out, the operation having been largely superseded by vagotomy and drainage procedures. Nevertheless, there are still significant numbers of patients with partial gastrectomy requiring medical advice and it is therefore important to understand both the nature of the small intestinal lesion after gastric operations, and the associated nutritional deficiencies which occur.

Consideration of the effects of gastric operations on the small bowel cannot be divorced from consideration of the effect of surgery on the stomach. The normal functions of the stomach include regulation of gastric emptying, breakdown of large particles of food into small particles, and mixing of the food with pepsin and acid. Disorder of any of these functions will indirectly affect small bowel function and they are usually disordered to some degree by any gastric operation. Furthermore, after a Billroth II type of reconstruction, or if a gastrojejunostomy has been performed, the mixing of the food with pancreatic and biliary secretions is also disturbed. Truncal vagotomy also affects small bowel function.

Effects on intestinal motility

The fasting motor activity of the small intestine is temporarily abolished by feeding (Chapter 4) and the duration of this abolition of activity is reduced after truncal vagotomy and drainage, particularly in patients with post-vagotomy diarrhoea (Thompson et al. 1982). The primary cause for this alteration in small bowel motor activity, however, may not be vagal denervation but rather the profound alteration in gastric emptying that has been produced. After truncal vagotomy and drainage, a much higher proportion than normal of ingested liquid and semi-solid food empties very rapidly from the stomach. This rapid early emptying is greatest in those patients with post-vagotomy diarrhoea or dumping symptoms (McKelvey et al. 1970, Colmer et al. 1973). Similar precipitous early gastric emptying is seen after Billroth II type partial gastrectomy (McGregor et al. 1977). The alterations in the pattern of gastric emptying probably affect the control of small bowel motility both directly, in terms of larger volumes of food reaching the bowel more rapidly, and also indirectly through alteration in the response of the controlling hormonal and neural mechanisms to the influx of food (Thompson et al. 1982). The premature return of fasting activity with migrating complexes (Phase III) in association with rapid gastric emptying may result in food products and bile acids being transported rapidly through the ileum into the colon before absorption is complete, and an increased amount of bile acids is therefore found in the faeces of patients with post-vagotomy diarrhoea (Allan et al. 1974). Dihydroxy bile acids in the colon cause a net secretion of water and electrolytes (Mekhjian et al. 1970) and bile acids also stimulate colonic motility (Galapeaux et al. 1938); both of these factors may contribute to the pathogenesis of post-vagotomy diarrhoea. Treatment with an oral bile salt-binding agent, such as cholestyramine, may be helpful in patients with this disorder.

Table 5.1. Dumping and diarrhoea 5–8 years after surgery.

Operation	No. of patients	Early dumping (%)	Diarrhoea (%) Mild	Severe
Subtotal Gastrectomy	107	21.5	5.6	0.9
TV + GE	119	17.9	21.2	5.1
TV + P	161	11.9	17.4	4.3

(from Goligher et al. 1972)

Whereas rapid gastric emptying seems to be the primary triggering mechanism for symptoms of dumping and diarrhoea, the response of the small bowel to the influx of food seems to be different depending upon whether or not it is innervated. The incidence of early dumping is probably greater after subtotal gastrectomy than after truncal vagotomy and drainage, whereas the incidence of diarrhoea is greatest after truncal vagotomy (Table 5.1).

After Billroth II gastrectomy rapid small intestinal transit seems largely confined to the jejunum (Glazebrook & Welbourn 1952, Stammers & Alexander-Williams 1963) and in patients who have diarrhoea after partial gastrectomy intestinal transit is similar to that in healthy controls, although gastric emptying is more rapid (Bond & Levitt 1977).

In the patients with diarrhoea after truncal vagotomy and drainage, overall intestinal transit is more rapid than in normal subjects (McKelvey 1970). Innervation of the small intestine, therefore, whilst not influencing the symptoms of early dumping, enables the bowel to slow down the rapid influx of food and therefore helps to prevent diarrhoea. Division of the coeliac branch of the posterior vagus is inherent to some techniques of partial gastrectomy; the hepatic branch of the vagus, however, is usually preserved and this is said to be the more essential nerve to preserve in an attempt to reduce the incidence of diarrhoea (Burge et al. 1961).

Rapid intestinal transit can be reduced by keeping the dietary intake of starches and sugars, particularly mono- and disaccharides, to a minimum. In the normal subject, sugars and other water-soluble materials are rapidly dissolved and the solution reduced to isotonicity in the jejunum by an inpouring of fluid. Unless absorption keeps pace with the input, however, an excessive amount of fluid accumulates in the upper jejunum and is moved on rapidly by peristaltic waves instead of by the slower normal process of progressive segmentation. A rapid conversion of starches to sugars and dextrins aggravates the osmotic effect and the stimulus to peristalsis may be enormous (Stammers & Alexander-Williams 1963). In the absence of the antral 'mill' and the pyloric 'filter', large boluses of food, for example orange pith or other fruit residues, may also provoke peristalsis and, under these circumstances, bolus obstruction can occur in the ileum.

Intestinal morphology

Radiological examination of the small bowel usually reveals a normal appearance. Gastric operations do not seem to produce any sustained effect on the dissecting or light microscopic appearances of the small bowel on biopsy. Both dissecting microscopy and the histological appearance of jejunum taken by peroral biopsy after partial gastrectomy are not different from those seen in normal controls. The morphological appearances do not correlate with the presence or absence of anaemia, increased frequency of bowel action, steatorrhoea, abnormal d-Xylose absorption or loss of weight (Stammers & Alexander-Williams 1963, Scott et al. 1964, Beno et al. 1970). Similarly, vagotomy in man does not appear to produce epithelial abnormalities (Cox 1969).

Latent coeliac disease

If asymptomatic coeliac disease has been present in a patient who has a partial gastrectomy then severe malabsorption is likely to follow the operation, probably due to the imposition of transit and mixing abnormalities onto the underlying defect (Hedberg et al. 1966). A jejunal biopsy should always be carried out to exclude the possibility of coeliac disease in an individual who suffers severe diarrhoea and steatorrhoea after either partial gastrectomy or vagotomy, since the stress of the operation may have precipitated the first symptoms of this disorder.

Bacteria and parasites

Bacterial overgrowth

As the afferent loop of a Billroth II partial gastrectomy contains no hydrochloric acid and has a pH of over 6, it may be the site of bacterial proliferation. Normally, however, the afferent loop is of the self-emptying type and significant bacterial overgrowth usually only occurs when there is an element of stasis due to mechanical obstruction. This is more likely to occur with longer than shorter afferent loops (Stammers & Alexander-Williams 1963). When bacterial growth occurs, the organisms may also colonize the jejunum and they are usually more akin to colonic flora than to flora that may be swallowed from the pharynx (Engstrom & Hellstrom 1973).

After vagotomy and pyloroplasty, the reduction in gastric acid production leads to colonization of the duodenal and jejunal juice with nasopharyngeal organisms, but colonic organisms are uncommon (McLoughlin 1978). The concentration of organisms found is similar in patients with and without post-vagotomy diarrhoea (McKelvey et al. 1973), indicating that bacterial overgrowth is not responsible for this problem. In general, bacterial overgrowth after gastric surgery is rarely of clinical significance, unless there is a blind loop due to mechanical obstruction or an associated condition causing the stagnant loop syndrome, as described in Chapter 15. Rarely, such patients may develop severe malabsorption and malnutrition.

IgA

The presence of intestinal IgA has been suggested to be of importance in keeping the upper small bowel free from bacterial growth (Heremans et al. 1966). In the uncommon state of primary IgA deficiency, patients who have a vagotomy for duodenal ulceration may develop significant overgrowth of colonic aerobic and anaerobic organisms in the jejunum, with an increased risk of associated diarrhoea (McLoughlin et al. 1978).

Parasites

Patients with partial gastrectomy may have an increased risk of parasitic infection. Parasitism of the small bowel by *Giardia lamblia* has been reported after partial gastrectomy, presenting with severe weight loss and fluid retention due to hypoalbuminaemia (Dawson 1982). *Isospora belli* infection has also been described, causing malabsorption, in individuals following partial gastrectomy who have visited areas of the world such as West Africa, where such infection is endemic.

Digestion and absorption

After gastric operations several factors contribute to impairment of the normal absorption of nutrients. Rapid transit reduces the time of contact between food and mucosa during which absorption can occur. Reduced mixing between food and biliary and pancreatic secretion has also been incriminated. A combination of these factors leading to malabsorption has been called pancreaticocibal asynchrony (Brain & Stammers 1951). In addition, after either truncal vagotomy and pyloroplasty, or Billroth II partial gastrectomy, the luminal concentrations of trypsin and bile salts found in the jejunum in response to a meal are reduced (McGregor et al. 1977). The main factor responsible for these reductions is rapid gastric emptying diluting the intraluminal contents but, after truncal vagotomy and pyloroplasty, there is also a depression of trypsin production. In patients after Billroth II gastrectomy, the levels of trypsin and bile salts in the jejunum approach normal 1 h or more after ingestion of the meal, presumably after initial sequestration of the secretions in the afferent loop (McGregor et al. 1977). Another factor contributing to malabsorption after Billroth II partial gastrectomy is autodigestion of other enzymes by trypsin which may occur in the afferent loop in the absence of competitive substrates in the form of food (Avakian 1961). Levels of enzymes such as lipase and amylase may, therefore, show an even greater reduction and the longer the afferent loop the more likely it is that auto-digestion will occur (Butler 1961).

Water, electrolytes, carbohydrates

After truncal vagotomy and drainage, the capacity of the jejunum to absorb water, electrolytes, or monosaccharides is normal (Bunch & Shields 1973, Cox 1962), and disaccharidase activity is also usually normal (Garcia-Paredes & Truelove 1971). After gastrectomy the capacity of the jejunum to absorb glucose is also normal (Bond & Levitt 1977). Milk intolerance, however, develops in some patients after partial gastrectomy. This may be due in part to the physical effects of the liquid milk. In the normal alimentary tract, milk is clotted into a semi-solid bolus in the gastric fundus and only passes through into the duodenum after it has been rendered more nearly isotonic and isothermic. After Billroth II gastrectomy, milk may pass directly into the jejunum where it stimulates peristalsis and rapidly passes through the small bowel (Stammers & Alexander-Williams 1963). Similar rapid liquid emptying occurs after vagotomy and drainage, as has already been discussed. In addition, lactose intolerance due to lactase deficiency may be more common after partial gastrectomy (Gryboski et al. 1963) and after vagotomy (Williams & Irvine 1966).

Fat and fat-soluble vitamins

Malabsorption of fat commonly occurs after partial gastrectomy and is more frequent following Billroth II or Polya gastrectomy than after Billroth I procedures. Steatorrhoea is rare, however, after vagotomy with pyloroplasty or gastroenterostomy. In many patients, steatorrhoea is mild and symptomless and it is relatively rare to encounter severe diarrhoea due to steatorrhoea after gastric operations.

Studies of absorption of fat-soluble vitamins have revealed conflicting results. Deficient absorption of vitamin A was reported in twenty-four out of twenty-seven cases studied after Billroth II gastrectomy (Althausen et al. 1960), but others have demonstrated normal absorption of vitamin A in the presence of steatorrhoea (Ellman & Irwin 1959).

Similarly, there may be normal absorption of vitamin D in the presence of steatorrhoea. Thompson et al. (1966a) studied the absorption of vitamin D using oral test doses of ^{3}H-labelled vitamin D_3 in patients following partial gastrectomy. Their results indicated that the operation is not a serious cause of malabsorption of vitamin D since, although two of four post-gastrectomy subjects without bone disease had steatorrhoea, they all absorbed vitamin D normally. Of five others with evidence of post-gastrectomy osteomalacia, four had a minor defect in vitamin D absorption, and the other with the most severe bone disease absorbed vitamin D normally. These observations suggest that defective absorption of vitamin D is not the major cause of osteomalacia after partial gastrectomy and that inadequate intake and lack of exposure to sunlight are more important factors. This is in striking contrast to studies of vitamin D absorption in patients with osteomalacia due to coeliac disease or intestinal lymphangectasia in whom absorption of ^{3}H vitamin D_3 is markedly reduced (Thompson et al. 1966b).

Iron

Absorption of crystalline iron is usually normal after gastric operations but there may be an inability to absorb iron from food, as well as a reduction in the normal capacity of the small intestine to respond to iron deficiency by enhancing absorption. This defect in absorption of iron from food may be due to a variety of factors, including hypochlorhydria, poor release of iron from food due to maldigestion, and possibly rapid passage of food through the proximal areas of the intestine which absorb iron most avidly.

Vitamin B_{12}

Malabsorption of vitamin B_{12} is not common

bacteria in inhibiting B_{12} absorption in this condition.

Folic acid

There is no evidence of malabsorption of folic acid after gastrectomy (Girdwood 1956) or after vagotomy with a drainage procedure (Cox et al. 1968), unless unsuspected coeliac disease is present.

Nutritional deficiency

Loss of weight

Loss of weight commonly occurs after partial gastrectomy but is not usually seen after vagotomy and drainage. It is usually due to inadequate dietary intake and malabsorption is rarely important. Occasionally, patients become extremely wasted, but even so they rarely develop hypoproteinaemia (Booth et al. 1964). They have total caloric undernutrition and, like the semi-starved people studied in Europe immediately after the Second World War, their serum albumin is usually normal or only slightly reduced (Beattie et al. 1948).

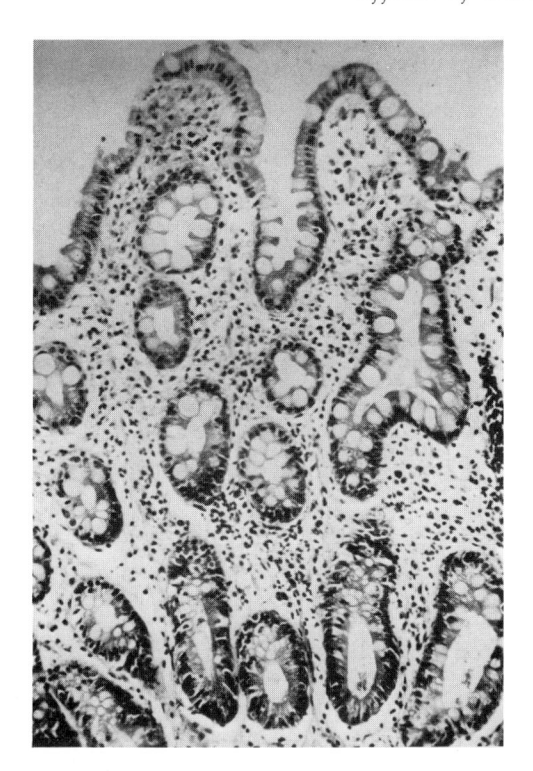

Fig. 5.1. Gastric mucosa from gastric remnant following partial gastrectomy. There is gastric atrophy and intestinal metaplasia. (H & E, × 250.)

after partial gastrectomy and there is only a slight and insignificant reduction in B_{12} absorption after vagotomy with pyloroplasty or gastroenterostomy (Cox et al. 1968).

When vitamin B_{12} absorption is reduced after partial gastrectomy, it is due to progressive gastric atrophy occurring in the gastric remnant (Fig. 5.1) which leads to intrinsic factor deficiency. This takes some years to develop. The defect in absorption therefore resembles that seen in Addisonian pernicious anaemia, malabsorption of a test dose of radioactive B_{12} being corrected by the addition of intrinsic factor.

In rare instances, B_{12} malabsorption may be caused by bacterial overgrowth in the small intestine. Under these circumstances, the defect in absorption is not corrected by intrinsic factor but absorption may improve following treatment with metronidazole (Toskes 1980) or other broad spectrum antibiotics. The response to metronidazole emphasizes the important of anaerobic

Hypoproteinaemia

Hypoproteinaemia is unusual after partial gastrectomy. When it occurs, it may cause oedema. It is not due to protein-losing enteropathy but is characteristically seen when there is either gross bacterial overgrowth in the small intestine or an associated lesion of the pancreas. Neale et al. (1967) described five patients with severe hypoproteinaemia after partial gastrectomy. All five patients were shown to have the clinical and biochemical features of a syndrome resembling kwashiorkor. The patients had severe protein depletion, together with disordered body protein synthesis. They were emaciated and oedematous. They showed a psychomotor state of irritable apathy and electroencephalograms were abnormal. Subnormal body temperature was found in three patients and there was loss of hair with total alopecia in one individual. This syndrome does not occur solely as a result of partial gastrectomy. A complicating factor is always present. In three of the patients described by Neale et al. (1967) there was an associated stagnant loop syndrome, as described in Chapter 15. In the other two patients there was chronic exocrine pancreatic insufficiency. Surgical correction of the blind loops, or pancreatic enzyme supplements where indicated, were dramatically successful in restoring these patients to health.

Anaemia

The prevalence of anaemia in thirty-four published series comprising 7222 patients who had undergone partial gastrectomy was 2078 (28.8%) (Chanarin 1979). The occurrence of anaemia, however, varies considerably, depending on the length of follow-up and the level of haemoglobin taken to be abnormal. The haemoglobin level falls progressively with time and the highest frequency of anaemia is in women who are still menstruating. In general, anaemia during the first 5 years after gastrectomy is due to iron deficiency and vitamin B_{12} deficiency usually only occurs after 5 years or more, usually in association with iron deficiency. Anaemia is more commonly seen after Billroth II partial gastrectomy than after Billroth I or vagotomy and drainage. Gastrojejunostomy as the drainage procedure carries an increased risk compared with pyloroplasty. Patients after gastric operation should have a haemoglobin estimation performed yearly to detect those individuals who become anaemic and therefore require treatment.

Iron deficiency

Iron deficiency develops insidiously after partial gastrectomy, usually becoming apparent within 3 or 4 years of the operation. It is most frequent in menstruating women before the age of 50. If iron deficiency is seen in the early years after gastrectomy, for example within the first year or two, it is important to exclude an alternative cause for this, such as an occult carcinoma. Occasionally, there may be occult haemorrhage from the operation site. When a gastrojejunostomy accompanies vagotomy, or when a gastrojejunal anastomosis has been performed as part of the Billroth II operation, increased blood loss from the stoma may be an important factor in the production of iron deficiency, even when no obvious pathological lesion is demonstrable (Stammers & Alexander-Williams 1963).

Patients with iron deficiency respond adequately to treatment with inorganic iron preparations so that either ferrous sulphate or ferrous gluconate are fully effective.

Vitamin B_{12} deficiency

The number of patients developing overt B_{12} deficiency up to 10 years after partial gastrectomy is approximately 5%, although the incidence of a low serum B_{12} level, without evidence of megaloblastic anaemia, is higher. Since B_{12} deficiency is so frequently associated with iron deficiency after gastrectomy, the characteristic signs of megaloblastic change in the bone marrow may be masked until the iron deficiency is corrected. Treatment with parenteral vitamin B_{12}, as in Addisonian pernicious anaemia, is fully effective.

Folic acid deficiency

Folic acid deficiency rarely occurs after partial gastrectomy and appears to be due to dietary deficiency rather than intestinal malabsorption, unless the folic acid deficiency is due to unsuspected coeliac disease. A jejunal biopsy should therefore be carried out in any patient with folic acid deficiency to exclude this possibility.

Bone disease

Thinning of bones is a late complication of partial gastrectomy occurring in as many as 15% of patients 10 years after the operation, but does not occur after vagotomy and drainage procedures. The bone lesion is frequently due predominantly to osteoporosis but signs of osteomalacia due to vitamin D deficiency are present in many patients if carefully sought. Serum values for

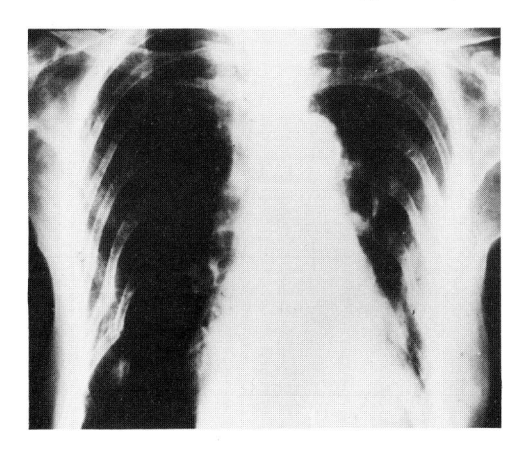

Fig. 5.2. Post-gastrectomy osteomalacia; chest radiograph showing multiple rib fractures in a post-menopausal woman who had a Polya partial gastrectomy 20 years previously.

calcium, phosphate and alkaline phosphatase are useful but insensitive markers of osteomalacia. Measurement of 25-hydroxycholecalciferol may indicate patients at risk but certain diagnosis can be made only by quantitative assessment of bone histology on biopsies taken from the iliac crest. The most severe bone disease appears to occur in post-menopausal women. With osteoporosis the patient develops an increasing kyphosis, and there may be bone pain due to vertebral crush fractures. When there is long-standing vitamin D deficiency, the characteristic myopathy may cause a waddling gait and muscle weakness and there may be bone pain due to fractures of ribs or, less frequently, long bones. Radiological studies usually reveal only evidence of bone thinning. In some instances, however, there may be signs of severe osteomalacia with pseudo-fractures, particularly to be seen in ribs and pelvis (Fig. 5.2). In rare cases there may be a triradiate pelvis and other deformities.

Serum alkaline phosphatase provides the most useful method of detecting vitamin D deficiency after gastrectomy. Although Paget's disease of bone or liver disease may cause an elevation of the serum alkaline phosphatase level, in the majority of patients the raised level is associated with abnormalities of bone and with vitamin D deficiency. Thompson *et al.* (1966c) screened 200 post-gastrectomy patients and found twenty-eight patients with an elevated alkaline phosphatase. Of these, three had had evidence of hepatic dysfunction, six had Paget's disease and the remainder had evidence of osteomalacia, either biochemically or on bone biopsy. Sections of undecalcified bone biopsies show the characteristic thickened osteoid seams and loss of calcification front, which are characteristic features of osteomalacia. Since the absorption of vitamin D is usually only marginally impaired in patients with post-gastrectomy osteomalacia, oral supplementation with vitamin D is a satisfactory method of treatment. At the same time, the diet should be supplemented with calcium salts.

References

Allan J.G., Gerskowitch V.P. & Russell R.I. (1974) The role of bile acids in the pathogenesis of post-vagotomy diarrhoea. *Brit. J. Surg.* **61**, 516–518.

Althausen T.L., Uyeyama K. & Loran M.R. (1960) Effects of alcohol on absorption of vitamin A in normal and in gastrectomised subjects. *Gastroenterol.* **38**, 942–945.

Avakian S. (1961) Current concepts in therapy, chymotrypsin and trypsin. *N. Engl. J. Med.* **264**, 764–765.

Beattie J., Herbert P.H. & Bell D.J. (1948) Famine oedema. *Brit. J. Nutr.* **2**, 47–65.

Beno I., Bucko A., Chorvathova V. & Babalu J. (1970) Absorption of d-Xylose and fat and histological changes of the small intestine in patients after partial gastrectomy. *Dig.* **3**, 97–104.

Bond J.H., and Levitt M.D. (1977) Use of breath hydrogen (H_2) to quantitate small bowel transit time following partial gastrectomy. *J. Lab. Clin. Med.* **90**, 30–36.

Booth C.C., Brain M.C. & Jeejeebhoy K.N. (1964) Hypoproteinaemia after partial gastrectomy. *Proc. Roy. Soc. Med.* **57**, 582–585.

Brain R.H. & Stammers F.A.R. (1951) Sequelae of radical gastric resections. *Lancet*, **i**, 1137–1140.

Bunch G.A. & Shields R. (1973) The effects of vagotomy on the intestinal handling of water and electrolytes. *Gut*, **14**, 116–119.

Burge H.W., Rizk A.R., Tompkin A.M.B., Barth, C.E., Hitchinson J.S.F., Longland C.J., McLennan I. & Miln D.C. (1961) Selective vagotomy in the prevention of post-vagotomy diarrhoea. *Lancet*, **ii**, 897–899.

Butler T.J. (1961) The effect of gastrectomy on pancreatic secretion in man. *Ann. R. Coll. Surg. Engl.* **29**, 300–327.

Chanarin I. (1979) *The Megaloblastic Anaemias.* 2nd ed., pp. 385–405, Blackwell Scientific Publications, London.

Colmer M.R., Owen G.M. & Shields R. (1973) Pattern of gastric emptying after vagotomy and pyloroplasty. *Brit. Med. J.* ii, 448–450.

Cox A.G., Hutchinson H.E. & Wordsop C.A.J. (1968) The blood changes eight years after vagotomy and gastrectomy compared with those following partial gastrectomy in the treatment of chronic duodenal ulcer. *Gut*, 9, 411–413.

Cox A.G. (1962) Small-intestinal absorption before and after vagotomy in man. *Lancet*, ii, 1075–1077.

Cox A.G. (1969) The small intestine. In *After Vagotomy*, pp. 68–76. (Ed. by J. Alexander-Williams and A.G. Cox). Butterworths, London.

Dawson J. (1982) Personal communication.

Ellman P. & Irwin D.B. (1959) Osteomalacia following gastrectomy. *Brit. Med. J.* I, 358–361.

Engstrom J. & Hellstrom K. (1973) Microflora of the small intestine and the incidence of liver disease, steatorrhoea and indicanuria, in patients subject to partial gastrectomy. *Acta. Chir. Scand.* 139, 539–545.

Galapeaux E.A., Templeton R.D. & Boolson E.L. (1938) The influences of bile on the motility of the dog's colon. *Amer. J. Physiol.* 121, 130–136.

Garcia-Paredes J. & Truelove S.C. (1971) Disaccharidase levels in the small intestine in patients with diarrhoea following vagotomy and pyloroplasty. *Gut*, 12, 107–109.

Girdwood R.H. (1956) The megaloblastic anaemias. *Quart. J. Med.* 25, 87–119.

Glazebrook A.J. & Welbourn R.B. (1952) Some observations on the function of the small intestine after gastrectomy. *Brit. J. Surg.* 40, 111–117.

Goligher J.C., Feather D.B., Hall R.A., Hopton D., Kenny T.E., Latchmore A.K.C., Matheson T., Shoesmith J.H., Smiddy F.E. & Willson-Pepper J. (1979) Several standard elective operations for Duodenal Ulcer: Ten to sixteen year clinical results. *Ann. Surg.* 189, 18–24.

Goligher J.C., Pulvertaft C.M., Irvin T.T., Johnston D., Walker B., Hall A., Willson-Pepper J. & Matheson T.S. (1972) Five to eight year results of truncal vagotomy and pyloroplasty for duodenal ulcer. *Br. Med. J.* i, 7–13.

Gryboski J.D., Thayer W.R., Gryboski W.N., Gabrielson I.W. & Spiro H.M. (1963) A defect in disaccharide metabolism after gastrojejunostomy. *N. Eng. J. Med.* 268, 78–80.

Hedberg C.A., Melnyk C.S. & Johnson C.F. (1966) Gluten enteropathy appearing after gastric surgery. *Gastroenterol.* 50, 796–804.

Heremans J.F., Crabbe P.A. & Masson P.L. (1966) Biological significance of exocrine gamma-A-immunoglobulin. *Acta. Med. Scand.* 445, Suppl. 84–88.

McGregor I.L., Martin P. & Meyer J.H. (1977) Gastric emptying of solid food in normal man and after subtotal gastrectomy and truncal vagotomy with pyloroplasty. *Gastroenterol.* 72, 210–211.

McKelvey S.T.D., Ferguson W.P. & Kennedy T.L. (1973) The bacterial flora of the upper gastrointestinal tract in relation to gastric secretion and to bowel habit following vagotomy and pyloroplasty. *Brit. J. Surg.* 60, 306–307.

McKelvey S.T.D. (1970) Gastric incontinence and post-vagotomy diarrhoea. *Brit. J. Surg.* 57, 741–747.

McLoughlin G.A., Hede J.E., Temple J.G. et al. (1978) The role of IgA in the prevention of bacterial colonization of the jejunum in the vagotomized subject. *Br. J. Surg.* 65, 437–437.

Mekhian H.S., Phillips S.F. & Hoffmann A.F. (1970) Colonic secretion of water and electrolytes induced by bile acids. Perfusion studies in man. *J. Clin. Invest.* 50, 1569–1577.

Neale G., Antcliffe A.C., Welbourn R.B., Mollin D.L. & Booth C.C. (1967) Protein malnutrition after partial gastrectomy. *Quart. J. Med. N.S.* 36, 469–494.

Scott G.B., Williams M.J. & Clarke C.G. (1964) Comparison of jejunal mucosa in post-gastrectomy states, idiopathic steatorrhoea, and consols using the dissecting microscope and conventional histological methods. *Gut*, 5, 553–561.

Stammers F.A.R. & Alexander-Williams J. (1963) *Partial Gastrectomy Complications and Metabolic Consequences*, pp. 241–245. Butterworths, London.

Thompson D.G., Ritchie H.D. & Wingate D.L. (1982) Patterns of intestinal motility in duodenal ulcer patients before and after vagotomy. *Gut*, 23, 517–523.

Thompson G.R., Lewis B. & Booth C.C. (1966a) Vitamin D absorption after partial gastrectomy. *Lancet*, i, 457–458.

Thompson G.R., Lewis B. & Booth C.C. (1966b) Absorption of vitamin D-^{3}H in control subjects and patients with intestinal malabsorption. *J. Clin. Invest.* 45, 94–102.

Thompson G.R., Neale G., Watts J.H. & Booth C.C. (1966c) Detection of vitamin D deficiency after partial gastrectomy. *Lancet*, i, 623–626.

Toskes P.P. (1980) Current concepts of Cobalamin (Vitamin B_{12}) absorption and malabsorption. *J. Clin. Gast.* 2, 287–297.

Williams E.J. & Irvine W.T. (1966) Functional and metabolic effects of total and selective vagotomy. *Lancet*, i 1053–1057.

Chapter 6
Intestinal Resection and Bypass

CHRISTOPHER C. BOOTH

Introduction 101
Conditions necessitating small intestinal resection 101
Adaptive response 101
Sites of absorption in the small intestine 105
Motility 107
Intestinal transit time 107
Distal small intestinal resection 107
Proximal small intestinal resection 111
Bacterial overgrowth after resection 112
Gastric hypersecretion 112
Nephrolithiasis after enteric resection 112
Other complications 112
Intestinal bypass operations 113

Introduction

Surgical resection of varying amounts of the small intestine has been carried out for more than 100 years. In 1880, Koeberle reported the successful removal of 2 m of small intestine, an operation followed by complete recovery. Since that time, there have been a large number of reports of successful resections of the small intestine in man, the extent of the resection in some instances leaving no more than a few inches of residual intestine (Haymond 1935, Meyer 1946, 1954, Cogswell 1948, Althausen et al. 1949, Schwartz et al. 1956, Kogan et al. 1957, Kinney et al. 1961, Anderson 1965, Parkinson & Walker-Smith 1973). Whereas the older literature is predominantly concerned with clinical and metabolic studies in small numbers of patients, recent studies have concentrated on the precise mechanisms involved in intestinal adaptation.

The results of small intestinal resection in man depend firstly on the site and extent of the resection and secondly on the degree of morphological and functional adaptation that may develop in the residual intestine. Since the small intestine has different functions in different parts of its length, resection of different segments may be followed by different results. The blanket term 'short bowel syndrome' is therefore inappropriate to describe the post-resection state. It has been known for many years that ileal resection is less well tolerated than jejunal resection, and in recent years, studies of the intestinal adaptive response following resection, both in experimental animals and in man, have revealed some of the reasons for this difference.

Conditions necessitating small intestinal resection

In Western Europe and the USA, resection of the small intestine is most frequently carried out for *regional enteritis*. In the elderly, *mesenteric vascular occlusion*, either as a result of thrombosis or embolism, may necessitate massive resection of the small intestine. *Volvulus* may result in intestinal infarction in the neonatal period, as well as occasionally in young inmates of institutions for the mentally ill or retarded. *Intussusception* is a rare cause of small intestinal resection in young children. *Gunshot wounds* of the abdomen, and *trauma following road traffic accidents* may also make it necessary to undertake small intestinal resection. Resection of areas of the small intestine involved by tumours is usually confined to relatively short lengths of intestine and often has no significant effect. *Radiation enteritis* (Chapter 25) and *intestinal pseudo-obstruction* may also sometimes necessitate extensive enteric resection.

Adaptive response

Quantitative studies of the morphological and functional response to partial small intestinal resection have been carried out predominantly in experimental animals, relatively few detailed observations having been made in man. In both animal models and in man, however, it is clear that proximal enteric resection is tolerated better than distal resection. This is partly because the adaptive response in the ileum following proximal resection is markedly greater than that of the jejunum following distal resection (Booth et al. 1959, Dowling & Booth 1967). In addition, the rate of transit of the luminal contents through the distal small intestine is slower than that through the jejunum, permitting more time for absorption in a distal than a proximal remnant.

Studies in experimental animals

Morphological adaptation

Compensatory adaptation of the small intestine following partial resection involves the entire bowel wall but is predominantly associated with hyperplasia of the enterocytes and enlargement of the villus (Williamson 1978). Figure 6.1 illustrates that the height of the villi in rat jejunum increases by approximately 15% after resection of the distal two-thirds of the small intestine (Dowling & Booth 1967). By contrast, the response in the ileum after proximal resection is much greater, the villus height increasing by more than 50%. Similar observations have been made in dog, guinea-pig and primate. In the rat, there is evidence suggesting that this response may be enhanced by prednisolone (Scott et al. 1979). The degree of villus enlargement after partial resection is proportional to the amount of intestine resected. In the case of proximal resection, the villus enlargement is greatest immediately distal to the resection and tapers off distally.

Microscopic studies confirm that the villus enlargement is due to a true hyperplasia of enterocytes. There is no hypertrophy, the size of the individual enterocytes remaining normal, but there is an increase in the number of cells per unit length of villus. Ultrastructural studies have been conflicting, some reports describing microvillus enlargement, whilst others have demonstrated either normal or shortened microvilli

(Genyk, 1971, Wilmore et al. 1971, Tilson & Wright 1972).

Cellular proliferation

Under normal circumstances, there is a constant rapid turnover of the cells of the small intestinal epithelium. Cells are produced in the crypts of Lieberkühn, where mitosis can be observed; they are then extruded onto the surface of the small intestine and they subsequently ascend the side of the villus as if on a moving staircase, to be shed at the villus tip. The whole process takes no more than 2 days in an experimental animal such as the rat or mouse, and perhaps 3 days in man. The small intestinal mucosa is therefore the most rapidly turning-over tissue in the human body.

The control of intestinal cell turnover must depend upon precise homeostatic mechanisms. The nature of these mechanisms is as yet uncertain but it is clear that cell turnover is an innate function of the intestinal mucosa

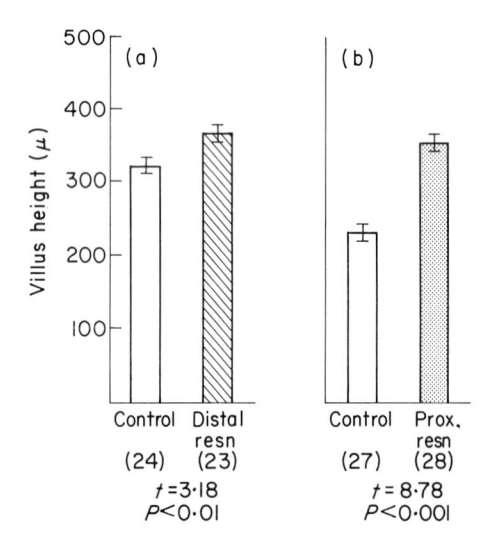

(a) Control (24), Distal resn (23); $t = 3.18$, $P < 0.01$
(b) Control (27), Prox. resn (28); $t = 8.78$, $P < 0.001$

Fig. 6.1. Villus height after two-thirds small intestinal resection in the rat (mean ± s.e. mean). (a) Jejunal villus height in control rats and in those after two-thirds *distal* resection, showing slight villus hyperplasia. (b) Ileal villus height in control rats and in those after two-thirds *proximal* resection, showing marked villus hyperplasia (Dowling & Booth 1966).

that is probably genetically determined. It is remarkable that, in spite of this extraordinarily rapid cell turnover, the villi of an individual may be maintained at the same height throughout an entire life span of more than three score years and ten.

After partial small intestinal resection, the villus hyperplasia is associated with an enhanced cell production rate as well as an increased migration rate of cells from the crypt to the villus tip. Since the villi are elongated, the total turnover time, in comparison with the normal situation, may not be increased. Overall, it seems likely that the cell turnover may be increased in the early weeks after resection but when adaptation is complete a steady state develops in which the increased villus height is maintained by an increased cell production rate and cell migration. The cellular changes may occur as soon as 2 days after an experimental resection in the rat (Williamson 1978).

Precise measurements of cell production rate may now be carried out using techniques developed by Wright (Wright et al. 1974, Wright 1982). Detailed quantitative studies of the cellular response after experimental resection have been reported by Hanson et al. (1977a & b). Within days of a partial intestinal resection the number of crypt cells increases. There is also an increase in the mass of proliferating calls and villus height increases, particularly in the ileum. There appears to be an increase in the number of intestinal stem cells (enteroblasts) and the proliferative characteristics of the mucosa shift to more rapid cycling.

Enzymes

Adaptive changes in the enzymes of the jejunal mucosa have been reported following experimental enteric resection, but the results have in some instances been conflicting (Weser & Hernandez 1971, McCarthy & Kim 1973). The disaccharidases, located in the brush border of the enterocyte, may be both increased or unchanged. The results for alkaline phosphatase, another brush border enzyme, have been similar. Peptide hydrolases, enterokinase and sodium potassium ATP-ase, however, are increased, and there may also be increases in enzymes responsible for lipid re-esterification. The enzymes associated with pyrimidine and DNA synthesis are increased, as might be expected in hyperplastic tissue.

Absorptive function

Perfusion studies, using glucose and other substances, have shown that after resection there is increased absorption per unit length of small intestine and that the increase of absorption is proportional to the degree of villus hyperplasia (Dowling & Booth 1967). If absorption by an adapted segment is corrected for the numbers of cells present in the tissue by expressing values per unit of mucosal weight, or per gram protein or DNA, then there is no apparent enhancement. This indicates that the absorptive capacity of the individual enterocytes is not increased and that the enhanced absorption per unit length of intestine is due to the increased number of enterocytes present on the elongated villi. Similar studies of adapted ileum have shown that the villus hyperplasia is associated with an increased capacity to absorb vitamin B_{12}, a substance specifically absorbed in the ileum. This enhancement is clearly achieved by the increased number of cells present rather than by any increase in the capacity of individual enterocytes to absorb this vitamin (Urban & Weser 1980).

Mechanisms of adaptation

One of the most important factors influencing the adaptive response to resection is the presence of nutrients within the lumen of the small intestine. Dowling & Booth (1967) originally showed that if the ileum is transposed to the position of the jejunum, and the jejunum retained distally (a situation in which no resection has been carried out), the ileum shows the same adaptive increase in villus height and bowel hyperplasia as when the jejunum is resected, indicating that the adaptive response is not due to resection alone. Furthermore, the remarkable adaptive response of the ileum following jejunal resection only occurs if feeding is carried out perorally; it does not occur if the experimental animals are fed intravenously, indicating the necessity for intraluminal nutrition to stimulate the adaptive response (Feldman et al. 1976).

There is also some evidence to suggest that pancreaticobiliary secretions may stimulate mucosal hyperplasia (Altman 1971, Hughes & Dowling 1978), but it remains uncertain whether this is due to a nutrient effect of such secretions or whether a specific trophic substance is secreted.

Other trophic substances of a hormonal nature may be involved in the adaptive response. In parabiotic rats or in paired animals with an established cross-circulation, DNA synthesis in the small intestinal mucosa of an animal without a resection may be stimulated if enteric resection is carried out in the other (Loran & Carbone 1968, Williamson et al. 1978). Sagor et al. (1983) have suggested that enteroglucagon may be involved in this response in experimental animals and in man there is evidence to suggest that enteroglucagon may be trophic to the small intestine. In a single case report villus hyperplasia in association with an endocrine tumour located in the kidney which secreted large amounts of enteroglucagon was described (Gleeson et al. 1971) (see Chapter 23). Glucagon itself has also been shown to stimulate intestinal transport in the rat (Rudo & Rosenberg 1973). Furthermore, there is a markedly greater elevation of plasma enteroglucagon levels following a meal in both animals and in man with distal intestinal resection than in control individuals (Besterman et al. 1982) (Chapter 23). Recent studies have also suggested that enteroglucagon may stimulate DNA synthesis in the intestinal mucosa *in vitro* (Uttental et al. 1982). Although these interesting observations suggest a role for enteroglucagon in the enteric adaptive response, the precise hormonal mechanism of enterocyte hyperplasia remains uncertain.

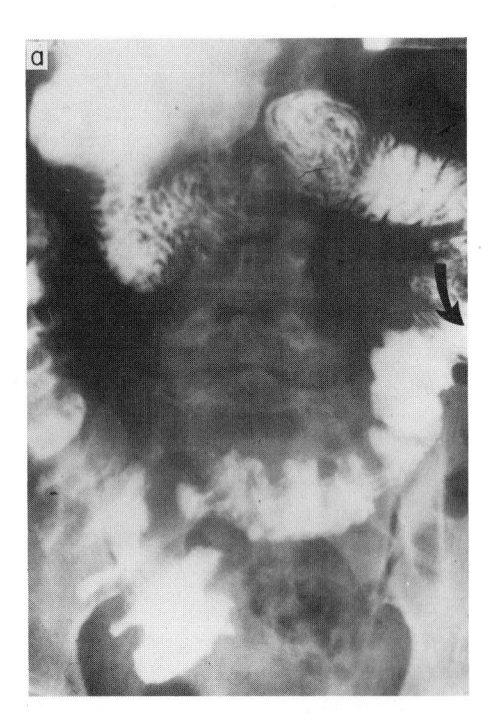

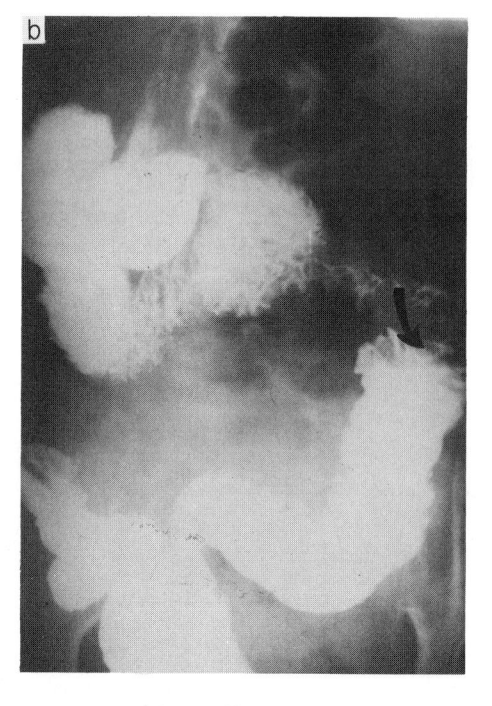

Fig. 6.2. Barium follow-through examination after extensive resection of the small intestine showing adaptive enlargement of the ileal remnant:
(a) 4 weeks postoperatively. (b) 4 years later. The arrows mark the site of the resection.

Studies in man

Morphological adaptation

Jejunal biopsies obtained from individuals with distal intestinal resection have shown increased numbers of enterocytes and increased height of villi, the hyperplastic response being similar to that shown in the rat. The jejunal response is relatively slight but quantitative studies have demonstrated a significant hyperplasia of jejunal enterocytes (Porus 1965, Dowling & Booth 1966).

There have been no significant studies of villus height in human ileum following jejunal resection, since this operation is carried out relatively infrequently in man. Radiological studies, however, suggest that an ileal response occurs in man similar to that in experimental animals subjected to jejunal resection. Figure 6.2 illustrates the radiological appearances of the ileum in an individual subjected to a massive jejunal resection for mesenteric vascular occlusion. Four years after the resection, there was a significant increase in the diameter of the ileum, an appearance similar to that seen in rats given barium meal examinations after jejunal resection (Booth et al. 1959).

Functional adaptation

Clinical studies have repeatedly suggested that functional adaptation occurs after enteric resection in man. In the immediate postoperative period, there are often massive losses of fluid, electrolytes and nutrients, yet after 4 weeks or so these gradually diminish, suggesting that adaptation is taking place. Direct studies of intestinal absorption by jejunal remnants after ileal resection, using perfusion techniques, have shown increased segmental absorption of glucose, water and electrolytes (Dowling & Booth 1966, Weinstein et al. 1969). Similar studies have been carried out in the ileum in a limited number of children with jejunal resection (Schmitz et al. 1980).

Sites of absorption in the small intestine

Figure 6.3 illustrates what has either been demonstrated or may safely be inferred as to the sites of absorption of different nutrients and other substances in the small intestine (Booth 1967). The jejunum is the major site of absorption of most substances. Carbohydrates, proteins and fat are predominantly absorbed in the proximal small intestine. The extent to which such substances are absorbed in the jejunum, however, depends also on the amount presented at any one time to the jejunal mucosa. If intestinal transport systems become increasingly saturated by increasing amounts of the substance to be transported, increasing amounts will be propelled distally before absorption is complete. The ileum therefore acts as a reserve area for absorption, becoming increasingly important as nutrient intake is increased, or taking over absorptive function if the jejunum is either resected or diseased (as in coeliac disease, cf. Chapter 9). Most vitamins and electrolytes are also absorbed in the jejunum.

The ileum, however, has other specific functions. There is a specific series of receptors in the ileal enterocytes which are involved in the intrinsic-factor-mediated absorption of vitamin B_{12}. It is, in fact, remarkable that the infinitesimally small requirement of vitamin B_{12} in man (approximately 0.000002–0.000004 g/day) should require both an intrinsic factor secreted by the stomach and a specific ileal receptor. The B_{12} receptors in the ileum are very easily saturated, and under physiological circumstances, absorption of B_{12} is limited to not more than 1–2 µg from a single orally ingested load.

The terminal ileum is also involved in the active transport of the conjugated bile salts (Lack & Weiner 1961, Hofmann 1978). A certain amount of conjugated bile salt absorption, however, may also occur by passive non-ionic diffusion in the jejunum. If the bile salts undergo deconjugation, as when there is significant bacterial overgrowth in the small intestine (Chapter 15), the deconjugated bile acids may be equally well absorbed in both jejunum and ileum.

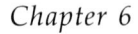

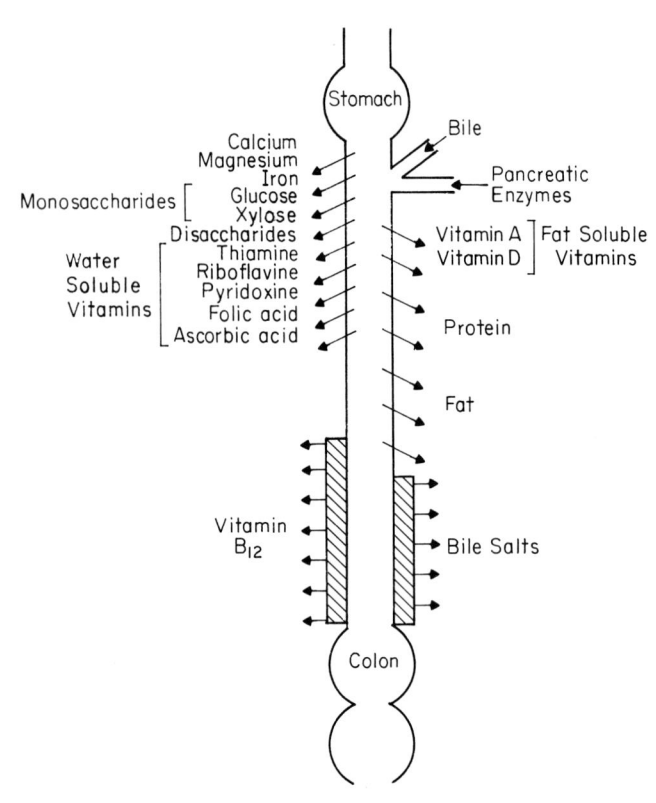

Fig. 6.3. Sites of absorption in the small intestine (Booth 1967).

The concept of intestinal reserve (Booth 1961)

Like other vital organs such as the liver and kidney, the small intestine has a remarkable functional reserve. The rat, for instance, is capable of absorbing more than 100 times its dietary requirement of pyridoxine and there appears to be virtually no limit to the absorption of this water-soluble vitamin in man. This capacity of the small intestine to absorb increasing and unlimited amounts of such water-soluble vitamins is a function of the jejunum, for even when very large doses of either pyridoxine or ascorbic acid are fed, the ileum plays little part in absorption.

The absorption of large amounts of fat, on the other hand, cannot be achieved entirely by the jejunum. When increasing amounts of fat are given to normal individuals, there is a progressive increase in absorption and even when diets containing as much as 350 g of fat are fed, more than 340 g are absorbed.

Although the jejunum plays an important part in absorbing such remarkable amounts of dietary fat, studies in both experimental animals and in man indicate that the ileum absorbs progressively more fat as the dietary fat is increased. The jejunum is undoubtedly of major importance and responds to an increased dietary load with an increased absorption, but as the dietary fat is increased more and more escapes the jejunum and passes on into the ileum to be absorbed there. The ileum is therefore an important part of the functional reserve of the small intestine for the absorption of fat.

Vitamin B_{12} behaves quite differently. In contrast to the substances already discussed, there is a striking limit to the amount of this essential nutrient which can be absorbed at any one time through the physiological intrinsic factor mechanism, the limitation being imposed by the limited amount of the ileal receptor available. Even when test doses of as much as 50 µg of vitamin B_{12} are given, absorption is limited to between 1 and 2 µg. Under physiological conditions the amount of B_{12} which can be absorbed by the intestinal transport mechanisms in the ileum is therefore only just enough to satisfy the daily requirements and there is virtually no functional reserve. It is possible, however, to overcome this limit to absorption by giving very large and unphysiological doses of crystalline B_{12}. Under these circumstances absorption probably occurs by diffusion and is not mediated by the physiological intrinsic factor mechanism. Absorption of such large and unphysiological amounts of crystalline B_{12} can occur from the jejunum in man and does not require the specialized transport mechanism in the ileum.

Motility

Few studies of intestinal motility have been carried out in patients following small intestinal resection. In a group of patients with extensive resection of the distal small bowel, Remington et al. (1983) demonstrated that during fasting the duration of the interdigestive motor complex was significantly shorter in patients with intestinal resection and the frequency of complexes was therefore increased. There was a marked reduction in Phase II activity but a normal feeding pattern. Loperamide therapy increased feeding activity while at the same time shortened its duration.

Intestinal transit time

Under normal circumstances, the transit of material through the small intestine is variable. Radiological studies, however, indicate that both in experimental animals and in man there is a difference in transit time between jejunum and ileum. The intestinal contents pass relatively rapidly through the jejunum but more slowly through the ileum. The rates of transit of barium through the residual small intestine after proximal or distal resection are therefore different. There are limitations to barium follow-through studies in assessing intestinal transit time, and although they have proved valuable for this purpose after resection in experimental animals (Booth et al. 1959), such studies should be interpreted with caution in man.

As might be expected, however, the transit of barium through the residual small intestine is more rapid in patients with distal resections and the rate of transit is usually most rapid in those with the most extensive resections. After resection of only 1.8 or 2.4 m of the terminal ileum, for instance, barium may take 2 h to reach the colon but when the resections are more extensive, leaving only 1.2 or 1.8 m of the proximal jejunum, the intestinal transit time is invariably more rapid, being as little as 20 or 30 min. In one patient in whom only 0.2 m of the proximal jejunum remained, barium appeared in the colon as early as 5 min after feeding. The relationship between intestinal transit and extent of resection is not invariably so direct, however, for another patient with a resection of only 1.8 m of the ileum has been described whose intestinal transit time was as fast as 15 min.

After resection of 2.4 m of the proximal jejunum, on the other hand, barium may take 4 h to reach the colon, a normal transit time; and in a child with only 0.4 m of the terminal ileum remaining, the transit time through the sluggish ileal segment was as long as 1¾ h (Booth 1961). The slower rates of transit observed in ileal remnants may therefore play a role in encouraging absorption, even though transport mechanisms are in general less active in ileum than in jejunum.

Distal small intestinal resection

The amount of intestine removed is of vital importance in determining the results of distal small intestinal resection. As already described, the residual intestine has a limited capacity to adapt following distal resection. Furthermore, the proximal small intestine does not appear to develop any of the specific functions of the ileum, such as the capacity to absorb vitamin B_{12}, or to transport the conjugated bile acids. In addition, partial colectomy is frequently performed in many patients undergoing distal enteric resection, which limits the colonic absorptive capacity for fluid and electrolytes and often exacerbates the degree of diarrhoea caused by malabsorption. Diarrhoea under these circumstances may be determined more by the amount of colon resected than small intestine (Cummings et al. 1973).

Malabsorption following distal resection may be classified as follows (Booth 1961).

Type 1: Malabsorption of B_{12} and bile acids

If the resection is limited to the ileum, resection of no more perhaps than 1–2 m being carried out, there may be malabsorption of vitamin B_{12} and conjugated bile salts, but no significant steatorrhoea, proximal small intestinal function remaining intact. The major symptom following such a resection is usually watery diarrhoea, as many as six to eight watery motions being passed daily, particularly in the early postoperative period. The diarrhoea is predominantly due to the deconjugation by bacteria in the colon of the conjugated bile salts, the resulting deconjugated bile salts inhibiting fluid and electrolyte absorption by the colonic mucosa.

The diarrhoea can usually be controlled by treatment with lomotil or codeine. In instances where such treatment is ineffective, cholestyramine, which binds the bile acids within the intestinal lumen, may relieve diarrhoea but this is rarely necessary. Nutrition is usually well maintained, electrolyte deficiencies only developing if there is significant diarrhoea. Vitamin B_{12} should, however, be given parenterally to prevent the subsequent development of B_{12} deficiency.

Type 2: Malabsorption of B_{12}, bile acids and steatorrhoea

If the distal resection is more extensive, leaving perhaps 1–1.5 m of residual jejunum only, there may be malabsorption of B_{12} and bile acids but there is, in addition, significant steatorrhoea. The degree of steatorrhoea depends on the fat intake, higher fat ingestion leading to greater degrees of steatorrhoea. It is also exacerbated by loss of bile salts in the stool. The liver has a limited capacity to compensate for this loss by increased bile acid synthesis and the concentration of bile salts in the upper jejunum may therefore fall below the critical level necessary for normal fat digestion and solubilization in micelles. Other aspects of proximal intestinal function may, however, be well maintained as indicated by normal absorption of xylose, glucose and folic acid.

In the immediate postoperative period, there may be severe malabsorption and watery diarrhoea, necessitating parenteral feeding during the first 2–4 weeks. Oral feeding, however, should be instituted at the earliest opportunity, small amounts being initially given frequently. Nutrition in solid form is usually better tolerated than fluid formula diets (Althausen et al. 1949). This is presumably because gastric emptying of solids is slower than for liquids, ensuring a slower presentation of food to the limited amount of residual proximal intestine.

One to 1.3 m of residual proximal small intestine is compatible with remarkably good health. The major nutritional deficiencies that may develop are of vitamin B_{12}, calcium and magnesium and vitamin D.

Vitamin B_{12} deficiency

In childhood, deficiency of vitamin B_{12} after distal intestinal resection may be associated with growth failure rather than classical megaloblastic anaemia (Clark & Booth 1960).

> Figure 6.4 illustrates the weight chart and response to treatment with parenteral vitamin B_{12} of a child in whom the distal two-thirds of the small intestine was resected at birth as a result of volvulus secondary to exomphalos. The child grew normally until 9 to 10 months of age, at which stage the supply of B_{12} stored in the liver and derived from her mother was exhausted and growth failure now developed. At 13 months, however, the haemoglobin concentration was 12 g/dl but the B_{12} level in the serum was so low as to be scarcely measurable. Treatment with vitamin B_{12} was dramatically effective. This individual has now been treated with a high protein, low fat diet and parenteral vitamin B_{12} until the age of 26 years and

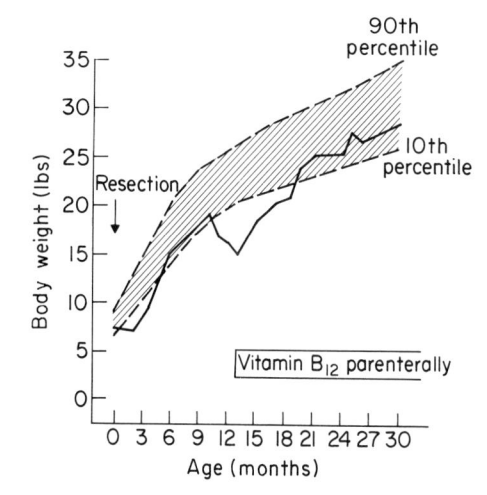

Fig. 6.4. Body weight and response to parenteral vitamin B$_{12}$ in a child in whom the distal two-thirds of the small intestine was resected at birth (Clark & Booth 1960).

she remains in good health, although she has recently suffered from attacks of erythema nodosum and arthritis similar to those sometimes seen after jejunoileal bypass.

In adults, vitamin B$_{12}$ deficiency develops 2–6 years after ileal resection, the delay again being due to the time required to exhaust the hepatic stores of vitamin B$_{12}$ (Booth et al. 1964). Anaemia is not usually severe and can be prevented by treatment with parenteral injections of vitamin B$_{12}$. In patients with a significant remnant of proximal small intestine, it is also possible to give vitamin B$_{12}$ in large and unphysiological doses by mouth. Between 1000 and 3000 µg orally in a single dose will significantly raise the serum level of vitamin B$_{12}$ (Booth 1967). Oral treatment may therefore be used in children if it is desired to avoid injections.

Consequences of bile acid malabsorption (Hofmann 1978)

Malabsorption of bile acids after ileal resection results in large quantities of unabsorbed, conjugated bile acids reaching the colon. Here they are deconjugated predominantly by anaerobic bacteria. Large amounts of free cholic acid and chenodeoxycholic acid are therefore formed which exacerbate diarrhoea by their effect in inhibiting colonic reabsorption of fluid and electrolytes. Dehydroxylation of bile salts, however, frequently does not occur so that patients with extensive distal small intestinal resection may have no deoxycholic acid in the stool. Since the capacity of the liver to resynthesize bile salts is severely limited, and can only compensate for as much as 30% of bile salt malabsorption, total malabsorption of bile salts due to ileal resection leads to a reduction in the total bile salt pool. The concentration of bile salts in the upper jejunum may therefore fall below the critical level necessary for normal micelle formation and fat absorption. This may exacerbate the steatorrhoea. Insufficiency of bile salts in the upper jejunum in patients with extensive small bowel resection tends to be less severe at the beginning of the day, becoming worse as the hours pass, when the repeated circulation of the bile salt pool in response to food leads to progressive depletion of bile salts as a result of ileal malabsorption.

Despite the loss of bile salt in the stool and reduction in the bile salt pool, there is paradoxically an increase in the total bile acid concentration of the blood. Under normal circumstances, there are significant quantities of free bile acid in the serum in addition to the conjugated bile acids (Setchell et al. 1982a) and these reflect the normal colonic deconjugation of bile salts by bacteria. After extensive ileal resection, however, the free bile acids in the serum are markedly increased, presumably as a result of increased absorption of free bile salts in the colon (Panveliwalla et al. 1970). The pattern of serum bile acid reflects the pattern in the stool and intestine, free deoxycholic acid being rarely found in the serum after ileal resection. There is a significant diurnal variation, particularly involving the unconjugated bile acids (Setchell et al. 1982b).

The reduction in the bile salt pool has a further important effect. Since the concentration of bile salts in the bile falls in relation to the concentration of cholesterol or phospholipid, the bile becomes lithogenic since cholesterol tends to precipitate out of solution. This leads to a significant increase in the incidence of gallstones after ileal resection as compared with control individuals.

Electrolyte deficiencies

In the early postoperative phase, deficiencies of sodium and potassium may develop as a result of the initial severe diarrhoea. In later months or years, hypomagnesaemia and hypocalcaemia may occur, and there may be frank tetany, with positive Chvostek's and Trousseau's signs. These abnormalities may be induced by high fat feeding. Patients may be encouraged to take very large amounts of fat in the diet in an attempt to 'put on weight' (Booth *et al.* 1964). The high fat intake results in severe steatorrhoea and the binding of divalent cations by fatty acids in the stool may lead to significant losses of magnesium and calcium. This is illustrated by the following case report.

> A 48-year-old housewife had a 19-year history of regional enteritis involving the distal small intestine. Repeated intestinal operations were carried out throughout her illness and her remaining intestine did not exceed 2 m. Following her last operation, when she was found to have no evidence of active regional enteritis, she was treated first with a low and then with a high fat diet in a vain attempt to increase her weight. On this regime, she had severe diarrhoea, passing eight to ten bulky stools daily. Her weight fell and she developed spontaneous tetany. At this stage serum calcium was 3.6 and magnesium 0.3 mEq/l. She also had severe B_{12} deficiency (serum B_{12} 15 pg/ml) and the haemoglobin was 6.7 g/dl. After initial treatment with calciferol (100,000 units daily for 5 days) and parenteral vitamin B_{12}, she was treated with a low fat, high protein diet. Her diarrhoea was immediately improved and her body weight, serum calcium and serum magnesium rose. Two years later she remained in good health with normal levels of serum calcium and magnesium (Booth *et al.* 1964).

Osteoporosis and osteomalacia

Both osteoporosis and osteomalacia may occur after distal small intestinal resection. Bone disease, however, is rarely severe and evidence of vitamin D deficiency is usually only present if the serum levels are measured or if biopsies are carried out and osteomalacia discovered (Compston & Creamer 1977a). The classical radiological picture of the bones with pseudofractures and subperiosteal bone erosions, seen after gastric resection or in coeliac disease, is not encountered. Serum 25-hydroxy vitamin D levels, however, may be subnormal (Compston & Creamer 1977b).

Treatment

The mainstay of treatment, as already indicated, is a low fat, high protein diet. The precise restriction to be placed on fat intake varies from one individual to another and may be between 30–60 g daily. Some individuals, however, may tolerate higher fat intakes. It is important to assess several levels of dietary fat and determine the effect on stool frequency. To compensate for reduction in fat intake, both protein and carbohydrate should be increased, the protein intake being maintained at more than 100 g daily. In order to compensate for the low fat diet, medium chain triglycerides may also be helpful. A recent study has suggested that a low fat diet is not necessary after distal small intestinal resection (Woolf *et al.* 1983). This study, however, was based on short-term studies of only 5 days and the fat intakes tested were not particularly high.

Supplementary fat-soluble vitamins, such as vitamin D, may be given by mouth, since sufficient intestine usually remains to achieve normal absorption. In addition, if iron supplements are required, as sometimes in regional enteritis, or if water-soluble vitamins are indicated, they too may be given orally. The only substance required parenterally is vitamin B_{12}.

Type 3: Massive distal small intestinal resection

The resection may be so severe that it involves all the functions of the proximal small intestine. This is illustrated by the following case report.

> An elderly lady who developed gangrene of the bowel as a result of mesenteric arterial thrombosis underwent resection of all but the proximal 0.2 m of jejunum which was anastomosed end-to-end to the transverse colon. The patient's resection was so severe that she not only had steatorrhoea and failure to absorb vitamin B_{12}, but also interference with the absorption of glucose, xylose and folic acid. Despite nutritional supplementation, her condition deteriorated steadily until her death 9 months later (Harrison & Booth 1960).

The minimum length of intestine necessary for maintaining life with oral nutrition is not known, but may vary with the age of the patient and the efficiency of adaptation of whatever remains of the small intestine. Survival with only duodenum and a 15 cm remnant of small intestine with oral nutrition has been successfully recorded (Anderson 1965). On the other hand, patients with similar amounts of residual small intestine have died after varying periods of time.

The treatment of such patients invariably requires a period of intravenous alimentation in the immediate postoperative period. Thereafter, attempts should be made to introduce oral feeding. In some instances, regular and frequent meals given by intragastric tube may be necessary. Although prognosis should be guarded, the remarkable examples of survival after massive resection of the intestine are an encouragement to persistent efforts to achieve oral alimentation. Furthermore, the results of continuous parenteral hyperalimentation in the home are now so good in specialist hands that this may be attempted if all else fails (Jeejeebhoy et al. 1973, Rault & Scribner 1977).

Surgical treatment of malabsorption following extensive resection

Reversal of short segments of small bowel has been used in an attempt to slow intestinal transit by creating a low grade obstruction due to an anti-peristaltic segment (Pertsemlidis & Kark 1974). In the authors' experience, this is rarely, if ever, necessary.

Hepatic failure

Although it is claimed that hepatic failure is a complication of jejunoileal bypass but does not occur after resection, there are reports of severe fatty infiltration of the liver in patients dying following massive resection of the intestine (Jackson 1958, Harrison & Booth 1960). In addition, jaundice of obscure cause may develop after massive resection and, in a single case, hepatic coma and death occurred with no demonstrable abnormality of hepatic histology in an individual with massive resection who also had oesophageal varices, due to portal vein thrombosis.

Proximal small intestinal resection

As already indicated, the adaptive response that occurs in the ileum after proximal resection, together with the slower transit of intestinal contents through the ileum, ensures that when the jejunum is resected the ileum, with its enormous reserve capacity, may take over the function of the resected jejunum. Resection of the proximal small intestine does not therefore cause any significant degree of malabsorption unless the resection is massive. Resection of as much as 2.4 m of jejunum may cause no malabsorption of glucose, folic acid, xylose, fat or vitamin B_{12} (Booth 1961), in contrast to the degree of malabsorption that a comparable distal resection would inevitably produce. Furthermore, even when only 0.4 m or so of terminal ileum remains after massive proximal resection, as in the patient described by Clayton & Cotton (1961) and

Booth (1961), there was only moderate steatorrhoea and the absorption of vitamin B_{12} was normal. After proximal resection, the ileal adaptive response ensures an enhancement in the absorption of vitamin B_{12}.

The question of whether the removal of the ileocaecal valve is important in patients with enteric resection remains uncertain. Regurgitation of colonic contents into the small intestine is more likely to occur if the ileocaecal valve is resected (Griffin et al. 1971). On the other hand, the better prognosis of patients in whom the ileocaecal valve has been preserved may be related more to the vital segment of adjacent ileum than to the valve itself.

Bacterial overgrowth after resection

Although it is frequently stated that significant bacterial overgrowth occurs in the residual small intestine after enteric resection, there have been remarkably few detailed studies of individual patients. Tabaqchali (1970) studied a single patient with a massive distal small intestinal resection, details of whose investigations are given in Chapter 15. Studies in this patient demonstrated that significant bacterial overgrowth occurred in the small intestine after extensive distal enteric resection and that this occurred particularly after a meal. By contrast, similar studies in a further patient in whom there was a massive jejunal resection with preservation of the ileocaecal valve and approximately 1.2 m of ileum showed no bacterial overgrowth and no bile salt deconjugation in the small intestinal lumen (Chapter 15).

Gastric hypersecretion

Gastric hypersecretion has been recorded following massive resection of the small intestine in man (Aber et al. 1967, Windsor et al. 1969) and in experimental animals (Landor 1969). This is not a universal phenomenon, however, and many patients with extensive resection show no evidence of gastric hypersecretion. Nevertheless, duodenal ulcer does appear to occur with greater frequency after resection. Removal of an inhibitor of gastric acid secretion by resecting a key segment of intestine is one possible explanation of this phenomenon. There may be elevation of the serum gastrin level (Buxton 1974) and experimental studies have shown an increase in gastric parietal cells after intestinal resection (Selig et al. 1977). The precise mechanism of increased gastric secretion is not yet established.

Nephrolithiasis after enteric resection

Renal stones occur with distressing frequency after resection of the small intestine. Patients with enteric resection develop hyperoxaluria and a proportion develop renal calculi which may be bilateral (Hofmann et al. 1970, Dowling et al. 1971, Smith et al. 1972). The cause of the hyperoxaluria appears to be enhanced absorption of dietary oxalate (Chadwick et al. 1973). Oxalate is normally absorbed from the diet by a passive process of non-ionic diffusion and most of the dietary oxalate is rendered insoluble as calcium oxalate. In steatorrhoea, from whatever cause, unabsorbed fatty acids bind with luminal calcium to form calcium soaps. Increasing amounts of dietary oxalate are therefore available for absorption. Tissue and bacterial production probably also contribute to hyperoxaluria. Hyperoxaluria may be reduced by dietary oxalate restriction, by a low fat diet or by the use of cholestyramine. Surgical removal of renal stones, however, may be necessary.

Other complications

Lactic acidosis, associated with severe metabolic disturbances, has been described in two patients with extensive resection of the small intestine (Satoh et al. 1982). Essential fatty acid deficiency has also been reported, resection patients having significantly less linoleate and more oleate in lecithin than controls or patients with other causes of malabsorption. In addition, in two out of five resection patients, an abnormal fatty acid, with the Rf of 8. 8. 11 eicosatrienoic acid (20;3 9) was also present. There were decreasing amounts of arachidonate in plasma lecithin and the linoleate content of cholesterol ester was also low (Shimoyama et al. 1973).

Intestinal bypass operations

During the past 20 years, small bowel bypass operations have been used to treat severe obesity (Payne & De Wind 1969, Scott et al. 1971). Although the results in terms of weight loss have been encouraging, a large number of undesirable side effects, together with an unacceptably high mortality, have led to a reappraisal of the type of operation (Finer & Pilkington 1980). A detailed review of the complications has been published by Juhl et al. (1979). In general, bypass operations are no longer considered justifiable and these have been superseded by other procedures such as jaw wiring or gastric bypass and plication. Nevertheless, the adaptive responses following bypass operations both in experimental animals and in man are worthy of consideration, as are the extraordinary variety of postoperative complications.

Bypass of the ileum alone, however, does not lead to the complications associated with major bypass operations for obesity. Ileal bypass induces loss of bile salts leading to reduction in serum levels of cholesterol. This operation is useful in the treatment of familial hypercholesterolaemia, and apart from diarrhoea has few complications.

Types of bypass operation for obesity

The original operation was Payne's end-to-side jejunoileostomy, leaving about 50 cm of small bowel in continuity. Other types of bypass have included jejunoileostomy end-to-end plus ileotransversostomy, and jejuno-ileostomy end-to-end plus ileocaecostomy. The complications of all these operations are broadly similar.

Adaptive response

The structural changes in the small bowel in continuity, whether in experimental animals or in man, shows similar changes to those after partial small intestinal resection. As after jejunal enterectomy, there is enterocyte hyperplasia and the villi become elongated. Functional adaptation also occurs. Increased absorption of glucose has been demonstrated directly by perfusion experiments 6 months after subtotal enteric bypass, and there may be enhancement of B_{12} absorption. The increased glucose absorption is proportional to the increase in villus height and there is also an increase in brush border disaccharidases.

By contrast, studies in experimental animals show that there is hypoplasia in defunctioned bowel which has been bypassed. There is reduction in the number of crypt cells, lower cell production and a reduced number of enterocytes to populate the villi. Villus height may therefore be reduced, although sometimes the degree of reduction is slight. At the same time, there may be progressive loss of function, absorption of glucose and aminoacids decreasing per unit length of bypassed intestine (Gleeson et al. 1972, Keren et al. 1975).

These observations are pertinent to the question whether luminal nutrition or hormonal factors are more important in inducing adaptive changes after resection or bypass. Since *hyperplasia* in the intestine in continuity and *hypoplasia* in the bypassed intestine may coexist after the operation, the adaptive response cannot be solely induced by hormonal changes. The presence of food or other substances within the intestinal lumen must be of greater importance.

In man, however, there have been conflicting reports of the state of the mucosa in the defunctioned segment following bypass, at least one study showing no mucosal atrophy (Tompkins et al. 1977).

Intestinal function

As would be expected, steatorrhoea is a constant feature of bypass operations and may be severe. There is also malabsorption of a wide range of other substances. Such is the nature of the reserve capacity of the small intestine, however, that it is the effect of the operation on reducing appetite that is more important than malabsorption in inducing weight loss (Pilkington et al. 1976).

Complications

The overall death rate following bypass operations is 5%. The major complications in 5000 patients treated for obesity with jejuno-ileal bypass between 1973 and 1977 were analysed by Juhl and his colleagues (1980).

Hepatic changes

The commonest abnormality is severe fatty liver, presumably as a result of triglyceride synthesis by the liver from fatty acids mobilized from fat stores during the initial period of intense weight loss. A similar fatty liver has been recorded after massive small intestinal resection. This condition is relatively benign. Many patients may show transient abnormalities of liver function tests in the early months after operation. Progressive liver disease, however, is a very much more serious complication and leads to hepatic failure and death in as many as 5% of patients. Initially the patient may develop anorexia, nausea and vomiting. There may be hepatomegaly and biochemical studies show a low serum albumin and abnormal transaminase and aminotransferase levels. Jaundice and ascites, followed by death from hepatic coma, may ensue. Cirrhosis may occur in rare instances but more often the liver at autopsy shows massive fatty infiltration and a lesion similar to that of acute alcoholic hepatitis. The cause of this complication is not fully understood but, although attempts have been made to incriminate bacterial toxins (Powell-Jackson et al. 1979), it is more likely to be the result of severe malnutrition.

Intestinal complications

Colonic pseudo-obstruction has been described, causing recurrent episodes of intestinal obstruction without obvious mechanical cause. Pneumatosis cystoides intestinalis has also been reported.

Joint symptoms

As many as 8% of patients develop arthralgia, polyarthritis, spondylitis, myalgia and occasionally erythema nodosum. These symptoms are frequently associated with the presence of circulating immune complexes but their precise pathogenesis is still uncertain.

Nutritional problems

Electrolyte deficiencies involving sodium and potassium occur in the early months of bypass before the initial diarrhoea has subsided. Later, calcium and magnesium deficiencies have been described. In some instances osteoporosis and osteomalacia may be found, although, as after resection, fractures of bone are not usually seen. Deficiency of vitamin D and vitamin A have been detected by measuring serum levels. Beri-beri, causing severe neurological disturbances, has also been described.

Lithiasis

Gallstones occur in 7% of patients postoperatively but, since obese patients have an increased incidence of gallstones, this may not necessarily be the result of the operation. Hyperoxaluria and renal stones, however, are a significant complication of bypass operations, as they are after intestinal resection.

Neuropathy

Severe peripheral neuropathy, unresponsive to treatment with vitamins or nutritional supplements, may be a crippling complication. The cause remains unknown.

Psychiatric complications

These may be related either to the pre-existing obesity or to an operation which has been followed by disastrous complications. The incidence of suicide following bypass in the 5000 patients reviewed by Juhl et al. (1980) was 0.4%.

References

Aber G.M., Ashton F, Carmalt M.H.B. & Whitehead T.P. (1967) Gastric hypersecretion following massive small bowel resection in man. *Amer. J. Dig. Dis.* **12**, 785–794.

Altman G.G. (1971) Influence of bile and pancreatic secretions on the size of the intestinal villi in the rat. *Amer. J. Anat.* **132**, 167–178.

Althausen T.L., Uyeyama K. & Simpson R.G. (1949) Digestion and absorption after massive resection of the small intestine: I. Utilization of food from a 'Natural' versus a 'Synthetic' diet and a comparison of intestinal absorption tests with nutritional balance studies in a patient with only 45 cm of small intestine, *Gastroenterol.* **12**, 795–807.

Anderson C. (1965) Long-term survival with six inches of small intestine. *Brit. Med. J.* **i**, 419–422.

Besterman H.S., Adrian T.E., Mallinson C.N., Christofides N.D., Sarson D., Pera A., Lombardo L., Modigliani R. & Bloom S.R. (1982) Gut hormone release after intestinal resection *Gut*, **23**, 854–861.

Booth C.C. (1967) Effect of location along the small intestine on absorption of nutrients. *Handbook of Physiology: Alimentary Canal*, vol. 3, pp. 1513–1527. Washington D.C. America Physiological Society.

Booth C.C. (1961) The metabolic effects of small intestinal resection in man. *Postgrad. Med. J.* **37**, 725–739.

Booth C.C., Evans K.T., Menzies T. & Street D.F. (1959) Intestinal hypertrophy following partial resection of the small bowel in the rat. *Brit. J. Surg.* **46**, 403–410.

Booth C.C., MacIntyre I. & Mollin D.L. (1964) Nutritional problems associated with extensive lesions of the distal small intestine in man. *Quart. J. Med.* **131**, 401–420.

Buxton B. (1974) Progress report. Small bowel resection and gastric acid hypersecretion. *Gut*, **15**, 229–238.

Chadwick V.S., Modha K. & Dowling R.H. (1973) Mechanism for hyperoxaluria in patients with ileal dysfunction. *N. Engl. J. Med.* **289**, 172–6.

Clark A.C.L. & Booth C.C. (1960) Deficiency of vitamin B_{12} after extensive resection of the distal small intestine in an infant. *Arch. Dis. Child.* **35**, 595–599.

Clayton B.E. & Cotton D.A. (1961) A study of malabsorption after resection of the entire jejunum and the proximal half of the ileum. *Gut*, **2**, 18–22.

Cogswell H.D. (1948) Massive resection of the small intestine. *Ann. Surg.* **127**, 377–382.

Compston J.E. & Creamer B. (1977a) The consequences of small intestinal resection. *Quart. J. Med.* **46**, 485–497.

Compston J.E. & Creamer B. (1977b) Plasma levels and intestinal absorption of 25-hydroxy vitamin D in patients with small bowel resection. *Gut*, **18**, 171–175.

Cummings J.H., James W.P.T. & Wiggins H. (1973) Role of the colon in ileal resection diarrhoea. *Lancet*, **i**, 344–347.

Dowling R.H. & Booth C.C. (1966) Functional compensation after small bowel resection in man. *Lancet*, **ii**, 146–147.

Dowling R.H. & Booth C.C. (1967) Structural and functional changes following small intestinal resection in the rat. *Clin. Sci.* **32**, 139–149.

Dowling R.H., Rose G.A., Sutor D.J. (1971) Hyperoxaluria and renal calculi in ileal disease. *Lancet*, **i**, 1103–1106.

Feldman E.J., Dowling R.H., McNaughton J. & Peters T.J. (1976) Effects of oral versus intravenous nutrition on intestinal adaptation after small bowel resection in the dog. *Gastroenterol.* **70**, 712–719.

Finer N. & Pilkington T.R.E. (1980) Obesity. Indications for surgery. *Brit. J. Hosp. Med.* **24**, 510–515.

Genyk S.N. (1971) Ultrastructure of the spiral part of the epithelial cells of the mucous membrane of the small intestine after extensive experimental enterectomy. *Bull. Exp. Biol. Med.* **72**, 964.

Gleeson M.H., Bloom S.R., Polak R.M., Henry K. & Dowling R.H. (1971) Endocrine tumour in kidney affecting small bowel structure, motility and absorptive function. *Gut*, **12**, 773–782.

Gleeson M.H., Cullen J. & Dowling R.H. (1972) Intestinal structure and function after small bowel by-pass in the rat. *Clin. Sci.* **43**, 731–742.

Griffin W.O., Richardson J.D. & Medley E.S. (1971) Prevention of small bowel contamination by ileo-caecal valve. *Southern Med. J.* **64**, 1056–1058.

Hanson W.R., Osborne J.W. & Sharp J.G. (1977a) Compensation by the residual intestine after intestinal resection in the rat. I. Influence of amount of tissue removed. *Gastroenterol.* **72**, 692–700.

Hanson W.R., Osborne J.W. & Sharp J.G. (1977b) Compensation by the residual intestine after intestinal resection in the rat. II. Influence of the post-operative time interval. *Gastroenterol.* **72**, 701–705.

Harrison R.J. & Booth C.C. (1960) Massive resection of the small intestine after occlusion of the superior mesenteric artery. *Gut*, **1**, 237–241.

Haymond H.E. (1935) Massive resection of small intestine: analysis of 257 collected cases. *Surg. Gyn. & Obst.* **61**, 693–705.

Hofmann A. (1978) The enterohepatic circulation of bile acids. In *Gastrointestinal Disease*, pp. 418–429. (Ed. by M. Sleisenger & J.S. Fordtran). W.B. Saunders, London.

Hofmann A.F. Thomas P.J., Smith L.H. & McCall J.T. (1970). Pathogenesis of secondary hyperoxaluria in patients with ileal resection and diarrhea. *Gastroenterol.* **58**, 960.

Hughes C.A., Bates T. & Dowling R.H. (1978) Cholecystokinin and secretin prevent the intestinal mucosal hypoplasia of total parenteral nutrition in the dog. *Gastroenterol.* **75**, 34–41.

Jackson W.P.U. (1958) Massive resection of the small intestine. In *Modern Trends in Gastroenterology*, ser. 2, p. 243. (Ed. by F. Avery Jones). Butterworths, London.

Jeejeebhoy K.N., Zohrab W.J., Langer B., Phillips M.J., Kuksis A. & Anderson G.H. (1973) Total parenteral nutrition at home for 23 months, without complication, and with good rehabilitation. A study of technical and metabolic features. *Gastroenterol.* **65**, 811–820.

Juhl E., Danø P. & Quaade F (1979) Shunt operations for obesity. *Clin. in Gastroenterol.* **8**, 386–397.

Keren D.F., Elliott H.L., Brown G.D. & Yardley J.H. (1975) Atrophy of villi with hypertrophy and hyperplasia of Paneth cells in isolated (Thiry-Vella) ileal loops in rabbits: light-microscopic studies. *Gastroenterol.* **68**, 83–93.

Kinney J.M., Goldwyn R.M., Barr J.S. & Moore F.D. (1961) Loss of the entire jejunum and ileum and the ascending colon. Management of a patient. *J. Amer. Med. Assoc.* **179**, 529–532.

Koeberle M. (1880) Resection de deux metres d'intestine grêle. *Bull. de l'Acad. Med.* **12**, 128–131.

Kogan E., Schapira A., Janomitz H.D. & Adlersberg D. (1957) Malabsorption following extensive small intestinal resection, including inadvertent gastroileostomy. *J. Mt. Sinai Hosp.* **24**, 399–424.

Lack L. & Weiner I.M. (1961) In vitro absorption of bile salts by small intestine of rats and guinea pigs. *Amer. J. Physiol.* **200**, 313–317.

Landor J.H. (1969) Intestinal resection and gastric secretion in dogs with antrectomy. *Arch. Surg.* **98**, 645–646.

Loran M.R. & Carbone J.V. (1968) The humoral effect of intestinal resection on cellular proliferation and maturation in parabiotic rats. *Gastrointestinal Radiation Injury*, pp. 127–139. (Ed. by M.F. Sullivan) Excerpta Medica, Amsterdam.

McCarthy D.M. & Kim Y.S. (1973) Changes in sucrase, enterokinase and peptide hydrolase after intestinal resection. The association of cellular hyperplasia and adaptation. *J. Clin. Invest.* **52**, 942–951.

Meyer H.W. (1946) Acute superior mesenteric artery thrombosis: Recovery following extensive resection of the small and large intestines. *Arch. Surg. (Chicago)* **53**, 298–303.

Meyer H.W. (1954) Discussion of paper by Kremen, Linner and Nelson (1954) *Ann. Surg.* **140**, 447.

Panveliwalla D., Lewis B., Wootton I.D.P. & Tabaqchali S. (1970) Determination of individual bile acids in biological fluids by thin layer chromatography and fluorimetry. *J. Clin. Path.* **23**, 309–314.

Parkinson R.S. & Walker-Smith J.A. (1973) Short small bowel syndrome. *Med. J. Australia* **2**, 205–210.

Payne J.H. & DeWind L.T. (1969) Surgical treatment of obesity. *Amer. J. Surg.* **118**, 141–147.

Pertsemlidis D. & Kark A.E. (1974) Anti-peristaltic segments for the treatment of short bowel syndrome. *Amer. J. Gastroenterol.* **62**, 526–530.

Pilkington T.R.E., Gazet J.C., Ang L., Kalucy R.S. Crisp A.H. & Day S. (1976) Explanations for weight loss after ileo-jejunal bypass. *Brit. Med. J.* **i**, 1504–1505.

Porus R.L. (1965) Epithelial hyperplasia following massive small bowel resection. *Gastroenterol.* **48**, 753–757.

Powell-Jackson P.R., Maudgal D.P., Sharp D., Goldie A. & Maxwell J.D. (1979) Intestinal bacterial metabolism of protein and bile acids: role in pathogenesis of hepatic disease after jejuno-ileal surgery. *Brit. J. Surg.* **66**, 772–775.

Rault R. & Scribner B.H. (1977) Parenteral nutrition in the home. In *Progress in Gastroenterology*, pp. 545–562. (Ed. by G.B.J. Glass). Grune & Stratton, New York.

Remington M., Malagelades J-R., Zinsmeister A. & Fleming C.R. (1983) Abnormalities in gastrointestinal motor activity in patient with short bowel: effect of a synthetic opiate. *Gastroenterol.* **85**, 629–636.

Rudo N.D. & Rosenberg I.H. (1973) Chronic glucagon administration enhances intestinal transport in the rat. *Proc. Soc. Exp. Biol. Med.* **142**, 521–525.

Sagor, G.R., Ghatei, M.A., Al-Mukhtar, M.V.T., Wright, N.A. & Bloom, S.R. (1983) Evidence for a humoural mechanism after small intestine resection. Exclusion of gastrin but not enteroglucagon. *Gastroenterol.* **84**, 902–906.

Satoh T., Narisawa K., Konno T., Katoh T., Fujiyama J., Tomoe A., Metoki K., Hayasaka K., Tada K., Ishibashi M., Yamana N., Mitsuoka T. & Benno Y. (1982) D-lactic acidosis in two patients with short bowel syndrome: bacteriological analyses of the faecal flora. *Eur. J. Pediat.* **138**, 324–326.

Schmitz J., Rey F., Bresson J.L., Ricour C. & Rey J. (1980) Etude par perfusion intestinale de l'absorption des sucres après résection étendue du grêle. *Arch. Francaises Pediatr.* **37**, 491–495.

Schwartz M.K., Medmid A., Roberts K.A., Sleisenger M. & Rondell H.T. (1956) Fat and nitrogen metabolism in patient with massive small bowel resection. *Surg. Forum*, **6**, 385–390.

Scott H.W., Sandstead H.H., Brill A.B., Burk O.H. & Younger R.K. (1971) Experience with a new technique of intestinal bypass in the treatment of morbid obesity. *Ann. Surg.* **174**, 560–572.

Scott J., Batt R.M. & Peters T.J. (1979) Enhancement of ileal adaptation by prednisolone after proximal small bowel resection in the rat. *Gut*, **20**, 858–864.

Selig L.L., Winborn W.B. & Weser E. (1977) Effect

of small bowel resection on the gastric mucosa in the rat. *Gastroenterol.* **72**, 421.

Setchell K.D.R., Lawson A.M., Blackstock E.J. & Murphy G.M. (1982a). Diurnal change in serum unconjugated bile acids in normal men. *Gut*, **23**, 637–642.

Setchell K.D.R., Worthington J., Smith S.M. & Murphy G.M. (1982) Diurnal variation of unconjugated bile acid concentrations in the peripheral circulation of patients with ileal resection. *Falk Symposium No. 33 VII Int. Bile Acid Meeting.* Basle, 1982. Lancaster M.T.P. Press.

Shimoyama T., Kikuchi H. Press M. & Thompson G.R. (1973) Fatty acid composition of plasma proteins in control subjects and patients with malabsorption. *Gut*, **14**, 716–722.

Smith L.H., Fromm H. & Hofmann A.F. (1972) Acquired hyperoxaluria, nephrolithiasis and intestinal disease. Description of syndrome. *N. Engl. J. Med.* **286**, 1371–1375.

Tabaqchali S. (1970) Case study of a patient with massive intestinal resection. *7th Int. Congr. Clin. Chem., Geneva, 1969*, pp. 119–123. Karger, Basle.

Tilson M.D. & Wright H.K. (1972) The effect of resection of the small intestine upon the fine structure of intestinal epithelium. *Surg. Gynecol. Obstet.* **134**, 992–994.

Tompkins R.K., Waisman J., Watts CM-H. et al. (1977) Absence of mucosal atrophy in human small intestine after prolonged isolation. *Gastroenterol.* **73**, 1406–1409.

Urban E. & Weser E. (1980) Intestinal adaptation to bowel resection. *Adv. Intern. Med.* **26**, 265–291.

Uttental L.O., Batt R.M., Carter M.W. & Bloom S.R. (1982) Stimulation of DNA synthesis in cultured small intestine by partially purified enteroglucagon. *Regul. Pept.* **3**, 84.

Weinstein L.D., Shoemaker C.P. & Hersh T. et al. (1969) Enhanced intestinal absorption after small bowel resection in man. *Arch. Surg.* **99**, 560–562.

Weser E. & Hernandez M.H. (1971) Studies of small bowel adaptation after intestinal resection in the rat. *Gastroenterol.* **60**, 69–75.

Williamson R.C.N. (1978) Intestinal adaptation. Structural, functional and cytokinetic changes. *New Engl. J. Med.* **298**, 1393–1402.

Williamson R.C.N., Buchholtz T.W. & Malt R.A. (1978) Humoral stimulation of cell proliferation in small bowel after transection and resection. *Gastroenterol.* **75**, 249–254.

Wilmore D.W., Dudrick S.J., Daly J.M. & Vars H.M. (1971) The role of nutrition in the adaptation of the small intestine after massive resection. *Surg. Gynecol. Obstet.* **132**, 673.

Windsor C.W.O., Fejfar J. & Woodward D.A.K. (1969) Gastric secretion after massive small bowel resection. *Gut*, **10**, 779–786.

Woolf G.M., Miller C., Kurian R. & Jeejeebhoy K.N. (1983) Diet for patients with a short bowel: High fat or high carbohydrate. *Gastroenterol.* **84**, 823–828.

Wright, N.A., Watson, A., Morly, A. Appleton D., Marks J. & Douglas A. (1974). The measurement of cell production rate in the crypts of Lieberkühn. *Virchows Archiv. Pathol. Anat. Histol.* **304**, 311–323.

Wright N.A. & Irwin M. (1982) The kinetics of villus cell populations in mouse small intestine. 1. Normal villi: the steady-state requirement. *Cell Tiss. Kinet.* **15**, 595–609.

Chapter 7
Food-Allergic Disorders

ANNE FERGUSON

Introduction and definitions 118
The intestinal immune system 119
Hypersensitivity reactions 123
Techniques for clinical investigation of
intestinal immunity and food allergy 125
Food-allergic diseases 127

Introduction and definitions

Whereas most of the cells of the body have a sterile environment, the luminal aspect of the gastrointestinal tract epithelium is continuously exposed to a large variety of living and non-living antigens, the majority of which are harmless. Active, vigorous immune responses to these antigens would be counter-productive and even potentially harmful, and so it is hardly surprising that in vertebrates the gut-associated lymphoid tissues have properties and functions quite distinct from the systemic immune apparatus. In health, there is substantial inhibition and suppression of immune responses in the wall of the gut. However, the individual does retain the capacity for many local and systemic, specific and non-specific immune responses to enteric pathogens.

The term 'allergy' was originally used by von Pirquet, to mean altered host reactivity to an antigen. This encompasses the whole spectrum of immune responses, but now allergy has a completely different meaning, and is used by immunologists as a synonym for 'hypersensitivity'. Hypersensitivity is defined as 'the state of a previously immunized body in which tissue damage results from the immune reaction to a further dose of antigen' (Herbert & Wilkinson 1977). Hypersensitivity may be antibody-mediated, as in immediate hypersensitivity or in the Arthus reaction, or it may be a reaction of cell-mediated immunity, as in delayed hypersensitivity.

Immunologically mediated tissue damage in the small intestine can be envisaged ultimately as the result of a disturbance in the normal inhibitory patterns of immune responses in the gut. An 'innocent bystander' effect causes damage of healthy tissues in association with the immune response to pathogens in many infectious diseases; immunological mechanisms mediate tissue damage in ulcerative colitis and Crohn's disease, two idiopathic inflammatory states in which no antigen has been identified; autoimmune damage to the small intestine is now being seriously considered as a cause of intractable diarrhoea; and immune responses to foods, and other enteric antigens are thought to be implicated in the pathogenesis of a variety of conditions loosely termed 'food allergic diseases'.

Immune reactions and allergy cannot be considered separately from the digestive functions of the intestine. The presence of proteins and other antigens within its lumen influence the digestive functions of motility, secretion, absorption and elimination; these in turn alter the amounts and distributions of antigen by dilution, neutralization and onward propulsion. Maldigestion and malabsorption increase the length of small intestine exposed to any food antigen and are likely therefore to influence the severity of disease in food protein-associated enteropathies. Finally, as discussed below in the section on hypersensitivity, local immune reactions have significant effects on the histopathology and function of the small intestinal mucosa.

Food intolerance and food allergy

A spectrum of disease mechanisms may be implicated when a patient complains that he or she is intolerant to food, or when a clinician suspects that a symptom or disease state is related to diet. There may be merely dislike or distaste of the substance concerned, although a pathological degree of food fadism occasionally exists. Many foods will precipitate symptoms of disease — for example a fatty meal may lead to the biliary colic of cholelithiasis; or gastrointestinal symptoms may be provoked by the ingestion of fats or carbohydrates in some patients with malabsorptive disorders. Allergic reactions to food antigens may cause disease, either in the gastrointestinal tract or systemically. Finally, toxic, allergic or biochemical events may be the result of adverse reactions to additives or contaminants in foodstuffs.

Considerable controversy and indeed scepticism surrounds the whole subject of food intolerance and food allergy. Symptoms reported by some patients and attributed to food intolerance, are often vague and unmeasurable and clinical descriptions are frequently anecdotal.

In order that doctors, paramedical personnel and patients can communicate about this emotive subject, it is essential that agreement be reached on working definitions which include clinical features, physical signs, results of laboratory investigations and pathogenetic mechanisms. The terminology that follows was proposed by participants at the First Food Allergy Workshop (Jackson 1980) and is strongly recommended.

Food intolerance

This is the term used to describe abnormal, adverse reactions to ingested foods. The term embraces both allergic and non-allergic adverse responses, and should always be used when the underlying mechanism is unknown.

Food idiosyncrasy

If the mechanism for food intolerance is known to be non-immunological (usually a biochemical defect), the term food idiosyncrasy should be used. The defect may be local as with deficiency of the enterocyte brush border enzyme lactase, which causes lactose intolerance; or systemic as with the deficiency of phenylalanine hydroxylase in patients with phenylketonuria. Reactions to certain foodstuffs which contain large amounts of histamine, or which produce direct liberation of histamine within the tissues of the gastrointestinal tract, should also be described as food idiosyncrasy.

Food-allergic disease

The adverse clinical response to ingestion of food shown to be the result of hypersensitivity may be classified as a food-allergic disease (or disorder). The interaction between antigen and antibody or lymphocyte may occur locally in the gut, or may be systemic. The hypersensitivity reaction may be mediated by antibody or immunocyte. Thus, the time course of the adverse reaction may range from hours to days, and the onset of symptoms or signs may be immediate or delayed. Rarely (coeliac disease is an example) weeks or months elapse between the time when the foodstuff is introduced into the diet and development of the typical intestinal lesion.

The intestinal immune system

In the early 1960s, two lines of evidence indicated the existence of a distinct mucosal immune system — the dimeric form of IgA in secretions (Tomasi *et al.* 1965) and the traffic of immunoblasts from the bloodstream to the lamina propria of the gut (Gowans & Knight 1964). The concept of a mucosal-associated lymphoid system has now been extended to encompass the gastrointestinal, respiratory, genital and urinary tracts, the eye, salivary glands and breast. The immune system of the small intestine comprises Peyer's patches and other follicles, with their associated epithelium; lymph nodes of the mesentery; intraepithelial and lamina propria lymphoid cells; and secretory immunoglobulins. In addition, the constituents of the systemic immune apparatus also contribute to intestinal immunity, particularly in disease and when there is inflammation. Small peripheral T and B lymphocytes, serum immunoglobulins and complement components are present in the blood which circulates in the capillaries of the gut. Immunoglobulins of the serum penetrate the extracellular fluid spaces of the lamina propria and epithelium and may ooze into the lumen of the intestine. It is not known whether luminal lymphocytes and macrophages survive or have any specific immunological role.

Antigens and intestinal permeability

The induction of intestinal immune responses depends on exposure of the mucosal lymphoid tissues to enteric antigen. *Antigens* are substances that elicit specific immune responses when introduced into the tissues of an animal. If an antigen is to stimulate an immune response in a human being it will normally be foreign to the person to whom it is administered, of molecular weight greater than 1000, and of protein or polysaccharide nature. An organism such as a bacterium will contain many hundreds of different antigens and even a single protein molecule may bear on its surface several different antigenic determinants. A *hapten* is a substance that can initiate an immune response only if it is bound to a carrier molecule before or after introduction into the body. Most haptens are small molecules of molecular weight less than 1000 and carry only one or two antigenic determinants. They can, however, combine with antibody even in the absence of a carrier. Clearly, in addition to the enormous variety of antigens present in foods, many foods and food additives also have the potential to act as haptens.

There are two main routes by which antigens cross the intestinal epithelium to enter the tissues of the body:
1 via the Peyer's patch epithelium, through the cytoplasm of specialized M cells of the follicle-associated epithelium, and
2 through the epithelium of the villi and crypts, intracellularly or intercellularly.

There is an increasing body of evidence that it is the antigen which crosses the follicle-associated epithelium to reach the organized lymphoid tissues of Peyer's patches, which is most relevant to induction of specific immune responses (Cebra *et al.* 1977). It is not yet known whether or how antigen absorbed across the villus epithelium may act in induction of immunity. Current clinical and experimental investigations of absorption of antigen can be criticized in that rarely is there differentiation between the Peyer's patch and mucosal routes, and little account is taken of potential changes in immunogenicity of absorbed protein, associated with digestion and absorption. Also, only a proportion of antigen which crosses the intestinal epithelium reaches the bloodstream. For example, in an already immunized animal, the development of immune reactions between antigen and pre-formed antibody or previously sensitized lymphocyte may occur within the gut lumen, in the vicinity of the epithelium, in the lamina propria of the gut, within the bloodstream and, after systemic absorption, in other organs such as skin and lung.

The magnitude of absorption of antigens is technically difficult to establish. However, studies in mammals of all ages, including human infants and adults, have shown that when proteins are placed within the lumen of a segment of intestine either *in vivo*, or in a gut sac *in vitro*, immunogenic material crosses the wall of the gut to be detected either in blood or lymph *in vivo*, or at the serosal site of the cultured intestine *in vitro*. Antigens crossing the intestinal mucosal barrier have been shown to elicit IgE-class systemic immune responses in rats (Jarrett 1978) and reduction in the quantity of antigen absorbed across a segment of intestine has been demonstrated in previously orally immunized rodents (Walker *et al.* 1972, Swarbrick *et al.* 1979). It has also been found that intestinal uptake of large molecules is enhanced in animals infected with a helminth parasite or subjected to mild systemic or gastrointestinal anaphylaxis (Bloch *et al.* 1979, Roberts *et al.* 1981).

Whereas in most experiments, absorption of material of the order of 0.1—1% of administered protein has been found, Hemmings and his colleagues have reported much greater access of dietary proteins across the gut mucosa. For example in adult rats they reported that up to 40% of a dose of bovine gammaglobulin with a molecular weight in the range of 20,000–50,000 daltons was absorbed, and they claimed that tissue cells throughout the body were loaded with foreign protein of dietary origin. Its ultimate fate was to be degraded over a protracted period (Hemmings & Williams 1978). These surprising findings have not been confirmed and it is likely that small isotope-labelled fragments of exogenous protein were bound to native proteins after absorption, and thus mimicked macromolecules in the assay system used (Udall et al. 1981).

Immune responses to enteric antigen

There are several different immune responses to orally administered antigen, some of which are illustrated in Fig. 7.1. These are not mutually exclusive, and include:
1 induction of secretory antibody responses;
2 induction of systemic tolerance — specific hyporesponsiveness for IgG, IgE and cell-mediated immunity;
3 induction of active systemic immunity (humoral and cellular), especially in infants and in disease;
4 induction of mucosal cell-mediated immunity. (CMI)

Experiments in rodents, using new methods of identifying subsets of lymphocytes and other immunocytes, have revealed complex immunoregulatory networks mediated by helper and suppressor cells and soluble products (Reinhertz & Schlossman 1981). This regulation may be non-specific, antigen-specific or isotype-specific. In general, the feeding of an antigen has been found to lead to induction of mainly suppressor mechanisms, including induction of suppressor T cells in Peyer's patches. Against this background of inhibition there is a 'window' of help for secretory IgA which may be due to helper T cells for IgA production (Elson et al. 1979).

Secretory antibodies

Within a few days of feeding of an antigen, antibodies of IgA and to a lesser extent IgM classes are present in the intestinal secretions. Dimeric IgA antibodies also appear in bile, although there is considerable species variation in this phenomenon. The upper intestinal secretions of healthy children and adults contain antibodies to many commensal micro-organisms and to foods (Ferguson 1976).

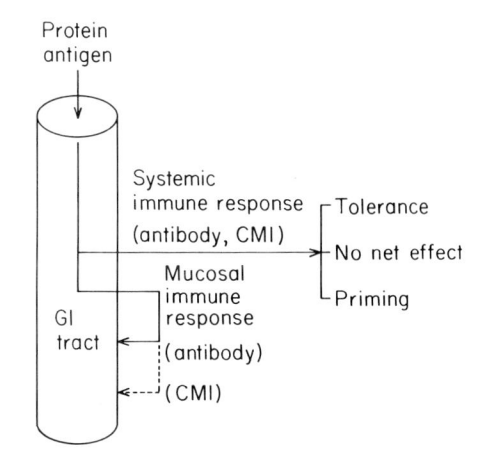

Fig. 7.1. Schematic diagram of the principal active and inhibitory immune responses to a fed protein antigen.

Serum antibodies

These are occasionally induced by the feeding of antigen but this is unusual. Exceptions include circulating antibodies to cow's milk antigens in the majority of young infants who have been bottle-fed; and circulating antibodies of IgG, A and M classes, to a variety of ingested foods in many patients with inflammatory gastrointestinal diseases (Ferguson 1976).

Cell-mediated immunity

By the usual techniques, such as skin tests, lymphocyte transformation and studies of leucocyte migration inhibition in the presence of antigen, tests of cell-mediated immunity to foods are usually negative in food allergic disorders. The detection of lymphocytes, sensitized to gluten, in patients with coeliac disease, is an important exception.

Immunological tolerance

It has been recognized for more than half a century that feeding of antigen may induce a state of systemic immunological tolerance (Wells & Osborne 1911). Tolerance is regularly produced by contact with antigen in early postnatal life or fetal life and by administration of very high or very low doses of certain antigens intravenously. Immunological reactions to unrelated antigenic substances are not affected by induction of tolerance. The induction and maintenance of oral tolerance are still incompletely understood. It is likely that more than one mechanism is involved in this important homeostatic function of the gut, and there is evidence to support roles of circulating antigen−antibody complexes (Andre et al. 1975), anti-idiotypic antibody (Kagnoff 1980) and specific suppressor T cells (Miller & Hanson 1979, Mowat et al. 1982).

Oral tolerance in man

All diseases due to food allergy can be envisaged as resulting from inefficient oral tolerance. There have been no definitive studies to document oral tolerance in the human species, but three published studies suggest that this probably does exist in man. These concern application of dinitrochlorobenzine to the buccal mucus membrane of prison volunteers (Lowney 1968), absence of an antibody response to parenterally injected milk protein in many adults (Korenblat et al. 1968) and poor response to tetanus vaccination in Indians, presumed to have chronic clostridial contamination of the small intestine (Dastur et al. 1981). The following report demonstrates the absence of an immune response to parenterally administered cow's milk in a British adult — circumstantial evidence of the existence of oral tolerance.

> A 34-year-old man was admitted to hospital with an exacerbation of duodenal ulcer, and treated with sedation, intravenous fluids and intermittent nasogastric suction. A 'milk drip' was ordered (the intention being to administer milk intragastrically). Inadvertently, the patient received 100 ml of pasteurized milk intravenously. The subsequent effects, including disseminated intravascular coagulation and fat embolism, were successfully treated with corticosteroids, antibiotics and heparin. Sera taken at intervals up to 2 months after this parenteral immunization with milk were examined for antibodies to cow's milk proteins, by precipitin and passive haemagglutination techniques. No antibodies were demonstrated.

Comment This patient appears to have immunological tolerance (specific non-reactivity) to cow's milk protein antigens — one of the few clinical documentations in man of oral tolerance (Wallace, Payne & Mack 1972).

T cells and immunoregulation

T cells are thought to originate from a common pluripotential haematopoietic stem cell, and their subsequent maturation depends on the environment of the thymus and on presentation of antigen. Systemic T cells are of three main types — helper (T_H), suppressor cytotoxic ($T_{S/CT}$) and those responsible for delayed type hypersensitivity (T_{DTH}). Although T cells are classified by function, different subsets can be recognized by cell surface markers (Reinherz & Schlossman 1981). Within Peyer's patches conditions are optimal for T-cell interactions with antigens. In addition to populations of gut-associated T cells, the Peyer's patches also contain precursors of lamina propria B lymphocytes. After antigenic stimulation, T and B cells pass via lymph and mesenteric lymph nodes into thoracic duct and bloodstream, and then home back to the intestinal mucosa where the B cells develop into IgA-secreting plasma cells (and perhaps plasma cells of other isotypes) and where the T cells can be recognized as mainly intraepithelial lymphocytes (Guy-Grand et al. 1974). Figure 7.2 outlines the known traffic routes of Peyer's patch T and B cells, and provides the basis for hypothetical immunoregulation of

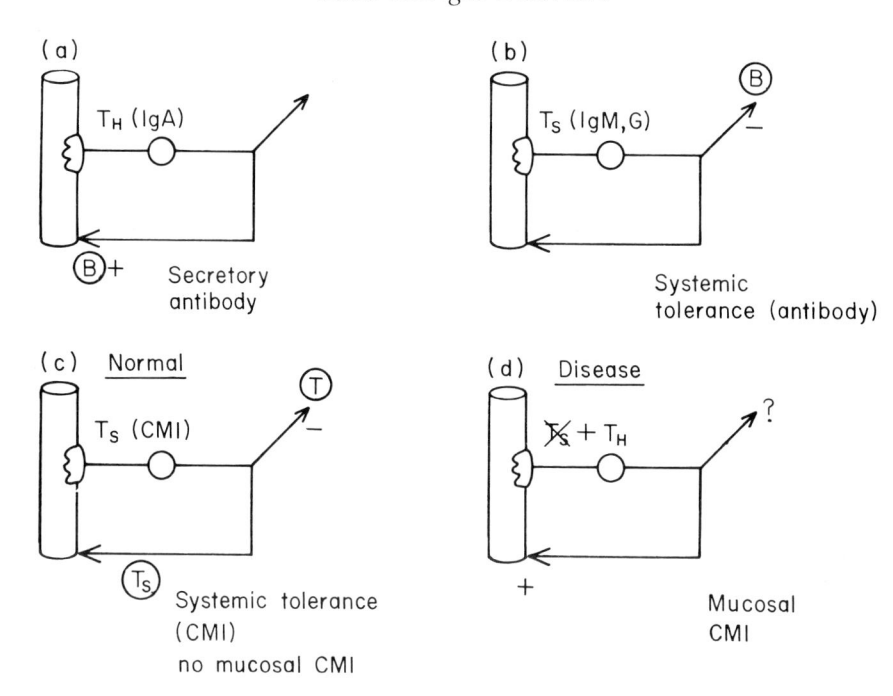

Fig. 7.2. Known and postulated traffic routes of T and B lymphocytes induced by the feeding of antigen. T_H—T helper lymphocyte; T_S—T suppressor lymphocyte; B—B lymphocyte. CMI—cell-mediated immunity.
(a) After antigenic stimulation precursors of lamina propria IgA-secreting plasma cells pass via the lymph into the thoracic duct, home back to the mucosa and develop into IgA-secreting plasma cells. At the same time antigen-specific T_H–IgA cells are activated, leading to induction of secretory IgA antibodies.
(b) Simultaneous with T_H–IgA induction there is specific T_S activation for IgG and IgM B cells and plasma cells. This is one of the mechanisms of specific systemic tolerance after feeding antigen.
(c) At the same time there is induction of specific T_S cells, responsible for suppression of CMI responses in the gut, thus, normally, protecting the gut from deleterious mucosal CMI with associated enteropathy.
(d) This illustrates likely events in intestinal disease. If induction of T_S is prevented, systemic immunization and mucosal CMI responses may result. The same net effect may occur if T_H for systemic or mucosal responses are activated.

mucosal and systemic immune responses by T lymphocytes. Antigen, presented to T cells by macrophages within the Peyer's patches (and possibly also mesenteric nodes) leads to induction of antigen specific T_H for the IgA system, and T_S for other immunoglobulin isotypes and for CMI, is the postulated mechanism of immunoregulation of all of the different types of immune response to fed antigen. Normal T-cell responses are the mechanism of protection against development of food allergic diseases and other intestinal mucosal hypersensitivity states. This is well illustrated by a report of a patient with immunodeficiency and evidence of defective T-suppressor functions, which was associated with auto- immune disease and enteropathy with diarrhoea and villous atrophy (Reinherz et al. 1979).

Hypersensitivity reactions

Tissue damage or disease, resulting from an immune reaction (hypersensitivity, allergy) may occur as an unavoidable side-effect of a protective immune response or as a primary pathological event. The reaction is triggered by the interaction of antigen with antibody or immunocyte, and the tissue damage is mediated either by soluble factors, by activated polymorphonuclear leucocytes, macrophages or by direct membrane effects between the immune cell and antigen on the membrane of another cell. The various types of hypersensitivity are not mutually exclusive since the time course of their development varies according to the type and to the antigen concerned. They may occur all at once or in sequence (Walker 1984).

The effects of humoral and cell-mediated immune reactions in the small intestinal mucosa have been studied in several experimental models, and results have been collated and are presented in detail elsewhere (Ferguson & Mowat 1980, Strobel & Ferguson, 1982).

Reaginic hypersensitivity

This is associated mainly with antibodies of the IgE class, although some IgG_4 antibodies may have a similar effect. The IgE antibodies are synthesized by plasma cells but the immunoglobulin is present in exceptionally small amounts in serum for IgE has a propensity to adhere to mast cells and basophils by a specialized area of the heavy chains. Mast cell granules are extruded into the extracellular space when an appropriate antigen interacts with two IgE molecules attached to the cell membrane. From these granules come the histamine, serotonin, slow-reacting substance of anaphylaxis and eosinophil chemotactic factor of anaphylaxis mediating the inflammatory reaction. Mast cell degranulation can be prevented pharmacologically by the use of drugs such as sodium cromoglycate.

Parasite infection is the commonest cause of reaginic hypersensitivity in the gut. Reaginic hypersensitivity has also been implicated in various syndromes associated with food allergy, with the malabsorption syndrome of cow's milk intolerance in children, in idiopathic protein-losing enteropathy and possibly in ulcerative colitis.

The inflammation associated with a Type 1, reaginic local reaction may be necessary to create the appropriate conditions for the further development of other types of hypersensitivity involving antigen–antibody complexes and cells.

Membrane reactive (cytotoxic) hypersensitivity

Antibody, interacting with antigen on the cell membrane, may occasionally have a cell stimulant effect. This is thought to be part of the pathogenesis of thyrotoxicosis. More frequently, interaction between antibody- and membrane-associated antigen causes cell lysis and local inflammation, with the involvement of complement components and polymorphs. In the gut it has been suggested that membrane reactive antibodies may cause the tissue damage of ulcerative colitis, antigens concerned being either auto-antigens or cell surface antigens which cross react with those of *Escherichia coli*.

Immune complex hypersensitivity

Normally, the combination of antigen with antibody results in destruction of the antigen, phagocytosis of the antigen–antibody complex and rapid clearance of both the antigen and the complexes from the circulation or from the tissue fluids. Under certain circumstances immune complexes may persist in the tissues and initiate a number of non-specific inflammatory reactions involving complement and polymorph activation. These harmful immune complexes form when there is antigen excess, if there is a persistent source of antigen or if the antibody has poor affinity so that the complexes are not taken up by cells of the reticuloendothelial system.

Immune complexes have been shown to appear in the tissues of the small bowel, and in the bloodstream when patients with cow's milk intolerance are challenged with cow's milk and when some patients with treated coeliac disease have been challenged with gluten. Tests for immune complexes in the circulation are frequently positive in a wide range of inflammatory small and large bowel diseases but the nature of the antigen within the complexes has not been defined. It is likely that in any situation where the intestinal tract is 'leaky', food and microbial antigens cross the mucosal barrier and form immune complexes with the appropriate antibodies in the circulation. From time to time these immune complexes are deposited in the tissues and this is the cause of iritis, uveitis, erythema nodosum and arthritis which may complicate the clinical course of some patients with inflammatory bowel disease.

T-cell hypersensitivity

T-cell hypersensitivity involves both direct cytotoxicity by the T cell in response to cell membrane antigens and the secretion of lymphocyte activation factors, lymphokines. Delayed hypersensitivity reactions develop in days rather than hours after challenge, and typical examples are the Mantoux reaction, contact dermal sensitivity and rejection of transplanted organs. The intestinal mucosa is the target of this type of reaction in graft-versus-host disease, and when an intestinal allograft is rejected. In animal models of both of these conditions, striking changes have been demonstrated in small intestinal architecture and lymphoid cell infiltrate (MacDonald & Ferguson 1977, Mowat & Ferguson 1982). The increased intraepithelial lymphocyte infiltrate and crypt hyperplasia with villous atrophy are indirect measures of the existence of a local delayed hypersensitivity reaction and this is of value in interpretation of jejunal biopsy changes after antigen challenge in patients investigated for possible food hypersensitivity (Ferguson 1978).

Techniques for clinical investigation of intestinal immunity and food allergy

The study of clinical immunology in the gastrointestinal tract has developed more slowly than that of systemic immunity. However, although in comparison to blood the secretions and tissues of the intestines are relatively inaccessible, there has recently been considerable progress in this facet of immunology, and several techniques are now available for investigation of gastrointestinal immune functions. It is, however, important to study intestinal immunity in parallel with an evaluation of systemic immunity.

Systemic immune status

Useful background information is obtained from the clinical interview and examination. For example there may be history of normal recovery from childhood infections and vaccinations, the existence of diseases in the patient or his family which are known to affect immunity, or conditions associated with aberrant immune function (sarcoidosis, autoimmune diseases, lymphoma, atopy). On clinical examination the presence of palpable lymph nodes, visible tonsils, a normal thymus on chest X-ray and a vigorous inflammatory response at the site of an infection, will all provide evidence of a normal, competent and protective systemic immune system.

General laboratory investigations are also useful. Simple tests such as absolute peripheral blood lymphocyte count and eosinophil count, or skin tests for delayed hypersensitivity, are often omitted but give valuable background information. The presence or absence of atopy can be established from the history and by skin tests with a battery of allergens.

Gastrointestinal immunity

Various tests which provide information on gastrointestinal immunity are summarized in Table 7.1. These must, however, be interpreted in the knowledge of the intestinal antigen exposure at the time of biopsy, venepuncture or collection of secretions — for example, jejunal biopsy is usually performed after an overnight fast, and evidence of immediate hypersensitivity reactions would be unlikely to be present. The rapid turnover of enterocytes, particularly in patients with crypt hyperplasia, means that the epithelium covering the surface of a flat, coeliac-like mucosa will have emerged from the crypts during the night and is unlikely to have been exposed to any food antigens. This factor is often ignored when mechanisms such as immune-complex-mediated

Table 7.1. Methods for investigation of intestinal immunity.

Investigation technique	Comments
Secretion immunoglobulins	Assays in salivary gastrointestinal secretions or faeces are technically difficult and require secretory IgA standards.
Specific antibodies in secretions	Techniques appropriate for serum antibodies may not be satisfactory,
Serum antibodies to antigens normally present in the lumen of the gut	High serum antibody titres to commensal gut bacteria or foods indicate the existence either of abnormal permeability of the intestinal mucosa or of abnormal immunoregulation. Changes in antibody titre can be used to monitor clinical and histological improvement in inflammatory diseases such as coeliac disease.
Cell-mediated immunity	No standard tests are available. Secretion of lymphokine-like substances by cultured intestinal biopsies has been documented in research studies in coeliac patients.
Histology of lymphoid constituents of biopsies	There are various techniques for staining and counting intraepithelial and lamina propria lymphocytes and other immunocytes. Patchy distribution of these cells within the mucosa may occur, so multiple sites should be sampled.
Distribution of plasma cells of major immunoglobulin classes	These can be counted by using immunofluorescence or immunoenzyme staining techniques.
Evidence of current immune reactions	This may be obtained from interpretation of conventional histology — oedema, eosinophil infiltration etc. — and immune complexes can be detected by electron microscopy or immunofluorescence.

damage are discussed in relation to coeliac disease and other enteropathies.

Static investigations, performed on a single occasion, are limited in the study of the dynamics of intestinal hypersenstivity reactions. Much more information accrues when serial studies are performed at intervals after antigen challenge or in the weeks after initiation of dietary or other treatment.

Diagnosis of food allergy

In order to establish the diagnosis of a food-allergic disease, it is necessary to show, by clinical means, that food intolerance exists. Only then can the mechanism, via an allergic reaction to the food in question, be confirmed. Unfortunately laboratory tests have proved of little value. Clinical diagnosis of food intolerance depends on objective measurements of symptoms and disease activity before and after withdrawal of the food in question, and before and after controlled re-introduction. Since alterations in the nature, quality and quantity of food have profound effects on gastrointestinal physiology it is essential to combine immuno-logical investigation of food intolerance with full, conventional assessment of gastrointestinal function.

Reagins — IgE class antibodies

The presence of reaginic antibodies can be inferred from positive *in vivo* prick tests, and can be demonstrated *in vitro* by the radioallergosorbent technique (RAST) applied to serum. Both of these depend, ultimately, on the quality and range of antigens available in commercial preparations. IgE anti-food antibodies are not normally found in the serum of children or adults. When they do occur, it is usual to find IgE antibodies to many foods, and often exceptionally high titres of IgE antibodies to inhalents such as house dust mite and animal danders (Barnetson *et al.* 1981). A high value for total serum IgE, and positive prick tests or RASTs to foodstuffs do increase the likelihood of food allergy but unfortunately the foods concerned in an individual patient cannot be predicted from the pattern of antibodies detected.

Anti-food antibodies of other immunoglobulin classes are present in low titres in the serum of normal children and adults, and are also present in intestinal secretions (Ferguson 1976). Although work continues, particularly in coeliac disease, in an attempt to correlate the presence of a specific anti-food antibody with the existence of disease, the presence of serum antibodies to foods is only of value as an index of the existence of some aberration in immunoregulation or in antigen exposure — for example the existence of inflammatory disease of the intestine such as coeliac disease or jejunal Crohn's disease. A high titre of serum anti-food antibody, whether detected by precipitin, haemagglutination, immuno-fluorescence or ELISA techniques, has no relationship to the presence or absence of allergy to the foodstuff concerned. Coeliac patients have high titres of antibodies to many antigens, to which they are completely tolerant, and after treatment of coeliac disease with a gluten-free diet, the serum antibodies to other foods such as eggs and milk drops significantly in titre despite their continuing ingestion (Ferguson & Carswell 1972, Carswell & Ferguson 1973).

Tests for cell-mediated immunity to foods may ultimately be of value in the diagnosis of malabsorption syndromes associated with food-allergic reactions, but are not yet available for clinical use.

Food-allergic diseases

There are many conditions in which, at least in some patients, a food-allergic reaction is likely to be the primary pathogenesis. Examples of food-allergic diseases are listed in Table 7.2. These can be grouped into a limited number of patterns of clinical presentation and, although the small intestine is likely to be involved in most patients, as the site of antigen penetration into the body, only a minority of patients with food-allergic diseases have symptoms and signs of involvement of the small intestine.

Acute food-related reactions

Many people are aware of a clear relation-

Table 7.2. Food-allergic diseases.

Systemic anaphylaxis
Rhinitis
Conjunctivitis
Asthma
Allergic alveolitis
Coeliac disease
Cow's milk protein enteropathy
Urticaria
Angio-oedema
Atopic eczema
Dermatitis herpetiformis

ship, on repeated occasions, between ingestion of small amounts of a specific food and the development of symptoms such as vomiting, diarrhoea, urticaria or headache. However, even when there are features to indicate that mast-cell-derived mediators are producing the clinical reaction, the diagnosis will not always be of food allergy, for some foods lead to mast cell degranulation directly, and other individuals are highly sensitive to the effects of histamine in ingested foods such as cheeses, shellfish and red wine. Where good test material is available and antigenic preparations are well standardized and validated, skin prick tests, RASTs and other immunological techniques may produce supporting evidence for allergy in a particular individual who has well-documented food intolerance.

Role of foods in patients with severe atopic disease

Patients with atopic diseases, such as eczema and asthma, often recognize a clear-cut clinical relationship between exposure to inhaled or ingested allergens and exacerbation of symptoms or the development of new, acute reactions. Although inhalants have been most extensively studied, there is limited evidence, from a few well-studied patients, that exacerbation of systemic atopic disease can be produced by ingestion of specific foods (Brostoff et al. 1979). Food allergy has been shown to be a major contributory factor in atopic eczema in children (Atherton 1981) and immune responses to foods are also strikingly abnormal in adult atopic eczema (Barnetson et al. 1981). Intractable asthma occasionally responds to treatment with an elimination diet (Hoj et al. 1981).

Malabsorption syndromes and idiopathic diarrhoea

Dietary protein intolerance has been clearly implicated as a cause of malabsorption, chronic diarrhoea and failure to thrive in infants and young children (Walker-Smith 1979). Evidence that this intolerance is due to allergy to food protein is still circumstantial but compelling, and includes the clear association of cow's milk protein sensitive enteropathy with atopy (Kuitunen et al. 1975), the fact that the features of intestinal pathology after antigen challenge are similar to those described above for intestinal delayed hypersensitivity reactions (Walker-Smith 1979) and the existence of similar dietary protein intolerance in large domestic animals, clearly associated with abnormal immune reactions to soya and other dietary proteins (Barratt et al. 1978, Kilshaw & Slade, in press).

Intolerance to cow's milk

The use of jejunal biopsy in the investigation of children with chronic diarrhoea is central to the recognition of dietary protein intolerance as a cause of malabsorption, as illustrated in the following case report. Since the clinical presentation and jejunal biopsy pathology are very similar to untreated coeliac disease, it is often only in retrospect that the diagnosis of transient food protein intolerance rather than permanent gluten intolerance is made.

> A female infant had been small for dates, weighing only 2.5 kg at birth with evidence of dysmaturity. She was bottle-fed from birth. At the age of 2 months she developed acute diarrhoea and vomiting after contact with two known cases of gastroenteritis. The diarrhoea lasted for 4 days and thereafter she failed to thrive, with intermittent vomiting and diarrhoea. Gluten-containing solids were introduced into her diet at the age of 3 months.
>
> On admission to hospital at the age of 4 months she had a protuberant abdomen, wasted buttocks and a provisional diagnosis of coeliac disease. However, small intestinal biopsy (Fig. 7.3a) showed short wide villi, lengthening of the crypts, columnar surface epithelium and normal numbers of intraepithelial lymphocytes. Serum immunoglobulins G, A and M were normal. Intradermal skin tests were positive to lactalbumin, casein and whole cow's milk.
>
> She was treated with nutramigen and a cow's milk-free diet, with immediate relief of symptoms and gain of weight. Four months later a repeat small intestinal biopsy (Fig. 7.3b) was normal, and while still on a cow's milk-free diet she had a cow's milk challenge. After 24 h there was profuse vomiting and diarrhoea, blood in the stools and a third small intestinal biopsy (Fig. 7.3c) showed severe mucosal damage with lengthening of the crypts and an abnormal surface epithelium. She was returned to a diet free of cow's milk.
>
> At the age of 1 year 6 months she was returned to a normal diet containing cow's milk, and thrived thereafter without symptoms.

Intolerance to soya protein

In 1972 Ament and Rubin demonstrated soya protein intolerance in a child who had malabsorption and a flat jejunal mucosa. After successful treatment with a soya-free diet, challenge produced a flat small intestinal mucosa indistinguishable from that seen in coeliac disease.

Idiopathic diarrhoea

Some children and adults with chronic diarrhoea have entirely normal intestinal histopathology, and investigations of intestinal absorption are also normal. This idiopathic diarrhoea is currently classified as part of the 'irritable bowel syndrome'. However, one of two trials of oral sodium cromoglycate therapy in idiopathic diarrhoea showed benefit from this drug (Bolin 1980, Ferguson & Gillon 1981). Occasionally, empirical elimination of allergens such as milk or eggs cures idiopathic diarrhoea in an atopic individual. A recent report from Holland suggests that counts of IgE containing plasma cells may be of value in identifying food-allergic patients (Rosekrans et al. 1980). Clearly, further investigation of intestinal immunity in patients with idiopathic diarrhoea is warranted.

Idiopathic inflammatory bowel disease

Food-allergic reactions can produce acute and chronic inflammation of the mucosa of the gastrointestinal tract, and may also exacerbate inflammation when the epithelium is ulcerated so that food antigens are in direct contact with tissue antibodies and lymphocytes. Elemental diet therapy and intravenous feeding are of clinical value in patients with Crohn's disease, and it is theoretically possible that at least part of the benefit is due to the hypoallergenic nature of such therapy (Logan et al. 1981). Nevertheless, food-allergic reactions are unlikely to be the primary pathogenetic mechanisms in patients with classical Crohn's disease or ulcerative colitis.

The apparent clinical benefit in some series, of oral sodium cromoglycate therapy in ulcerative colitis, led to a reappraisal of the evidence for intestinal allergic reactions in this disease. If, in a minority of patients, a diffuse inflammatory state involving both the small and large intestine is produced by allergic reactions to enteric contents including foods, sodium cromoglycate treatment or elimination diet may be likely to be of benefit, and clinical investigations might well lead to a diagnosis of idiopathic inflammatory bowel disease, based on the usual criteria of histopathology of a rectal biopsy and findings on examination by barium enema. The following illustrates a patient who fulfilled diagnostic criteria for ulcerative colitis but in whom jejunal biopsy

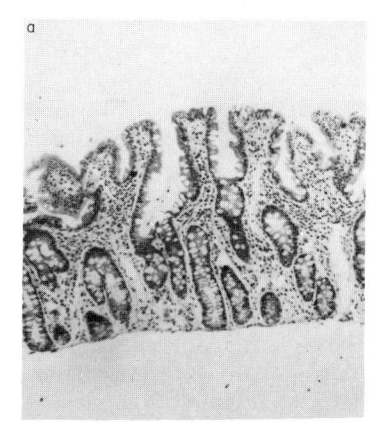

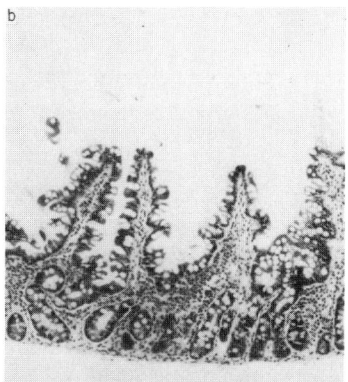

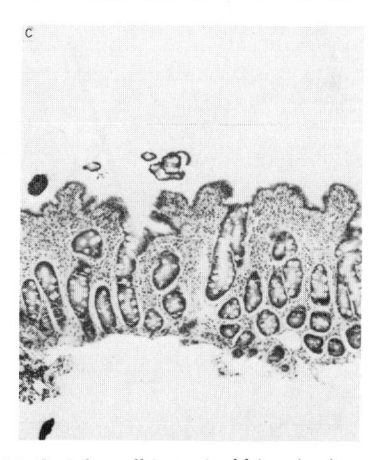

Fig. 7.3. Serial small intestinal biopsies in cow's milk intolerance (a) at diagnosis; (b) after a period on cow's milk-free diet; and (c) 24 h after cow's milk challenge. (Illustrations provided by Dr J.A. Walker-Smith.) (× 87)

pathology was abnormal in having an excess of intraepithelial lymphocytes, and whose subsequent clinical course supports the diagnosis of a diffuse allergic low grade enterocolitis.

> A 13-year-old boy had a history of atopic disease dating from infancy. He was adopted, and bottle-fed. Eczema had been present since age 7 weeks. Multi-system atopic disease had been present since then and included atopic eczema, asthma, hay fever, vernal conjunctivitis and corneal ulcers. There was also a history of school refusal with fears of the aggressive behaviour of other school children. He presented as a gastrointestinal emergency with a 4-week history of abdominal pain, nausea, vomiting, intermittent diarrhoea, the stools containing mucus and blood. Relevant investigations included barium enema (Dr G.M. Fraser) which showed a granular appearance affecting the whole colon down to the proximal sigmoid. Barium follow-through was normal. At sigmoidoscopy the rectal mucosa appeared visually normal but histopathology showed erosion of surface epithelium, distorted and hyperchromatic crypts with marked loss of mucin, a heavy inflammatory cell infiltrate in the lamina propria with prominent lymphoid follicles. Jejunal biopsy was minimally abnormal, with an apparent reduction in the height of the villi with respect to the basal portion of the mucosa, excess intraepithelial lymphocyte infiltrate and a mild excess of lamina propria cells.
>
> A clinical diagnosis of idiopathic ulcerative colitis was made. He was initially treated with oral sodium cromoglycate with immediate relief of symptoms and normal growth, increasing his centiles from below the 25th to above the 50th. His systemic allergic diseases substantially improved within a month of starting sodium cromoglycate treatment.

Food intolerance and general malaise

Patients, and some doctors, believe without scientific evidence that a wide variety of rather vague but very common symptoms are due to food allergy. These include persistent fatigue, overweight, underweight, puffiness of hands, face and abdomen, palpitations, sweating, depression, anxiety states and confusion. Similarly it has been suggested that hyperactivity and enuresis in children are the result of allergy to ingested foods. Although symptoms such as irritability or bed-wetting in a child may be a non-specific response to ill health, and will improve when the primary disease state, such as atopic eczema, is improved by an elimination diet, there is no conclusive evidence that food allergy is a widespread and unrecognized condition. A sympathetic approach is necessary, however, in the management of the patient who has made a self-diagnosis of food allergy, if only to ensure that ultimately the patient is ingesting a nutritionally adequate diet. The uncertainty surrounding the concept of food intolerance highlights the importance in maintaining strict diagnostic criteria for food allergy.

Food intolerance in clinical practice

The importance of the various syndromes and symptom patterns described above can be put in perspective by summarizing the results of two recent reports, concerning children and adults investigated for possible food allergy.

Bock and colleagues (1978), from Denver USA, reported the results of their clinical investigation of sixty-eight children, aged between 5 months and 15 years. All of these had a history of adverse reaction to ingestion of one or more of the fourteen foods which were used in the study. Ninety-four double-blind food challenges were carried out with one or more of the fourteen foods concerned. Of children aged 3 years or more, only sixteen of forty-three had adverse reactions. All these reactions were precipitated by peanuts or other nuts, milk, egg and soya. Of twenty-five children aged less than 3 years, thirteen manifested adverse reactions during double-blind food challenges. Skin tests with locally prepared food extracts, applied by a puncture technique, were positive in the older group of children but in only ten of the children under 3 years. As a result of their experience these workers recommended that double-blind challenge should remain the indispensable tool for reaching an unequivocal diagnosis of food hypersensitivity in children.

Lessof et al. (1980), from Guy's Hospital in London, studied 100 patients who reacted adversely to one or more specific foods. In selecting patients they excluded a number with an identifiable non-allergic cause of food intolerance such as lactase deficiency, effects of caffeine in coffee drinkers, gallstones in an egg-intolerant patient. They also excluded a number of patients who had psychoneurotic illness and food fads. In 93 of 100 patients there were symptoms suggestive of an allergic reaction outside the intestinal tract — in sixty-four the features included asthma, eczema or both and in twenty-two the principal component was angio-oedema or urticaria. The remaining fourteen patients had predominantly abdominal symptoms and/or food-related paroxysms of rhinorrhoea. There were six patients with headaches, three with cough and one with joint pains. The range of foods which was found to be capable of causing symptoms on repeated challenge included milk (46% of the patients), egg (40%), nuts or peanuts (22%), fish or shellfish (22%). Less than 10% of the patients reacted to wheat, chocolate, artificial colourings, pork or bacon, chicken, tomato, soft fruits, cheese or yeast. The timecourse of a development of symptoms after food ingestion varied. Early manifestations included lip swelling, vomiting, rhinorrhoea and urticaria whereas diarrhoea, asthma and eczema tended to develop after a few hours. These authors found that a high proportion of patients who were intolerant to egg, fish or nuts had positive skin prick tests or RAST results whereas only 30% of the patients with milk intolerance had positive tests. This suggested that either methods for detection of IgE anti-milk antibodies were inadequate, or that there was a non-allergic cause for milk intolerance in many patients. Of particular interest, in relation to non-IgE-mediated food hypersensitivity, were five patients who were milk-intolerant, had negative skin and RAST tests, but who had fully documented milk-induced asthma.

Table 7.3. Diagnostic process in food-allergic disease.

1 Full clinical assessment and relevant investigations

2 Personal and family features of atopy, allergy, immune status

3 Elimination diet

4 Clinical decision — has there been complete symptomatic and pathological remission after a period of elimination diet?

5 Open food reintroduction, in food groups with subjective and objective measurements of disease activity

6 Establish a maintenance diet of tolerated foods, with nutritional adequacy checked by a dietitian

7 If appropriate, double-blind challenges to be performed, assessed by objective measurements of disease activity or pathology

Diagnosis of food-allergic disease and food intolerance

Since the response to elimination and reintroduction of foods is part of the diagnostic process, manipulation of diet is relevant both in the diagnosis and management of food-allergic diseases (Table 7.3). In the UK, gluten-free and cow's milk protein free-diets are widely used. When multiple foods may be implicated, a number of different approaches can be followed. None has so far proved universally applicable.

Elemental diet

In order to eliminate all allergens completely, the patient may fast, drinking only water, or may take an elemental diet, such as Vivonex. Elemental diets are unpalatable and few patients can tolerate such substances for more than 3 or 4 weeks. Since elemental diets reduce the bulk of intestinal secretions, dramatic relief of symptoms may result if factors such as intestinal obstruction contribute to symptomatology, as may occur in Crohn's disease.

Oligoallergenic diets

Several diet regimens, each of which exposes

the patient to only a small number of food allergens, have been developed by interested dietitians in hospitals around the UK. If after 3–4 weeks on an oligoallergenic diet the patient is no better, then food intolerance is most unlikely to be the cause of his disease. Rarely, he may in fact be allergic to one of the antigens provided in the diet, and it may be worth substituting beef for lamb, apple for rhubarb, etc.

Empirical diets

Under some circumstances, particularly when food additives are suspected to be the relevant antigenic substances, empirical diets, free of preservatives, colouring and additives can be prescribed; where one or a few substances are suspected, diets free of milk and eggs, or avoidance of shellfish, fish, tomatoes, etc. may be appropriate.

Provocation of symptoms

If foodstuffs are reintroduced in a controlled way, on an open basis, clinical reaction to a recently introduced foodstuff can readily be demonstrated. If practicable, measurement of disease activity should be made, for example by studies of respiratory function. Occasionally it will be appropriate to conduct double-blind challenges by using either a specially prepared, masked foodstuff, or by administering antigen by stomach tube or opaque capsules.

Management of food-allergic diseases and food intolerance

Even when there is reasonably good evidence of food allergy or food intolerance, symptomatic treatment for asthma, diarrhoea or eczema, may be all that is necessary. If a foodstuff has been clearly shown to be harmful, strict avoidance can usually be achieved by a motivated patient assisted by a dietitian. Care must be taken to ensure that the maintenance diet is nutritionally adequate. It is important to achieve a balance between clinical care and obsessive concern by the patient regarding diet.

In some food-allergic patients, the mast-cell-stabilizing agent, sodium cromoglycate, has been valuable in management. Research continues on the optimal dosage regimes, and in techniques of identifying patients who are likely to benefit. Nevertheless, this drug, taken by mouth, has been used successfully as an adjuvant to a restricted diet in order to allow more dietary freedom; and as the sole therapy in long term management of some cases (Edwards 1980).

Acknowledgements

I am grateful to Dr Walker-Smith for permission to publish the case history and illustrations as mentioned in the text. In the section on clinical immunology. I have drawn heavily on discussions with Dr Stephan Strobel.

References

Ament, M.E. & Rubin, C.E. (1972) Soy protein — another cause of the flat intestinal lesion. *Gastroenterol.* **62**, 227.

Andre C., Heremans J.F., Vaerman J. & Cambiaso C.L. (1975) A mechanism for the induction of immunological tolerance by antigen feeding: antigen-antibody complexes. *J. Exp. Med.* **142**, 1509–1519.

Atherton D.J. (1981) Allergy and atopic eczema. *Clin. Exp. Dermatol.* **6**, 317–325.

Barnetson R. StC., Merrett T.G. & Ferguson A. (1981) Studies on hyperimmunoglobulinaemia E in atopic diseases with particular reference to food allergens. *Clin. Exp. Immunol.* **46**, 54–60.

Barratt M.E.J., Strachan P.J. & Porter P. (1978) Antibody mechanisms implicated in digestive disturbances following ingestion of soya protein in calves and piglets. *Clin. Exp. Immunol.* **31**, 305–312.

Bloch K.J., Bloch D.B., Stearns M. & Walker W.A. (1979) Intestinal uptake of macromolecules. VI Uptake of protein antigen *in vivo* in normal rats and in rats infected with *Nippostrongylus brasiliensis* or subjected to milk systemic anaphylaxis. *Gastroenterol.* **77**, 1039–1044.

Bock S.A., Lee W.Y., Remigio L.K. & May C.D. (1978) Studies of hypersensitivity reactions to foods in infants and children. *J. Allergy Clin. Immunol.* **62**, 327–334.

Bolin T.D. (1980) Use of oral sodium cromoglycate in persistent diarrhoea. *Gut*, **21**, 848–850.

Brostoff J., Carini C., Wraith D.G. & Johns P. (1979) Production of IgE complexes by allergen challenge in atopic patients and the effect of sodium cromoglycate. *Lancet*, **i**, 1268–1270.

Carswell F. & Ferguson A. (1973) Plasma food antibodies during the withdrawal and reintroduction of dietary gluten in children with coeliac disease. *Arch. Dis. Child.* **48**, 583–586.

Cebra J.J., Kamat R., Gearhart P., Robertson S.M. & Tseng J. (1977) The secretory IgA system of the gut. *Ciba Foundation Symposium No. 46*, pp. 5–28. Elsevier North-Holland Inc., Amsterdam.

Dastur F.D., Awatramani V.P. & Dixit S.K. (1981) Response to single dose of tetanus vaccine in subjects with naturally acquired tetanus antitoxin. *Lancet*, **ii**, 219–221.

Edwards A. (1980) Drug management. In *Proceedings of the First Food Allergy Workshop*, pp. 95–101. (Ed. by W. Jackson). Medical Education Services, Oxford.

Elson C.O., Heck J.A. & Strober W. (1979) T-cell regulation of murine IgA-synthesis. *J. Exp. Med.* **149**, 632–643.

Ferguson A. (1976) Coeliac disease and gastrointestinal food allergy. In *Immunological Aspects of the Liver and Gastrointestinal Tract*, pp. 153–202. (Ed. by A. Ferguson & R.N.M. MacSween). MTP Press Ltd, Lancaster.

Ferguson A. (1978) Lymphocytes and cell-mediated immunity in the small intestine. In *Advanced Medicine*, 14, pp. 278–293. (Ed. by D. Weatherall). Pitman Medical, Tunbridge Wells.

Ferguson A. & Carswell F. (1972) Precipitins to dietary proteins in the serum and upper intestinal secretions of coeliac children. *Br. Med. J.* **i**, 75–77.

Ferguson A. & Mowat A.McI. (1980) Immunological mechanisms in the small intestine. In *Recent Advances in Gastrointestinal Pathology*, pp. 93–103 (Ed. by R. Wright). W.B. Saunders, Eastbourne.

Ferguson A. & Gillon J. (1981) Clinical aspects of food allergy. In *Food Allergy*, pp. 31–38. (Ed. by C. Zanussi, C. Ortolani & P. Torzuoli). Masson Italia Editori, Milan.

Gowans M.L. & Knight E.J. (1964) The route of recirculation of lymphocytes in the rat. *Proc. R. Soc. Lond. (Biol.)* **159**, 257–282.

Guy-Grand D., Griscelli C. & Vassalli P. (1974) The gut-associated lymphoid system: nature and properties of the large dividing cells. *Europ. J. Immunol.* **4**, 435–443.

Hemmings W.A. & Williams E.W. (1978) Transport of large breakdown products of dietary protein through the gut wall. *Gut*, **19**, 715–723.

Herbert W.J. & Wilkinson P.C. (1977) *A Dictionary of Immunology*, pp. 84. Blackwell Scientific Publications, Oxford.

Hoj L., Osterballe O., Bundgaard A., Weeke B. & Weiss M. (1981) A double-blind controlled trial of elemental diet in severe, perennial asthma. *Allergy*, **36**, 257–262.

Jackson W. (1980) Definitions and terminology: workshop summary. In *Proceedings of the First Food Allergy Workshop*, pp. 7–8. (Ed. by W. Jackson) Medical Education Services, Oxford.

Jarrett E.E.E. (1978) Stimuli for the production and control of IgE in rats. *Immunol. Rev.* **41**, 52–76.

Kagnoff M.F. (1980) Effects of antigen feeding on intestinal and systemic immune responses. IV Similarity between the suppressor factor in mice after erythrocyte-lysate injection and erythrocyte feeding. *Gastroenterol.* **79**, 54–61.

Kilshaw P.J. & Slade H. 1982 Villus atrophy and crypt elongation in the small intestine of preruminant calves fed with heated soyabean flour or wheat gluten. *Res. Vet. Sci.* **33**, 305–308.

Korenblat P.E., Rothberg R.M., Minden P. & Farr R.S. (1968) Immune responses of human adults after oral and parenteral exposure to bovine serum albumin. *J. Allergy* **41**, 226–235.

Kuitunen P., Visakorpi J.K., Savilahti E. & Pelkonen P. (1975) Malabsorption syndrome with cow's milk intolerance. Clinical findings and course in 54 cases. *Arch. Dis. Child.* **50**, 351–356.

Lessof M.H., Wraith D.G., Merrett T.G., Merrett J. & Buisseret P.D. (1980) Food allergy and intolerance in 100 patients — local and systemic effects. *Quart J. Med.* **49**, 259–271.

Logan R.F.A., Gillon J., Earnshaw P., Ferrington C. & Ferguson A. (1981) Elemental diets in treatment of acute Crohn's disease. *Br. Med. J.* (letter) **282**, 144–145.

Lowney E.D. (1968) Immunologic unresponsiveness to a contact sensitizer in man. *J. Invest. Dermatol.* **51**, 411–417.

MacDonald T.T. & Ferguson A. (1977) Hypersensitivity reactions in the small intestine. 3 The effects of allograft rejection and of graft-versus-host disease on epithelial cell kinetics. *Cell Tiss. Kinet.* **10**, 301–312.

Miller S. & Hanson D. (1979) Inhibition of specific immune responses by feeding protein antigens. IV Evidence for tolerance and specific active suppression of cell-mediated immune responses to ovalbumin. *J. Immunol* **123**, 2344–2350.

Mowat A.McI. & Ferguson A. (1982) Intraepithelial lymphocyte count and crypt hyperplasia measure the mucosal component of the graft-versus-host reaction in mouse small intestine. *Gastroenterol.* **83**, 417–423.

Mowat A.McI., Strobel S., Drummond H.E. & Ferguson A. (1982) Immunological responses to fed protein antigens in mice 1 Reversal of oral tolerance to ovalbumin by cyclophosphamide. *Immunol.* **45**, 105–113.

Reinherz E.L. & Schlossman S.F. (1981) Characterization and function of human immunoregulatory T lymphocyte subsets. *Immunol. Today*, **2**, 69–75.

Reinherz E.L., Rubinstein A., Geha R.S., Strelkauskas A.J., Rosen F.S. & Schlossman S.F. (1979) Abnormalities of immunoregulatory T cells in disorders of immune function. *N. Engl. J. Med.* **301**, 1018–1022.

Roberts S.A., Reinhardt M.C., Paganelli R. & Levinsky R.J. (1981) Specific antigen exclusion and non-specific facilitation of antigen entry across the gut in rats allergic to food proteins. *Clin. Exp. Immunol.* **45**, 131–136.

Rosekrans P.C.M., Meijer C.J.L.M., Cornelisse C.J., Van der Wal A.M. & Lindeman J. (1980) Use of morphometry and immunohistochemistry of small intestinal biopsy specimens in the diagnosis of food allergy. *J. Clin. Path.* **33**, 125–130.

Strobel S. & Ferguson A. 1982 Immunbiologische grundlagen der gastrointestinalen abwehr. In *Wissenschaftliche Information*. Milupa A.G., Friedrichsdorf.

Swarbrick E.T., Stokes C.R. & Soothill J.F. (1979) Absorption of antigens after oral immunisation and the simultaneous induction of specific systemic tolerance. *Gut*, **20**, 121–125.

Tomasi J.B., Tan E.M., Solomon A. & Prendergast R.A. (1965) Characteristics of an immune system common to certain external secretions. *J. Exp. Med.* **121**, 101–124.

Udall J.N., Bloch K.J., Fritze L. & Walker W.A. (1981) Binding of exogenous protein fragments to native proteins: possible explanation for the over estimations of uptake of extrinsically labelled macromolecules from the gut. *Immunol.* **42**, 251–257.

Walker W.A., Isselbacher K.J. & Bloch K.J. (1972) Intestinal uptake of macromolecules: effect of oral immunization. *Sci.* **177**, 608–610.

Walker W.A. (1984) Immunoregulation of small intestinal function *Gastroenterol.* **86**, 577–579.

Wallace J.R., Payne R.W. & Mack A.J. (1972) Inadvertent intravenous infusion of milk. *Lancet*, **i**, 1264–1266.

Walker-Smith J. (1979) Dietary protein intolerance. In *Diseases of the Small Intestine in Childhood*, 2nd ed., pp. 139–170. Pitman Medical Bath.

Wells H.G. & Osborne T.B. (1911) The biological reaction against vegetable proteins. I Anaphylaxis. *J. Infect. Dis.* **8**, 66–124.

Chapter 8
Immune Deficiency

A.D.B. WEBSTER

The gut-associated lymphoid tissue and immunoglobulins 135
Antibody deficiency disorders 136
Cellular immune deficiency 144
Cl esterase inhibitor deficiency 147
Immunodeficiency secondary to gut disease 148

The alimentary and respiratory systems are repeatedly exposed to antigenic material from commensal bacteria, food, and occasionally pathogenic organisms. It is therefore not surprising that both these systems have acquired a specialized lymphoid apparatus. Current evidence, however, suggests that the primary role of the gut-associated lymphoid tissue (GALT) is to protect against infections such as typhoid, cholera and parasitic infestation.

Although animal experiments have contributed much knowledge about the detailed morphology of GALT, very little is known about its importance in protecting man against intestinal infections. This reflects the very different susceptibility of man and animals to various organisms. However, we have some insight into the importance of antibody in the gut from studies of patients with antibody deficiency syndromes, although much of this research has involved patients living in relatively hygienic environments. Clinical observations in patients with the very rare primary defects in macrophage and neutrophil function have demonstrated the importance of such cells in the gut. However, little is known of the relevance of cell-mediated immunity to gut disease, despite extensive work trying to link disorders of cellular immunity with Crohn's and coeliac disease. A classification of primary immunodeficiency syndromes, together with diagnostic screening tests, is given in Table 8.1.

The gut-associated lymphoid tissue and immunoglobulins

There are numerous plasma cells in the lamina propria of the small intestine. Most numerous are those secreting IgA, although IgG- and IgM-secreting cells are plentiful (Crabbe & Heremans 1966). The IgA and IgM produced by these plasma cells binds to secretory piece on the basal aspect of the epithelial cells. The complex (S−IgA or S−IgM) is pinocytosed by the epithelial cells and then extruded into the lumen (Brandtzaeg 1977). Secretory piece is not only a receptor for IgA, but when combined with IgA protects the immunoglobulin molecule from proteolytic enzymes in the small bowel juice, thus prolonging the half-life (Brandtzaeg & Baklien 1976). The binding of the secretory piece to IgM, however, is not so stable and is easily cleaved by enzymes in the intestinal juice (Richman & Brown 1977). IgG will not bind to secretory piece and is therefore thought to have a relatively short half-life in the intestine, although this has not yet been formally demonstrated. Nevertheless, there is a higher concentration of IgG in duodenal juice than either IgA or IgM, this IgG apparently entering the intestine by diffusion from the circulation (Lebenthal et al. 1980).

Most mammals are also able to concentrate IgA in the bile, the hepatic cells synthesizing secretory piece which binds IgA from the plasma, and then transporting S−IgA into the bile by a similar mechanism to that used by intestinal epithelial cells (Hall et al. 1980, Nagura et al. 1981).

Scattered throughout the small intestine are the specialized lymphoid structures, Peyer's patches, which are more common in the terminal ileum than the jejunum. These structures consist of between ten and 900 nodules (Fig. 8.1) and number about 300 in children, diminishing to about 100 in old age. The epithelium overlying the Peyer's patch is modified and contains specialized phagocytic cells (M cells). The rest of the structure is similar to the germinal centre of a lymph node, with T lymphocytes encircling a less densely packed central zone of B lymphocyte and macrophage-like cells (Waksman & Ozer 1976). However, the Peyer's patch is unusual in having no afferent lymphatic system so that cells can only enter via blood vessels. Cells can leave the Peyer's patch via efferent lymphatics which drain into the thoracic duct via the mesenteric lymph nodes. Experiments in rats and sheep have shown that most of the lymphoblasts leaving the Peyer's patch end up in the lamina propria of the small intestine, where they presumably become immunoglobulin-secreting plasma cells (Hall et al. 1977). The receptor responsible for 'capturing' these lymphocytes in the gut is not known. There are T lymphocytes between the epithelial cells, most of which have the suppressor phenotype (Selby et al. 1981). These T cells may play some part in suppressing immune reactions to food antigens and commensal bacteria. There is controversy over whether they actually increase in number in chronic inflammatory bowel disorders such as coeliac disease (Guix et al. 1979).

Antibody deficiency disorders

Selective IgA deficiency

Incidence

It is useful to distinguish between serum levels of IgA below the limit of detection by radial immunodiffusion (about 1 mg/100 ml), hereafter referred to as 'IgA deficiency'; and

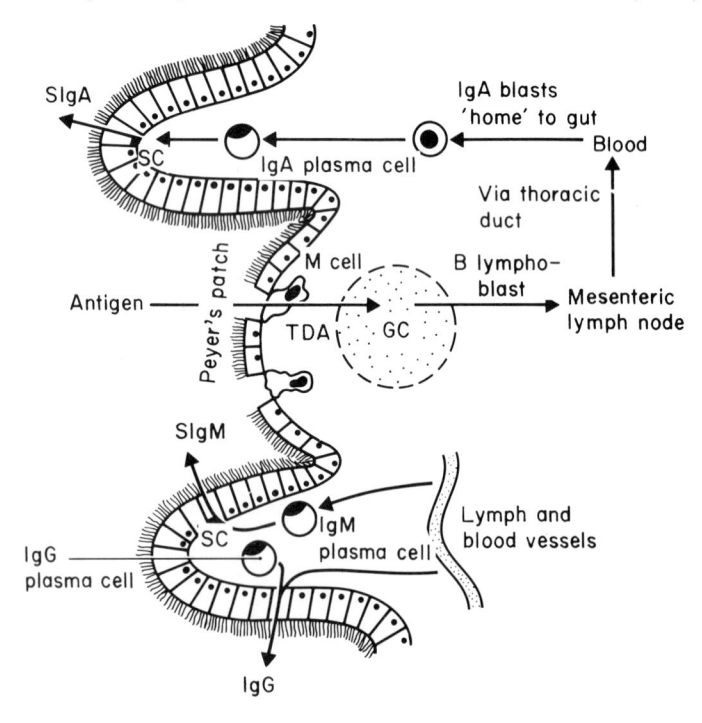

Fig. 8.1. Diagrammatic representation of antigen entering Peyer's patch and inducing sensitized lymphocytes which enter the circulation. Those B cells destined to synthesize IgM and IgA eventually home to the lamina propria. SC, secretor piece; SIgA, secretory IgA; M cell, specialized phagocytic cell; TDA, thymic dependent area of Peyer's patch; GC, germinal centre of Peyer's patch.

'low serum IgA' which refers to detectable levels which are below the 2.5 percentile. The prevalence of IgA deficiency varies in different countries but on average is about 1:800 of the population (Koistinen 1975, Holt et al. 1977, Gudmundsson & Jensson 1977). There is a similar prevalence of low serum IgA. IgA deficiency is sometimes familial, the inheritance being autosomal dominant or recessive. It is not yet known whether the gene coding for alpha chain is missing in these patients or whether the defect is in regulating IgA production. Environmental factors, possibly viral infections, are probably important in some cases since very low levels were found in only one of a pair of identical twins (Lewkonia et al. 1976). There are also a few inherited syndromes where IgA deficiency is prominent (Asherson & Webster 1980). Some drugs will reversibly induce IgA deficiency or lower serum IgA, but this has not been associated with gastrointestinal problems. There are, however, some gastrointestinal diseases which are associated with an increased frequency of IgA deficiency.

The incidence of IgA deficiency in underdeveloped countries, particularly in the tropics, is unknown but it is very rarely encountered in hospitalized Negro patients (Lawton et al. 1972). This may mean that IgA deficiency predisposes to fatal intestinal infections in African children.

Symptoms

Surveys of 'healthy' blood donors with IgA deficiency in Western countries show that they only have a slightly increased incidence of recurrent diarrhoea as compared to subjects with normal IgA levels (Koistinen 1975). No long-term follow-up of blood donors with IgA deficiency has yet been published, but it is assumed that in most the IgA deficiency is permanent and has been present since birth.

Jejunal mucosa

Jejunal biopsies are usually morphologically normal in selective IgA deficiency. Immunofluorescent studies show either an absence or a severe reduction in IgA plasma cells. On the other hand, there is a compensatory increase in IgM-secreting cells. Since IgM binds to secretory piece, this adaptive response may be important in providing an alternative immune mechanism.

Table 8.1. Classification and diagnosis of primary immunodeficiency.

Disease	Screening tests
Children and adults	
Primary hypogammaglobulinaemia	
Late onset	Very low serum IgG and IgA. Variable IgM
X-linked	
Functional antibody deficiency	No antibody reponse to immunization with Tet. Tox. or pneumococcal polysaccharides
Selective IgA deficiency	
Inherited (dominant, recessive)	Absent serum and secretory IgA (often high S−IgM)
Sporadic	
Drug-induced (penicillamine, phenytoin, gold)	Low or absent serum IgA
Infants and children	
Selective T-cell deficiencies	
Thymic aplasia	Very low numbers of circulating T cells
Purine nucleoside phosphorylase deficiency	Normal antibody response to immunization
Severe combined immunodeficiency	
Auto-recessive	Very low numbers of circulating T cells
X-linked	No antibody response to test immunization
Neutrophil defects	
Primary neutropenia	Low neutrophil count
Chronic granulomatous disease	Nitroblue tetrazolium (NBT) test
Chemotactic defects	(Refer to specialized laboratory)
Complement defects	Depressed total haemolytic complement

IgA in allergic disease

IgA may play some part in preventing macromolecules from crossing the small intestine, since animals pre-immunized with bovine serum albumin absorb much less of this substance when compared to un-immunized controls (Walker et al. 1975). This view is supported by the high incidence of serum antibodies to milk in IgA deficient subjects, although this is not associated with gastrointestinal symptoms of milk intolerance (Koistinen & Sarna 1975, Buckley & Dees 1969). Many patients with IgA deficiency also have serum antibodies to human IgA, IgM and IgG, as well as to thyroglobulin and collagen (Wells et al. 1973). This can either be explained by a defect in immune regulation or to increased absorption from the gut of antigens which stimulate cross-reactive autoantibodies. None of these autoantibodies are clinically relevant, with the exception of anti-IgA antibodies in the rare patient who may develop an anaphylactic reaction when given plasma or whole blood.

It is suggested that IgA deficiency might predispose to the production of IgE antibodies to food antigens entering the circulation. This would only occur in genetically susceptible subjects who were capable of producing a brisk IgE response. This hypothesis has been tested by following up a group of infants of atopic parents and sequentially measuring their serum IgA. Eight of twenty-two infants developed infantile eczema and twelve showed positive immediate skin tests to milk protein. The serum IgA was significantly lower at 3 months in those with eczema, but not subsequently. A further study by the same group showed a correlation between a low serum IgA at 3 months and positive immediate prick tests to milk protein at 1 year (Taylor et al. 1973, Soothill et al. 1976). They subsequently showed that a similar group of infants can be protected from developing eczema by exclusively feeding on breast milk (Matthew et al. 1977).

There are two sub-classes of IgA, IgA2 being predominantly secreted into the gut. The IgA level in the serum bears no relation to that in the gut, the latter reaching adult levels by the third month of life while the former may still be unrecordable (Lebenthal et al. 1980, Isaacs et al. 1983). Serum IgA levels may therefore be misleading, and it could be argued that the low serum IgA in eczematous infants is secondary to the atopic state. By analogy with the finding in patients with allergy to pollens (Platts-Mills 1982), minute quantities of food protein should be capable of inducing a brisk IgE response. It is now well established, however, that large amounts of potentially antigenic material can cross the gut, and this presumably explains why many normal infants produce a transient IgG response to milk protein (Parish 1971).

Association with coeliac disease

IgA deficiency occurs in about 2% of patients with coeliac disease (Asquith 1974, Savilahti et al. 1971). Patients with either coeliac disease or selective IgA deficiency have a raised incidence of the DR3 histocompatibility marker, so that a direct relationship between these two disorders is unlikely (Keuning et al. 1976, Hammarstrom & Smith 1983). The common factor is probably the DR3 marker, but it is also possible that IgA deficiency makes coeliac disease more overt.

Post-vagotomy diarrhoea

McLoughlin et al. (1976) found IgA deficiency in six out of fourteen patients with severe diarrhoea in a survey of over 2000 patients who had had gastroenterostomy and truncal vagotomy. They also had unrecordable serum IgM but normal IgG levels; this pattern of immunoglobulin deficiency is extremely unusual. The same patients had altered gastrointestinal motility, achlorhydria and bacterial overgrowth in the jejunal juice with raised urinary indican. On the other hand, a subsequent study showed that the combination of IgA deficiency and achlorhydria did not lead to gastrointestinal symptoms, indicating that a disturbance of motility was an important factor (McLoughlin et al. 1978). This suggests that IgA may play some part in preventing the adherence of bacteria to the gastrointestinal mucosa, but is relatively unimportant when there is normal movement of the intestinal contents. From a practical point of view, serum immunoglobulin levels should be measured routinely as a preliminary to gastric surgery, and procedures likely to affect small bowel motility avoided in patients with a very low serum IgA level.

Treatment

There might be a case for giving replacement IgA by mouth to IgA-deficient patients with intractable diarrhoea following vagotomy and gastroenterostomy. IgA concentrates can be easily prepared from plasma but will not be bound to secretory piece. Although this material will pass undegraded through the achlorhydric stomach, it will probably be cleaved by proteolytic enzymes in the intestine. Nevertheless, such treatment is worth considering in difficult cases. It is likely that IgG concentrates would be just as effective since this has been shown to reduce the incidence of rotavirus enteritis in low birth weight infants (Barnes *et al.* 1982). This protective effect is probably due to specific IgG antibody coating the pharynx, oesophagus and the achlorhydric stomachs of these neonates, rather than having an effect in the small intestine.

Theoretically, an S—IgA concentrate would be the best orally administered treatment for intractable intestinal infections, and may have helped two immunodeficient patients (Matsumoto *et al.* 1983). It would probably be advantageous to give cimetidine before each treatment to prevent acidification of the immunoglobulin.

Primary hypogammaglobulinaemia

The lifetime prevalence of primary hypogammaglobulinaemia in the UK is about fifteen per million of the population for males, and four per million for females. The commonest form of the disease can occur at any age ('common variable' hypogammaglobulinaemia) but there is a peak incidence in the third decade of life. There is an X-linked variety (Bruton's agammaglobulinaemia) which is much rarer. The T and B lymphocytes have an 'immature' phenotype in both the familial and non-familial forms of the disease, although the cause of the maturation arrest is unknown. Large series of these patients have now been described in the USA and UK, but few patients have been reported in Africa or India, suggesting either that patients in these countries die early from respiratory or gastrointestinal infections or that natural selection has eliminated any genetic predisposition to these diseases. All affected patients are prone to recurrent upper respiratory tract infections with *H. influenzae* and pneumococci, and to joint and urinary infections with mycoplasmas (Asherson & Webster 1980). Gastrointestinal complications also occur and are reviewed below. About 25% of patients have gastric atrophy and achlorhydria. In contrast to patients with Addisonian pernicious anaemia, who have antral G-cell hyperplasia and raised serum gastrin levels, there is atrophy of the entire stomach in hypogammaglobulinaemia and the serum gastrin levels are normal.

Parasites

Giardiasis is probably the commonest cause of diarrhoea in hypogammaglobulinaemic patients in the USA, although it is much rarer in British patients (Ament *et al.* 1973, Asherson & Webster 1980). Steatorrhoea usually occurs and with prolonged infection patients lose weight and develop deficiencies of calcium and folate. Oocysts are often found in the stool, but if not it may be necessary to look for giardia trophozoites in intestinal juice or on the surface of a Giemsa-stained jejunal biopsy. The jejunal biopsy may show partial villous atrophy with a chronic inflammatory infiltrate, although this is usually patchy.

The high incidence of giardiasis in primary hypogammaglobulinaemia clearly shows that antibodies are important in the defence against this organism. However, it is unclear which class of antibody is involved. Since there is no clear evidence that patients with selective IgA deficiency are prone to giardiasis, it seems likely that IgG antibody is protective (Ridley & Ridley 1976, Owen 1980). This is supported by work in guinea-pigs which shows that IgG antibody to trophozoites will enhance opsonization by macrophages and also agglutinate the organisms (Radulescu & Meyer 1981). S—IgA antibodies are probably also effective since suckling mice are protected from giardia infection (Andrews & Hewlett 1981). Nevertheless, patients on intramuscular gammaglobulin replacement therapy, which produces a rise in the serum IgG to about 25% of the lower limit of the normal range, are not always protected. There are presumably other defence mechanisms, particularly since immunocompetent patients and susceptible strains of mice with chronic giardiasis usually have high titres of IgG-specific antibody (Owen 1980, Anders et al. 1982). There are a number of surface antigens on the giardia parasite, however, and it is not known which is crucial for the parasite to survive in the intestine. It is therefore possible that an isolated failure to produce antibody to this component leads to chronic infection. The newer types of intravenous gammaglobulin, which can raise the serum IgG to within the normal range, may be expected to prevent giardiasis in hypogammaglobulinaemic patients living in endemic areas.

Giardiasis in hypogammaglobulinaemic patients can be effectively treated with either a course of mepacrine (100 mg three times daily for 7 days) or metronidazole (7 day course of 2 g daily). There is no tendency for these patients to relapse when treatment is discontinued.

Cryptosporidiosis is a very rare complication in patients with hypogammaglobulinaemia, and is also occasionally seen in patients on immunosuppressive therapy for other diseases (Lasser et al. 1979, Meisel et al. 1976, Weisburger et al. 1979). It may cause death in the acquired immunodeficiency syndrome (AIDS). It has also been reported in apparently immunocompetent subjects, where it can present as a self-limiting diarrhoeal illness (Nime et al. 1976). It appears to be a common cause of traveller's diarrhoea in Finland (Jokipii et al. 1983). The organism belongs to the sub-order Eimeriina, which includes *Isospora*, *Toxoplasma* and *Sarcocystis*. These organisms are collectively referred to as Coccidia (Bird & Smith 1980). Cryptosporidiosis is common in farm animals such as calves, lambs and goats. Cats and dogs do not seem to be affected. The disease is therefore probably a zoonosis although very little is known about the life cycle outside the human intestine. It is also not known whether humans are prone to a particularly virulent strain of the organism. Affected patients suffer from chronic malabsorption with steatorrhoea. The disease may last for up to 6 years with the patient slowly wasting from 'malnutrition'. There are often acute episodes of profuse watery diarrhoea similar to cholera, probably caused by rapid multiplication of organisms in the large bowel. This may necessitate emergency admission to hospital for correction of water and electrolyte loss. The following case history is typical (Sloper et al. 1982).

A 6-year-old boy presented with steatorrhoea and growth retardation. He was already known to have primary hypogammaglobulinaemia with residual IgM production, and for some years had been on treatment with intramuscular gammaglobulin. There was an eosinophilia and the jejunal biopsy showed partial villous atrophy. Investigations over the subsequent few years excluded bacterial overgrowth in the small bowel, dissaccharide intolerance, gastrinoma and pancreatic disease. He was given a variety of antibiotics and anti-parasite drugs without effect. Various dietary restrictions also failed to help. At 10 years of age he was admitted to intensive care for treatment of water and electrolyte loss after 24 h of profuse watery diarrhoea. This improved within a few days. At 12 years he was again admitted for emergency treatment with cholera-like diarrhoea which persisted despite treatment with steroids. By this time he was severely malnourished and died shortly afterwards from pneumonia and pancreatitis. A jejunal biopsy shortly before his death showed numerous parasites which were confirmed as cryptosporidia by electron-microscopy (Fig. 8.2). A review of the numerous previous jejunal biopsies

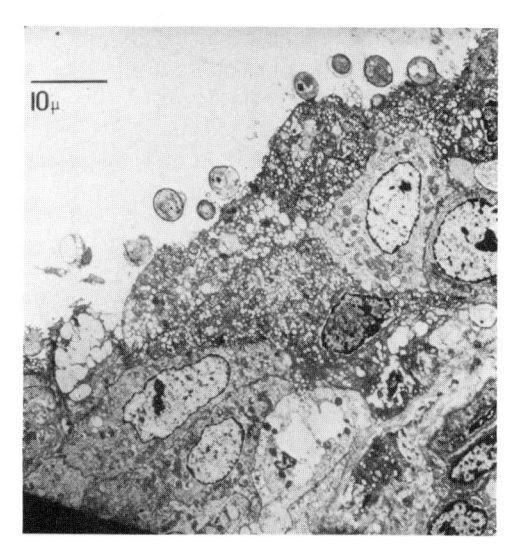

Fig. 8.2. Electron micrograph showing cryptosporidia attached to the jejunal mucosa (× 2500).

showed the presence of a few cryptosporidia which had been overlooked.

Oocysts can be seen by experienced observers in the stools with a modified Ziehl–Neelsen stain (Garcia et al. 1983). The disease can also be transmitted to new-born lambs or mice by intragastric inoculation of stools from affected patients (Tzipori et al. 1982). The diagnosis, however, usually depends on identifying the organisms in a jejunal biopsy. This should be divided, one piece being sent for histology and staining with Giemsa, and the other fixed for electronmicroscopy. If light microscopy shows suspicious organisms on the villous brush border, then electronmicroscopy is required to identify the organism. Further biopsies may be required if the first is negative, since the degree of intestinal infestation seems to vary from time to time.

Treatment is unsatisfactory and there are no known drugs which will affect the course of the disease. Even drugs used by veterinarians to treat animal coccidiosis are ineffective. Intramuscular gammaglobulin therapy does not help but it would be reasonable to try high doses of the newer types of gammaglobulin intravenously, and perhaps even by mouth.

Campylobacter

The majority of hypogammaglobulinaemic patients in England complaining of diarrhoea have *Campylobacter* species in their stools. Since no other causative organism can usually be found, and because most patients improve on erythromycin, it is reasonable to assume that they have a campylobacter enteritis. A few patients have persistent diarrhoea despite erythromycin therapy, and continue to excrete the organism. Such patients probably have campylobacter colonization of the gall bladder. The following case illustrates the difficulty in managing this complication.

A-50-year-old lady with late onset hypogammaglobulinaemia developed watery diarrhoea. She had been on treatment with weekly intramuscular gammaglobulin for 3 years. There was a previous history of autoimmune thrombocytopenia requiring splenectomy, and more recently autoimmune haemolytic anaemia controlled with prednisolone. The diarrhoea persisted for 5 years, although this improved whenever the prednisolone was increased to control exacerbations of the haemolytic anaemia. There was no significant malabsorption or steatorrhoea, although the Schilling test showed moderate B_{12} malabsorption. The urinary indicans and ^{14}C deoxycholate breath tests were normal. Barium follow-through and sigmoidoscopy were normal. *Campylobacter jujuni* was isolated from small bowel juice and stools, the latter also containing high concentrations of primary bile acids. Prolonged courses of oral erythromycin failed to eradicate the campylobacter and had no effect on the diarrhoea. This year she developed an acute uveitis in the left eye which responded to an increased dose of prednisolone. She eventually became asymptomatic after the infection was eradicated with a 6 day course of intravenous erythromycin (600 mg three times daily).

Campylobacter jejuni is the species which causes diarrhoea in both immunocompetent and immunodeficient subjects. *Campylobacter fetus fetus* can cause systemic disease, including cholangitis, in patients who have cirrhosis, are on immunosuppressive drugs, or have primary hypogammaglobulinaemia (Targan et al. 1976, Lawrence et al. 1971, Wyatt et al. 1977, Webster 1973).

Animals vary widely in their susceptibility to campylobacter, with primates often being asymptomatic excretors of the organism and chicks developing a severe and often fatal ileitis (Newell 1984). The diarrhoea in man is probably due to an enterotoxin similar to that produced by *V. cholera* (Ruiz-Palacios et al. 1983). The susceptibility of hypogammaglobulinaemic patients to campylobacter-associated diarrhoea suggests that antibodies are important in eliminating the organism.

Isolates from the stools of our immunodeficient patients have always been erythromycin-sensitive. The diarrhoea in most patients subsides in about 10 days of starting oral erythromycin (500 mg q.d.s.). It is our practice to continue treatment for at least 3 weeks to minimize the chances of relapse. However, since the incidence of erythromycin-resistant strains varies between countries, it is important to check the sensitivity of the organism before starting treatment.

We have recently studied two hypogammaglobulinaemic patients with chronic watery diarrhoea and mild steatorrhoea. No pathogens could be cultured from the stools which nevertheless contained numerous organisms which reacted with an antiserum raised against *C. jejuni*. One of the patients became asymptomatic after the organism was eradicated with a course of intravenous erythromycin. The other patient remains symptomatic after erythromycin failed to eradicate the organism. It is likely that the diarrhoea in both these patients was caused by a *Campylobacter* species which cannot yet be cultured *in vitro*.

Miscellaneous intestinal disorders

In more than seventy patients with primary hypogammaglobulinaemia followed for up to 10 years at the Clinical Research Centre, about a third have complained of one or more episodes of prolonged diarrhoea. Only about 40% of these patients had steatorrhoea, with most of these only excreting between 5–10 g fat/day. The majority of those with steatorrhoea had giardiasis and responded to a course of mepacrine or metronidazole. However, five patients developed chronic malabsorption not apparently related to infections. Two of these patients had coeliac disease. The first was a 63-year-old HLA–DR3 positive man with no other unusual complications; the other a 40-year-old woman who also had steroid-responsive fibrosing alveolitis. The diagnosis was confirmed in the first case, demonstrating that coeliac disease can occur in the virtual absence of plasma cells and immunoglobulin in the small intestine (Webster et al. 1981). The second case has responded on two occasions to gluten withdrawal while relapsing on a normal diet. These cases suggest that there may be a 3% incidence of coeliac disease in patients with hypogammaglobulinaemia, in contrast to the 0.1% incidence suggested for the general population. Unlike selective IgA deficiency, primary panhypogammaglobulinaemia is not associated with a high incidence of the HLA–DR3 histocompatibility marker, and this raises the possibility that lack of antibody increases the mucosal damage in coeliac patients and produces more overt disease.

Commensal bacteria in antibody-deficient patients

Mild asymptomatic steatorrhoea is common in patients with primary hypogammaglobulinaemia. Only a moderate increase in commensal bacteria (about 10^5 organisms/ml) is usually found in their jejunal juice, and no unusual strains of bacteria are identified. As a result of the gastric atrophy so frequently present, many of these patients also have achlorhydria which is known to be associated with a slight increase in small bowel commensal bacteria (Parkin et al. 1972, Webster 1976). A raised faecal fat excretion, however, rarely occurs in classical pernicious anaemia, and this slight increase in the jejunal flora cannot therefore be the explanation for the mild steatorrhoea in hypogammaglobulinaemic patients. Similar numbers of bacteria to those found by Tomkins et al. (1975) in patients with tropical sprue were cultured from washed jejunal biopsies taken from hypogammaglobulinaemic patients complaining of diarrhoea (Webster 1976). However gastric mucosa from achlorhydric patients with either Addisonian pernicious anaemia or primary hypogammaglobulinaemia contained the same number and variety of bacteria (Dolby et al. 1984). These findings show that local antibody production plays little part in controlling the numbers of intestinal bacteria in patients in the Western world. The situation may be different in developing countries where a larger number and variety of bacteria are ingested in the diet.

There is no convincing evidence that bacterial overgrowth in the small bowel ever causes steatorrhoea in hypogammaglobulinaemic patients. There are a few patients, however, with >10^7 organisms/ml in their jejunal juice who improve on antibiotics such as tetracycline and metronidazole.

Nodular lymphoid hyperplasia (NLH)

Hypertrophy of the gut-associated lymphoid tissue occurs in about 20% of patients with primary adult onset hypogammaglobulinaemia (Hermans et al. 1966, Webster et al. 1977). Patients with X-linked agammaglobulinaemia do not seem to be affected. The lymphoid nodules are most prominent in the small bowel although they can occur in the large bowel, and more rarely in the stomach (Cowling et al. 1974). They have a similar structure to the Peyer's patch with a central follicle containing large macrophage-like cells and lymphoblasts, which is surrounded by densely packed small lymphocytes (Adjukiewicz et al. 1972). The overlying epithelium, however, is not specialized (Fig. 8.3). They can sometimes be seen on the duodenal mucosa at endoscopy and usually show a characteristic nodular appearance on a barium follow-through (Fig. 8.4). Some of

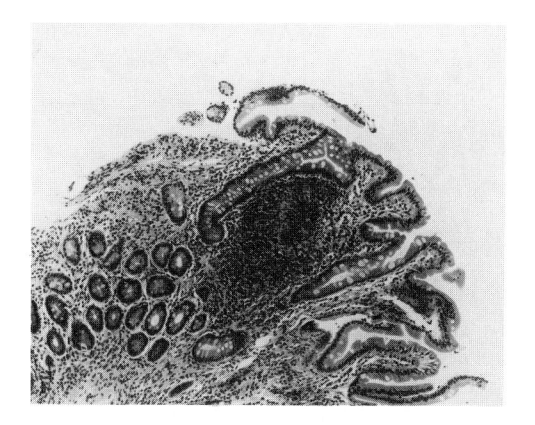

Fig. 8.3. Histological section of a lymphoid nodule in a jejunal biopsy from a patient with adult onset primary hypogammaglobulinaemia (H & E, × 150).

the cells in the centre of the nodules contain IgM immunoglobulin (Nagura et al. 1979), and most patients with NLH have some IgM in their jejunal secretions and some IgM-containing cells in the lamina propria of the small bowel (Webster et al. 1977). This may explain why patients with X-linked agammaglobulinaemia, who have a complete failure to make any class of antibody, do not develop NLH.

There are a few reports of similar nodules in apparently immunocompetent subjects in whom small intestinal lymphoma has developed (Kahn & Novis 1974). The evidence that NLH may be a premalignant condition is reviewed in Chapter 10. A similar more localized and self-limiting nodular lymphoid hyperplasia, probably involving Peyer's patches, occurs in the terminal ileum of 'healthy' children where it is associated with abdominal pain (Fieber & Schaefer 1966). Recently, Ward et al. (1983) reported patients with NLH of the small bowel in southern India. These patients were being investigated for chronic malabsorption and diarrhoea and many had giardiasis. None of the patients had hypogammaglobulinaemia, although a functional antibody deficiency was not critically excluded. The NLH in many of these patients disappeared after they were given antibiotics and antigiardial drugs, and after their nutritional status was improved. It is possible that there was a failure of the normal local antibody

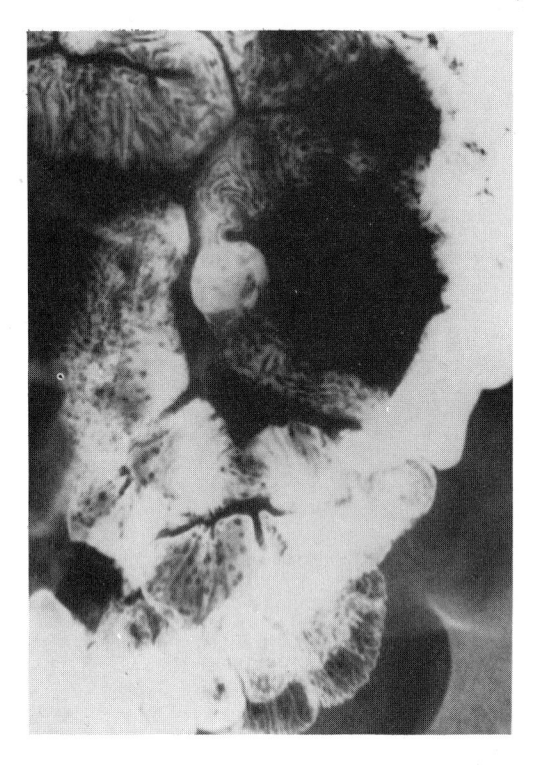

Fig. 8.4. Barium follow-through examination in a patient with nodular lymphoid hyperplasia and adult onset hypogammaglobulinaemia. Multiple nodules are seen in the intestinal mucosa.

response to the causative organism, either because of some subtle primary defect in antibody production, or more likely because of secondary immunodeficiency due to chronic illness and poor nutrition.

The aetiology of NLH is unknown but it probably represents hypertrophy of the lymphoid apparatus in response to organisms in the gut. Ament et al. (1973), suggested that there was an association of NLH with giardiasis, but we have failed to find giardia infestation in the majority of our patients. It is likely that commensal intestinal bacteria are also capable of stimulating this response, which in the absence of specific antibody and possibly other regulatory mechanisms, continues unchecked. The condition is uninfluenced by treatment with intramuscular gammaglobulin therapy, although it will be interesting to see whether treatment with the newer intravenous gammaglobulin preparations will have an effect.

Cellular immune deficiency

Primary defects

Primary defects in cellular immunity are rare and most affected patients have a combination of antibody deficiency and cellular immune defects. Twenty or more patients with selective T-lymphocyte defects have been reported. These patients either have thymic aplasia (Di George's syndrome) caused by a non-inherited failure of the third and fourth fetal pharyngeal pouch to develop, or an inherited deficiency of the enzyme purine nucleoside phosphorylase. Gastrointestinal complications are unusual in this group of patients, suggesting that T lymphocytes do not play a major role in protecting the small intestine from infection. On the other hand, infants with severe combined immunodeficiency, who have a profound deficiency of both T- and B- lymphocyte function, commonly suffer from diarrhoea and malabsorption. Jejunal biopsy in such infants often shows partial villous atrophy and numerous PAS positive macrophages in the lamina propria (Horowitz et al. 1974). These children are also prone to vaccine-related poliomyelitis, generalized candidiasis and aspergillosis, *Pneumocystis carinii* pneumonia and systemic BCGitis (Hitzig et al. 1979). By analogy with T-cell deficient animals, they should also be prone to giardiasis and coccidiosis (Asherson & Webster 1982). Nowadays, such infants rapidly receive a bone marrow transplant so that the natural course of the disease is rarely seen.

Secondary defects

Immunosuppressive and cytotoxic drugs are commonly used to treat a variety of lymphoreticular malignancies and connective tissue disorders. Patients with leukaemia and lymphomas are particularly prone to infections while on such drugs, probably because the disease itself also depresses immunity. There are no good surveys of the frequency of gastrointestinal complications in such patients, although anecdotal cases show that they are prone to strongyloidiasis, coccidiosis and bacterial infection of the small bowel, the latter sometimes presenting as pneumatosis cystoides intestinalis (Henry et al. 1974, Powell et al. 1980, Kleinman et al. 1980). Moreover, patients on immunosuppressive therapy following bone marrow transplantation are prone to Coxsackie, rotavirus and adenovirus gastroenteritis (Yolken et al. 1982). Children with severe malnutrition are particularly at risk for gut infections, since both epithelial cell turnover and immunity are depressed (Brunser 1977).

Acquired immunodeficiency syndrome (AIDS)

This syndrome has reached epidemic proportions during the past 2 years in the USA. Nearly all affected patients have been promiscuous male homosexuals, although a few apparently heterosexual male Haitians and haemophiliacs treated with Factor VIII concentrates have developed the disease (Gottlieb et al. 1981, Vieira et al. 1983, MMWR 1982a). The occurrence in haemophiliacs is strong evidence that the disease is caused by a transmissible agent, probably a virus. This is supported by the isolation of a retrovirus from the lymph nodes and blood lymphocytes of patients with AIDS (Barré-Sinoussi et al. 1983, Gallo et al. 1983). This virus selectively infects the T_4 subset of lymphocytes, which explains some of the immunological features of this dread disease. It is possible that this agent is directly responsible for the high frequency of Kaposi's sarcoma in these patients. The condition clinically resembles severe combined immunodeficiency with affected patients developing protozoal, fungal, viral and bacterial infections. *Pneumocystis carinii* pneumonia and wasting from chronic malabsorption and diarrhoea are common. The latter is frequently due to cryptosporidiosis (MMWR 1982b), a finding which has stimulated much research into this previously rare condition.

The underlying defect in host defence appears to involve cellular immunity. There is usually a severe lymphopenia, with very low relative numbers of T_4 (helper) cells in the circulation. There is a relative increase in circulating T_8-suppressor cells; these are cells that can be recognized with specific markers and which suppress immunoglobulin and antibody production in various *in vitro* systems. These T-cell changes are not unique to AIDS and occur in many other conditions. Despite the increased T-suppressor cells, most patients are hypergammaglobulinaemic and can produce antibodies to organisms like cryptosporidia (Campbell & Current 1983). This is puzzling because the only previously reported fatal cases of cryptosporidiosis have occurred in hypogammaglobulinaemic patients who appear to have normal T-cell function. This suggests that both T cells and antibodies are required to eliminate cryptosporidial infestation.

Graft-versus-host disease (GVHD)

GVH disease occurs when 'mis-matched' bone marrow, and occasionally blood transfusions, are given to patients who either have a severe primary defect in cellular immunity (e.g. severe combined immunodeficiency) or have been irradiated and treated with cytotoxic drugs to prevent graft rejection. Most patients in the latter category have aplastic anaemia although it is becoming increasingly popular to graft patients with leukaemia. There is a wide spectrum of severity of GVH disease, ranging from a very mild disease characterized by fever and skin rash when a histocompatible sibling is used as donor, to a potentially fatal condition when the donor bone marrow is taken from an unrelated donor. The severe disease is characterized by an exfoliating skin rash, bone marrow depression with neutropenia and thrombocytopenia, hepatosplenomegaly, diarrhoea and malabsorption. The gut lesion is due to infiltrating donor T lymphocytes which may release factors (lymphokines) which damage the enterocytes (Ferguson & Mowat 1980). Focal dilatation and degeneration of small bowel mucosal glands occurs in the early stages, followed by villous atrophy and finally sloughing of the mucosa (Lerner et al. 1974) (Fig. 8.5).

Mild GVHD can be effectively treated with cyclosporin A and the gut is never significantly damaged (Storb et al. 1983). Severe

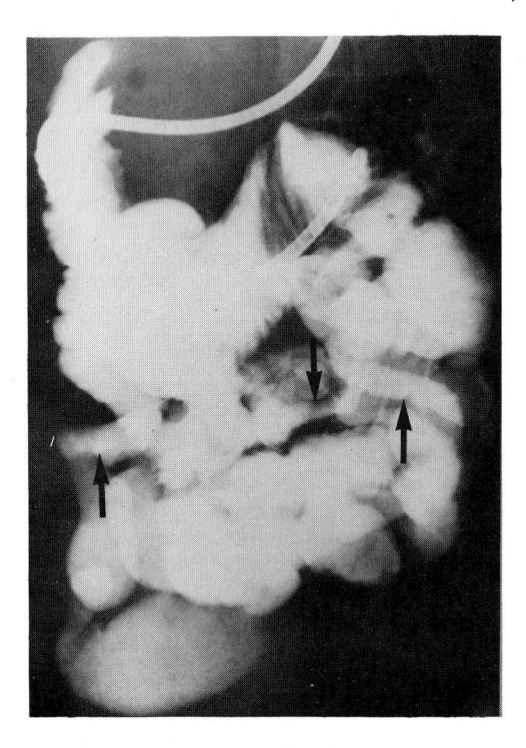

Fig. 8.5. Barium follow-through in a patient with graft-versus-host disease following bone marrow transplantation. The arrows indicate narrowed segments of intestine. (Courtesy of Dr Sue Barter.)

GVHD is usually fatal.

Defects of neutrophil function

Severe primary neutropenia invariably leads to a fatal outcome in early infancy, usually from septicaemia and pneumonia. Primary functional neutrophil defects are very rare, and usually involve either neutrophil chemotaxis or bactericidal killing. Disorders of chemotaxis are not well characterized, but there is a syndrome manifested by severe eczema, recurrent staphylococcal abscesses and a grossly elevated serum IgE where the neutrophils frequently fail to show *in vitro* chemotaxis towards various attractants. Gastrointestinal complications, however, are not a recognized feature of this disease. On the other hand, patients with defective bactericidal killing (chronic granulomatous disease — CGD) do suffer from granulomatous gut changes, intestinal perforations with fistulas, and salmonellosis (Ament & Ochs 1973). Jejunal biopsies show characteristic pigmented lipid-laden macrophages in the lamina propria of both symptomatic and asymptomatic patients. It is useful to fix the biopsy in osmium, otherwise these macrophages may not be noticed. Affected patients are prone to episodes of steatorrhoea and malabsorption, the ileum probably being mainly involved since B_{12} malabsorption is common. Salicylazosulphapyridine is the treatment of choice for patients with diarrhoea, but antibiotics which penetrate cells (e.g. rifampicin) should be considered in severe cases.

Patients with CGD are also prone to severe Salmonella gastroenteritis and septicaemia, this being a common cause of death in countries where Salmonella infection is endemic. This is illustrated by the following cases (Matamoros *et al.* 1982).

> A previously healthy 5-year-old girl living in Majorca developed fever, diarrhoea and abdominal swelling. *Salmonella typhimurium* was isolated from the stools and she improved with amoxycillin. Over the next 2 years she suffered from recurrent salmonella enteritis and septicaemia and finally died during such an episode. CGD was diagnosed 1 year before death. Her only brother developed fever, diarrhoea and abdominal swelling at 16 months. He had a laparotomy and multiple abscesses were found on the peritoneum with enlarged abdominal lymph nodes. He developed a pneumonia and an osteomyelitic lesion in a rib at 2 years. Pleural fluid grew *Aspergillus fumigatus*. At 4 years he developed *Salmonella typhimurium* enteritis and septicaemia but responded to cotrimoxazole. However, despite prophylactic cotrimoxazole, he developed further episodes of salmonella infection and died of salmonella septicaemia 1 year later.

The underlying defect in CGD is a failure to initiate the burst of oxidative metabolism which occurs during the phagocytosis of bacteria. These events are crucial for the killing of certain catalase-negative organisms, such as staphylococci and *Serratia marcescens*. Such organisms therefore survive inside the macrophage, causing a chronic granulomatous reaction. Despite obvious parallels, no abnormalities have yet been demonstrated in the neutrophils and macrophages of patients with Whipple's and Crohn's disease. A summary of the different types of small intestinal disease occuring in the various syndromes of immunodeficiency is set out in Table 8.2.

C1 esterase inhibitor (C1−INH) deficiency

Clinical features

This is the only known disorder of the complement system in which gastrointestinal symptoms are a prominent feature. Affected patients present with recurrent episodes of angioedema of the extremities, face and throat, the latter being potentially fatal (Frank *et al.* 1976). Most patients also suffer from colicky abdominal pain, often with vomiting, due to oedema of the intestine. This may lead to an increase of the intraluminal fluid and watery diarrhoea. Hypotension and 'shock' have occurred when there is massive fluid retention in the bowel. An oedematous segment of bowel may also rarely cause intussusception. The attacks of angioedema may last from to 4 h to several days. Unlike urticaria, the skin lesions are non-pruritic and painless.

The angioedema is often precipitated by trauma, particularly dental manipulation, but exercise and psychological factors may also provoke attacks. Sex hormones may also modulate attacks which often decrease in frequency during the latter part of pregnancy but are worse during menstruation.

The abdomen in patients with intestinal angioedema is tender to palpation but not rigid, and the bowel sounds are often increased. Barium follow-through during attacks may show a 'stacked coin' appearance characteristic of mucosal oedema.

Aetiology

The autosomal dominant form of the disease has two phenotypes. In the more common variety there is a low but detectable level of functional C1−INH in the serum; while in the rarer 'variant' type the level of C1−INH protein is normal but functionally inactive. The disease may also be acquired in patients with lymphoreticular malignancy, paraproteinaemia, autoimmune disease and more rarely in non-lymphoid malignancy (Gelfand *et al.* 1979). The low C1−INH in these cases, however, is due to increased consumption by C1 which is excessively activated by an autoantibody, paraprotein or cryoglobulin. Angioedema is also one of the manifestations of a systemic lupus erythematosus-like syndrome, the other features being arthralgia, erythema-multiforme vasculitis and a high titre of antibodies to single stranded DNA. In these cases the classical complement pathway appears to be excessively activated by immune complexes (Sissons *et al.* 1974).

Activated C1 becomes inactivated when it forms a tightly bound complex with C1−INH. There seems to be little reserve in this system since half normal levels of C1−INH are not sufficient to protect patients with hereditary angioedema. However, since there is no relationship between the level of

Table 8.2. Small intestinal disease in immunodeficiency disorders.

Primary hypogammaglobulinaemia
   Campylobacter enteritis
   Giardiasis
   Coccidiosis
   Coeliac disease ⎫ late onset cases
   Nodular lymphoid hyperplasia ⎭ only

Selective IgA deficiency
   Bacterial overgrowth after gastric surgery
   Coeliac disease

Combined T and B lymphocyte deficiency
(including patients with lymphoreticular disease ± cytotoxic therapy)
   Viral gastroenteritis
   Candidiasis
   Strongyloidiasis
   Giardiasis
   Coccidiosis

Chronic granulomatous disease
   Granulomatous enteritis
   Salmonellosis

serum C1–INH and the severity of symptoms, other factors are probably involved. The failure to inactivate C1 causes consumption of C4 and C2 with low serum levels. The mechanism of the angioedema is not known but it is suggested that vasoactive kinins are produced by the action of cleaved C2 on plasmin or by Hageman factor-dependent pathways which are also inactivated by C1–INH (Frank 1982).

Diagnosis

Patients with the hereditary and acquired form usually have a low serum C2, C4 and functional C1–INH level during and sometimes between attacks of angioedema. The level of C1–INH protein is also low in patients with the common type of hereditary disease, but is normal in the minority of patients with the 'variant' form. C1 levels are usually normal in both types of hereditary disease but are usually very low (<10% normal mean) in patients with acquired C1–INH deficiency. A low C1q level, measured by immunodiffusion, is therefore a useful indicator of acquired disease. The angioedema associated with the SLE-like syndrome is characterized by low levels of C1, C4, C2 and C3 during attacks, although the C1–INH level is usually normal. These patients have circulating immune complexes and low total haemolytic complement activity.

There is therefore no difficulty in distinguishing between these different types of angioedema since commercially available 'kits' are available for measuring the serum levels of the various complement proteins.

Treatment

Androgens with low virilizing capacity have now superseded Epsilon aminocaproic acid as the treatment of choice for patients with hereditary angioedema. Gelfand et al. (1979) showed that Danazol produced a rise in the level of C1–INH activity in both types of hereditary disease. More recently, Warin et al. (1980) have shown that very low doses of danazol (200 mg/day) or stanozolol (5 mg twice a week) are sufficient to prevent attacks. Affected patients should also be given fresh frozen plasma before dental extractions or other surgery. The treatment of attacks is far from satisfactory but injections of purified C1–INH have been successful (Gadek et al. 1980). There is argument over whether fresh frozen plasma should be given during attacks as this will supply further C1 for activation. Antihistamines are not helpful and it is unclear whether steroids are beneficial.

Danazol is also effective in preventing attacks in patients with acquired C1–INH deficiency. The angioedema often improves, however, when the primary condition is treated with immunosuppressive drugs. Plasmaphoresis should be considered in acute situations when a cryoglobulin or paraprotein is causing C1 activation.

Immunodeficiency secondary to gut disease

Although chronic inflammatory bowel disease can cause a significant protein-losing enteropathy, the most florid cases of secondary hypogammaglobulinaemia are due to either congenital lymphatic abnormalities or lymphatic obstruction in the intestine (Chapter 21). Such patients often have low numbers of circulating T lymphocytes due to leakage from the bowel (Stoelinga et al. 1963). The serum IgG is usually the most severely depressed; but some patients can be mistaken for having primary immunodeficiency when the serum IgA and IgM are also low. Primary hypogammaglobulinaemia can be excluded by showing that such patients produce normal specific antibody responses when test immunized with tetanus toxoid or pneumococcal polysaccharide, or by the presence of normal numbers and classes of plasma cells in a rectal or jejunal biopsy (Table 8.3). Furthermore, nearly all patients with a significant protein-losing enteropathy have hypoalbuminaemia which very rarely occurs in primary immunodeficiency states. Patients with intestinal lymphangiectasia (Chapter 21) often have depressed delayed hypersensitivity skin reactions due to the low numbers of circulating T cells (Strober et al. 1967). However, neither the partial depression of cellular immunity nor the

Table 8.3. Differential diagnosis of primary hypogammaglobulinaemia and protein-losing enteropathy.

	Primary	Protein-losing enteropathy
Serum albumin	Normal	Usually low
Blood lymphocyte count	Often low % T cells normal	Low in lymphangiectasia % T cells low
Serum immunoglobulins	IgG < 200 mg/100 ml IgA < 5 mg/100 ml IgM variable	IgG 200–500 mg/100 ml IgA > 10 mg//100 ml IgM variable
Intestinal plasma cells	Scanty (IgM) or none	Normal numbers of IgG, IgA and IgM cells
Response to test immunization	No antibodies	Normal
IgG half-life	Prolonged	Short
^{51}Cr transferrin excretion in stools	Normal	Raised

moderate hypogammaglobulinaemia makes these patients prone to recurrent infections.

References

Ajdukiewicz A.B., Youngs G.R. & Bouchier I.A.D. (1972) Nodular lymphoid hyperplasia with hypogammaglobulinaemia. *Gut*, **13**, 589.

Ament M.E., Ochs H.D. & Davis S.D. (1973) Structure and function of the gastrointestinal tract in primary immunodeficiency disorders: a study of 39 patients. *Medicine (Baltimore)*, **52**, 227.

Ament M.E. & Ochs H.D. (1973) Gastrointestinal manifestations of chronic granulomatous disease. *New Engl. J. Med.* **288**, 382.

Anders R.F., Roberts-Thomson I.C. & Mitchell G.F. (1982) Giardiasis in mice: analysis of humoral and cellular immune responses to *Giardia muris*. *Parasite Immunol.* **1**, 47–57.

Andrews J.S. & Hewlett E.L. (1981) Protection against infection with *Giardia muris* by milk containing antibody to giardia. *J. Inf. Dis.* **143**, 242–246.

Anton A.T. (1961) Agammaglobulinaemia complicating Whipple's disease — Case Report. *Ohio State Med. J.* **57**, 650.

Asherson G.L. & Webster A.D.B. (1980) *Diagnosis and Treatment of Immunodeficiency Diseases*. Blackwell Scientific Publications, London.

Asquith P. (1974) Immunology of coeliac disease. *Clin. Gastroenterol.* **3**, 213.

Barnes G.L., Hewson P.H., McLellan J.A., Doyle L.W., Knoches A.M.L., Kitchen W.H. & Bishop R.F. (1982) A randomised trial of oral gammaglobulin in low birth weight infants infected with rotavirus. *Lancet*, **i**, 1371.

Barré-Sinoussi F., Chermann J.C., Rey F., Nugeyre M.T., Chamaret S., Gruest J., Daugvet C., Axler-Blin C., Vézinet-Brun F., Rouzioux C., Rozenbaum W. & Montagnier L. (1973). Isolation of a T-lymphotropic retrovirus from a patient at risk for acquired immune deficiency syndrome (AIDS). *Science* **220**, 868–871.

Bird R.G. & Smith M.D. (1980) Cryptosporidiosis in Man. Parasite life cycle and fine structural pathology. *J. Pathol.* **132**, 217–33.

Brandtzaeg P. (1977) Human secretory component VI immunoglobulin-binding properties. *Immunochem.* **14**, 179.

Brandtzaeg P. & Baklien K. (1976) Immunoglobulin-producing cells in the intestine in health and disease. *Clin. Gastroenterol.* **5**, 251.

Brunser O. (1977) Effects of malnutrition on intestinal structure and function in children. *Clin. Gastroenterol.* **6**, 341–353.

Buckley R.H. & Dees S.C. (1969) Correlation of milk precipitins with IgA deficiency. *New. Engl. J. Med.* **281**, 465.

Campbell P.N. & Current W.C. (1983) Demonstration of serum antibodies to *Cryptosporidium sp.* in normal and immunodeficient humans with confirmed infections. *J. Clin. Microbiol.* **18**, 165–169.

Cochran M., Cook M.G., Gallagher J.C., & Peacock M. (1973) Hypogammaglobulinaemia with Whipple's disease. *Postgrad. Med. J.* **49**, 355.

Cowling D.C., Strickland R.G., Ungar B., Whittingham S. & Rose W.M. (1974) Pernicious anaemia-like syndrome with immunoglobulin deficiency. *Med. J. Aust.* **1**, 15.

Crabbe P.A. & Heremans J.F. (1966) The distribution of immunoglobulin-containing cells along the human gastrointestinal tract. *Gastroenterol.* **51**, 305.

Dobbins W.O. (1981) Is there an immune deficit in Whipple's Disease. *Dig. Dis. Sci.* **26**, 247–252.

Dolby J.M., Webster A.D.B., Boriello S.P., Barclay F.E., Bartholomew B.A. & Hill M.J. (1984) Bacterial colonisation and nitrite concentration in the achlorhydric stomachs of patients with primary hypogammaglobulinaemia or classical pernicious anaemia. *Scand. J. Gastroenterol.* **19**, 105–110.

Eggert R.C., Wilson I.D. & Good R.A. (1969) Agammaglobulinaemia and regional enteritis. *Ann. Intern. Med.* **71**, 581.

Ferguson A. & Mowat A. (1980) Immunological mechanisms in the small intestine. *Clin. Gastroenterol.* **9**, Suppl. 1, 93–103.

Fieber S.S. & Schaefer H.J. (1966) Lymphoid hyperplasia of terminal ileum — a clinical entity? *Gastroenterol.* **50**, 83.

Frank M.M., Gelfand J.A. & Atkinson J.P. (1976) Hereditary angioedema: the clinical syndrome and its management. *Ann. Intern. Med.* **84**, 580–593.

Frank M.M. (1982) The C1 esterase inhibitor and hereditary angioedema. *J. Clin. Immunol.* **2**, 65–68.

Gadek J.E. Hosea S.W., Gelfand J.A., Santaella M. Wickerhauser M., Triantaphyllopoulos D.C. & Frank M.M. (1980) Replacement therapy in hereditary angioedema. *N. Engl. J. Med.* **302**, 542.

Gallo R.C., Sarin P.S., Gelmann E.P., Robert-Guroff M., Richardson E., Kalyanaraman V.S., Mann D., Sidhu G.D., Stahl R.E., Zolla-Pazner S., Leibowitch J. Popovic M. (1983). Isolation of human T-cell leukaemia virus in acquired immune deficiency syndrome (AIDS). *Science* **220**, 865–867.

Garcia L.S., Bruckner D.A., Brewer T.C., Shimizu R.Y. (1983) Techniques for the recovery and identification of Cryptosporidiosis oocysts from stool specimens. *J. Clin. Microbiol.* **18**, 185–190.

Gelfand J.A., Boss G.R., Conley C.L., Reinhart R. & Frank M.M. (1979) Acquired C1 esterase inhibitor deficiency and angioedema: a review. *Medicine.* **58**, 321–328.

Goebel K.M., Goebel F.D. & Baier R. (1982) Impaired cell-mediated immunity among HLA-B27 related rheumatoid variants responding to Yersinia antigen. *J. Clin. Lab. Immunol.* **8**, 75–81.

Gottlieb M.S., Schroff R., Schanker H.M., Weisman J.D., Peng Phim Fan, Wolff R.A. & Saxon A. (1981) *Pneumocystis carinii* pneumonia and mucosal candidiasis in previously healthy homosexual men; evidence of a new acquired cellular immunodeficiency. *N. Engl. J. Med.* **305**, 1425-31.

Gudmundsson S. & Jensson O. (1977) Frequency of IgA deficiency in blood donors and Rh negative women in Iceland. *Acta Path. Microbiol. Scand (C)* **85**, 87.

Guix M., Skinner J.M., & Whitehead R. (1979) Measuring intraepithelial lymphocytes, surface area, and volume of lamina propria in the jejunal mucosa of coeliac patients. *Gut,* **20**, 275–8.

Hall J.G., Gyure L.A. & Payne A.W.R. (1980) Comparative aspects of the transport of immunoglobulin A from blood to bile. *Immunol.* **41**, 899.

Hall J.G., Hopkins J. & Orlans E. (1977) Studies on the lymphocytes of sheep III. Destination of lymph-borne immunoblasts in relation to their tissue of origin. *Europ. J. Immunol.* **7**, 30.

Hammarstrom L. & Smith C.I.E. (1983) HLA-A,B,C and DR antigens in immunoglobulin A deficiency. *Tiss. Antigens,* **2**, 75.

Henry K., Bird R.G. & Doe W.F. (1974) Intestinal coccidiosis in a patient with Alpha-chain disease. *Br. Med. J.* **1**, 542–543.

Hermans P.E., Huizenga K.A., Hoffman H.N., Brown A.L. & Markowitz H. (1966) Dysgammaglobulinaemia associated with nodular lymphoid hyperplasia of small intestine. *Amer. J. Med.* **40**, 78.

Hitzig W.H., Dooren L.J. & Vossen J.M. (1979) Severe combined immunodeficiency diseases. In: *Immune Deficiency,* p. 49. (Ed. by M.D. Cooper, A.R. Lawton, P.A. Miescher & H.J. Mueller-Eberhard). Springer-Verlag, New York.

Holt P.D.J., Tandy N.P. & Anstee D.J. (1977) Screening of blood donors for IgA deficiency; a study of the donor population of south-west England. *J. Clin. Path.* **30**, 1007.

Horowitz S., Lorenzsonn V.W., Olsen W.A., Albrecht R., Hong R. (1974) Small intestinal disease in T-cell deficiency. *J. Pediat.* **85**, 457–462.

Isaacs D., Altman D.G., Tidmarsh G.E., Webster A.D.B. & Valman H.B. (1983) Serum immunoglobulin levels in pre-school children. Reference ranges for IgG, IgA and IgM. *J. Clin. Pathol* **36**, 1193–1196.

Jokipii L., Pohjola S. & Jokipii A.M.M. (1983) Cryptosporidium: a frequent finding in patients with gastrointestinal symptoms. *Lancet* **ii**, 358–360.

Jones C.C. & Pugsley S.O. (1981) Persistent excretion of *Campylobacter fetus* (subsp. jejuni.) *Can. Med. Ass. Jnl.* **125**, 247.

Kahn L.B. & Novis B.H. (1974) Nodular lymphoid hyperplasia of the small bowel associated with primary small bowel reticulum cell lymphoma. *Cancer,* **33**, 837.

Keuning J.J., Pena A.S., Van Leeuwen A., Van Hooff J.P., & Van Rood J.J. (1976) HLA-DW3 associated with coeliac disease. *Lancet,* **i**, 506.

Kleinman P.K., Brill P.W. & Winchester P. (1980) Pneumatosis intestinalis. *Amer. J. Dis. Child.* **134**, 1149–1151.

Koistinen J. (1975) Selective IgA deficiency in blood donors. *Vox. Sang.* **29**, 192.

Koistinen J. & Sarna G. (1975) Immunological abnormalities in the sera of IgA-deficient blood donors. *Vox. Sang.* **29**, 203.

Lasser K.H. Lewin K.J. & Ryning F.W. (1979) Cryptosporidial enteritis in a patient with congenital hypogammaglobulinaemia. *Human Pathol.* **10**, 234–40.

Lawrence R., Nibbe A.F. & Levis S. (1971) Lung abscess secondary to *Vibrio fetus,* malabsorption syndrome and acquired agammaglobulinaemia. *Chest,* **60**, 191.

Lawton, A.R., Royal S.A., Self K.S. & Cooper M.D.

(1972) IgA determinants on B-lymphocytes in patients with deficiency of circulating IgA. *J. Lab. Clin. Med.* **80**, 26.

Lebenthal E., Clark B.A. & Kim O. (1980) Immunoglobulin concentrations in duodenal fluid of infants and children. *Amer. J. Dis. Child.* **134**, 834–837.

Lerner K.G., Kao G.F., Storb R., Buckner C.D., Clift R.A. & Thomas E.D. (1974) Histopathology of graft-vs-host reaction (GVHR) in human recipients of marrow from HLA matched sibling donors. *Transplant. Proc.* **6**, 367–371.

Lewkonia R.M., Gairdner D. & Doe W.F. (1976) IgA deficiency in one of identical twins. *Br. Med. J.* **i**, 311.

McLoughlin G.A., Bradley J., Chapman D.M., Temple J.G., Hede J.E. & McFarland J. (1976) IgA deficiency and severe post-vagotomy diarrhoea. *Lancet*, **i**, 168.

McLoughlin G.A., Hede J.E., Temple J.G., Bradley J.B., Chapman D.M. & McFarland J. (1978) The role of IgA in the prevention of bacterial colonization of the jejunum in the vagotomized subject. *Br. J. Surg.* **65**, 435.

Matamoros N., North M.E., Ciria L. & Webster A.D.B. (1982) Chronic granulomatous disease with normal neutrophil glutathione peroxidase activity in a brother and sister. *Acta Paediatr. Scand.* **71**, 327–328.

Matsumoto S., Watanabe T., Chiba S., Abo W. & Nakao T. (1983) Oral administration of secretory IgA and its clinical benefits. *Birth defects* **19**, 229.

Matthew D.J., Norman A.P., Taylor B., Turner M.W., Soothill J.F. (1977) Prevention of eczema. *Lancet*, **i**, 321–324.

Meisel J.L., Perera D.R., Meligro B.S., Rubin C.E. (1976) Overwhelming watery diarrhoea associated with a *Cryptosporidium* in an immunosuppressed patient. *Gastroenterol.* **70**, 1156–50.

MMWR (1982a) Update on acquired immunodeficiency syndrome (AIDS) among patients with haemophilia A. *Morbid. Mortal. Weekly Rep.* **31**, 644–646.

MMWR (1982b) Cryptosporidiosis: Assessment of chemotherapy in males with acquired immune deficiency syndrome (AIDS). *Morbid. Mortal. Weekly Rep.* **31**, 589–592.

Nagura H., Kohler P.F. & Brown W.R. (1979) Immunocytochemical characterisation of lymphocytes in nodular lymphoid hyperplasia of the bowel. *Lab. Invest.* **40**, 66.

Nagura H., Smith P.D., Nakane P.K. & Brown W.R. (1981) IgA in human bile and liver. *J. Immunol.* **126**, 587–595.

Newell D.G. (1984) Experimental studies of campylobacter enteritis. In *Campylobacter Infection in Man and Animals*. (Ed. by J.-P. Butzler). CRC Press Inc., Boca Raton.

Nime F.A., Burek J.D., Page D.L., Holscher M.A., Yardley J.H. (1976) Acute enterocolitis in a human being infected with the protozoan *Cryptosporidium*. *Gastroenterol.* **70**, 592–596.

Owen R.L. (1980) The immune response in clinical and experimental giardiasis. *Trans. Roy. Soc. Trop. Med. Hyg.* **74**, 443–445.

Parish W.E. (1971) Detection of reaginic and short term sensitising anaphylactic or anaphylactoid antibodies to milk in sera of allergic and normal persons. *Clin. Allergy*, **1**, 369.

Parkin D.M., McLelland D.B.L., O'Moore R.R., Percy-Robb I.W., Grant I.W.B. & Shearman D.J.C. (1972) Intestinal bacterial flora and bile salt studies in hypogammaglobulinaemia. *Gut*, **13**, 182.

Platts-Mills T.A.E. (1982) Type I or immediate hypersensitivity: hay fever and asthma. In: *Clinical Aspects of Immunology*. (Eds. Lachmann P.J. & Peters D.K.) p.579. Blackwell Scientific Publications, Oxford.

Powell R.W., Moss J.P., Nagar D., Melo J.C., Boram L.H., Anderson W.H. & Cheng S.H. (1980) Strongyloidiasis in immunosuppressed hosts. Presentation as massive lower gastrointestinal bleeding. *Arch. Intern. Med.* **140**, 1061–1063.

Radulescu S. & Meyer E.A. (1981) Opsonisation *in vitro* of *Giardia lamblia* trophozoites. *Inf. Immunity*. **32**, 852–856.

Richman L.K. & Brown W.R. (1977) Immunochemical characterization of IgM in human intestinal fluids. *J. Immunol.* **119**, 1515–1519.

Ridley M.J. & Ridley D.S. (1976) Serum antibodies and jejunal histology in giardiasis associated with malabsorption. *J. Clin. Path.* **29**, 30–34.

Ruiz-Palacios G.M., Torres J., Torres N., Escamilla E., Ruiz-Palacios B. & Tamayo J. (1983) Cholera-like enterotoxin produced by *Campylobacter jejuni*. *Lancet*, **ii**, 250–252.

Savilahti E., Pelkonen P. & Visakorpi J.K. (1971) IgA deficiency in children. A clinical study with special reference to intestinal findings. *Arch. Dis. Child.* **46**, 665.

Selby W.S., Janossy G., Goldstein G. & Jewell D.P. (1981) T lymphocyte subsets in human intestinal mucosa. *Clin. exp. Immunol.* **44**, 453.

Sissons J.G.P., Peters D.K. Williams D.G., Boulton-Jones J.M. & Goldsmith H.J. (1974) Skin lesions, angioedema and hypocomplementemia. *Lancet*, **ii**, 1350–1352.

Sloper K.S., Dourmashkin R.R., Bird R.B., Slavin G. & Webster A.D.B. (1982) Chronic malabsorption due to cryptosporidiosis in a child with immunoglobulin deficiency. *Gut*, **23**, 80–82.

Soothill J.F., Stokes C.R., Turner M.W., Norman A.P. & Taylor B. (1976) Predisposing factors and the development of reaginic allergy in infancy. *Clin. Allergy*, **6**, 305.

Stoelinga G.B.A., van Munster P.J.J. & Slooff J.P. (1963) Chylous effusions into the intestine in a patient with protein-losing gastroenteropathy. *Pediat.* **31**, 1011.

Storb R., Prentice R.L., Buckner C.D., Clift R.A., Appelbaum F., Deeg J., Doney K., Hansen J.A., Mason M., Sanders J.E., Singer J., Sullivan

K.M., Witherspoon R.P. & Thomas E.D. (1983) Graft-versus-host disease and survival in patients with aplastic anaemia treated by marrow grafts from HLA-identical siblings. *New Eng. J. Med.* **308**, 302–307.

Strober W., Wochner R.D., Carbone P.P. & Waldmann T.A. (1967) Intestinal lymphangiectasia: a protein-losing enteropathy with hypogammaglobulinaemia, lymphocytopenia and impaired homograft rejection. *J. Clin. Invest.* **46**, 1643.

Targan S.R., Chow A.E. & Guze L.B. (1976) Spontaneous peritonitis in cirrhosis due to *Campylobacter fetus*. *Gastroenterol.* **71**, 311.

Taylor B., Norman A.P., Orgel H.A., Stokes C.R., Turner M.W. & Soothill J.F. (1973) Transient IgA deficiency and pathogenesis of infantile atopy. *Lancet*, **ii**, 111.

Tomkins A.M., Drasar B.S. & James W.P.T. (1975) Bacterial colonisation of jejunal mucosa in acute tropical sprue. *Lancet*, **i**, 59.

Tzipori S., Angus K.W., Campbell I. & Gray E.W. (1982) Experimental infection of lambs with Cryptosporidium isolated from a human patient with diarrhoea. *Gut*, **23**, 71.

Tzipori S. (1983) Cryptosporidiosis in animals and humans. *Microbiol. Rev.* **47**, 84–96.

Vieira J., Frank E., Spira T.J. & Landesman S.H. (1983) Acquired immune deficiency in Haitians: opportunistic infections in previously healthy Haitian immigrants. *N. Eng. J. Med.* **308**, 365–367.

Waksman B.H. & Ozer H. (1976) Specialised amplification elements in the immune system. The role of nodular lymphoid organs in the mucous membranes. *Prog. Allergy.* **21**, 1.

Walker W.A., Wu M. Isselbacher K.J. Bloch K.J. (1975) Intestinal uptake of macromolecules. III. Studies on the mechanism by which immunization interfers with antigen uptake. *J. Immunol.* **115**, 854.

Ward H., Jalan K.N., Maitra T.K., Agarwal S.K. & Mahalanabis D. (1983) Small intestinal nodular lymphoid hyperplasia in patients with giardiasis and normal serum immunoglobulins. *Gut* **24**, 120–126.

Warin A.P., Greaves M.W., Gatecliff M., Williamson D.M. & Warin R.P. (1980) Treatment of hereditary angioedema by low dose attenuated androgens: disassociation of clinical response from levels of C1 esterase inhibitor and C4. *Brit. J. Dermatol.* **103**, 405–409.

Webster A.D.B. (1973) Spirillum hepatitis in 'acquired' hypogammaglobulinaemia with thyroiditis, pernicious anaemia and possible dermatitis herpetiformis. *Proc. Roy. Soc. Med.* **66**, 1126.

Webster A.D.B. (1976) The gut and immunodeficiency disorders. *Clin. Gastroent.* **5**, 323.

Webster A.D.B., Kenwright S., Ballard J., Shiner M., Slavin G. Levi A.J., Loewi G. & Asherson G.L. (1977) Nodular lymphoid hyperplasia of the bowel in primary hypogammaglobulinaemia: a study of *in vivo* and *in vitro* lymphocyte function. *Gut*, **18**, 264.

Webster A.D.B., Slavin G., Shiner M., Platts-Mills T.A.E. & Asherson G.L. (1981) Coeliac disease with severe hypogammaglobulinaemia. *Gut*, **22**, 153–157.

Wells J.V., Michaeli D. & Fudenberg H.H. (1973) Antibodies to human collagen in subjects with selective IgA deficiency. *Clin. Exp. Immunol.* **13**, 203.

Weisburger W.R., Hutcheon D.F., Yardley J.H., Roche J.C., Hillis W.D. & Charache P. (1979) Cryptosporidiosis in an immunosuppressed renal transplant recipient with IgA deficiency. *Amer. J. Clin. Path.* **72**, 473–478.

Wyatt R.A., Younoszai K., Anuras S. & Myers M.G. (1977) *Campylobacter fetus* septicaemia and hepatitis in agammaglobulinaemia. *J. Pediat.* **91**, 441.

Yolken R.H., Bishop C.A., Townsend T.R., Bolyard E.A., Bartlett J., Santos G.W., Saral R. (1982) Infectious gastroenteritis in bone marrow transplant recipients. *New. Eng. J. Med.* **306**, 1009–1013.

Chapter 9
Coeliac Disease

ANTHONY M. DAWSON AND PARVEEN KUMAR

History 153
Definition 153
Pathology 153
Genetics 156
The role of gluten 157
Aetiology 159
Clinical features 161
Conditions associated with coeliac disease .. 167
Malabsorption non-responsive to treatment
    with a gluten-free diet 168
Complications of coeliac disease 169
Dermatitis herpetiformis 170

History

The first description of malabsorption is attributed to Arataeus the Cappadocian in the second century A.D. (Adams 1856). He described a chronic condition in adults who were emaciated, starved, pallid and feeble with foul-smelling eructations and rumblings with 'emission of flatulent material which is thick, liquid and looks like white clay'. In 1888, Samuel Gee gave the first clear description of coeliac disease, a condition of 'chronic indigestion' with steatorrhoea which occurred at all ages but particularly in children aged 1 to 5 years. He concluded perceptively that if a patient can be cured at all, it must be 'by means of diet'. In 1932 Thaysen gave a classic description of the adult form of disease, which became known as idiopathic steatorrhoea. During and after the Second World War, Dicke (1950) established the role of flour in this disease. He observed that children improved during the war years when wheat and rye flour were unobtainable in Holland, and that they relapsed when wheat flour became freely available after the war. Subsequently van der Kamer et al. (1953) and van der Kamer & Weijers (1955) showed that gluten, the water-insoluble protein of wheat, was the substance which damaged the small intestine of these patients. In 1954, Paulley noted the characteristic histological features of this disease on operative biopsies of the small intestine. Since then, the development of the peroral biopsy technique has greatly facilitated the diagnosis of the condition and encouraged investigations into its aetiology (Royer et al. 1955, Shiner 1956a, b, Crosby & Kugler 1957).

Definition

Coeliac disease is a common cause of malabsorption in Britain and North America. The diagnosis is based on an abnormal jejunal biopsy which improves on gluten withdrawal, and the use of the descriptive term 'gluten-sensitive enteropathy' therefore avoids the confusion of older terminologies such as idiopathic steatorrhoea, non-tropical sprue or Gee—Herter disease. The disorder may be defined as *a condition in which there is an abnormal jejunal mucosa which improves morphologically when treated with a gluten-free diet and which again shows abnormalities when gluten is re-introduced.* Although reintroduction of gluten is frequently necessary to establish the diagnosis in childhood (Meeuwisse 1970), it is rarely practical or necessary in adults.

Pathology

Coeliac disease affects the mucosa of the small intestine. The proximal small bowel is severely affected and the lesion decreases distally, the ileum either being normal or less severely involved than the jejunum (Rubin et al. 1960, Stewart et al. 1967). The lesion may occasionally be patchy (Scott et al. 1976) and the less affected areas are likely to be in the furrows between the valves of Kerkring.

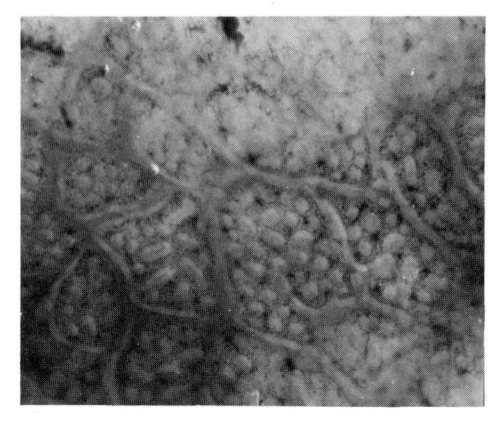

Fig. 9.1. Flat coeliac mucosa on dissecting microscopy (× 44). (Courtesy of Dr J.S. Stewart.)

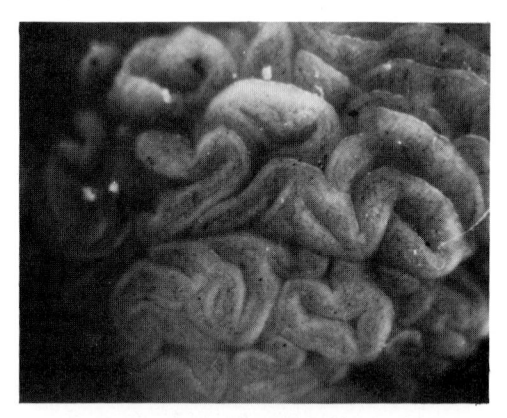

Fig. 9.2. Convoluted coeliac mucosa on dissecting microscopy (× 70). (Courtesy of Dr. J.S. Stewart.)

Stereomicroscopic examination

The characteristic finding in untreated coeliac disease is a pale 'flat' mucosal surface without villi; the crypt orifices open onto tiny depressions on the surface. Frequently the flat surface has a mosaic or cobble-stone pattern (Fig. 9.1). A convoluted pattern, resembling the convolutions on the surface of the brain (Fig. 9.2), is less often present (Stewart et al. 1967).

Scanning electron microscopy

Scanning electron microscopy also shows the flat mucosal surface, the mucosa often forming a mosaic pattern and the orifices of the crypts can be seen opening onto the surface. At higher power the individual crypts can be visualized with a rim of cells around the orifice of the crypt (Fig. 9.3). At even higher power the individual enterocytes can be seen end on. By contrast with the normal regular hexagonal pattern of enterocytes seen in control subjects, the enterocytes in coeliac disease show variation in size and shape (Marsh et al. 1970).

Histology

The main histological features are an absence of villi, crypt hyperplasia and infiltration of the *lamina propria* with chronic inflammatory cells (Fig. 9.4). The total thickness of the mucosa is normal or only slightly reduced, as hypertrophy of the crypts compensates for the absence or shortening of the villi. The mucosa is therefore in a hyperkinetic state, the increased rate of cell production by the crypts compensating for damage to the surface enterocytes. A small percentage of patients have partial villous atrophy; here the villi are shortened with crypt hyperplasia and infiltration of the lamina propria with inflammatory cells (Fig. 9.5), an appearance corresponding to the convoluted mucosa already described.

The enterocytes (Booth 1970) are reduced in height and become cuboidal. The cytoplasm is more basophilic and the basal polarity of the nuclei is lost. On electron microscopy, there is increased vacuolation, mitochondrial swelling, an excess of free-lying ribosomes and an increase in lysosomes. The microvilli on the surface of the cells are irregular, shortened and often fused. The fibres of the basement membrane and the reticulin network supporting the epithelial cells may be normal or show gross thickening (Shiner 1974). A reduction in mucosal enzymes (disaccharidases, peptidases, alkaline phosphatase, adenosine triphosphatase and esterase) has been described (Padykula et al. 1961, Douglas & Booth 1970, Peters et al. 1975). The reduction of brush border enzymes may be shown both by histochemistry and biochemical analysis.

Interspersed between the enterocytes are intraepithelial lymphocytes. These originate

Coeliac Disease

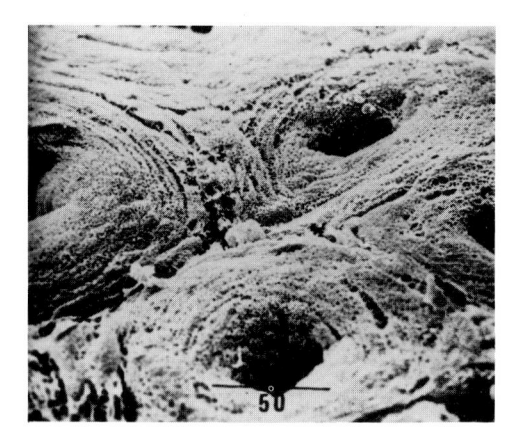

Fig. 9.3. Scanning electron microscopy showing enterocytes heaping up around crypt orifices in coeliac disease (× 1500) (Courtesy of Dr. M.N. Marsh.)

in the lamina propria and enter the space between the enterocytes through a break in the basal lamina of the epithelium. The ratio of the lymphocytes to epithelial cells is increased in coeliac disease (Ferguson & Murray 1971), although the total number of lymphocytes per unit length of intestine may not be increased (Marsh 1980, 1981). The normal range of intraepithelial lymphocytes is six to forty for every 100 epithelial cells whilst most untreated coeliac patients have counts in excess of forty (Ferguson & Murray 1971).

The undifferentiated crypt cells are increased in number, causing a lengthening of the crypts. The mitoses per crypt are increased mainly in the lower third (Padykula et al. 1961, Yardley et al. 1962). The cytology and histochemistry of the crypt cells are normal by both light and electron microscopy (Rubin et al. 1966). The goblet cells are usually normal although occasionally increased in number. The exact role of the Paneth cells at the crypt fundus is still unknown (Thurlbeck et al. 1960, Lewin 1969, Peeters & van Trappen 1975). Crypt enterochromaffin cells may be increased in number (Dawson 1976).

The *lamina propria* has an increased cellular infiltrate, consisting of lymphocytes,

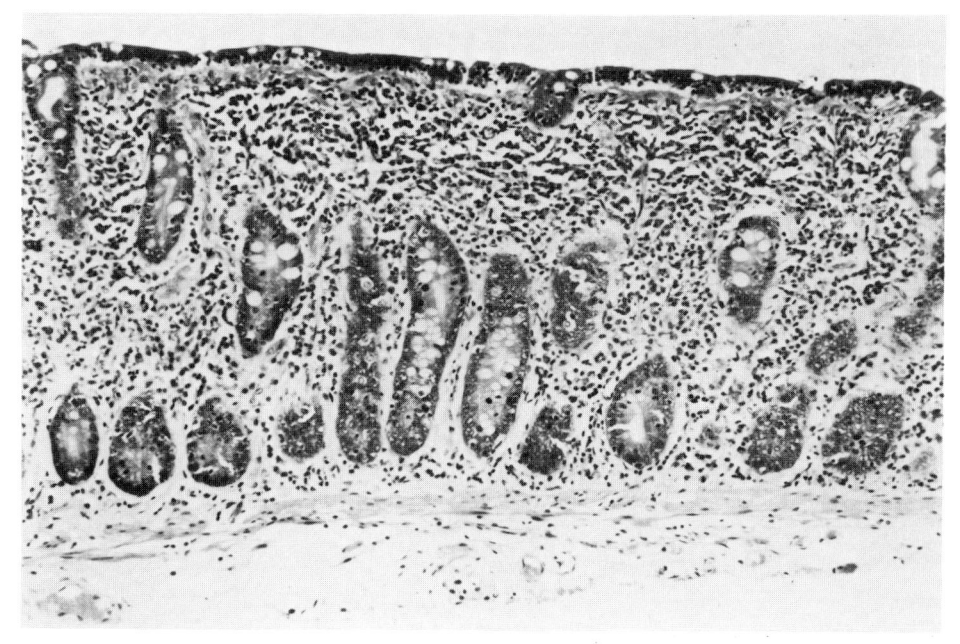

Fig. 9.4. Histological appearance of subtotal villous atrophy with a lack of villi, cuboidal epithelial cells, an increase in intraepithelial lymphocytes, hypertrophy of the crypts and an increased cellular infiltrate in the lamina propria.

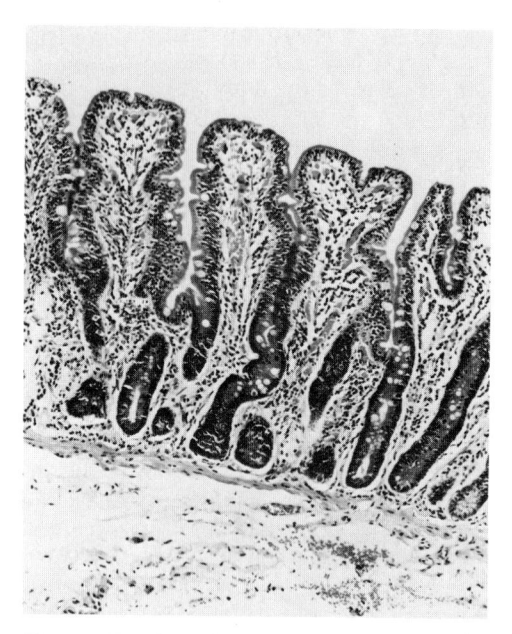

Fig. 9.5. Histological section showing partial villous atrophy with stunting of villi, increase in intraepithelial lymphocytes, and increase in the cellular infiltrate in the lamina propria.

plasma cells, macrophages, mast cells and eosinophils. The plasma cells and lymphocytes produce immunoglobulins and, although IgA-producing cells are most abundant in normal individuals, IgM-containing cells predominate in the untreated coeliac patient (Douglas et al. 1970, Soltoft 1970, Lancaster-Smith et al. 1974). The basement membrane of the surface epithelial cells may be irregular and thickened. Some degree of subepithelial collagenization in biopsies with villous atrophy is seen in 36% of patients (Bossart et al. 1975). The term 'collagenous sprue' was coined by Weinstein et al. (1970) to indicate a lack of response to a gluten-free diet in severely ill patients with a poor prognosis whose biopsies showed a thick pale-staining subepithelial hyaline collagenous zone and minimal crypt hyperplasia. However, other patients with heavy collagenous infiltrate have been noted to respond well to a gluten-free diet (Bossart et al. 1975).

Specificity of a flat mucosa

There are conditions other than coeliac disease which may be associated with a flat or otherwise abnormal mucosa. In childhood, these include gastroenteritis (Walker-Smith 1972), cow's milk intolerance (Visakorpi & Imonen 1967), sensitivity to soya protein (Ament & Rubin 1972) and protein−calorie malnutrition (Brunser et al. 1966). In adults, the mucosa may be abnormal in tropical sprue but only rarely shows the flat mucosa typical of coeliac disease, partial villous atrophy being characteristic of the tropical condition (Chapter 19). Hypogammaglobulinaemia and parasitic disease are described in Chapters 8 and 17. In addition, there is a rare type of malabsorption associated with a flat mucosa in which there is no response to a gluten-free diet. This condition is considered in more detail at the end of this chapter and in Chapter 12.

Cytokinetics

Although the mucosa is flattened it is highly proliferative, as shown by raised mitotic indices (Padykula et al. 1961, Yardley et al. 1962, Wright et al. 1973). The raised mitotic index is mainly due to an increased rate in cell division as the cell cycle time is more than halved when compared with control mucosa; it is also partly due to an increase in the mitotic duration. The cell production rate per crypt is greatly increased from the normal rate of 25 cells/crypt per hour to 155 cells/h in adult coeliacs (Wright et al. 1973, Watson & Wright 1974). Similar increases are seen in childhood coeliac disease and in the flattened mucosa in dermatitis herpetiformis: the crypts are not only increased in length, but also in girth. The mechanism compensating for cell loss is therefore a decrease in cell cycle time, a three-dimensional enlargement of the proliferative compartment in the crypt and an upward movement of the cut-off point where the cells stop proliferating and start maturation.

Genetics

The prevalence of coeliac disease in the general population varies between 1 in 300 in the West of Ireland (Mylotte et al.

1973), 1 in 1850 in Scotland (McCrae et al. 1970) to 1 in 960 in Sweden (Hallert et al. 1983). There are few reports of coeliac disease occurring in Japanese or black Africans, suggesting a genetic basis for the disease. In addition, if jejunal biopsies are carried out in asymptomatic first degree relatives, as many as 10% may be shown to have coeliac disease (MacDonald et al. 1965). The increased incidence of the HLA B8 antigen in approximately 80% of patients, compared with 20% of the general population, emphasizes the importance of genetic factors in coeliac disease (Falchuk et al. 1972, Stokes et al. 1972, Keuning et al. 1976). As the genes controlling the HLA antigens are closely linked on the same chromosome, they tend to be inherited together. Coeliac disease is strongly associated not only with the haplotype B8, but also −CW7, −DR3/AW24, −BW59, −DR3 and less strongly with the haplotype −AX, −B12−DR7 (Betuel et al. 1980). Coeliac disease is primarily associated with HLA−DR3 as the association with B8 is due to the linkage disequilibrium that normally exists between B8 and DR3. A similar analysis performed for the two antigens DR3 and DR7 showed a strong association with both antigens in Spain whereas in the Netherlands there was an association only with DR3 (Pena 1981). Several population and family studies have also shown that coeliac disease is primarily associated with DR3 and DR7 (Albert 1978, Marchi et al. 1979).

The exact mode of inheritance is still unknown. A dominantly inherited autosomal gene with low penetrance was suggested by MacDonald et al. (1965). The results of HLA studies in multiple case families, however, support the concept that a recessive gene within the HLA system is implicated. Only 60% of HLA identical siblings manifest the disease and as many as 30% of identical twins are discordant for coeliac disease (Pena 1981). Mann et al. (1976) screened sera from mothers of patients with coeliac disease and found antibodies directed against the B-cell antigens which were strongly associated with the disease. Pena (1978) found that the sera reacted independently of HLA, A1, B8 and DR3 antigens and suggested that coeliac patients were homozygous for the coeliac-associated B-cell antigen.

The role of gluten

Gluten is toxic to the small intestinal mucosa of patients with coeliac disease and is contained in wheat, rye and barley. Whether oats are invariably toxic remains controversial (Dicke et al. 1953, Dissanayake et al. 1974a). In most coeliac individuals, oats may be taken with impunity. There may, however, be occasional patients who are sensitive to oats although this has not yet been clearly documented.

Gluten is contained in wheat grain, a cross section of which is shown in Fig. 9.6. The endosperm is composed of starch (70−75%) and protein (7−15%) as well as lipids and other minor components. During milling the endosperm is separated from the bran and germ and ground to produce flour. An aqueous extraction of flour gives rise to a soluble portion, consisting of starch, albumin and globulin, and an insoluble fraction containing gluten. Gluten can be further fractionated either by partial digestion with pepsin and trypsin to produce Fraser's fraction III or by an alcoholic extraction to produce gliadin. The latter is a complex mixture of peptides separated into the classes of α, β, γ and ω on account of decreasing relative mobility on starch gel electrophoresis (Woychik et al. 1961).

Fraser et al. (1959), seeking the toxic fraction, took whole gluten with its myriads of peptides and made a peptic−tryptic digest which was toxic. Complete digestion with fresh hog mucosa (Fraser et al. 1959), complete acid hydrolysis, deamidation by acid (Alvey et al. 1957) and treatment with papain (Krainick & Mohn 1959), however, abolished this toxicity. Krainick & Mohn (1959), using provocation tests in patients in whom faecal fat excretion was measured, found that ultrafiltrates of the peptic−tryptic digest with molecular weights as low as 900 were toxic and this was later confirmed by Bronstein et al. (1966).

Subsequently gluten was fractionated using 70% ethanol water extraction, produc-

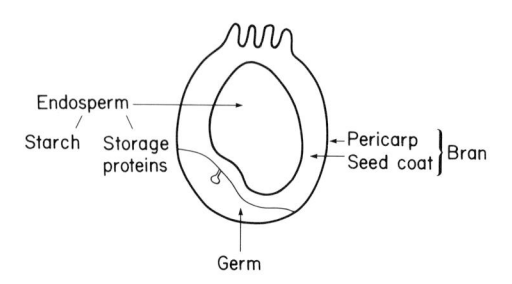

Fig. 9.6. A cross-section of a wheat grain.

ing an insoluble (glutenin) and a soluble (gliadin) component. Gliadin, the parent toxic fraction, accounts for approximately 40% of the total protein from wheat and is still toxic after peptic–tryptic digestion. The search over recent years has been to separate pure fractions of α, β, γ and ω gliadins. Each class, however, comprises a complex group of proteins which have a high glutamine and proline content (Autran et al. 1979). For example, Mecham et al. (1978) found at least thirty to fifty bands on two-dimensional electrophoresis of A gliadin which has a molecular weight of 50,000 (Bernardin et al. 1967). On further degradation, substances with molecular weights as small as 2000–10,000 have been described as toxic (Jos & Rey 1975, Dissanayake et al. 1974). Attempts have also been made to separate gliadins on ion exchange and gel filtration chromatography (Patey & Evans 1973). The precise nature of the toxic fraction of gluten remains to be determined. A suggestion that the toxicity of gluten is due to a carbohydrate side chain (Phelan et al. 1978, Stevens et al. 1978) has not been confirmed and other workers have failed to demonstrate glycoproteins in gliadin (Bernadin et al. 1976).

Test systems for gluten fractions

The search for the toxic fraction in gluten has been carried out in the past by studying the effect of a test substance in a patient with coeliac disease in whom treatment has been successful. Tests of absorption have largely been replaced by tests using repeated jejunal biopsy in such subjects *in vivo*. Recently, however, the attempt has been made to develop *in vitro* techniques.

In vivo techniques

These techniques can be used in the course of a normal challenge for the confirmation of coeliac disease. Challenges with a normal diet (Visakorpi 1974, Kumar et al. 1979a), with gluten or gliadin or short term challenges with toxic fractions may be undertaken. It takes a variable length of time for the mucosa to become abnormal when patients in remission are put on gluten-containing diets and the results of challenges may therefore be different. Some observations have indicated that gluten induces an Arthus type reaction, abnormalities being induced within 8–12 h of the installation of gluten either into the normal ileum of individuals with active disease in the jejunum (Rubin et al. 1960) or into the jejunum of individuals who have a normal mucosa following successful treatment (Booth et al. 1977). Damage within 24 h after a gluten challenge, however, has varied from subepithelial changes on electron microscopy (Shiner 1973), to changes in intraepithelial lymphocyte counts and immunoglobulin-containing plasma cells (Lancaster-Smith et al. 1976a, b) or even to gross structural change (Anand et al. 1981, Ciclitera et al. 1981). In our experience, however, gross mucosal damage has not occurred following gluten challenge using large doses within 24 h. Present evidence suggests that α fractions of gliadin are toxic and the role of other fractions is contentious.

In vitro techniques

In order to avoid the necessity of performing repeated jejunal biopsies in patients, as required by *in vivo* techniques, attempts have been made to develop *in vitro* methods of testing the toxicity of gluten and its fractions using jejunal mucosa obtained by biopsy. Organ culture techniques using pieces of intestinal mucosa were originally described by Browning & Trier (1969) and Trier et al. (1970) and subsequent modifications have been developed (Hirondel et al. 1976, Autrup et al. 1978). Cell death at varying rates under similar laboratory conditions is high and the technique is therefore not sufficiently sensitive to assess toxicity.

Falchuk and his colleagues (1974a) measured brush border enzymes and found an inhibitory effect of gluten on biopsies from untreated patients. Surprisingly, however, they showed that this inhibition depended on the activity of the disease as gluten had no effect on biopsies from treated patients. Gluten was therefore not directly toxic but the susceptibility of the mucosa to gluten was only induced by recent exposure to gluten *in vivo*. In a further set of co-culture experiments, where biopsies from treated and untreated patients were cultured together with gluten, the treated mucosa could now be made susceptible. This led to the suggestion that toxic substances, possibly lymphokines, were produced by the mucosa of the untreated patient. The results of testing fractions *in vitro*, like those *in vivo*, suggest that the α fraction of gliadin is the toxic factor.

Nullisomic 6 A variants

As a gliadin peptide appears to be the agent toxic to patients with coeliac disease, attempts have been made to breed a wheat free of toxic gliadin. Bread wheats belong to a hexaploid species containing three genomes A B and D, each contributing seven pairs of chromosomes. Genes on chromosomes 6 A code for some of the alpha gliadins and in particular are thought to code for the components of A gliadin (Kasarda *et al.* 1976). A variety of Chinese spring wheat lacking this 6 A chromsome has been developed. Sadly, feeding experiments have shown this wheat to produce histological damage in coeliac patients (Ciclitira *et al.* 1980).

Aetiology

Enzyme deficiency

Fraser (1956) suggested a congenital absence of a peptidase in the intestinal mucosa so that gluten was not fully digested and toxic peptides might then damage the mucosa. Current evidence, however, suggests that peptidase deficiency in coeliac disease is secondary to enterocyte damage (Douglas & Booth 1970, Peters *et al.* 1975, 1978). Although Townley and his colleagues (1973) and Cornell & Townley (1973) have challenged this view, the discordance for coeliac disease in as many as 30% of identical twins is strongly against a primary enzyme deficiency.

Enterocyte membrane defect

This postulates a membrane defect which would expose a sugar residue interacting with a lectin (Adair & Kornfeld 1974) in wheat gluten, and this combination could have a toxic effect on the intestinal epithelial cell (Weiser & Douglas 1976).

Immunological hypothesis (Fig. 9.7)

An immunological response to the toxic factor in gluten is the likeliest explanation for the intestinal lesion in coeliac disease. The association of HLA−DR3 with the disorder suggests the possibility of an abnormal immune response, as is the case in other conditions associated with HLA−DR3. Corticosteroids improve both the clinical symptoms and histological abnormality in untreated patients (Wall *et al.* 1970, Kumar *et al.* 1973b), further supporting the hypothesis that the damage is produced by immunological mechanisms.

Does gluten enter the intestinal mucosa?

In order to induce an immunological response, it might be expected that gluten in some way enters the mucosa. Macromolecules have been shown to gain entry through intact mucosa (Walker *et al.* 1972, Swarbrick *et al.* 1979, Hemmings & Williams 1978) (Chapter 7). Alternatively it has been suggested that there may be a specific surface receptor for gluten. This could be an HLA gene or a B-cell receptor or there may be a hitherto undiscovered binding site. HLA−B8/DR3 antigens are thought to be associated with a general facilitation of immunological responses. Indeed, HLA−B8 positive individuals have been shown to

Chapter 9

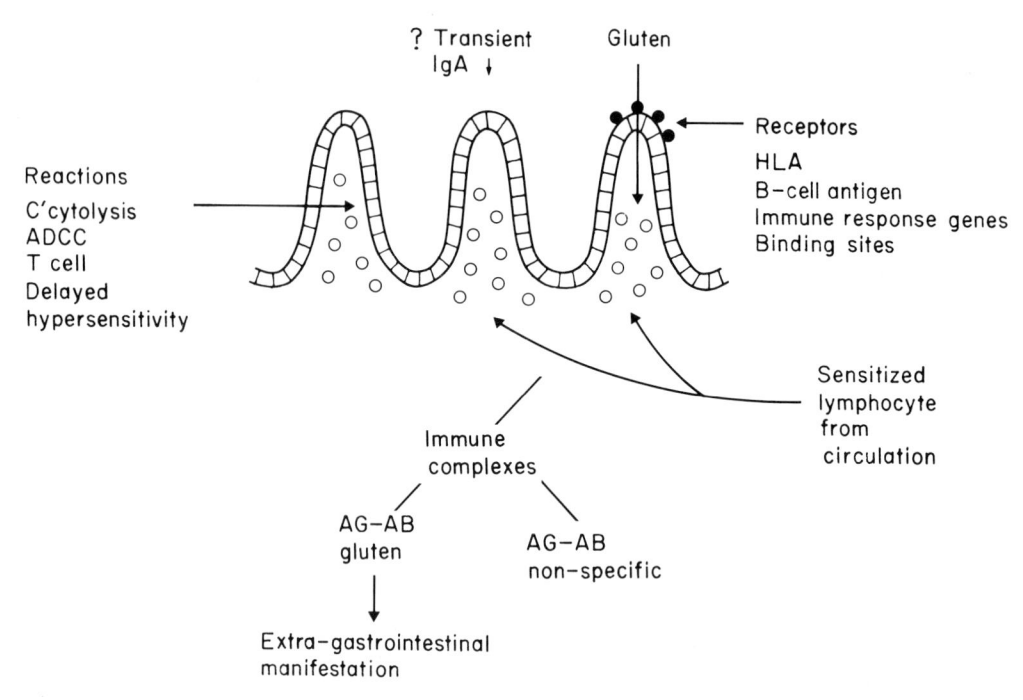

Fig. 9.7. Diagram of small intestinal mucosa showing possible immunological mechanisms that may play a part in the pathogenesis of the flattened mucosa.

respond more vigorously to gluten than B8 negative controls in mixed leucocyte cultures (Osoba & Falk 1976) and their lymphocytes are said to be more sensitive to gluten in transformation experiments (Cunningham–Rundles et al. 1978). Alternatively, a B-cell antigen may be present on the surface of the mucosa and initiate a response. If the epithelial cell is the target of immunocytotoxicity, then one would expect gluten to bind to it, and Rubin et al. (1965) were unable to find any binding to enterocytes, other than crypt cells.

Immunological response

It has been known for many years that antigen-sensitized lymphocytes will migrate from the lamina propria to the thoracic duct and general circulation (Gowans & Knight 1964). Such sensitized lymphocytes home back to the lamina propria where they differentiate into plasma cells. It is therefore possible that gluten-sensitive lymphocytes producing antigluten antibody are present in the lamina propria. At a histological level, gluten challenge can be shown to induce a proliferation of plasma cells secreting immunoglobulin (Lancaster-Smith et al. 1974). Furthermore, Loeb & colleagues (1971), using labelled amino acid incorporation in jejunal culture, showed that the newly synthesized immunoglobulin resulting from gluten challenge *in vivo* had a specificity for gluten. These observations support the theory that the immunocytes in the gut in coeliac disease may be producing a humoral antibody.

Mechanism of enterocyte damage

The exact way in which enterocytes are damaged may involve several immunological processes. Firstly antigen–antibody immune complexes with gluten specificity may be formed and deposited in the lamina propria, as suggested by Shiner & Ballard (1972) and by Doe et al. (1974), causing enterocyte damage. Other immunological mechanisms causing damage may include complement-mediated cytotoxicity, antibody-dependent cell-mediated cytotoxicity or direct cellular cytotoxicity (Doe et al. 1974, Ezeoke et al.

1974). Cell-mediated mechanisms may also play a part as it has been shown that lymphokines are released in organ culture on the addition of gluten (Ferguson et al. 1975). Whether delayed hypersensitivity reactions are important is uncertain. Interaction between the intraepithelial lymphocytes, thought to be T cells, and dietary antigens, is another possible mechanism of enterocyte damage.

Clinical features

The clinical presentation of coeliac disease varies greatly and patients may present to a variety of specialists. Most commonly, the recognition of a nutritional deficiency caused by malabsorption leads to the diagnosis. In some cases gastrointestinal symptoms may predominate whilst in others they are negligible. Symptoms do not appear to be related to the severity of the mucosal lesion (Rubin 1960, Samloff et al. 1964) but may be related to its extent (Rubin 1960). Many cases remain undiagnosed as evidenced by the numbers of asymptomatic relatives, already referred to, who have flattened jejunal biopsies (MacDonald et al. 1965, Robinson et al. 1971, Mylotte 1972, Shipman et al. 1973, Rolles et al. 1974, Asquith 1974, McCarthy et al. 1974, Rosekrans et al. 1978).

Childhood coeliac disease

The age of *presentation* is variable but symptoms often appear between the ages of 1 and 5 years, with a predominance in the second year (Young & Pringle 1971). The age at which gluten-containing cereals are introduced into the diet may be important, for Anderson et al. (1972) found that if the age at which cereals were introduced was reduced, the mean age at presentation also fell. The earlier introduction of cereals, however, does not increase the incidence of coeliac disease (Walker-Smith 1975). The 'latent interval' between the introduction of gluten and the development of symptoms varies from a few months to years but in one series 19.6% of coeliac children, as well as 4.3% of their unaffected siblings, had symptoms on their first contact with gluten (Walker-Smith 1975).

Table 9.1. Symptoms present at the time of diagnosis in fifty-two coeliac children.

Symptoms	Percentage
Diarrhoea	45
Abdominal distension	23
Vomiting	32
Lassitude	32
Weight loss	31
Irritability	30
Anorexia	25
Abdominal pain	23
Respiratory infection	14
Failure to thrive	14
Sleep disturbance	9
Appetite increased	8
Oedema	7
Muscle wasting	7
Pallor	7
Constipation	3
Mouth ulceration	3
Rectal prolapse	2
Skin infections	2

(Courtesy of Dr. J.A. Walker-Smith.)

Diarrhoea, vomiting, weight loss and a failure to thrive are common childhood presentations (Table 9.1). Diarrhoea may be acute, insidious or recurrent and a child may pass either two to three fatty stools per day or just one large bulky motion. Alternatively, there may be constipation which rarely may be so severe as to be confused with Hirschsprung's disease (Bennett et al. 1932, Walker-Smith 1975). Abdominal pain, when present, is not severe. Emotional symptoms are common and the child may be 'extremely irritable, fretful, capricious or peevish' (Gibbons 1889). There is often a 'clingingness' of the child to his mother, who herself may become depressed, anxious and abnormally preoccupied with her child (Gardner et al. 1973).

On *examination*, the classical picture of a miserable child with a distended abdomen, wasted buttocks and shoulder girdle may be seen; alternatively the child may look well. There may be a history of delay in motor milestones and measurements of height and weight may show a drop below the 10th percentile.

The *diagnosis*, as in adults, should be based on the characteristic jejunal biopsy with clinical and morphological response to a gluten-free diet. It is now usual to rechallenge a child with gluten later and show mucosal deterioration to exclude transient gluten intolerance (Walker-Smith 1970). As this may take a long time, the child should be followed for up to 4 years after gluten reintroduction (Visakorpi 1974, McNicholl et al. 1974).

Complications in childhood coeliac disease include rickets and growth and developmental retardation, often with delayed onset of puberty (Gee 1888, Prader et al. 1963, 1969). Several observations suggest that there may be hypothalamic hypofunction. Studies of growth hormone have shown that coeliacs have reduced levels after intravenous tolbutamide and oral Bovril when compared to control children (Day et al. 1973). However, using insulin tolerance tests Vanderschueren-Lodeweycky and her colleagues (1973) found that the fall in blood glucose after insulin was the same in coeliacs and controls but the subsequent response of blood glucose levels to induced hypoglycaemia was reduced in coeliacs. This abnormality was corrected after a gluten-free diet. The majority of patients also had a reduced response of plasma growth hormone.

Coeliac disease in teenagers

Coeliac disease presenting in the second decade is unusual. There appears to be a natural tendency for the childhood disease to remit during this period. Many children, however, who have discontinued their diets relapse in early adult life. In untreated patients puberty may be delayed and Lindsay et al. (1956) found that the age of menarche was 1–2 years later than in normal girls. Some patients may present with primary amenorrhoea (Gent 1973).

Adult coeliac disease

Presentation

Adult patients can present at any age, the peak incidence being in the third and fourth decades; there is a female preponderance. Symptoms are variable (Cooke et al. 1953, Benson et al. 1964, Barry et al. 1974). In general, however, presentation may be either with gastrointestinal symptoms and diarrhoea, or with symptoms of malnutrition caused by malabsorption, particularly iron and folic acid deficiency, and less frequently hypocalcaemia and bone disease.

Table 9.2. Symptoms at diagnosis in 168 adult patients with coeliac disease.

Symptom	Percentage
Malaise	79
Diarrhoea	70
Steatorrhoea	58
Weight loss	62
Anorexia	41
Abdominal pain	42
Oral ulceration	28
Childhood history	46 (14)[*]
Distension	23
Wind	19
Nausea vomiting	18
Muscle pain	7
Tetany	4
Bone joint pains	8
Ankle oedema	10
Dyspnoea	9

( )[*]Diagnosed in childhood

The characteristic features are diarrhoea and weight loss, or symptoms from anaemia (Table 9.2). The onset may be acute with diarrhoea, weight loss, vomiting, anorexia and abdominal distension, or may be so insidious that a patient may drift into chronic ill health. Some patients may give a history of recurrent iron deficiency anaemia, or of megaloblastic anaemia. As many as two-thirds of patients had been misdiagnosed at the onset of symptoms in one series and this accounts for the delay in diagnosis experienced by some patients. Diarrhoea may be continuous, or recurrent, or alternating with constipation. It is usually not severe, the patient passing loose, pale or watery stools three or four times a day. Rarely, there may be torrential diarrhoea with over twenty stools a day. On the other hand, there may be only one fatty stool a day and some patients present with constipation; one third of the patients whose symptoms are listed in Table 9.2 did not have diarrhoea, and diarrhoea was absent in nearly two-thirds of the patients described by Swinson & Levi (1980). Weight loss is variable; most patients have lost a few kilograms, but a few may present with severe weight loss and emaciation, predominantly as a result of anorexia rather than malabsorption. Abdominal distension is common. Secondary lactase deficiency may also lead to diarrhoea and abdominal discomfort after milk ingestion. Abdominal pain occurs in about a third of patients. Mouth ulceration may be persistent or intermittent. Less frequent symptoms include tetany, bone pain and muscle weakness. Many patients are asymptomatic and are detected by blood tests showing mild anaemia with iron or folate deficiency, sometimes with Howell–Jolly bodies on the blood film. A few patients present with infertility.

Physical examination

There may be few signs and these are often non-specific. The patient may be thin with dry hair and hyperpigmented skin. Mucous membranes may be pale due to anaemia. Atrophic glossitis, apthous ulceration, angular stomatitis or koilonychia may be seen due to iron or folate deficiency. Bruising may be due to vitamin K malabsorption. Dependent ankle oedema due to hypoproteinaemia is unusual. Abdominal distension is common. Finger-clubbing is rare, but latent tetany due to low calcium may be demonstrated by a positive Trousseau or Chvostek test. There may be bony tenderness and a myopathy if there is vitamin D deficiency. Rarely a peripheral neuropathy due to unknown factors may be demonstrated.

Investigations

Haematology

The incidence of anaemia varies from 40–84% (Cooke et al. 1963, Kumar 1976, Hoffbrand 1974) and is mainly due to iron and folate deficiency, a reflection of jejunal malabsorption (cf. Fig. 6.3). Fifty per cent of patients are iron deficient (Kumar 1976) although Badenoch & Callender (1960) found all their patients had abnormal iron absorption when tested. Excessive intestinal loss of iron may also contribute to deficiency (Sutton et al. 1970). Iron deficiency may mask macrocytosis if reliance is put on a Coulter counter, and, if a blood smear is not performed, macrocytes and hypersegmented polymorphs, indicating folate deficiency, and Howell–Jolly bodies may be missed. Folate deficiency is virtually universal and a low red cell folate measured by microbiological assay is the best haematological screening test (Magnus 1966, Hoffbrand et al. 1966, Cooke 1968, Kumar 1976). Low serum levels of vitamin B_{12} occur in a third to a fifth of patients (Mollin et al. 1957, Stewart et al. 1967, Cooke 1968, Kumar 1976) but these do not usually indicate B_{12} deficiency. Subacute combined degeneration of the cord due to B_{12} deficiency has not been described in coeliac disease. Bone marrow examination may show megaloblastic changes, mixed iron and megaloblastic changes or iron deficiency changes (Hoffbrand 1974, Kumar 1976). There may be a raised erythrocyte sedimentation rate in about 20% of patients (Kumar 1976).

Rarer haematological manifestations include a prolonged prothrombin time, which may lead to the patient presenting with bleeding (Benson et al. 1964). Vitamin B_6 deficiency may cause a sideroblastic anaemia (Dawson et al. 1964) and vitamin E deficiency may be associated with anaemia in infants (Binder et al. 1965). Riboflavin deficiency (Monro 1972) has also been described.

Biochemical findings

Total serum protein and albumin are reduced in a third to a half of the patients (Cooke 1963, Kumar 1976), due to a combination of a protein-losing enteropathy and decreased albumin synthesis. A low serum calcium may be present (Cooke et al. 1953) with low vitamin D levels (Moss et al. 1965) but osteomalacia on bone biopsy is much less frequent. Alkaline phosphatase may be raised and although it is usually of bony origin it may be associated with abnormal liver function. Low serum zinc and serum magnesium have been reported in severely ill patients (Jones & Peters 1981).

Immunological abnormalities

1 Serum immunoglobulins: Serum IgA is usually normal. Selective IgA deficiency has been reported in one in seventy patients with coeliac disease which is ten times the incidence in the general population (Hobbs & Hepner 1968). A reduced level of IgM is seen in 60% of untreated coeliac patients (Hobbs & Hepner 1968) but this reverts to normal with gluten exclusion. The overall synthesis rate of IgM is reduced (Brown et al. 1969), reflecting the decreased lymphoreticular dysfunction in these patients. Reports of increased IgG in patients with coeliac disease vary from 15–37% in coeliac patients (Blecher et al. 1969).

2 Lymphoreticular dysfunction: The presence of Howell–Jolly bodies on blood films indicates splenic atrophy (Blumgart, 1923, McCarthy et al. 1966, Blecher et al. 1969, Pettit et al. 1972, Marsh & Stewart 1970, Bullen & Losowsky 1979). Spleen scans and studies using radioactive scans suggest that as many as two-thirds of patients have splenic atrophy (Pettit et al. 1972). Treatment with a gluten-free diet does not reverse this (Trewby et al. 1981).

3 Circulating dietary antibodies: Dietary protein antibodies, including antibodies to gluten (Berger 1958) have been described in the serum in this disease (Taylor et al. 1961, Heiner et al. 1962, Kenrick & Walker-Smith 1970, Carswell & Ferguson 1973, Kumar et al. 1973a). These antibodies are, however, non-specific as they occur in other conditions with intestinal mucosal damage such as Crohn's disease (Alp & Wright 1971) and they are probably due to an increased permeability of dietary macromolecules.

Circulating antibodies to gluten and its fractions are present in approximately a third of patients with coeliac disease as compared with 5% of controls (Ferguson & Carswell 1972). Unsworth and his colleagues (1981) using a tissue pre-prepared with gliadin have shown an increased incidence of anti-gliadin antibodies in the serum of patients. Benson et al. (1972) found 40% of coeliac patients had positive avian precipitins to budgerigar, pigeon and hens as compared to negative results in control patients. As there was no correlation with the presence or absence of dietary gluten, autoantibodies or immunoglobulin level, these abnormalities are probably also the result of mucosal damage.

4 Circulating autoantibodies and immune complexes: Increased autoantibodies to reticulin, anti-nuclear factor, gastric parietal cells and thyroid have been described in patients with coeliac disease (Seah et al. 1971, Lancaster-Smith et al. 1971, Amman & Hong 1971, Lancaster-Smith et al. 1975). The most consistently found antibody is that against reticulin. The exact significance of this antibody is not known but there is a correlation with the presence of dietary gluten (Seah et al. 1971). It has been suggested that there is a cross-reactivity between reticulin and gliadin or that anti-reticulin antibody production is stimulated indirectly by the damaged jejunal mucosa produced by gluten during the pathogenesis of the intestinal lesion. Alternatively, it could merely be a non-specific response to absorption of dietary reticulin. Anti-reticulin antibodies have been demonstrated in 25% of patients with Crohn's disease (Alp & Wright 1971) but not in patients with cow's milk intolerance or tropical sprue who also have an intestinal lesion similar to that seen in coeliac disease. An increased incidence of circulating immune complexes have been found in coeliac patients and there is a significant reduction after starting a gluten-free diet (Doe et al. 1974). Cryoglobulinaemia and cutaneous vasculitis have also been described in coeliac disease (Doe et al. 1972), possibly a further reflection of the presence of immune complexes in the serum of these patients.

Anatomical abnormalities of the small intestine

The diagnosis is made on jejunal biopsy, which shows the characteristic features illustrated in Figs 9.1–9.5. As already stated, the ileum is either normal or less severely involved than the jejunum. In view of the severe proximal small intestinal abnormality, which in functional terms resembles that of proximal small intestinal resection, an adaptive ileal hypertrophic response might be expected to occur, as has been described after resection in Chapter 6. No hyperplasia of enterocytes has, however, been reported in the ileum in coeliac disease, although there is a significant augmentation of absorptive function in the ileum.

A barium follow-through examination will exclude gross anatomical causes of malabsorption such as diverticula and complications such as neoplasia and strictures. Jejunal dilatation and changes of fold pattern in coeliac disease are non-specific and may be seen in other gut disorders. Some of the changes in fold pattern may be related to hypoalbuminaemia. Transient intussusception may also be seen.

X-rays may show bone-thinning, with pseudofractures and sub-periosteal bone erosion if osteomalacia is severe.

Gastrointestinal function tests

Jejunum

Tests of intestinal absorption reflect the pathological changes in the intestine in coeliac disease. There are defects in the absorption of many substances normally absorbed in the jejunum, such as glucose, xylose, folic acid, iron and vitamin D. These absorption defects may lead to the nutritional deficiencies of folic acid, iron and vitamin D which are seen in coeliac disease.

Further absorption abnormalities have been shown by using jejunal perfusion techniques. Patients with untreated coeliac disease have a depressed water absorption and may actually secrete water when the jejunum is perfused with solutions containing glucose and bicarbonate (Schedl & Clifton 1963, Holdsworth & Dawson 1965, Fordtran et al. 1967, Schmid et al. 1969). These abnormalities reverse on treatment. The secretory state in untreated patients may account for some of the diarrhoea they experience.

Ileum

Since the ileum has so great a reserve capacity for absorption and for adaptation (Chapter 6), it is not surprising that absorption in coeliac disease is determined more by ileal than jejunal function (Stewart et al. 1967). The absorption of vitamin B_{12} may be abnormal in a proportion of patients, particularly those with significant steatorrhoea, but a defect in B_{12} absorption is of minor significance in coeliac disease and subacute combined degeneration of the cord has not been described in this condition. This contrasts with the B_{12} malabsorption that is associated with bacterial overgrowth (Chapter 15) or with chronic long-standing tropical sprue (Chapter 19) where neurological lesions due to B_{12} deficiency have been recognized.

The primary absorptive abnormality in many individuals with coeliac disease is jejunal malabsorption associated with ileal hyperabsorption. The adaptive response of the ileum in coeliac disease was first clearly demonstrated by Schedl & Clifton (1963, 1967) who showed, using perfusion techniques, that although there was jejunal malabsorption of both glucose and aminoacids, there was enhanced absorption of these substances in the ileum. Similar observations have been made by Silk et al. (1975). Furthermore, Mackinnon et al. (1975) have shown that the absorption of vitamin B_{12} may be enhanced in individuals with coeliac disease with good ileal function. This ileal adaptive response, a reflection of the reserve capacity of the small intestine, ensures that absorption may be well maintained in the presence of even severe jejunal disease and explains why so many coeliacs may be either asymptomatic or have little or no diarrhoea.

The explanation for this functional adaptation in the ileum is uncertain. (Besterman et al. 1978) have shown that coeliac patients in relapse may show an enhanced serum enteroglucagon response after a meal similar to that seen after resection of the small intestine (Chapter 23) and it is tempting to speculate that enteroglucagon may in some way enhance absorption in the ileum in coeliac disease.

Intestinal permeability

The permeability of the small intestine

appears to be altered in coeliac disease. This allows the more ready passage of water-soluble molecules such as disaccharides (for example, lactulose, cellobiose) and Chromium-EDTA (Menzies et al. 1979, Cobden et al. 1980, Bjarnason et al. 1983). If the test substance cannot be metabolized, it may be recovered quantitatively from the urine and this provides another means of testing intestinal function in coeliac disease. The defect in permeability may persist in the treated patient (Bjarnason et al. 1983).

In contrast the monosaccharides (e.g. mannitol) and polyethylene glycol with a wide range of molecular weights (40–4000) are less readily transferred across the mucosa of the small intestine in coeliac disease (Chadwick et al. 1977, Cobden et al. 1980). These findings indicate that there is more than one transfer mechanism for inert molecules.

Changes in permeability may also be partly responsible for the loss of divalent cations (iron, calcium, magnesium) into the intestine of patients with untreated coeliac disease (Creamer, 1970; Melvin et al. 1970).

The diagnostic value of intestinal absorption tests

Tests of gastrointestinal function are of little importance in the diagnosis of coeliac disease. They may be used as screening tests and for follow-up but the morphological appearance of the jejunal mucosa on biopsy is the key investigation. A raised faecal fat is no longer a *sine qua non* of the disease and normal fat excretion was seen in 43% of fifty-four patients in our series (Kumar 1976). Xylose absorption, a test of jejunal function, is frequently abnormal and is a good screening test. Rolles and his colleagues (1973) have found a 1 h blood xylose level a useful investigation in children.

Pancreatic function

Exocrine pancreatic insufficiency has been reported in coeliac disease. It was suggested that this was due to a presumed impaired release of cholecystokinin from the atrophic jejunal mucosa. A stimulation test may be normal (Berg et al. 1979). Regan & Di Magno (1980), however, showed mild to moderate pancreatic insufficiency in 42% of thirty-one patients and in three patients the deficiency was so severe as to necessitate pancreatic supplements. Ansaldi and his colleagues (1981) have also shown a pancreatic deficiency using the secretin–CCK test in children which improved on treatment with a gluten-free diet.

Treatment

A strict gluten-free diet should be recommended for life. It is arguable, however, whether the asymptomatic older patient presenting with minor nutritional abnormalities requires a gluten-free diet in addition to dietary supplements of iron, folate or vitamin D (Cooke et al. 1953). Nevertheless, many patients are unaware of the extent of their ill health and only notice the difference after starting a diet.

There are, however, some urgent reasons for a diet. The ill patient undoubtedly improves clinically and any gastrointestinal symptoms may be controlled. Secondly, if there are problems over infertility or recurrent abortion, a diet should be recommended. Thirdly, in childhood, a strict diet is essential for growth and development. The most important reason for putting patients on gluten-free diets is the risk of developing a malignancy. Initially it was suggested that a gluten-free diet would reduce the risk of malignant complications to that of the normal population but this has not yet been established (Stokes & Holmes 1974).

A gluten-free diet implies the withdrawal of wheat, rye, barley and, in those few patients who are sensitive, oats. The grains of rice and corn are not toxic to coeliac patients. Initially, if anaemia or osteomalacia are prominent, oral supplements of iron, folic acid, calcium and vitamin D may be necessary. Troublesome steatorrhoea may be helped by a low fat diet for a short while.

A diet is not difficult if the patient is instructed by a dietician about the pitfalls. The obvious foods of bread, cakes, biscuits, pasta are easy to avoid but care must be taken over substances where flour may have been used, for example, soups, tinned foods, mustard. Cornflour is gluten-free and may be used as a thickening agent. Gluten-free bread, flour, bread mixes, biscuits, pasta etc. can be obtained in the UK on prescription. Patients vary in their ability to keep a strict diet; children are usually strict due to parental influences, but adolescents and adults often find a strict diet more difficult. The Coeliac Society provides help and encouragement. It is a co-operative run by patients and parents and distributes information, handbooks and diet sheets. There are local branches throughout the UK (Head Office, P.O. Box 181, London NW2 2QY). They have introduced a symbol showing a crossed sheaf of wheat, which some manufacturers are now using on their gluten-free products.

Follow-up

The continual follow-up of patients is important. Children are assessed on weight and height percentile charts. It is useful to see the patients after 3 weeks to assess clinical problems and dietary compliance. Continued assessment should be made on clinical grounds, weight, serum and red cell folate levels, serum alkaline phosphatase and albumin levels. After treatment with the gluten-free diet, the jejunal biopsy should be repeated at 3 months and 1 year, when there should be an increase in villous and enterocyte height, a decrease in intraepithelial lymphocyte counts and a decrease in inflammatory cells in the lamina propria. Once the patients are well and have normal jejunal biopsies, they should be seen at yearly intervals. Paediatricians usually confirm the diagnosis with a gluten challenge, but this is not a common practice in adult patients, in whom challenge is only necessary if there is doubt about the diagnosis. The prognosis is excellent as most patients show an improvement with a gluten-free diet.

Conditions associated with coeliac disease

Joint abnormalities

No specific arthritis has been found in association with coeliac disease. Two of our patients, however, presented with arthralgia which improved on gluten withdrawal and in one case reappeared on gluten challenge.

Infertility

Morris *et al.* (1970) reported infertility in three patients diagnosed in childhood but treated only with a low fat diet. Rapid conception followed the introduction of a gluten-free diet. Infertility in males may also reverse on a gluten-free diet (Baker & Read 1975). The exact relationship between coeliac disease and infertility is uncertain and is not always related to ill-health (Smith 1946). Green *et al.* (1977) have shown a reversible insensitivity to androgens in men with untreated coeliac disease with elevated plasma testosterone and reduced dihydrotestosterone levels. Farthing *et al.* (1982) have suggested impaired hypothalamic–pituitary function and have also shown increased numbers of abnormal spermatozoa and impaired sperm motility in coeliac patients. They found clinical evidence of hypogonadism in 7% and impotence in 18% of male coeliacs. Infertile marriages occurred in 19% of coeliacs — a value higher than expected in the general population.

Bacterial overgrowth

Some workers have found increased bacterial counts in jejunal aspirates in coeliac disease, thought to be secondary to decreased intestinal motility and stasis. Occasionally this may be clinically significant (Hamilton *et al.* 1970).

Hepatic abnormalities

A raised alkaline phosphatase of liver origin is common in grossly malnourished patients and the liver biopsy may show fatty change.

Jaundice in coeliac disease is rare, but it is a serious prognostic feature in the unresponsive patient. Cirrhosis has been described, especially primary biliary cirrhosis (Logan *et al.* 1978, Kumar *et al.* 1981).

Neurological disorders

Sencer (1957) described a neuropathy under

the term 'progressive neuromyeloradiculitis' or 'pseudotabes' and Cooke et al. (1963) described four such patients whose features superficially suggested a subacute combined degeneration of the cord. This syndrome was unrelated to vitamin B_{12} deficiency and the neuropathy was not prevented by a gluten-free diet. Other neurological disturbances have been described, including peripheral neuropathies, epileptiform attacks, parasthesia, Wernicke's encephalopathy and psychiatric disturbances (Cooke & Smith 1966, Binder et al. 1967, Hall 1968). A central pontine demyelination has also been described in association with malabsorption (Pallis & Lewis 1974). Once established, these disorders are not helped by gluten restriction.

Alveolar diffusion defect

Fibrosing alveolitis has been described, presenting as dyspnoea, but this is rare (Hood & Mason 1970).

Immunological disorders

A variety of disorders thought to have an immunological basis has been reported in association with coeliac disease. These include thyroid disease, inflammatory bowel disease and diabetes mellitus. There is no evidence that the co-existence of any of these diseases is more than a chance association.

Malabsorption non-responsive to treatment with a gluten-free diet

According to the definition of coeliac disease given at the beginning of this chapter, patients who do not show a histological response to treatment with a gluten-free diet should not be classified as coeliacs. Non-responsiveness to a gluten-free diet, however, is initially a clinical diagnosis and the commonest cause of a persistently flattened jejunal biopsy is non-adherence to a gluten-free diet. True non-responders can only be diagnosed after extensive discussion with both patient and dietician. Very small amounts of gluten may occasionally damage the intestinal mucosa. The ingestion of wafers at Mass by Catholic patients may be sufficient to inhibit response.

The patient who is truly unresponsive to treatment is rare. The jejunal mucosa may have the appearance of coeliac mucosa with crypt hyperplasia and decreased enterocyte height. It is not known whether this persisting lesion represents a reaction to some other dietary constituent or whether it was initiated by gluten sensitivity, but has subsequently become self-perpetuating.

In some patients a clinical and morphological improvement may be induced by corticosteroid therapy (Wall et al. 1970). Unfortunately, not all patients respond to this treatment and, even with intravenous alimentation, may deteriorate and die (Neale 1968). Immunosuppressive agents may be an alternative to corticosteroids (Hamilton et al. 1976, Hillman 1972) as illustrated by the following patient.

> N.C., a female aged 68, presented at the age of 62 with diarrhoea, weight loss and tiredness. She was found to be anaemic and a jejunal biopsy showed subtotal villous atrophy with crypt hyperplasia as seen in coeliac disease. Over the next 2 years, despite a strict gluten-free diet, she continued to feel unwell with diarrhoea, passing more than 500 g stool/day. Blood tests now showed a normal haemoglobin, albumin, calcium and phosphate, and immunoglobulins. Because of her extremely poor clinical state, she was started on prednisolone 20 mg/day. There was a dramatic improvement, diarrhoea being completely relieved. A repeat jejunal biopsy showed considerable improvement. The steroids were discontinued, she deteriorated again and the jejunal biopsy showed subtotal villous atrophy. Steroids again induced clinical improvement but she became unwell after cessation. She was now given steroids and azathioprine at a dose of 2 mg/kg. She remained well on azathioprine alone and had a normal jejunal biopsy 9 months later (Fig. 9.8).

Another very rare group of patients with flattened mucosa may show an initial response to gluten withdrawal but subsequently, after inadvertent gluten ingestion, run a persistently downhill course (Neale 1968); the reasons for this are unknown.

Some severe non-responsive cases have a deposition of a thick layer of subepithelial collagen in the jejunal mucosa (Neale 1968, Weinstein et al. 1970) and the term collagenous sprue was coined to describe these patients. Subepithelial collagen, however, is simply a non-specific marker of an inflammatory process and is seen in 36% of patients with untreated coeliac disease in whom it may disappear on treatment (Bossart et al. 1975, Cluysenaer & van Tongeren 1977).

In another group of patients the jejunal mucosa is hypoplastic. The enterocytes may be severely abnormal and there is a relative absence of crypts, unlike the characteristic hyperplastic crypt lesion seen in coeliac disease (Barry & Read 1973, Jones & Peters 1977). It is probable that these patients do not have coeliac disease. Furthermore, the lesion may not be limited to the jejunum in these patients and the ileum may show similar severe changes (Hourihane 1963, Cluysenaer & van Tongeren 1977, Booth 1981). Ulceration, stricture formation and terminally very severe and total malabsorption may ensue (see Chapter 12). At autopsy, the small intestine is found to be severely atrophic and there is frequently extensive ulceration. On detailed pathological examination of the ulcers, it has been shown that some of these patients are suffering from malignant histiocytosis (Isaacson & Wright 1978).

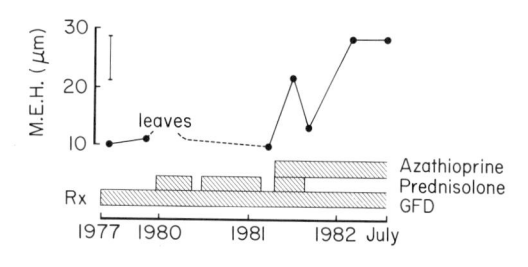

Fig. 9.8. Mean epithelial heights (MEH) of patient N.C. showing the effects on the jejunal enterocytes of treatment with a gluten-free diet, prednisolone and azathioprine.

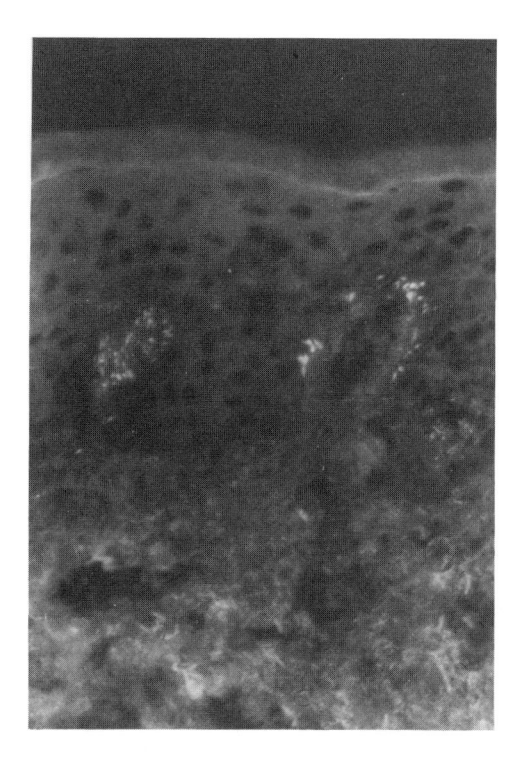

Fig. 9.9. IGA deposits shown by immunofluorescence in the dermal papillae from the uninvolved skin of a patient with coeliac disease and dermatitis herpetiformis. (Courtesy of Dr Lionel Fry.)

Complications of coeliac disease

Malignancy

That small intestinal malignant lymphoma might complicate coeliac disease was first suggested in a report from Bristol in 1962 (Gough et al. 1962). A later report from the same centre established that carcinomas, particularly of the fore- and midgut, were also associated with coeliac disease. Subsequent studies from Birmingham (Harris et al. 1967) indicated that malignancy might develop in as many as 14% of patients with coeliac disease. Approximately half the malignancies were lymphomas, but there was also a raised incidence of other malignancies, particularly carcinomas of the gastrointestinal tract. Further studies (Holmes et al. 1974) confirmed these findings and indicated that in men in the Birmingham area carcinoma of the pharynx and oesophagus were particularly associated with coeliac disease. Perhaps surprisingly, no case of primary small intestinal carcinoma occurred in the Birmingham patients. Subsequently a report from Australia (Selby & Gallaghan 1979) confirmed the increased incidence of oesophageal carcinomas in coeliac patients and suggested an increased incidence of small intestinal adenocarcinomas. Four cases of small intestinal adenocarcinoma were later reported in coeliac patients attending clinics in Birmingham or Derby (Holmes *et al.* 1980).

The histological type of lymphoma most frequently associated with coeliac disease was initially described as either Hodgkin's disease or reticulum cell sarcoma. More recently it has been suggested that the lymphoma associated with malabsorption should be classified as a malignant histiocytosis and may present with intestinal ulceration (Isaacson & Wright 1978).

A recent nationwide study in the UK has established the types of malignant tumour associated with coeliac disease and has confirmed that the malignant 'lymphoma' is most frequently a malignant histiocytosis. Of 259 histologically confirmed malignancies in 235 patients with histologically proven coeliac disease, 133 were malignant lymphomas, the predominant histological type being malignant histiocytosis and the commonest site of this lesion the small intestine. Patients with coeliac disease also had a greatly increased risk for the development of small intestinal adenocarcinomas. Among 116 invasive non-lymphomatous malignancies there were 19 small intestinal adenocarcinomas, compared with 0.23 expected from national cancer registrations adjusted for sex and age. There were also more oesophageal and pharyngeal squamous carcinomas than expected (Swinson *et al.* 1983). The malignant lymphoma of coeliac disease is discussed in greater detail in Chapter 10.

Ulceration and strictures

Ulceration of jejunum and stricture formation may occur in untreated coeliac disease but are rare (Bayless *et al.* 1967).

Dermatitis herpetiformis

Patients with this blistering skin eruption also have a gluten-sensitive enteropathy. Dermatitis herpetiformis was first described by Duhring in 1884 as a clinical entity distinct from other blistering eruptions (Alexander 1975). There are itchy blisters mainly on the knees, elbows, buttocks and shoulders but they can occur at any site. Because of the intense irritation, excoriated papules rather than blisters are usually seen. It can occur at any age and runs a chronic course. Clinically it should be differentiated from pemphigus, pemphigoid and bullous impetigo. Histologically there are characteristic subepidermal blister cavities and infiltration with neutrophils and eosinophils. Immunofluorescence shows IgA basement membrane staining of either a granular or continuous pattern (Seah *et al.* 1972, Cormane 1967) in the uninvolved skin (van de Meer 1969). These IgA deposits (Fig. 9.9) are thought to be diagnostic of dermatitis herpetiformis (Fry *et al.* 1973) and do not occur in coeliac disease (Seah *et al.* 1972). In addition to IgA, IgG and IgM deposits are also seen (van de Meer 1969, Chorzelski *et al.* 1971, Seah *et al.* 1972).

The small intestinal lesion was first reported by Smith (1966) and by Marks *et al.* (1966). Marks and her colleagues found nine of twelve patients had an abnormality of the small intestinal mucosa. This has since been confirmed (Fraser *et al.* 1967, Fry *et al.* 1967, van Tongeren *et al.* 1967, Shuster *et al.* 1968). Using multiple biopsies, however, a jejunal lesion has been found to be much more common (twenty-one of twenty-two patients) and the lesion may be patchy (Brow *et al.* 1971, Scott *et al.* 1976). The intestinal lesion is milder than in coeliac disease, but if intraepithelial lymphocytes are counted, 95% have an abnormality (Fry *et al.* 1972). A flattened biopsy is seen in a small percentage but, despite this, clinical malabsorption is rare.

Dermatitis herpetiformis (DH) has many features similar to coeliac disease (Fry *et al.* 1967, Petit *et al.* 1972, Kumar 1976) including an improvement of the intestinal lesion with gluten withdrawal (Fry et al. 1968, Shuster et al. 1968, Marks & Whittle 1969, Fry et al. 1982). Curiously there is a greater frequency of immunological abnormalities and autoimmune diseases than in the more severely affected coeliac patients. Nevertheless, levels of serum autoantibodies (Fraser 1970, Seah et al. 1971, Lancaster-Smith et al. 1975) antireticulin antibody (Seah et al. 1971, Alp & Wright 1971, Von Essen et al. 1972, Brown et al. 1973, Seah et al. 1973, 1971) circulating immune complexes (Mowbray et al. 1973), splenic atrophy (Fry et al. 1967, Pettit et al. 1972) gastric atrophy (O'Donoghue et al. 1976) and HLA B8 and DR3 status (Stokes et al. 1972, Falchuk et al. 1972, Katz et al. 1972, White et al. 1973). All occur with similar frequencies to those in coeliac disease. It is possible that DH and coeliac disease are the same condition but polarizing to either the skin or gut.

The skin lesion is controlled with dapsone (Esteves & Brandas 1950) but sulphapyridine is also effective (Costello 1940). Dapsone only improves the skin lesion but a gluten-free diet improves the skin lesion as well as the gastrointestinal abnormality (Fry et al. 1973). Most DH patients present with the irritative rash but a few (5%) may present with the malabsorption of coeliac disease. The concensus of opinion now supports the conclusion that the skin lesion may be controlled by treatment with a gluten-free diet (Fry et al. 1973, Heading et al. 1976, Reunala et al. 1977, Frodin et al. 1981, Fry et al. 1982).

References

Adair W.L. & Kornfelds (1974) Isolation of receptors for wheat germ agglutinin 'risinus communis' lectins from human erythrocytes using affinity chromatography. *J. Biol. Chem.* **249**, 4696–4704.

Adams F. (1856) Arataeus the Cappadocian: Extant works. In *The Malabsorption Syndrome*, p. 3. (Ed. by D. Aldersberg). Grune & Stratton, New York (1957).

Albert E., Harms K., Bertele R., Andreas A., McNicholas A., Kuntz B., Scholz S., Schiessly B., Wetzmüller H., Rerssinger P. & Wesser-Krell Ch. (1978) In *Perspectives in Coeliac Disease*, pp. 123–130 (Ed. by B. McNicholl, C.F. McCarthy & P.F. Fottrell). MTP Press, Leicester.

Alexander J. O'D. (1975) *Dermatitis Herpetiformis*. W.B. Saunders Co. Ltd. London.

Alp M.H. & Wright R. (1971) Autoantibodies to reticulin in patients with idiopathic steatorrhoea, coeliac disease and Crohn's disease and their relation to immunoglobulins and dietary antibodies. *Lancet*, **ii**, 682–685.

Alvey C., Anderson C.M. & Freeman M. (1957) Wheat gluten and coeliac disease. *Arch. Dis. Child.* **32**, 434–437.

Ament M.E. & Rubin C.E. (1972a) Soya protein — another cause of a flat intestinal lesion. *Gastroenterol.* **62**, 227.

Amman A.J. & Hong R. (1971) Unique antibody to basement membrane in patients with selective IgA deficiency and coeliac disease. *Lancet*, **i**, 1264–1266.

Anand B.S., Piris J., Jerrome D.W., Offord R.E. & Truelove S.C. (1981) The timing of histological damage following a single challenge with gluten in treated coeliac disease. *Quart. J. Med. N.S.* **50**, 83–94.

Anderson C.M., Gracey M. & Burke V. (1972) Coeliac disease. Some still controversial aspects. *Arch. Dis. Child.* **47**, 292–298.

Ansaldi N. & Oderda G. (1981) Exocrine pancreatic insufficiency in coeliac sprue. *Gastroenterol.* **80**, 883.

Asquith P. (1974) Family study in coeliac disease In *Coeliac Disease*, pp. 322–325. (Ed. by W.T. Hekkens & A.S. Pena). Stenfert Kroese, Leiden.

Autran J.C., Lew E.J. J-L., Nimmo C.C. & Kasarda D.D. (1979) N-terminal amino acid sequencing of prolamines from wheat and related species. *Nature*, **282**, 527–529.

Autrup H., Barrett L.A., Jackson F.C., Jesudason M.L., Stoner G., Phelps P., Trump B.F. & Harris C.C. (1978) Explant culture of human colon. *Gastroenterol.* **74**, 1248–1257.

Badenoch J. & Callender S.T. (1960) Effect of corticosteroids and gluten-free diet on absorption of iron in idiopathic steatorrhoea and coeliac disease. *Brit. J. Haematol.* **23**, Suppl., 135–146.

Baker P.G. & Read A.E. (1975) Reversible infertility in male coeliac patients. *Brit. Med. J.* **ii**, 316–7.

Barry R.E. & Read A.E. (1973) Coeliac disease and malignancy. *Quart. J. Med. N.S.* **42**, 665–675.

Barry R.E., Baker P. & Read A.E. (1974) The clinical presentation. *Clin. in Gastroenterol.* **3**, 55–69.

Bayless T.M., Kapelowitz R.F., Shelley M.W. Ballinger W.G. & Hendrix T.R. (1967) Intestinal ulceration — a complication of coeliac disease. *New Engl. J. Med.* **276**, 996–1002.

Benardin J.E., Kasarda D.D. & Mecham D.K. (1967) Preparation and characterisation of α-gliadin *J. Biol. Chem.* **242**, 445–450.

Bennett T., Hunter D. & Vaughan J.M. (1932) Idiopathic steatorrhoea (Gee's disease): a nutritional disturbance associated with tetany, osteomalacia & anaemia. *Quart. J. Med.* **1**, 603–677.

Benson G.D., Kowlessar O.B. & Schleisenger M.H. (1964) Adult coeliac disease with emphasis on the response to a gluten-free diet. *Medicine (Baltimore)*, **43**, 1–40.

Benson M.K., Lancaster-Smith M.I. & Perrin J. (1972) Serum immunoglobulins, autoantibodies and avian precipitins in adult coeliac disease and avian antigen inhalation provocation tests in patients with adult coeliac disease and diffuse intestinal lung disease. *Arch. fracaises des maladies de L'appareil digestif* p. 398. 9th Congress Internationale de Gastroenterology, Paris.

Berg N.O., Dahlquist A. & Lindberg T. (1979) Exocrine pancreatic insufficiency, small intestinal dysfunction & protein intolerance. A chance occurrence or a connection? *Acta Paediatr. Scand.* **68**, 275–276.

Berger E. (1958) Zur allerguchen pathogenese der coliakie nut versuchen aber die spalburg pathogenes antigene durch fermente. *Bibl. paediat.* **67**, 1–55.

Besterman H.S., Bloom S.R., Sarsen D.L., Blockburn A.M., Johnstone D.I., Patel H.R., Stewart J.S., Modigliani R., Guerin S. & Mallinson C.N. (1978) Gut hormone profile in coeliac disease. *Lancet*, **i**, 785–788.

Betuel H., Gebuhrer L., Descos L., Percebois H., Minaire Y. & Bertrand J. (1980) Adult coeliac disease associated with HLA-DRW3 & DRW7. *Tiss. Antig.* **15**, 231–238.

Binder H.J., Herting D.C., Hurst V., Finch S.C. & Spiro H.M. (1965) Tocopherol deficiency in man. *New Engl. J. Med.* **273**, 1289–1297.

Binder H.J., Solitaire G.B. & Spiro H.M. (1967) Neuromuscular disease in patients with steatorrhoea. *Gut*, **8**, 605–611.

Bjarnason I., Peters T.J. & Veall N. (1983) A persistent defect in intestinal permeability in coeliac disease demonstrated by a ^{51}Cr-labelled EDTA absorption test. *Lancet*, **i**, 323–325.

Blecher T.E., Brzechwa-Ajdukiewicz A, McCarthy C.F. & Read A.E. (1969) Serum immunoglobulins & lymphocyte transformation studies in coeliac disease. *Gut*, **10**, 57–62.

Blumgart H.L. (1923) Three fatal adult cases of malabsorption of fat. *Arch. Intern. Med.* **32**, 113–128.

Booth C.C. (1970) Enterocyte in coeliac disease. *Brit. Med. J.* **3**, 725–731 & **4**, 14–17.

Booth C.C. (1981) Malabsorption unresponsive to treatment with a gluten-free diet. In *Topics in Gastroenterology*, vol. 9, pp. 83–84. (Ed. by D.P. Jewell & E. Lee). Blackwell Scientific Publications, Oxford.

Booth C.C., Peters T.J. & Doe W.F. (1977) Immunopathology of coeliac disease. *Ciba Foundation Symposium* No. 46.

Bossart R., Henry K., Booth C.C. & Doe W.F. (1975) Subepithelial collagen in intestinal malabsorption. *Gut*, **16**, 18–22.

Bronstein H.D., Haeffner L.J. & Kowlessar D. (1966) Enzymatic digestion of gliadin: the effect of the resultant peptides in adult coeliac disease. *Clin. Chim. Acta.* **14**, 141–155.

Brow J.R., Parker F., Weinstein W.M. & Rubin C.E. (1971) The small intestinal mucosa in dermatitis herpetiformis. I. Severity & distribution of the small intestinal lesion & associated malabsorption. *Gastroenterol.* **60**, 355–361.

Brown D.L., Cooper A.G. & Hepner G.W. (1969) IgM metabolism in coeliac disease. *Lancet*, **i**, 858–861.

Brown I.L., Ferguson A., Carswell F., Horne C.H.W. & MacSween R.N.M. (1973) Autoantibodies in children with coeliac disease. *Clin. Exp. Immunol.* **13**, 373–382.

Browning T.H. & Trier J.S. (1969) Organ culture of mucosal biopsies of human small intestine. *J. Clin. Invest.* **48**, 1423–1432.

Brunser O., Reid A., Monckeberg F., Maccioni A. & Contreras I. (1966) Jejunal biopsies in infant malnutrition with special reference to mitotic index. *Paediat.* **38**, 605.

Bullen A.W. & Losowsky M.S. (1979) Consequences of impaired splenic function. *Clin. Sci.* **57**, 129–37.

Carswell F. & Ferguson A. (1973) Plasma food antibodies during withdrawal & re-introduction of dietary gluten in coeliac disease. *Arch. Dis. child.* **48**, 583–586.

Chadwick V.S., Phillips S.F. & Hofmann A.F. (1977) Measurement of intestinal permeability using low molecular weight polyethylene glycols (PEG 400). II. Application to normal and abnormal permeability states in man and animals. *Gastroenterol.* **73**, 247–251.

Chorzelski T.P., Beutner E.H., Jablonska S., Blaszezyk M. & Triffshauser C.B. (1971) Immunofluorescence studies in the diagnosis of dermatitis herpetiformis and its differentiation from bullous pemphigoid. *J. Invest. Derm.* **56**, 373–80.

Ciclitira P.J., Hunter J.O. & Lennox E.S. (1980) Clinical testing of bread made from nullisomic 6A wheats in coeliac patients. *Lancet*, **ii**, 234–237.

Ciclitira P.J., EVans D.J., Lennox E.S. et al. (1982) The toxic effects of gliadin fractions on the small bowel mucosa of patients with coeliac disease. *Clin. Sci.* **62**, 48.

Cluysenaer O.J.J. & van Tongeren J.H.M. (1977) *Malsorption in Coeliac Sprue*, p. 228. Martinus Nijhoff, The Hague.

Cobden I., Rothwell J. & Axon A.T.R. (1980) Intestinal permeability and screening tests for coeliac disease. *Gut*, **21**, 512–518.

Cooke W.T., Peeney A.L.P. & Hawkins C.F. (1953) Symptoms, signs & diagnostic features of idiopathic steatorrhoea. *Quart J. Med.* **22**, 59–77.

Cooke W.T., Fone D.J., Cox E.V., Meynell M.J. & Gaddie R. (1963) Adult coeliac disease. *Gut*, **4**, 279–291.

Cooke W.T. & Smith W.T. (1966) Neurological disorders in adult coeliac disease. *Brain*, **89**,

683–722.

Cooke W.T. (1968) Adult coeliac disease. In *Progress in Gastroenterology*, pp. 299–338. (Ed. by G.B. Jerzy Glass) Grune & Stratton, New York.

Cormane R.H. (1967) Immunofluorescent studies of the skin in lupus erythematosus and other diseases. *Pathol. Europa.* **2**, 170–180.

Cornell H.J. & Townley R.R.W. (1973) Investigation of possible intestinal peptides deficiency in coeliac disease. *Clin. Chim. Acta*, **43**, 113–127.

Costello M.J. (1940) Dermatitis herpetiformis with sulfapyridine. *Arch. Dermatol. Syphil.* **64**, 684–687.

Creamer B. (1970) Loss from the small intestine. *J. Roy. Coll. Phys.* **5**, 323–332.

Crosby W.H. & Kugler H.W. (1957) Intraluminal biopsy of the small intestine: The intestinal biopsy capsule. *Amer. J. Dig. Dis.* **2**, 236–241.

Cunningham-Rundles S., Cunningham-Rundles C., Pollack M.S., Good R.A. & Dupont B. (1978) Response to wheat antigen in *in vitro* lymphocyte transformation among HLA-B8 positive normal donors. *Transpl. Proc.* **10**, 977–979.

Dawson A.M., Holdsworth C.D. & Pitcher C.S. (1964) Sideroblastic anaemia in adult coeliac disease. *Gut*, **5**, 304–308.

Dawson I.M.P. (1976) The endocrine cells of the gastrointestinal tract and the neoplasms which arise from them. *Curr. Top. Pathol.* **63**, 221.

Day G., Evans K. & Wharton B. (1973) Abnormalities of insulin and growth hormone secretion in children with coeliac disease. *Arch. Dis. Child.* **48**, 41–46.

Dicke W.K. (1950) Coeliac disease. Investigation of harmful effects of certain types of cereal on patients with coeliac disease. Doctoral thesis. Univ. of Utrecht, Netherlands.

Dicke W.K., Weijers H.A. & van de Kamer J.H. (1953) Coeliac disease, presence in wheat of a factor having deleterious effect in cases of coeliac disease. *Acta. Paediat.* **42**, 34–42.

Dissanayake A.S., Jerrome D.W., Offord R.E., Truelove S.C. & Whitehead R. (1974a) Identifying toxic fractions of wheat gluten and their effect on the jejunal mucosa in coeliac disease. *Gut*, **15**, 931–946.

Dissanayake A.S., Truelove S.C. & Whitehead R. (1974) Lack of harmful effect of oats on small intestine mucosa in coeliac disease. *Brit. Med. J.* **i**, 189–191.

Doe W.F., Evans D, Hobbs J.R. & Booth C.C. (1972) Coeliac disease, vasculitis and cryoglobulinaemia. *Gut*, **13**, 112–123.

Doe W.F., Booth C.C. & Brown D.L. (1973) Evidence for complement binding immune complexes in adult coeliac disease, Crohn's disease and ulcerative colitis. *Lancet*, **i**, 402–404.

Doe W.F., Henry K. & Booth C.C. (1974) Complement in coeliac disease. In *Coeliac Disease*, pp. 189–196. (Ed. by W. Hekkens & A.S. Pena). Stenfert Kroese, Leiden.

Douglas A.P. & Booth C.C. (1970) Digestion of gluten peptides by normal human jejunal mucosa and by mucosa from patients with adult coeliac disease. *Clin. Sci.* **38**, 11–25.

Duhring L.A. (1893) Duhring's papers on dermatitis herpetiformis. In *Selected Monographs on Dermatology*, pp. 196–297. New Sydenham Society, London.

Esteves J. & Brandao F.N. (1950) Au sujet de l'action des sulfamides et des sulfones dans la maladie de Duhring. *Trabal. Socied. Portug. Dermatol. Venereol.* **8**, 209.

Ezeoke A., Ferguson M., Fakhri O., Hekkens W. Th. J. M. & Hobbs J.R. (1974) Antibodies in the sera of coeliac patients which can co-opt K cells to attack gluten labelled targets. In *Coeliac Disease*, p. 176. (Ed. by W. Hekkens & A.S. Pena). Stenfert Kroese, Leiden.

Falchuk Z.M., Rogentine G.N. & Strober W.J. (1972) Predominance of histocompatibility antigen HLA-A8 in patients with gluten — sensitive enteropathy. *J. Clin. Invest.* **51**, 1602–1605.

Falchuk Z.M., Gebhard R.L., Sessoms C. & Strober W. (1974a) An *in vitro* mode of gluten-sensitive enteropathy. Effect of gliadin on intestinal epithelial cells of patients with gluten-sensitive enteropathy in organ culture. *J. Clin. Invest.* **53**, 487–500.

Farthing M.J.G., Edwards C.R.W., Rees L.M. & Dawson A.M. (1982) Male gonadal function in coeliac disease. I. Sexual dysfunction, infertility and semen quality. *Gut* **23**, 608–614.

Ferguson A. & Murray D. (1971) Quantitation of intraepithelial lymphocytes in human jejunum. *Gut*, **12**, 988–994.

Ferguson A., MacDonald T.T., McClure J.P. & Holden R.J. (1975) Cell-mediated immunity to gliadin within the small intestinal mucosa in coeliac disease. *Lancet*, **i**, 895–897.

Fordtran J.S., Rector F.C., Locklear T.W. & Ewton M.F.E. (1967) Water and solute movement in the small intestine of patients with sprue. *J. Clin. Invest.* **46**, 287–298.

Fraser A.C. (1956) Discussion on some problems of steatorrhoea and reduced stature. *Proc. Roy. Soc. Med.* **49**, 1009–1013.

Fraser A.C., Fletcher R.F., Ross C.A.C., Shaw B., Sammons H.G. & Schneider R. (1959) Gluten-induced enteropathy. The effect of partially digested gluten. *Lancet*, **ii**, 252–255.

Fraser N.G., Murray D. & Alexander J. O'D. (1967) Structure and function of the small intestine in dermatitis herpetiformis. *Brit. J. Derm.* **79**, 509–518.

Fraser N.G. (1970) Autoantibodies in dermatitis herpetiformis. *Brit. J. Dermatol.* **83**, 609–613.

Frodin T., Gotthard R., Hed J., Molin L., Norrby K. & Walan A. (1981) Gluten-free diet for dermatitis herpetiformis, the long-term effect on cutaneous immunological and jejunal manifestations. *Acta. Derm. Vencrol. (Stockh.)* **61**, 405–411.

Fry L., Kier P., McMinn R.M.H., Cowan J.O. & Hoffbrand A.V. (1967) Small intestinal structure and function and haematological changes in dermatitis herpetiformis. *Lancet*, **ii**, 739–734.

Fry L., McMinn R.M.H., Cowan J.D. & Hoffbrand A.V. (1968) Effect of a gluten-free diet on dermatological intestinal and haematological manifestations of dermatitis herpetiformis. *Lancet*, **i**, 557–561.

Fry L., Seah P.P., McMinn R.R.M. & Hoffbrand A.V. (1972) Lymphocyte infiltration of epithelium in diagnosis of gluten-sensitive enteropathy. *Brit. Med. J.* **3**, 371–374.

Fry L., Seah P.P., Riches D.J. & Hoffbrand A.V. (1973) Clearance of skin lesions in dermatitis herpetiformis after gluten withdrawal. *Lancet*, **i**, 288–291.

Fry L., Leonard J.N., Swain F., Tucker W.F.E., Haffenden G., Ring N. & McMinn R.M.H. (1982) Long-term follow-up of dermatitis herpetiformis with and without dietary gluten withdrawal. *Brit. J. Dermatol.* **107**, 631–640.

Gardner A.J., Mutton K.J. & Walker-Smith J.A. (1973) A family study of coeliac disease. *Aust. Paediat. J.* **9**, 18.

Gee S.J. (1888) On the coeliac affection. *St. Bartholomew's Hospital Reports*, **24**, 17–20.

Gent A.E. (1973) Coeliac primary amenorrhoea *Dig.* **8**, 509–12.

Gibbons R.A. (1889) The coeliac affection in children. *Edin. Med. J.* **35**, 321.

Gough K.R., Read A.E., Naish J.M. (1962) Intestinal reticulosis as a complication of idiopathic steatorrhoea. *Gut*, **3**, 232–239.

Gowans J.L. & Knight E.T. (1964) The route of recirculation of lymphocytes in the rat. *Proc. Roy. Soc. B.* **159**, 257.

Green J.R.B., Goble H.L., Edwards C.R.W. & Dawson A.M. (1977) Reversible insensitivity to androgens in men with untreated gluten enteropathy. *Lancet*, **i**, 280–282.

Hall W.H. (1968) Proximal muscle atrophy in adult coeliac disease. *Amer. J. Dig. Dis.* **13**, 697–704.

Hallert C., Gotthard R., Jansson G., Norby K. & Walen A. (1983) Similar prevalence of coeliac disease in children and middle-aged adults in a district of Sweden. *Gut*, **24**, 389–391.

Hamilton J.D., Dyer N.H., Dawson A.M., O'Grady F.W., Vincé A., Fenton J.C. & Mollin D.L. (1970) Assessment and significance of bacterial overgrowth in the small bowel. *Quart. J. Med. N.S.* **29**, 265–285.

Hamilton J.D., Chambers R.A. & Wyn-Williams A. (1976) Role of gluten, prednisolone and azathioprine in non-responsive coeliac disease. *Lancet*, **i**, 1213–1215.

Harris O.D., Cooke W.T., Thompson M. et al. (1967) Malignancy in adult coeliac disease and idiopathic steatorrhoea. *Amer. J. Med.* **49**, 899–912.

Heading R.C., Paterson W.D., McClelland D.B.L., Barnetson R.St.C. & Murray M.S.W. (1976) Clinical response of dermatitis herpetiformis skin lesions to a gluten-free diet. *Brit. J. Dermatol.* **94**, 509–514.

Heiner D.C., Lahey M.E., Wilson J.F., Gerrard J.W., Shwachman H. & Khaw K.T. (1962) Precipitins to antigens of wheat and cow's milk in coeliac disease. *J. Paediat.* **61**, 813–830.

Hemmings W.A. & Williams E.W. (1978) Transport of large breakdown products of dietary protein through the gut wall. *Gut*, **19**, 715–723.

Hillman H.S. (1972) Intestinal malabsorption with subtotal villous atrophy unresponsive to a gluten-free diet but responding to immunosuppressive therapy. *Med. J. Aust.* **2**, 82–84.

Hirondel C., Doe W.F. & Peters T.J. (1976) Biochemical and morphological studies on human jejunal mucosa maintained in culture. *Clin. Sci., Mol. Med.* **50**, 425–429.

Hobbs J.R. & Hepner G.W. (1968) Immunoglobulins and alimentary disease. *Lancet*, **ii**, 47.

Hoffbrand A.V., Newcombe B.F.A. & Mollin D.L. (1966) Method of assay of red cell folate and the value of the assay as a test for folate deficiency. *J. Clin. Path.* **19**, 17–28.

Hoffbrand A.V. (1974) Anaemia in adult coeliac disease. *Clin. in Gastroenterol.* **3**, 71–89.

Holdsworth C.D. & Dawson A.M. (1965) Glucose and fructose absorption in idiopathic steatorrhoea. *Gut*, **6**, 387–391.

Holmes G.K.T., Stokes P.L., McWalter R. Walerhouse J.A.M. & Cooke W.T. (1974) Coeliac disease, malignancy and a gluten-free diet. *Gut*, **15**, 339.

Holmes G.K., Dunn G.I., Cockel, R. & Brookes V.S. (1980) Adenocarcinoma of the upper bowel complicating coeliac disease. *Gut*, **21**, 1010–1016.

Hood J. & Mason A.M. (1970) Diffuse pulmonary disease with transfer defect occuring with coeliac disease. *Lancet*, **i**, 445–447.

Hourihane D. O'B. (1963) The histology of intestinal biopsies. *Proc. Roy. Soc. Med.* **56**, 1073–1077.

Isaacson P. & Wright D.H. (1978) Intestinal lymphoma associated with malabsorption. *Lancet*, **i**, 67–70.

Jones P.E. & Peters T.J. (1977) DNA synthesis by jejunal mucosa in responsive and non-responsive coeliac disease. *Brit. Med. J.* **1**, 1130–1131.

Jones P.E. & Peters T.J. (1981) Oral zinc supplements in non-responsive coeliac syndrome: effect on jejunal morphology, enterocyte production and brush border disaccharidase activities. *Gut*, **22**, 194–198.

Jos J. & Rey J. (1975) L'apport de la culture organotypique à l'etude pathogenique de la maladie coeliaque. *Arch. Fr. Mal. App. Dig.* **64**, 461.

Kasarda D.D., Bernardin J.E. & Qualset C.C. (1976) Relationship of gliadin protein components to chromasomes in hexaploid wheats (Triticum aestrivum L) *Proc. Nat. Acad. Sci. USA*, **73**, 3646.

Katz S.I., Falchuk Z.M., Dahl M., Rogentine G.N. & Strober W. (1972) H1-A8: a genetic link between dermatitis herpetiformis and gluten sensitive enteropathy. *J. Clin. Invest.* **51**,

2977–2980.

Kenrick K.G. & Walker-Smith J.A. (1970) Immunoglobulins and dietary protein antibodies in childhood coeliac disease. *Gut*, **11**, 635–640.

Keuning J.T., Pena A.S., van Leeuwen A., van Hoof J.P. & van Rood J.J. (1976) HLA-DW3 associated with coeliac disease. *Lancet*, **i**, 506–507.

Krainick H.G. & Mohn G. (1959) Weitre Unterschungen uber den schadlichen weizemmehleffek bei der coliakie. 2 Die wirkung der enzymatischen. Abbauproukte des Gliadin. *Helv. Paed. Acta.* **14**, 124–140.

Kumar P.J., Ferguson A., Lancaster-Smith M.L. & Dawson A.M. (1973a) Relationship between dietary food. Antigen and jejunal mucosal morphology. *Gut*, **14**, 829–830.

Kumar P.J., Silk D.B.A., Marks P., Clark M.L. & Dawson A.M. (1973b) Treatment of dermatitis herpetiformis with corticosteroids and a gluten-free diet: a study of jejunal morphology and function. *Gut*, **14**, 280–283.

Kumar P.J. (1976) Adult coeliac disease and dermatitis herpetiformis: a comparison. MD Thesis, University of London.

Kumar P.J., O'Donoghue D.P., Stenson K. & Dawson A.M. (1979) Re-introduction of gluten in adults and children with treated coeliac disease. *Gut*, **20**, 743–749.

Kumar P.J., Oliver R.T.D., O'Donoghue D.P., Cudworth A., Lancaster-Smith M., NG AH Foong L. & Pillam A. (1981) The relationship of HLA-A, B status to the clinical findings and autoimmunity in coeliac disease. In *The Genetics of Coeliac Disease*, pp. 173–180. R.B. McConnell MTP Press Ltd, Lancaster.

Lancaster-Smith M.J., Benson M.K. & Strickland I.D. (1971) Coeliac disease and diffuse intestinal lung disease. *Lancet*, **i**, 473.

Lancaster-Smith M., Kumar P.J., Marks R., Clark M.L. & Dawson A.M. (1974) Jejunal mucosal immunoglobulins containing cells and jejunal fluid immunoglobulins in adult coeliac disease and dermatitis herpetiformis. *Gut*, **15**, 371–376.

Lancaster-Smith M.L., Kumar P.J., Clark M.L., Marks R. & Johnson G.D. (1975) Anti-reticulin antibodies in dermatitis herpetiformis and adult coeliac disease. *Brit. J. Dermatol.* **92**, 37–42.

Lancaster-Smith M., Packer S., Kumar P.J. & Harries J.T. (1976a) Cellular infiltrate of the jejunum after re-introduction of dietary gluten in children with treated coeliac disease. *J. Clin. Path.* **29**, 587–591.

Lancaster-Smith M., Packer S., Kumar P.J. & Harries J.T. (1976b) Immunological phenomena in the jejunum and serum after re-introduction of dietary gluten in children with treated coeliac disease. *J. Clin. Path.* **29**, 592–597.

Leonard J.N., Tucker W.F., Fry J.S. *et al.* (1983) Increased incidence of malignancy in dermatitis herpetiformis. *Brit. Med. J.* **286**, 16–18.

Lewin K. (1969) The Paneth cell in disease. *Gut*, **10**, 804–811.

Lindsay M.K.M., Nordin B.E.C. & Norman A.P. (1956) Late prognosis in coeliac disease. *Brit. Med. J.*, **i**, 14–18.

Loeb P.M., Strober W., Falchuk Z.M. & Laster L. (1971) Incorporation of Leucine — ^{14}C into immunoglobulins by jejunal biopsies of patients with coeliac sprue and other gastrointestinal diseases. *J. Clin. Invest.* **50**, 559–569.

Logan R.F.A., Ferguson A., Finlayson N.D.C. & Weir D.G. (1978) Primary biliary cirrhosis and coeliac disease. *Lancet*, **i**, 230–233.

McCarthy C.F., Fraser I.D., Evans K.T. & Read A.E. (1966) Lymphoreticular dysfunction in idiopathic steatorrhoea. *Gut*, **7**, 140–148.

McCarthy C.F., Mylotte M., Stevens F., Egan-Mitchell B., Fottrell P.F. & McNicholl B. (1974) Family studies on coeliac disease in Ireland. In *Coeliac Disease*, p. 311. (Ed. by W. Hekkens & A.S. Pena). Stenfert Kroese, Leiden.

McCrae W.M. (1970) The inheritence of coeliac disease. In *Coeliac Disease*, pp. 55–62. (Ed. by C.C. Booth & R.H. Dowling). Churchill Livingstone, Edinburgh.

MacDonald W.C., Dobbins W.O. & Rubin C.E. (1965) Studies of the familial nature of coeliac sprue using biopsy of the small intestine. *New Engl. J. Med.* **272**, 448–456.

Mackinnon A.M., Short M.D., Elias E. & Dowling R.H. (1975) Adaptive changes in vitamin B_{12} absorption in coeliac disease and after proximal small bowel resection in man. *Amer. J. Dig. Dis.* **20**, 835–840.

McNicholl B., Egan-Mitchell B. & Fottrell P.F. (1974) Varying gluten susceptibility in coeliac disease. In *Coeliac Disease*, pp. 413–420. (Ed. by W. Hekkens & A.S. Pena). Stenfert Kroese, Leiden.

Magnus E.M. (1966) Low serum and red cell folate activity in adult coeliac disease. *Amer. J. Dig. Dis.* **11**, 314–319.

Mann D.L., Katz S.I., Nelson D.L. Abelson L.D. & Strober W. (1976) Specific B-cell antigens associated with gluten sensitivity enteropathy and dermatitis herpetiformis. *Lancet*, **i**, 110–111.

Marchi M de., Borelli I., Olivetti E., Richiardi P., Wright P., Ansaldi N., Barbera C. & Santini B. (1979) Two HLA-D and -DR alleles are associated with coeliac disease. *Tiss. Antig.* **14**, 309.

Marks J., Shuster S. & Watson A.J. (1966) Small bowel changes in dermatitis herpetiformis. *Lancet*, **ii**, 1280–1282.

Marks R. & Whittle M.W. (1969) Results of treatment of dermatitis herpetiformis with a gluten-free diet after 1 year. *Brit. Med. J.* **II**, 772–775.

Marsh G.W. & Stewart J.S. (1970) Splenic function in adult coeliac disease. *Brit. J. Haematol.* **19**, 445–457.

Marsh M.N., Brown A.C.T. & Swift J.A. (1970) The surface ultrastructure of the small intestinal mucosa of normal subjects and of patients with untreated and treated coeliac disease using the scanning electron microscope. In *Coeliac*

Disease, pp. 26–44. (Ed. by C.C. Booth & R.H. Dowling). Churchill Livingstone, London.

Marsh M.N. (1980) Studies of intestinal lymphoid tissue. III Quantitative analyses of epithelial lymphocytes in the small intestine of human control subjects and of patients with coeliac sprue. *Gastroenterol.* **79**, 481–492.

Marsh M.N. (1981) The small intestine: Mechanisms of local immunity and gluten sensitivity. *Clin. Sci.* **61**, 497–503.

Mecham D.K., Kasarda D.D. & Qualset C.O. (1977) Genetic aspects of wheat gliadin proteins. *Biochem. Gent.* **16**, 831.

Meeuwisse G.W. (1970) Diagnostic criteria in coeliac disease. *Acta Paediat. Scand.* **59**, 461–463.

Melvin K.E.W., Hepner G.W., Bordier P., Neale G. & Joplin G.F. (1970) Calcium metabolism and bone pathology in adult coeliac disease. *Quart. J. Med.* **39**, 83–113.

Menzies I.S., Pounder R., Heyer S., Laker M.F., Bull J., Wheeler P.G. & Creamer B. (1979) Abnormal intestinal permeability to sugars in villous atrophy. *Lancet*, **ii**, 1107–1109.

Mollin D.L., Booth C.C. & Baker S.J. (1957) The absorption of vitamin B_{12} in control subjects, in Addisonian pernicious anaemia and in the malabsorption syndrome. *Brit. J. Haematol.* **3**, 412–428.

Monro J. (1972) Pantothenic acid and coeliac disease. *Brit. Med. J.* **iv**, 112.

Morris J.S., Ajdukiewicz A.B. & Read A.E. (1970) Coeliac infertility: an indication for dietary gluten restriction? *Lancet*, **i**, 213–214.

Moss A.J., Waterhouse C. & Terry R. (1965) Gluten-sensitive enteropathy with osteomalacia but without steatorrhoea. *New Engl. Med. J.* **272**, 825–834.

Mowbray J.F., Hoffbrand A.V., Holborrow E.J., Seah P.P. & Fry L. (1973) Circulating immune complexes in dermatitis herpetiformis. *Lancet*, **i**, 400–402.

Mylotte M.J. (1972) Familial coeliac disease. *Quart. J. Med.* **164**, 527–528.

Mylotte M.J., Egan-Mitchell B., McCarthy C.F. & McNicholl B. (1973) Incidence of coeliac disease in the West of Ireland. *Brit. Med. J.* **i**, 703–705.

Neale G. (1968) A case of adult coeliac disease resistant to treatment. *Brit. Med. J.* **ii**, 678–684.

O'Donoghue D.P., Lancaster-Smith M., Johnson G.D. & Kumar P.J. (1976) Gastric lesion in dermatitis herpetiformis. *Gut*, **17**, 185–188.

Osoba D. & Falk J. (1976) HLA genes regulating the magnitude of the mixed leucocyte reaction (MLR) *Fed. Proc.* **35**, 712.

Padykula H.A., Strauss E.W. Ladman A.J. & Gardner F.H. (1961) A morphologic and histochemical analysis of the human jejunal epithelium in non-tropical sprue. *Gastroenterol.* **40**, 735–765.

Pallis C.A. & Lewis P.D. (1974) The neurology of gastrointestinal disease, pp. 138–156. W.B. Saunders, London.

Patey A.L. & Evans D.J. (1973) A large-scale preparation of gliadin protein. *J. Sci. Fd. Agri.* **24**, 1229–1233.

Paulley L.W. (1954) Observations on the aetiology of idiopathic steatorrhoea. *Brit. Med. J.* **ii**, 1318.

Peeters T. & van Trappen G. (1975) The Paneth cell: A source of intestinal lysozyme. *Gut*, **16**, 553–558.

Pena A.S., Mann D.L., Hague N.E., Heck J.A., van Leeuwen A., van Rood J.J. & Strober W. (1978) B-cell alloantigens and the inheritance of coeliac disease. In *Perspectives in Coeliac Disease*, pp. 131–136. (Ed. by B. McNicholl, C.F. McCarthy & P.F. Fottrell). MTP Leicester.

Pena A.S. (1981) Genetics of coeliac disease In *Topics in Gastroenterology*, vol. 9. (Ed. by D.P. Jewell & E. Lee). Blackwell Scientific Publications, Oxford.

Peters T.J., Heath J.R., Wansbrough-Jones M.H. & Doe W.F. (1975) Enzyme activities and properties of lysosomes and brush borders in jejunal biopsies from control subjects and patients with coeliac disease. *Clin. Sci. Mol. Med.* **48**, 259–267.

Peters T.J., Jones P.E., Jenkins W.J. & Nicholson J.A. (1978) Analytical subcellular fractionation of jejunal biopsy specimens from control subjects and patients with coeliac disease. In *Perspectives in Coeliac Disease*, pp. 423–436. (Ed. by B. McNicholl, C.F. McCarthy & P.F. Fottrell). MTP Leicester.

Pettit J.E., Hoffbrand, A.V., Seah P.P. & Fry L. (1972) Splenic atrophy in dermatitis herpetiformis. *Brit. Med. J.*, **2**, 438–440.

Phelan J.J., Stevens F.M., Cleere W.F. McNicholl B., McCarthy C.F. & Fottrell P.F. (1978) The detoxification of gliadin by the enzymic cleavage of a side chain substituent. In *Perspectives in Coeliac Disease*. pp. 33–39. (Ed. by B. McNicholl, C.F. McCarthy & P.F. Fottrell). MTP, Leicester.

Prader A., Tanner J.M. & von Harnack G.A. (1963) Catch-up growth following illness and starvation. *J. Paediat.* **62**, 646–659.

Prader A., Shmerling D.H., Zachmann M. & Biro Z. (1969) Catch-up growth in coeliac disease. *Acta Paediat. Scand.* **58**, 311.

Regan P.T. & Di Magno E.P. (1980) Exocrine pancreatic insufficiency in coeliac sprue: a cause of treatment failure. *Gastroenterol.* **78**, 484–488.

Reunala T., Blomquist K., Tarpila S., Halme H. & Kangas K. (1977) Gluten-free diet in dermatitis herpetiformis. 1 Clinical response of skin lesion in 81 patients. *Brit. J. Dermatol.* **97**, 473–480.

Robinson D.C., Watson A.J., Wyatt E.H., Marks J.M. & Roberts F. (1971) Incidence of small intestinal mucosal abnormalities and of clinical coeliac disease in the relatives of children with coeliac disease. *Gut*, **12**, 789–793.

Rolles C.J., Kendall M.J., Nutter S. & Anderson C.M. (1973) One hour blood xylose screening test for coeliac disease. *Lancet*, **ii**, 1043–1044.

Rolles C.J., Kyaw-Myint T.O. & Sin W.K. (1974) Family study of coeliac disease. In *Coeliac Disease*, pp. 320–321. (Ed. by W. Hekkens & A.S. Pena). Stenfert Kroses, Leiden.

Rosekrans P.C.M., Pena A.S., Hekkens W.Th.J.M., Vries R.R.P. de & Haex A.J.Ch. (1978) Coeliac disease. A family study in the Netherlands. In *Perspectives in Coeliac Disease*, pp. 147–154. (Ed. by B. McNicholl, C.F. McCarthy & P.F. Fottrell). MTP, Leicester.

Royer M., Croxatto O., Biempica L. & Balcazar Morrison A.J. (1955) Biopsie duodenal por aspiracion bajo control radio-scopico. *Pren. Med. Argent.* **42**, 2515–2519.

Rubin C.E. (1960) Coeliac disease and idiopathic sprue. Some reflections on reversibility, gluten and the intestine. *Gastroenterol.* **39**, 260–261.

Rubin C.E., Brandborg L.L., Flick A.L., Parmentier C.M., Phelps P. & van Niel S. (1960) Studies of Coeliac Sprue III. The effect of repeated wheat instillation into the proximal ileum of patients on a gluten-free diet. *Gastroenterol.* **43**, 621–641.

Rubin C.E., Brandburg L.L., Phelps P.C. & Taylor H.C. jr. (1960) Studies in coeliac disease, 1. The apparent identical and specific nature of the duodenal and proximal jejunal lesion in coeliac disease and idiopathic sprue. *Gastroenterol.*, **38**, 29–49.

Rubin W., Fauci A.S., Sleisenger M.N. & Jeffries G.H. (1965) Immunofluorescent studies in adult coeliac disease. *J. Clin. Invest.* **44**, 475–485.

Samloff I.M., Kelly M.L., Logan V.W. & Terry R. (1964) Severe histopathological lesion of sprue of a patient with minimal evidence of malabsorption. *Annal. Int. Med.* **60**, 637–679.

Schedl H.P. & Clifton J.A. (1963) Solute and water absorption by the human small intestine. *Nature (Lond.),* **199**, 1264–1267.

Schmid W.C., Phillips S.F. & Summerskill W.H. J. (1969) Jejunal secretion of electrolytes and water in non-tropical sprue. *J. Lab. Clin. Med.* **73**, 772–783.

Scott B.B. & Losowsky M.S. (1976) Patchiness and duodenal-jejunal variation of the mucosal abnormality in coeliac disease and dermatitis herpetiformis. *Gut*, **17**, 984–987.

Seah P.P., Fry L., Rossiter M.A., Hoffbrand A.V. & Holborrow E.J. (1971) Anti-reticulin antibodies in childhood coeliac disease. *Lancet*, **ii**, 681–682.

Seah P.P., Fry L., Stewart J.S., Chapman B.L., Hoffbrand A.V. & Holborrow E.J. (1972) Immunoglobulins in the skin in dermatitis herpetiformis and coeliac disease. *Lancet*, **i**, 611–614.

Seah P.P., Fry L., Holborrow E.J. Rossiter M.A., Doe W.F., Megalhaes A.F. & Hoffbrand A.V. (1973) Antireticulin antibody: Incidence and diagnostic significance. *Gut*, **14**, 311–315.

Selby W.S. & Gallagher N.D. (1979) Malignancy in a 19-year experience of adult coeliac disease. *Dig. Dis. Sci. Sept.* **24**, 684–688.

Sencer W. (1957) Neurologic manifestations in the malabsorption syndrome. *J. Mt. Sinai. Hosp.* **24**, 331–345.

Shiner M. (1956a) Duodenal biopsy. *Lancet*, **i**, 17–19.

Shiner M. (1956b) Jejunal biopsy tube. *Lancet*, **i**, 85.

Shiner M. & Ballard J. (1972) Antigen–antibody reactions in jejunal mucosa in childhood coeliac disease after gluten challenge. *Lancet*, **i**, 1202–1205.

Shiner M. (1973) Ultrastructural changes suggestive of immune reactions in the jejunal mucosa of coeliac children following gluten challenge. *Gut*, **14**, 1–12.

Shiner M. (1974) Electron microscopy of jejunal mucosa. *Clin. in Gastroenterol.* **3**, 33–53.

Shipman R.T., Williams A.L., Kay R. & Townley R.R.W. (1973) A family study of coeliac disease. *Aust. N.Z. J. Med.* **1975**, 250.

Shuster S., Watson A.J. & Marks J. (1968) Coeliac syndrome in dermatitis herpetiformis. *Lancet*, **i**, 1101–1106.

Silk D.B.A., Kumar P.J., Webb J.P.W., Lane A.E., Clark M.L. & Dawson A.M. (1975) Ileal function in patients with untreated adult coeliac disease. *Gut*, **16**, 261–267.

Smith C.A. (1946) The effects of maternal undernutrition upon the newborn infant in Holland 1944–1945. *J. Paediat.* **30**, 229–243.

Smith E.L. (1966) The diagnosis of dermatitis herpetiformis. *Trans. St John's Hosp. Derm. Soc.* **52**, 176–196.

Soltoft J. (1970) Immunoglobulin-containing cells in non-tropical sprue. *Clin. Exp. Immunol.* **6**, 413–420.

Stevens F.M., Phelan J.J. McNicholl B., Comerford F.R., Fottrell P.F. & McCarthy C.F. (1978) Clinical demonstration of the reduction of gliadin toxicity by enzymic clearage of a side chain substituent. In *Perspectives in Coeliac Disease.* (Ed. by B. McNicholl, C.F. McCarthy & P.F. Fottrell). MTP, Leicester.

Stewart J.S., Pollock D.J., Hoffbrand A.V., Mollin D.L. & Booth C.C. (1967) A study of proximal and distal intestinal structure and absorptive function in idiopathic steatorrhoea. *Quart. J. Med. N.S.* **26**, 425–445.

Stokes P.L., Asquith P., Holmes G.K.T., McKintosh P. & Cooke W.T. (1972) Histocompatibility antigens associated with adult coeliac disease. *Lancet*, **ii**, 162-164.

Stokes P.L. & Holmes G.K.T. (1974) Malignancy. *Clin. in Gastroenterol.* **3**, 159–170.

Sutton D.R., Baird I.M., Stewart J.S. & Coghill N.F. (1970) Free iron loss in atrophic gastritis, postgastrectomy states and adult coeliac disease. *Lancet*, **ii**, 387–391.

Swarbrick E.T., Stokes C.R. & Soothill J.F. (1970) The absorption of antigens after oral immunization and the simultaneous induction of systemic tolerance. *Gut*, **20**, 121–125.

Swinson C.M. & Levi A.J. (1980) Is coeliac disease

underdiagnosed? *Brit. Med. J.*, **2**, 1258–1260.

Swinson C., Slavin G., Coles E.C. & Booth C.C. (1983) Coeliac disease and malignancy. *Lancet*, **i**, 111–114.

Taylor W.H. (1959) Gastric proteolysis in disease. The proteolyte activity of gastric juice in chronic hypochronic anaemia and in idiopathic steatorrhoea. *J. Clin. Path.* **12**, 473–476.

Taylor K.B., Truelove S.C., Thomson D.L. & Wright R. (1961) An immunological study of coeliac disease and idiopathic steatorrhoea. Serological reaction to gluten and milk proteins. *Brit. Med. J.* **ii**, 1727–1731.

Thaysen T.E.H. (1932) *Non-Tropical Sprue*. Oxford University, Press, London.

Thurlbeck W.M., Benson J.A.Jr. & Dudley Jr.H.R. (1960) The histopathologic changes of sprue and their significance. *Amer. J. Clin. Path.* **34**, 108–117.

Townley R.R.W., Cornell H.J., Bhathal P.S. & Mitchell J.D. (1973) Toxicity of wheat gliadin fractions in coeliac disease. *Lancet*, **i**, 1363–1365.

Trewby P.N., Chipping P.M., Palmer S.J., Roberts P.D., Lewis S.M. & Stewart J.S. (1981) Splenic atrophy in adult coeliac disease: Is it reversible? *Gut*, **22**, 628–32.

Trier J.S. & Browning T.H. (1970) Epithelial cell renewal in cultured duodenal biopsies in coeliac sprue. *New Engl. J. Med.* **283**, 1245–1364.

Unsworth D.J., Manuel P.D., Walker-Smith J.W., Campbell C.A., Johnson G.A. & Holborrow J. (1981) New immunofluorescent blood test for gluten. *Arch. Dis. Child.* **58**, 864–86.

van der Kamer J.H., Weijers H.A. & Dicke W.K. (1953) Coeliac disease IV. An investigation into the injurious constituents of wheat in connection with their action on patients with coeliac disease. *Acta Paediat.* **42**, 223–231.

van der Kamer J.H. & Weijers H.A. (1955) Coeliac disease: some experiments on the cause of the harmful effects of wheat gliadin. *Acta Paediat.* **44**, 465–469.

van de Meer J.B. (1969) Granular deposits of immunoglobulins in the skin of patients with dermatitis herpetiformis; an immunofluorescent study. *Brit. J. Derm.* **81**, 493–503.

Vanderschueren-Lodeweycky M., Wolter R., Molla A., Eggermont E. & Eeckels R. (1973) Plasma growth hormone in coeliac disease. *Helvet. Paediat. Acta*, **28**, 349–357.

van Tongeren J.H.M. van der Staak W.J.B.M. & Schillings P.H.M. (1967) Small bowel changes in dermatitis herpetiformis. *Lancet*, **i**, 218.

Visakorpi J.K. & Immonen P. (1967) Intolerance to cow's milk and wheat gluten in the primary malabsorption syndrome in infancy. *Acta Paediat. Scand.* **56**, 49.

Visakorpi J.K. (1974) Definition of coeliac disease in children. In *Coeliac Disease* (Ed. by W. Hekkens & A.S. Pena). Stenfert Kroese, Leiden.

Von Essen R., Savilahti E. & Pelkonen P. (1972) Reticulin antibody in children with malabsorption. *Lancet*, **i**, 1157–1159.

Walker W.A., Cornell R.K., Davenport L.M. & Isselbacher K.J. (1972) Macromolecular absorption. Mechanism of HRP uptake and transport in adult and neonatal rat intestine. *J. Cell. Biol.* **54**, 195–205.

Walker-Smith J.A. (1970) Transient gluten intolerance. *Arch. Dis. Child.* **45**, 523–6.

Walker-Smith J.A. (1972) Gastroenteritis. *Med. J. Aust.* **1**, 329–332.

Walker-Smith J.A. (1975) *Diseases of the Small Intestine in Children* p. 65. Pitman Medical, London.

Wall A.J., Douglas A.P. Booth C.C. & Pearce A.G.E. (1970) Response of the jejunal mucosa in adult coeliac disease to oral prednisolone. *Gut*, **11**, 7–14.

Watson A.J. & Wright N.A. (1974) Morphology and cell kinetics of the jejunal mucosa in untreated patients. *Clin. in Gastroenterol.* **3**, 11–31.

Weinstein W.M., Saunders D.R., Tytgat G.N. & Rubin C.E. (1970) Collagenous sprue — an unrecognized type of malabsorption. *New Engl. J. Med.* **283**, 1297–1301.

Weiser M.M. & Douglas A.S. (1976) An alternative mechanism for gluten toxicity in coeliac disease. *Lancet*, **1**, 567–569.

White A.G., Barnetson R.St. C., Dacosta J.A.G. & McClelland D.B.L. (1973) The incidence of HLA antigens in dermatitis herpetiformis and gluten sensitive enteropathy. *Brit. J. Dermatol.* **89**, 133–136.

Woychik A.C., Boundy J.A. & Dinker R.J. (1961) Starch-gel electrophoresis of wheat gluten proteins with concentrated urea. *Arch. Biochem.* **94**, 477–482.

Wright N., Watson A., Morley A., Appleton D. & Marks J. & Douglas A. (1973) Cell kinetics in flat (villous) mucosa of the human small intestine. *Gut*, **14**, 701–710.

Yardley J.H., Bayless T.M. Norton J.H. & Hendrix T.R. (1962) A study of jejunal epithelium before and after a gluten-free diet. *New Engl. J. Med.* **267**, 1173.

Young W. & Pringle E.M. (1971) 110 children with coeliac disease. *Arch. Dis. Child.* **46**, 421–436.

Chapter 10
Lymphoma and Alpha-chain Disease

WILLIAM F. DOE

Introduction 179
Primary Western lymphomas 179
Secondary intestinal lymphomas 184
Immunoproliferative small intestinal disease
 (IPSID) 185

Introduction

Lymphoma is defined as a malignant tumour arising from lymphoid tissue, characterized by proliferation and abnormal growth with local invasion and a propensity to widespread distant metastases and to multi-focal involvement. In Western countries, lymphomas arising primarily in the intestine are rare, representing 1% of all gastrointestinal neoplasms. They usually affect patients in the fifth or sixth decade of life and are characteristically localized to a segment of bowel which is more commonly the ileum than the jejunum (Rosenberg et al. 1961, Naqvi et al. 1969, Fu & Perzin 1972). Coeliac disease (Austad et al. 1967, Cooper et al. 1980), immunodeficiency states (Lamers et al. 1980) and immunosuppressive therapy (Kapadia 1979) predispose to the development of primary lymphomas. Intestinal lymphomas are commonly an unsuspected finding at laparotomy performed for surgical emergencies arising from bowel obstruction, perforation, intussusception or bleeding (Green et al. 1979). There is a second type of intestinal lymphoma called immunoproliferative small intestinal disease (IPSID), which forms a distinct clinicopathological entity and is remarkably prevalent in developing countries, particularly those around the Mediterranean basin. In contrast to the primary intestinal lymphoma found in the Western world, there is a premalignant phase involving diffuse plasmacytoid infiltration of the wall of the small intestine which progresses to frank lymphoma. Young adults develop abdominal pain, weight loss and a severe malabsorption syndrome. Low socio-economic status and poor hygiene, together with genetic factors, may predispose to this condition (Seligmann et al. 1971). The characteristics of the two types of primary lymphomas affecting the small intestine are set out in Table 10.1.

Primary Western lymphomas

Lymphomas arising in the small intestine and mesenteric nodes in the absence of superficial lymphadenopathy, liver or spleen involvement are termed primary lymphomas of the small intestine.

Clinical features

Retrospective surveys show that primary intestinal lymphomas are uncommon. They comprise some 42% of all lymphomas and represent only the third most common small intestinal malignancy after adenocarcinoma and carcinoid tumours. Their frequency has been estimated as 12–13% of all small intestinal malignancies in Western specialist referral hospitals (Mittal & Bodzin 1980). A more accurate view of their frequency and presentation may be given by an epidemiological survey of gastrointestinal lymphomas which was performed over a 6-year period in an unselected population in the north-east of Scotland and which included all the hospitals in the region. Forty-five cases of gastrointestinal lymphomas were diagnosed, of which fifteen (33%) were primary small intestinal lymphomas. Forty per cent of these presented as surgical emergencies with intestinal perforation or obstruction. Constitutional symptoms, hepatosplenomegaly or peripheral lymphadenopathy were rare and a preoperative diagnosis was seldom made. A

Table 10.1. Characteristics of primary small intestinal lymphomas.

	Western lymphomas	Lymphomas of developing countries Immunoproliferative small intestinal disease (IPSID)
Frequency	Rare	Relatively common
Patient's age	5th or 6th decade	2nd or 3rd decade
Predisposing factors	Coeliac disease Immunosuppression Immunodeficiency states	?Poor hygiene and low socio-economic status ?Intestinal parasitic infestation ?Genetic predisposition

Presentation	Abdominal catastrophe common in unsuspected lymphomas
	  perforation
	  obstruction
	  intussusception
	  bleeding
	Weight loss
	Abdominal pain
	Diarrhoea
		Diarrhoea & steatorrhoea
		Weight loss
		Abdominal pains } common
		Finger clubbing
		Abdominal catastrophe (presentation uncommon)
		  perforation
		  obstruction
		  intussusception
		  bleeding

Localization	Usually segmental Ileum predominates	Diffuse proximal involvement (may affect entire length of small intestine)
Histological types	Malignant histiocytosis Histiocytic lymphoma Lymphocytic lymphoma	Plasmacytoid progressing to an immunoblastoma comprising immature plasma cells derived from the same defective clone which synthesizes α-chain disease polypeptide

palpable abdominal mass was present in seven of the fifteen patients. In two of the fifteen patients in whom there was an antecedent history of coeliac disease, steatorrhoea was a presenting symptom (Green et al. 1979). The defined population of 475,000 provides a reasonably accurate estimate for the incidence of primary small intestinal lymphomas as five cases/1,000,000 population. A second retrospective survey covering a period of 11 years in Hong Kong showed that the small intestine was involved in 35% of forty-six Chinese patients suffering from primary gastrointestinal lymphoma. Malabsorption was present in two cases, one as a result of a jejunocolic fistula while the second case showed the diffuse intestinal involvement which is characteristic of the lymphoma of developing countries (Ho & Gibson 1979).

Predisposing factors

Coeliac disease

Although the association of malabsorption and infiltrative disease of the small intestine accompanied by mesenteric node enlargement was first reported in 1855 by Gull, the recognition that intestinal lymphomas were a complication of coeliac disease was not made until 1962 (Gough et al. 1962). Subsequent studies conducted in a large series of coeliac patients in Birmingham demonstrated that there was a statistically significant increase in intestinal lymphoma in coeliac disease (Harris et al. 1967). A prospective survey of the same coeliac population has confirmed this finding (Holmes et al. 1976). A similar association has been reported in patients suffering from dermatitis herpetiformis (Anderson et al. 1971, Freeman et al. 1977), a condition closely linked to coeliac disease (Fry et al. 1968, Weinstein et al. 1974). Of 259 histologically confirmed malignancies reported in 235 coeliac patients, 133 (51.4%) were malignant lymphomas (Swinson et al. 1983a).

Although the Birmingham survey of 385 coeliac patients began in 1946, and therefore includes a number of patients diagnosed on clinical grounds without histological confirmation, it represents a valuable long-term study because the great majority of patients have regularly attended clinics following their diagnosis. Twenty-seven of the 385 coeliac patients (7%) developed intestinal lymphoma, mainly in the fifth and sixth decades of life (mean age 55 years). The age range is similar for gastrointestinal lymphoma occurring in Western subjects without coeliac disease. The condition carries a bad prognosis and was responsible for 23% of the 118 recorded deaths in this series (Cooper et al. 1980).

The presentation of intestinal lymphoma complicating coeliac disease may be that of an acute abdominal emergency due to intestinal perforation, peritonitis, obstruction or bleeding, particularly if the coeliac disease was previously undiagnosed. In the more common insidious presentation, the lymphoma may occur after an established response to a gluten-free diet and present with symptoms such as weight loss, lethargy, diarrhoea, muscle weakness, fever and abdominal pain. Alternatively, the development of lymphoma may manifest itself as progressive deterioration in a recently diagnosed patient despite a gluten-free diet. A palpable abdominal mass and lymphadenopathy are often present. The time lapse between the onset of symptoms attributable to coeliac disease and the development of lymphoma, ranged widely between 6 months and 60 years and averaged 29 years (Cooper et al. 1980). The case reported below illustrates the insidious development of intestinal lymphoma in a coeliac patient under regular follow-up whose lymphoma presented as an obstruction of the small bowel.

A female canteen worker presented at the age of 35 in 1945 complaining of fatigue, malaise, sore tongue and pruritus vulvae. There was a past history of rickets, growth retardation and episodic diarrhoea. Facial pigmentation, glossitis, vulvovaginitis, mild hepatomegaly and a hypochromic anaemia of 9.7 g/l were noted. Pellagra was diagnosed and, following treatment with nicotinic acid, iron and vitamin B, the symptoms improved. Over the next 19 years, however, recurrent episodes of chest infection and chronic anaemia required frequent hospital admissions. In 1968 bone pain and tenderness developed in the tibiae and radii. Investigation showed macrocytosis and microcytosis on the blood film, a marginal value for serum folate (4.8 ng/ml), a raised alkaline phosphatase (19 KAU/dl) and steatorrhoea (25 g fat/24 h). Jejunal biopsy showed a loss of villus architecture and measurement of the serum immunoglobulins revealed selective IgA deficiency.

The diagnoses of selective IgA deficiency and adult coeliac disease causing osteomalacia were made and treatment was commenced with parenteral vitamin D and a gluten-free diet. The patient was admitted to hospital repeatedly for treatment of megaloblastic anaemia and steatorrhoea, probably related to dietary indiscretions.

In 1973, the patient developed dysphagia due to a tumour narrowing the upper third of the oesophagus. Biopsy showed the appearances of a squamous cell carcinoma which was treated by irradiation. Six months later the patient complained of right-sided abdominal pain. Abdominal X-ray showed dilated loops of small bowel. The patient deteriorated suddenly and died of pulmonary embolism aged 63.

Autopsy confirmed the presence of small intestinal lymphoma causing a stricture in proximal jejunum.

The diagnosis of intestinal lymphoma is usually made in only two-thirds of cases during life, the remaining third being discovered at autopsy. Barium meal and follow-through examination is frequently abnormal but changes suggesting lymphomatous involvement of the intestine were found in only four of fifteen patients studied by Cooper et al. (1980). Endoscopy now provides access to the proximal jejunum and terminal ileum and mutiple biopsies may be taken along the length of the small intestine using hydraulic multiple biopsy techniques. These advances, together with recent developments in organ imaging, may substantially improve the chances of diagnosing intestinal lymphomas during life and computed tomography may be particularly useful for staging and follow-up (Blackledge 1981).

Although the initial impression gained from the Birmingham survey suggested that adherence to a gluten-free diet decreased the risk of malignancy in coeliac patients (Harris et al. 1967), further analysis failed to support this view. The diagnosis of coeliac disease was made long before the development of lymphoma in the majority of patients who had been maintained on a gluten-free diet, and reviewed several times a year, for many years. Indeed, lymphoma was observed to complicate patients shown to be in virtually complete remission as judged by the morphological appearances along the length of the small intestine (Cooper et al. 1980). Nor is there strong evidence to suggest that patients who respond poorly to gluten withdrawal from the diet are more liable to develop malignancy than those who are good responders (Holmes et al. 1976, Swinson et al. 1983a).

Ulcerative jejunitis, formerly thought to be a non-malignant complication of coeliac disease, appears to predispose to, or be a manifestation of, intestinal lymphoma (Isaacson & Wright 1978, Baer et al. 1980). The presentation is often similar to that found for overt lymphomas, i.e. unexplained malabsorption and abdominal pain in a patient taking a gluten-free diet, or the development of complications including bleeding, perforation or obstruction. The diagnosis is usually made at surgery where resection of ulcerated segments appears to be the best hope of cure (Baer et al. 1980).

Why patients suffering from coeliac disease should develop malignancy, particularly intestinal lymphoma, is not clear. There is persistent antigenic stimulation to the exposed and inflamed intestinal mucosa which becomes heavily infiltrated with lymphoid cells. Moreover, loss of integrity of the surface epithelium results in increased antigen entry and lymphoid hyperplasia which may increase the risk of lymphoma. The immaturity of the enterocyte monolayer in untreated coeliac disease may also result in a decreased ability to detoxify potential carcinogens. The atrophy of lymph nodes and spleen which occurs in a high proportion of coeliac patients suggest that diminished immune surveillance may also be a factor. On the other hand, while hyposplenism is a well recognized feature of coeliac disease, no association has been found between splenic atrophy and the development of malignant lymphoma in coeliac disease (Robertson et al. 1982). In addition-genes linked to those for the known histocompatibility markers of coeliac disease, HLA-B8 and DrW3, may predispose patients to the expression of the oncogenes which cause intestinal lymphomas, but there are no HLA genetic markers associated specifically with the development of malignancy in coeliac disease (Swinson et al. 1983b).

Immunodeficiency

Evidence from a large series of patients suffering from congenital (Spector et al. 1978) and idiopathic, late-onset immunoglobulin deficiency (Hermans et al. 1976) suggests that the incidence of generalized lymphomas in this disorder is significantly higher than that found in the general population. Whether the incidence of intestinal lymphomas is increased in immunodeficiency patients, however, is less certain. Jejunal lymphoma complicating late-onset hypogammaglobulinaemia and nodular lymphoid hyperplasia has been reported (Lamers et al. 1980). In a review of fifty cases of idiopathic late-onset hypogammaglobulinaemia, lymphoma developed in two patients and in one of these there was a primary lymphoma affecting the rectum and sigmoid in association with nodular lymphoid hyperplasia of the small intestine (Hermans et al. 1976). Small intestinal lymphoma has also been reported in patients shown to have nodular lymphoid hyperplasia of the small intestine but in whom serum immunoglobulin levels were normal (Kahn & Novis 1974, Matuchansky et al. 1980). This provides evidence that nodular lymphoid hyperplasia itself may predispose to malignancy. In one of these cases, both the lymphomatous cells in the jejunum and the lymphocytes present in nearby lymphoid hyperplastic nodules, were part of a monoclonal expansion of B lymphocytes of IgM−K type, whereas staining of the lymphoid hyperplastic nodules in intestinal tissue far distant from the lymphomatous involvement showed polyclonal B lymphocytes in the germinal centres. This finding suggests that the jejunal lymphoma had arisen as a malignant transformation of the nodular lymphoid hyperplasia (Matuchansky et al. 1980).

Autoimmune disorders

In addition to primary immunodeficiency syndromes, autoimmune disorders such as systemic lupus erythematosus and Sjögren's syndrome (Zulman et al. 1978) and disseminated viral infections, such as those in association with the Epstein−Barr virus (Magrath et al. 1975), predispose to the development of lymphomas. Iatrogenic immunosuppression to prevent rejection of renal transplants or arising as a side-effect of chemotherapy given for another malignancy, such as multiple myeloma (Kapadia 1979), may also predispose to intestinal lymphomas. The incidence of malignancies in imunosuppressed recipients of renal transplants, for example, is estimated to be 100 times that of an age-matched population and involves a relatively greater proportion of lymphomas than that found in the malignancies affecting the general populations (Penn 1979).

Histopathology

Several factors conspire to limit the data base from which a rational classification of Western intestinal lymphomas may be developed. The condition is relatively rare and frequently presents as an abdominal emergency in which the diagnosis is unsuspected preoperatively. Rapid autolysis and poor fixation of intestinal specimens make morphological examination difficult. Moreover, the tradition of limiting the basis for classification to morphological appearances rather than to studies related to cell function or to antigenic markers has resulted in schemes which are contradictory. In recent years the standard lymphoma classification has divided non-Hodgkin's lymphomas into nodular or diffuse groups which are further classified by cytological characteristics viewed by light microscopy (Rappaport 1966). The use of electron microscopy, immunohistochemistry and surface markers has shown that lymphomas classified as histiocytic are in fact lymphocytic in origin. It is not surprising, therefore, that the classification of Western intestinal lymphomas, as with lymphomas in general, is in a state of confusion (Dorfman 1977) and that new attempts at classification have been attempted (Lennert & Stein 1981, Non-Hodgkin's Lymphoma Pathologic classification project 1982). These classifications may improve with the recognition of cell markers that identify the different types of immune-related cells and their subsets, using monoclonal antibodies and immunohistochemical techniques such as the peroxidase−antiperoxidase (PAP) methods.

Isaacson et al. (1979) have made use of this approach in a retrospective study of sixty-six cases of primary gastrointestinal lymphoma of which forty involved the small intestine. Using morphologic techniques, particularly the demonstration of phagocytosis, and the PAP system to detect lysozyme, α 1-antitrypsin, the presence of polyclonal antibody and the third component of complement within tumour cells, 50% of the lymphomas were classified as histiocytic. Eleven cases with variable morphology were classified as histiocytic lymphomas on the basis of their immunochemical features. In the latter group the villus architecture in the uninvolved small intestine was normal, and the tumour formed solid masses in a similar manner to lymphocyte-derived tumours. A much more pleomorphic tumour that diffusely infiltrated the lamina propria with histiocytes, often in bizarre multinucleated giant forms and with an associated polyclonal plasma cell infiltrate, was classified as malignant histiocytosis. Whereas α 1-antitrypsin stains were very weak or negative in histiocytic lymphomas, those in tumour cells in malignant histiocytosis were clearly positive. In this condition the villus height in uninvolved mucosa was markedly reduced. There was spread to lymph nodes, spleen and liver suggesting that malignant histiocytosis of the intestine is part of the systemic condition classified as malignant histiocytosis or histiocytic medullary reticulosis (Byrne & Rappaport 1973) and behaves as an extra-nodal lymphoma. Of the remaining intestinal lymphomas in the series, 41% were classified by morphologic appearances as lymphocyte-derived lymphomas and the immunohistochemical studies were negative. Further improvements in technique and prospective studies of intestinal lymphomas are needed to confirm these unexpected findings (Lightdale 1980).

In patients with lymphoma complicating coeliac disease, histological and immunohistochemical studies also indicate that the tumour is predominantly a malignant histiocytosis (Isaacson & Wright 1978, Swinson et al. 1983a). There is a characteristic early lesion comprising aggregations of histiocytes which invade the epithelium of the surface and the crypts. These appearances have been reported in 'uninvolved' jejunal mucosa in the presence or absence of obvious lymphoma. In the latter instance this lesion may pre-date the diagnosis of frank malignant histiocytosis of the intestine by many years (Issacson 1980).

In contrast to the frequency of plasmacytoid intestinal lymphomas found in the developing countries, intestinal plasmacytomas appear to be rare in Western countries. In a review of 272 extramedullary plasmacytomas in Britain, only ten were found to involve the intestinal tract (Wiltshaw 1976). Although a retrospective survey of Western intestinal lymphomas reported that 39% were predominantly of plasma cell type, the study was based exclusively on morphologic criteria (Henry & Farrer-Brown 1977) and is at variance with a recent survey which found that only 8% of lymphomas showed plasmacytoid changes which were classified as a distinct sub-group of the parent lymphoma (Lewin et al. 1976). It has been suggested that the majority of the lymphomas decribed as plasma cell type would be shown to be histiocytic if immunochemical studies had been performed (Isaacson et al. 1979).

Course and treatment

The clinical course of untreated primary lymphoma of the intestine is one of a rapid progression to death. Where possible, the primary lesion should be widely excised and regional lymph nodes removed *en bloc* (Naqvi et al. 1969, Loehr et al. 1969, Herbsman et al. 1980). The place of adjuvant radiotherapy following an apparently complete resection is unclear but radiotherapy is indicated in cases of unresectable or palliatively resected intestinal lymphoma (Treadwell & White 1975). The place of modern chemotherapy for both localized and unresectable lesions has yet to be fully evaluated.

Prognosis is related to the morpholgical features of the small bowel lymphoma as well as to its extent (Fu & Perzin 1972). The ulcerative type of tumour has a significantly worse prognosis than the polypoid lymphomas and tumours over 10 cm in size have a poor outlook. Nodal involvement and multi-centre lesions are also poor prognostic features. The lymphocytic cell type and the giant follicular pattern appear to be associated with a better prognosis. Fifty per cent of patients with nodular lymphomas, but only 25% of patients suffering from diffuse lymphomas, survive 5 years. The overall 5-year survival rate following wide resection or resection plus radiotherapy varies from 30–48% (Herbsman et al. 1980, Fu & Perzin 1972).

Secondary intestinal lymphomas

The involvement of the intestine in a generalized lymphomatous process which began elsewhere in the body is termed secondary intestinal lymphoma. This is diagnosed in 5–13% of patients (Sugarbaker & Craver 1940, Gall & Mallory 1942, Rosenberg et al. 1961) although at autopsy the incidence is more than 50% and is especially high in children.

The location of the tumour, its gross

appearance and its histological features are like those of primary intestinal lymphomas. Similarly it often presents as an abdominal catastrophe due to bleeding, perforation, intussusception or obstruction. Alternatively, there may be the insidious development of anorexia, weight loss and abdominal pain. Diarrhoea is infrequent and steatorrhoea rare. Diagnosis is largely dependent on careful radiological examination of the small intestine.

The management of secondary intestinal lymphomas follows similar lines to that for the primary lymphomas, and involves surgical resection with or without radiotherapy. The prognosis of secondary intestinal lymphomas is strikingly worse than that for primary lymphomas reflecting the increased frequency of lymph node involvement and of multi-centric lesions (Fu & Perzin 1972).

Immunoproliferative small intestinal disease (IPSID)

Diffuse primary intestinal lymphomas associated with malabsorption were first described in the Middle East and Mediterranean region (Azar 1962, Ramot et al. 1965, Eidelman et al. 1966, Al-Bahrani et al. 1983). These 'Mediterranean lymphomas' display clinical and pathological features which clearly distinguish them from the Western type of primary intestinal lymphoma (Table 10.1). More recently, the condition has been described in many countries outside the Mediterranean area including Pakistan (Doe et al. 1972), South Africa (Novis et al. 1973), Cambodia and Argentina (Seligmann 1975), Nigeria (Whicher et al. 1977) and the Soviet Union (Chernokhvostova & German 1980). Clinical studies suggest evolution from a diffuse, premalignant plasmacytoid infiltrate of the small intestine to frank lymphoma involving more primitive immunoblasts. Immunoglobulin fragments comprising incomplete heavy chains of IgA, have now been detected in the sera and secretions of the majority of patients, giving rise to the term α-chain disease (αCD) (Seligmann et al. 1968, Rambaud et al. 1968). Although αCD is mainly localized to the small intestine, cases of primary lung involvement have been described (Stoop et al. 1971, Florin-Christensen et al. 1974). This observation, together with the geographical diversity of the disorder and the evidence for a premalignant phase characterized by plasma cell infiltration, have led to the intestinal condition being renamed immunoproliferative small intestinal disease (IPSID) (WHO 1976).

Although evidence from formal epidemiological surveys is lacking, reviews of large numbers of cases indicate that IPSID is a remarkably common condition, especially in the Mediterranean region and the Middle East. Young adults from under-privileged backgrounds develop a syndrome which results from extensive and diffuse infiltration of the wall of the small intestine, predominantly by plasma cells.

Clinical features

The clinical features of IPSID are markedly uniform. The major symptoms are diarrhoea with steatorrhoea, generalized colicky abdominal pain and weight loss (Doe et al. 1972, Salem et al. 1977). In those with heavy protein-losing enteropathy, ankle-swelling and ascites may develop. Sustained electrolyte loss may lead to symptoms of polyuria due to kaliopenic nephropathy (Inunberry et al. 1970, Laroche et al. 1970, Manousos 1974) and hypocalcaemic tetany (Doe et al. 1972, Bonomo et al. 1972). At an advanced stage of the disease when frank lymphoma supervenes, bleeding, intestinal obstruction, perforation or intussusception may be presenting features (Bognel et al. 1972, Doe 1975, Lewin et al. 1976).

Physical signs are usually limited to wasting, marked clubbing of fingers and toes and ankle oedema. In some instances abdominal lymphoid masses are palpable but the liver and spleen are not clinically enlarged. Peripheral lymphadenopathy is not a feature of IPSID except in the terminal stages. A nasopharyngeal lymphoid tumour was present in a patient who had a history of blood in his saliva (Doe et al. 1970). At laparotomy the wall of the small intestine is often thickened and mesenteric nodes are enlarged (Laroche et al. 1970). Haematological studies show that iron and folic acid deficiency are common but the haemoglobin levels are usually near normal. Morphologically abnormal plasma cells have been found in the peripheral blood (Doe et al. 1972). Biochemical investigations show reduced levels of plasma potassium, calcium, and magnesium. Hypoalbuminaemia associated with protein-losing enteropathy is a common finding. One striking biochemical feature is the marked increase of circulating alkaline phosphatase of intestinal origin (Ramot & Streifler 1966, Rambaud et al. 1968, Doe et al. 1972).

Radiological examination of the small intestine reveals diffusely abnormal changes. The proximal bowel is typically more severely affected than distal small intestine. The mucosal pattern is coarse and nodular and the contour of the bowel may be irregular. Strictures leading to obstruction may also become apparent (Ramot et al. 1965, Nasr et al. 1970, Doe et al. 1976). Hypertrophic osteoarthropathy is an occasional finding (Doe et al. 1976).

Tests of intestinal function reveal malabsorption in both jejunum and ileum, together with steatorrhoea, suggesting diffuse involvement of the whole length of the small intestine. Parasitic infection is common. Hookworm, *Trichuris trichuria*, *Trichomonas hominis*, *Giardia lamblia* and coccidia are among many of the parasites reported (Doe et al. 1972, Novis et al. 1973, Henry et al. 1974, Salem et al. 1977). No particular parasitic or bacterial pathogen, however, has been isolated consistently from the stools of IPSID patients. Overgrowth of aerobes and anaerobes has been demonstrated in jejunal fluid in several patients in whom steatorrhoea, vitamin B_{12} absorption and ^{14}C-glycocholate breath test improved following oral antibiotic therapy (WHO 1976). These findings suggest that a stagnant loop syndrome may contribute to the malabsorption in some IPSID patients. In other studies, however, no evidence for a stagnant loop syndrome was observed (Chernov et al. 1972).

Protein studies

A characteristic immunoglobulin abnormality is found in the serum, urine and jejunal fluid of the majority of IPSID patients. The aberrant protein comprises incomplete α-heavy chains devoid of light chains (Seligmann et al. 1968) (Fig. 10.1). Antigenic analysis (Seligmann et al. 1969) and chemical studies of the αCD polypeptide (Wolfenstein-Todel et al. 1974) indicate that the C terminus sequence is identical to that of the normal subclass 1 α-heavy chains and that the heavy-light peptide is absent. Thus the entire Fc fragment is included in the αCD polypeptide which also binds the secretory piece. The molecular weight of the monomeric αCD polypeptide varies between 29,000 and 34,000 (Dorrington et al. 1970). The missing portion of the α-heavy chain is located in the Fd segment and involves both V_H and C_H1 domains. The N-terminal sequences performed on several αCD polypeptides show marked heterogeneity suggesting that some post-synthetic intracellular proteolysis occurs (Seligmann et al. 1971). Failure of light chain synthesis by cells synthesizing the αCD polypeptides has been confirmed by biosynthetic studies of nascent immunoglobulin subunits (Buxbaum & Preud'homme 1972).

Although some 30–40% of normal secretory IgA belongs to subclass 2, all fifty αCD

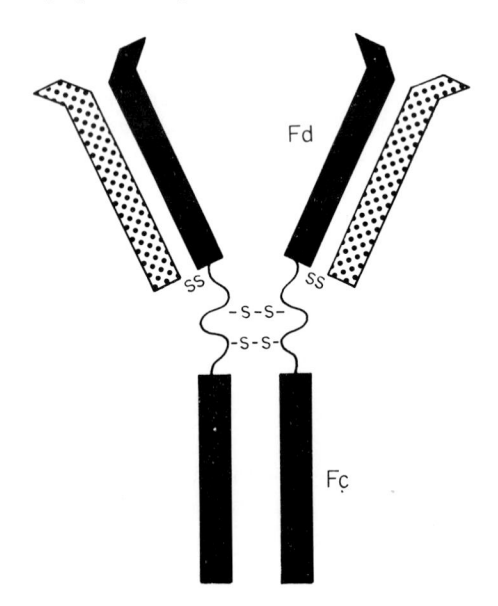

Fig. 10.1. Diagram showing the basic structure of immunoglobins. ■ = heavy chain; ▨ = light chain (κ, λ). In α-chain disease the Fc fragment is synthesized by the abnormal plasma cells but the associated light chains and most of the Fd fragment of the heavy chain are absent.

polypeptides studied so far have been typed as subclass 1 (Seligmann 1975). This finding lends further support to the view that αCD polypeptides are monoclonal proteins.

The detection of αCD polypeptide in serum, urine and jejunal fluid depends on immunochemical analysis. Serum protein electrophoresis is abnormal in only 50% of cases with an abnormally broad band in the α_2 or β region. The characteristic narrow band of a monoclonal immunoglobulin abnormality is not seen. Where no abnormal electrophoretic band is seen, the only changes present are those of a reduced serum albumin and hypogammaglobulinaemia.

Testing by immunoelectrophoresis using antisera monospecific for IgA, usually reveals an abnormal precipitin arc extending from the α_1 to the β_2 region which often has a faster electrophoretic mobility than normal IgA. The inability of αCD polypeptide to precipitate with antisera to light chains can also be used as the basis for a diagnostic test but the failure of some IgA myeloma proteins to precipitate with anti-light chain antisera may produce false positive results. An immunoselection technique in which the test serum is electrophoresed into agarose containing an antiserum which recognizes the conformational specificities of the Fab fragment of IgA provides the most sensitive technique for detecting αCD polypeptide (Doe & Spiegelberg 1979). This step results in the precipitation of normal IgA present in the serum close to the origin. The αCD polypeptide, which lacks Fab α determinants and is therefore unaffected by the presence of anti-Fab antibody in the agarose, migrates unimpeded. The αCD polypeptide can then be detected by an antiserum which is monospecific for IgA (Fig. 10.2) (Doe et al. 1979). In most IPSID patients, αCD polypeptide can also be detected at low levels in concentrated urine and jejunal fluid (Seligmann et al. 1968).

Histopathology

The small intestinal mucosa presents a characteristic appearance. Villi are shortened and broadened giving the appearance of total or partial obliteration of villus architecture. There is a diffuse, dense, mononuclear infil-

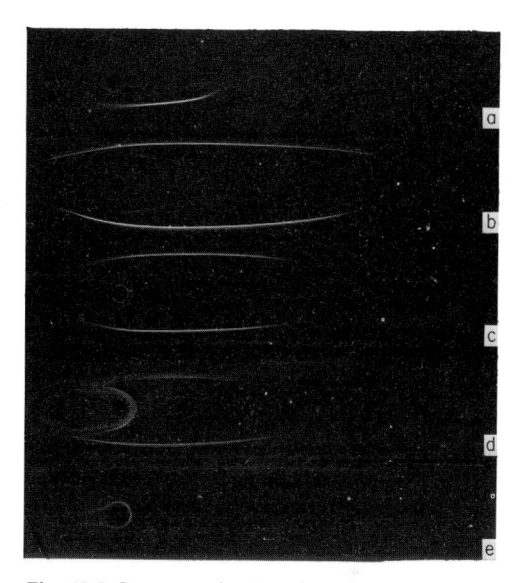

Fig. 10.2. Immunoselection plates for detecting αCD polypeptide, showing the appearances seen in normal control serum (a) and the positive findings in an IPSID serum (b), jejunal fluid (c) and concentrated urine (d). No αCD polypeptide is seen in the patient's saliva (e).

trate of the lamina propria causing wide separation of the crypts of Lieberkühn and effacement of villus structure without significant impairment of the integrity of the surface epithelium (Fig. 10.3). The cellular infiltrate consists mainly of plasma cells (Fig. 10.4) of varying degrees of maturity. Topographically the infiltrate usually begins in the jejunum and then extends often to involve the entire length of the small intestine. The distribution contrasts with the Western-type intestinal lymphomas which, with the exception of malignant histiocytosis, are typically solitary and show a predeliction for the ileum (Table 10.1). In early cases of IPSID, the cellular infiltrate is confined to the lamina propria and bears none of the histological stigmata of malignancy — a finding consistent with the view that there is a pre-malignant stage of the disease. The proliferating cells may invade the submucosa, destroy the architecture of mesenteric lymph nodes and spread to the rectum (Laroche et al. 1970, Bognel et al. 1972), post-nasal space (Doe et al. 1970), bone marrow (Rambaud et al. 1968, Doe et al. 1970), and blood (Doe et al. 1972, Bognel et al. 1972). This clearly establishes the malignant potential of IPSID.

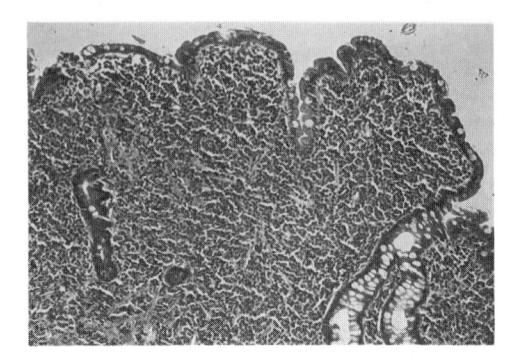

Fig. 10.3. Jejunal biopsy from an IPSID patient, showing flat deformed villi, sparse crypts, preservation of luminal epithelium and a very dense cellular infiltrate (H & E × 60).

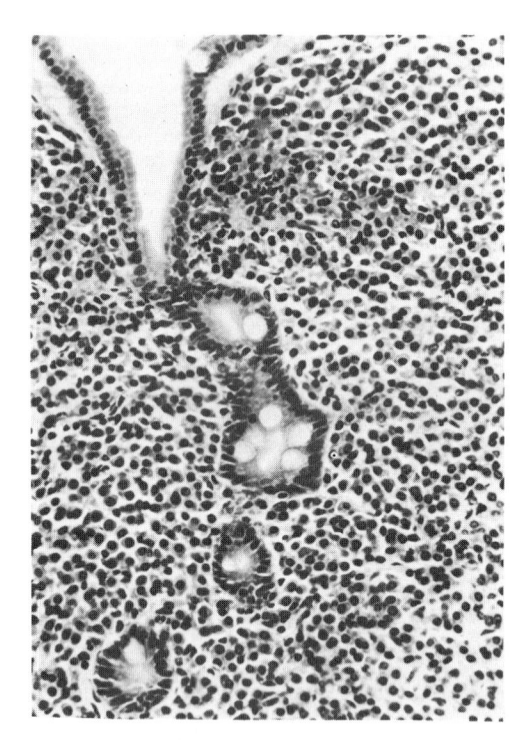

Fig. 10.4. Detail from an IPSID jejunal biopsy showing the relatively normal surface epithelium and the dense cellular infiltrate which is composed largely of immature plasma cells (H & E × 360).

Ultrastructural studies have confirmed that the plasma cells, or a cell intermediate between the plasma cell and the lymphocyte, is the proliferating cell type in the early phase of IPSID (Fig. 10.5). The rough endoplasmic reticulum is prominent in all but the most immature plasma cells and cisternae are often distended with granular material and electron dense secretory products (Fig. 10.6 and 10.7) (Scotto et al. 1970, Doe et al. 1972). Amyloid deposits have not been seen.

The relationship between the apparently benign plasma cell infiltrate which characterizes the premalignant phase of IPSID, the secretion of αCD polypeptides by these cells and the development of frank lymphoma affecting the intestine and mesenteric nodes, is becoming clearer. There is strong evidence that the lymphoma that supervenes in IPSID results from malignant transformation of the same clone of proliferating plasma cells which constituted the premalignant phase. Biosynthetic studies of cells from a lymphoma which developed in the intestine of a patient suffering from IPSID, showed that both the benign-appearing plasma cell infiltrate and the lymphoma cells synthesized αCD polypeptide, strongly indicating that the immunoblastic tumour cells arose by dedifferentiation from the same defective clone and not from a separate clone of pathological cells (Ramot et al. 1977, Preud'homme et al. 1979). These findings are supported by immunoelectron-microscopic studies of lymphoma tissue from IPSID patients which show an αCD polypeptide in the cytoplasm and on the membranes of the large immunoblasts which constitute the lymphoma (Brouet et al. 1977).

Clinical variants

Several variants of IPSID have been described. Two patients presenting with the typical clinicopathological features of IPSID were shown to have complete monoclonal IgA gammopathy (Chantar et al. 1974, Tangun et al. 1975) and in a third patient γ-heavy chain protein was demonstrated in serum and in the plasma cells of the intestinal infiltrate (Seligmann 1975). A Finnish boy developed involvement of distal jejunum, ileum and colon as part of αCD and associated with selective IgA deficiency. Synthesis of αCD polypeptide by the colonic cellular infiltrate was demonstrated (Savilahti et al. 1980). A polypoid lymphoma

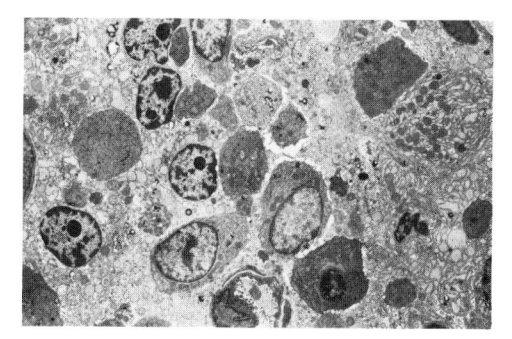

Fig. 10.5. Low-power view of proliferating plasma cells, the majority showing immature nuclei with prominent nucleoli. Note the abundant cytoplasm, often with ill-defined contours (TEM × 2500). (Courtesy of Professor Kristen Henry.)

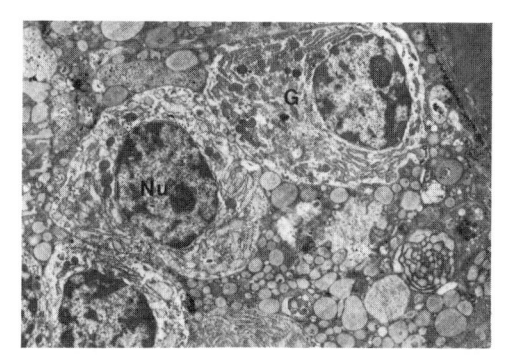

Fig. 10.6. Three immature plasma cells. There is an abundance of rough endoplasmic reticulum containing electron-dense secretory products (TEM × 5800). Nu, nucleus; G, golgi. (Courtesy of Professor Kristen Henry.)

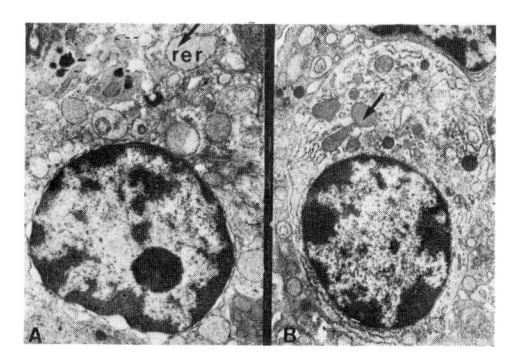

Fig. 10.7. (A) High-power view of plasmablast in alpha-chain disease, showing the nuclear and cytoplasmic details. (B) Mature reactive plasma cell from a patient with coeliac disease for comparison. Rough endoplasmic reticulum (rer) containing electron-dense secretory products (arrows). (TEM × 8000) (Courtesy of Professor Kristen Henry.)

affecting the stomach, small intestine and colon has been reported in a North American patient whose serum contained αCD polypeptide. There was no evidence of malabsorption and the areas of intestine between the lymphomatous polyps showed normal histological appearances (Cohen et al. 1978). In this instance, there was no direct evidence that the lymphoma cells synthesized αCD polypeptide. In a second North American case of αCD, there was lymphomatous involvement of the colon and later the stomach. The small intestine was unaffected and no malabsorption was observed. Stains of the involved tissue suggested that the tumour cells contained αCD polypeptide and appeared to be the source of the serum αCD polypeptide (Cho et al. 1982).

A non-secretory variant of IPSID has also been described. In this case the small intestine was diffusely infiltrated by plasma cells but no αCD polypeptide was detectable in serum, urine or concentrated jejunal fluid. The presence of αCD polypeptide was, however, indicated in the cytoplasm of the infiltrating plasma cells by direct immunofluorescence (Rambaud et al. 1983). This finding suggests that there may be a non-secretory variant of IPSID in which αCD polypeptide is not detectable in the serum.

Course of disease

IPSID is initially characterized by a diffuse infiltrate of the small intestine comprising mainly plasma cells. During this apparently premalignant phase, the infiltrate remains confined to the lamina propria. Whether this phase is truly benign, is open to question. There is a monoclonal expansion of aberrant plasma cells which secrete substantial quantities of an abnormal immunoglobulin fragment. The appearances of differentiation in the cells comprising the cellular infiltrate and the scarcity of mitoses does not necessarily indicate a benign disorder. Chronic lymphatic leukaemia and Waldenstrom's macroglobulinaemia show similar features. Karyotyping of the plasma cells present in the 'premalignant' infiltrate of IPSID may help resolve this question. To date, direct tissue karyotyping has been confined to studies of IPSID at an advanced stage. In these studies, aneuploidy was found in the mucosal infiltrate of one αCD patient and in another a small G member similar to the Philadelphia chromosome was observed. Studies in two other cases, however, revealed a normal karyotype (Nassar et al. 1978). Recently the marker D_{14} chromosome ($D_{14}q+$) has been reported in 10% of the bone marrow cells of an αCD patient (Gafter et al. 1980). This abnormality of the D_{14} chromosome has been previously shown to occur in lymphoid B-cell neoplasia such as plasma cell leukaemia, multiple myeloma, acute lymphoblastic leukaemia, and malignant lymphoma (Oshimura et al. 1977) and may represent a marker for malignancy in B lymphocytes.

The following case report illustrates the progressive course of the disease with the ultimate development of primitive plasma cell tumours of the alimentary tract.

> L.M., a 32-year-old Bengali factory worker, developed cramping abdominal pains, fever, weight loss and diarrhoea with the features of steatorrhoea, 12 months after his arrival in London from Bangladesh. Initial investigations revealed a non-specific colitis, hookworm and *Trichuris trichuria* infestation. There was no response to treatment with anti-helminthics. One month later, clinical examination revealed an emaciated man (45 kg) whose fingers and toes showed marked clubbing. Investigations showed a normal haemoglobin, reduced serum folate (2.9 ng/ml) and albumin (24 g/l) and marked increases in serum globulins and in the intestinal isoenzyme of alkaline phosphatase. There was malabsorption of D-Xylose (2.3 g/5 h), vitamin B_{12} (Schilling test with intrinsic factor 4.5%), and fat (11 g/24 h). Barium examination (Fig. 10.8) revealed duodenal narrowing and a diffuse coarse nodularity of the small intestinal mucosa. Jejunal biopsy was flat and there was a dense infiltrate of mature plasma cells confined to the lamina propria and sparsity of the crypts (Figs 10.3 and 10.4). Abnormal plasma cells were found in the bone marrow and biopsy of a lymphoid mass in the nasopharynx showed an increase in mature plasma cells.

Electrophoretic analysis of serum proteins showed a broad band in the α_2 to β_2 region. An abnormal precipitin arc developed against anti-IgA antiserum in the serum, urine and jejunal fluid. αCD polypeptide was detected in serum, urine and jejunal fluid by immunoselection.

Treatment was begun with intermittent melphalan. Twelve months later, after ceasing treatment, there was a recurrence of abdominal pain, weight loss and steatorrhoea. Melphalan and prednisone were given with some symptomatic improvement. Twelve months later, right-sided hypochondrial pain, vomiting, anorexia and weight loss developed. A hard mass was palpable in the right hypochondrium and there was a rectal polypoid mass. At laparotomy there were tumours in duodenum and

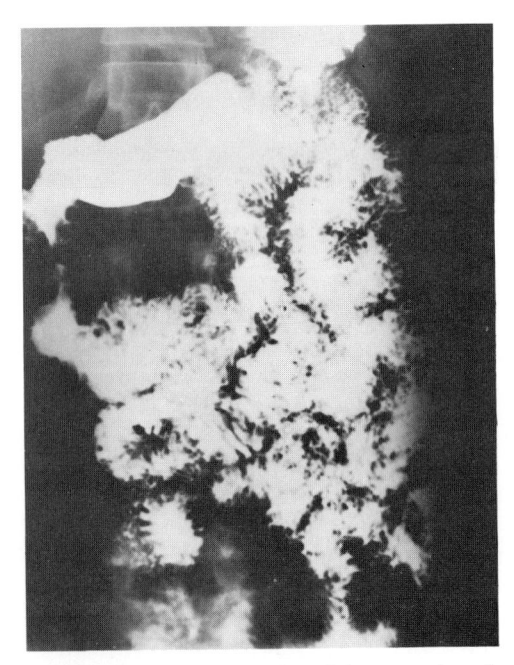

Fig. 10.8. Barium examination of the stomach and proximal small bowel showing some narrowing of the second part of the duodenum, nodularity of the mucosal pattern and the combination of scalloping and spikiness of its contours with thickening of circular folds.

ileum. The mesenteric nodes were enlarged but liver and spleen size appeared normal. Histological examination of the duodenal and rectal tumours showed the appearances of a primitive plasma cell tumour. Despite intensive cytotoxic therapy the patient deteriorated and he died 6 years after the onset of his illness.

Prognosis and therapy

The prognosis of IPSID depends upon the stage of progression of the disease at diagnosis. In the initial 'premalignant' stage where the plasma cell infiltrate is confined to the lamina propria of the small intestine, remission of the clinical, histological and immunological features has been reported in seven of seventeen patients. Treatment with broad spectrum antibiotics and/or a chemotherapy regime comprising prednisone and melphalan or cyclophosphamide, may give remission of more than 5 years (Galian et al. 1977). In one instance, after an initial remission sustained for 2 years (Manousos et al. 1974), the patient developed a plasmacytoma confined to the ileum (Skinner et al. 1976).

In IPSID patients suffering from more advanced disease, no clear therapeutic guidelines are available. When the cellular infiltrate is clearly invading into the submucosa but there is no clinical evidence of overt lymphoma, chemotherapy with broad spectrum antibiotics has occasionally induced remission. When the immunoblastoma is clinically evident and confined to the abdomen, radiotherapy has produced prolonged remission in three cases (Galian et al. 1977). Recently several complete and prolonged remissions have been achieved using chemotherapy according to the CHOP protocol (Rambaud et al. 1983).

Predisposing factors

The clear predilection of IPSID for underprivileged populations of low socioeconomic status suggests that enviromental factors may be implicated in its pathogenesis. Since ingested micro-organisms are a powerful proliferative stimulus to the secretory IgA system (Crabbé et al. 1970), the early stage of IPSID could represent an aberrant immune response following sustained antigenic stimulation of the mucosa in populations exposed to an environment of poor hygiene (Seligmann et al. 1971). Bacteriological, parasitic and virological studies, however, have as yet revealed no specific agent.

Several other pathogenic mechanisms have been suggested. Cells synthesizing the αCD polypeptide may be present in small numbers in normal subjects and be predisposed to proliferation when there is intense, chronic intestinal exposure to microorganisms. The presence of an oncogenic virus which interferes with IgA synthesis has also been suggested (Rambaud & Matuchansky 1973).

The importance of genetic predisposition is unknown. Although limited family studies have failed to provide evidence for a heritable trait for IPSID (Novis et al. 1973), little data are available on genetic markers including those represented in the major histocompatibility complex. The finding of the intestinal isoenzyme of alkaline phosphatase in the serum of IPSID patients and their relatives (Ramot & Streifler 1966, Doe et al. 1972) could form the basis for a prospective study of the natural history of IPSID.

References

Al-Bahrani Z.R., Al-Mondhiry H., Bakir F. & Al-Saleem T. (1983) Clinical and pathologic subtypes of primary intestinal lymphoma. *Cancer* 52, 1666–1672.

Anderson H., Dotevall G. & Mobacken H. (1971) Malignant mesenteric lymphoma in a patient with dermatitis herpetiformis. *Scand. J. Gastroenterol.* 6, 397.

Austad W.I., Cornes J.C., Gough K.R., McCarthy C.F. & Read A.F. (1967) Steatorrhoea and malignant lymphoma. The relationship of malignant tumors of lymphoid tissue and coeliac disease. *Amer. J. Dig. Dis.* 12, 475–490.

Azar H.A. (1962) Cancer in Lebanon and the Near East. *Cancer*, 15, 66–78.

Baer A.N., Bayless T.M. & Yardley J.H. (1980) Intestinal ulceration and malabsorption syndromes. *Gastroenterol.* 79, 754–65.

Blackledge G., Mamtora H., Crowther D., Isherwood I. & Best J.J.K. (1981) The role of abdominal computed tomography in lymphoma following treatment. *Brit. J. Radiol.* **54**, 955–960.

Bognel J.C., Rambaud J.C. Modigliani R. Matuchansky C., Bognel C., Bernier J.J., Scotto J., Hautefeuille P., Mihaesco E., Hurez E., Preud'Homme J.L. & Seligmann M. (1972) Etude clinique, anatomo-pathologique et immunochimique d'un nouveau cas de maladie des chaines alpha suivi pendant cinq ans. *Rev. Europ. d'Etud. Clin. Biolog.* **17**, 362–374.

Bonomo L., Dammaco F., Marano R. & Bonomo G.M. (1972) Abdominal lymphoma and alpha chain disease. *Amer. J. Med.* **52**, 73–86.

Brouet J.C., Mason D.Y., Danon F., Preud'homme J.L., Seligmann M., Reyes F., Navab F., Galian A., Rene E. & Rambaud J.C. (1977) Alpha-chain disease: Evidence for common clonal origin of intestinal immunoblastic lymphoma and plasmacytic proliferation. *Lancet*, **i**, 861.

Buxbaum J.N. & Preud'homme J.L. (1972) Alpha and gamma heavy chain diseases in man: intracellular origin of the aberrant polypeptides. *J. Immunol.* **109**, 1131–1137.

Byrne G.E. & Rappaport H. (1973) Malignant histiocytosis. In *Malignant Diseases of the Haemopoeitic System.* (Ed. by K. Akazaki, H. Rappaport & C.W. Bernard. University Park Press, Baltimore.

Chantar C., Escartin P. & Plaza A.G. (1974) Diffuse plasma cell infiltration of the small intestine with malabsorption associated to IgA monoclonal gammopathy. *Cancer*, **34**, 1620–1630.

Chernokhvostova E.v. & German G.P. (1980) Immunochemical study in two cases of alpha chain disease. *Folia Haematol.* **107**, 757–771.

Chernov A., Doe W.F. & Gompertz D. (1972) Intrajejunal volatile fatty acids in the stagnant loop syndrome. *Gut*, **13**, 103–106.

Cho C., Linscheer W.G., Bell R. & Smith R. (1982) Alpha chain disease without malabsorption. *Gastroenterol.* **83**, 121–126.

Cohen H.J., Gonzalvo A., Krook J., Thompson T.T. & Kremer W.B. (1978) New presentation of alpha heavy chain disease: North American polypoid gastrointestinal lymphoma. *Cancer*, **41**, 1161–1169.

Cooper B.T., Holmes G.K.T., Ferguson R. & Cooke W.T. (1980) Coeliac disease and malignancy. *Medicine*, **59**, 249–261.

Crabbé P.A., Nash D.R., Bazin H., Eyssen H. & Heremans J.F. (1970) Immunohistochemical observations on lymphoid tissues from conventional and germ-free mice. *Lab Invest.* **22**, 448–457.

Doe W.F. (1975) Alpha chain disease clinicopathological features and relationship to so-called Mediterranean lymphoma. *Brit. J. Cancer*, **31**, Suppl. 2, 350–355.

Doe W.F., Danon F. & Seligmann M. (1979) Immunodiagnosis of alpha chain disease. *Clin. Experi. Immunol.* **36**, 189–197.

Doe W.F., Henry K. & Doyle F.H. (1976) Radiological findings in six patients with alpha-chain disease. *Brit. J. Radiol.* **49**, 3–11.

Doe W.F., Henry K., Hobbs J.R., Avery Jones F., Dent C.E., & Booth C.C. (1972) Five cases of alpha chain disease. *Gut*, **13**, 947–957.

Doe W.F., Hobbs J.R., Henry K. & Dowling R.H. (1970) Alpha chain disease. *Quart. J. Med.* **39**, 619–620.

Doe W.F. & Spiegelberg H.L. (1979) Characterization of an antiserum specific for the Fabα fragment. Its use for detection of α-heavy chain disease protein by immunoselection. *J. Immunol.* **122**, 19–23.

Dorfman R.F. (1977) Pathology of the non-Hodgkin's lymphoma: new classifications. *Cancer Treat. Rep.* **61**, 945–951.

Dorrington K.J., Mihaesco E. & Seligmann M. (1970) Molecular size of 3 alpha chain disease proteins. *Biochim. Biophys. Acta*, **221**, 647–649.

Eidelman S., Parkins A. & Rubin C. (1966) Abdominal lymphoma presenting as malabsorption. A clinical pathologic study of 9 cases in Israel and a review of the literature. *Medicine*, **45**, 111–137.

Florin-Christensen A., Doniach D. & Newcomb P.B. (1974) Alpha chain disease with pulmonary manifestations. *Brit. Med. J.* **2**, 413–415.

Freeman H.J., Weinstein U.M. & Shnitka T.K. (1977) Primary abdominal lymphoma. *Amer. J. Med.* **63**, 585–594.

Fry L., McMinn R.M.H., Cowan J.D. & Hoffbrand A.V. (1968) Effect of a gluten-free diet on dermatological intestinal and haematological manifestations of dermatitis herpetiformis. *Lancet*, **i**, 557.

Fu Y.S. & Perzin K.H. (1972) Lymphosarcoma of the small intestine: a clinicopathological study. *Cancer*, **29**, 645–659.

Gafter U., Kessler E., Shabtay F., Shaked P. & Djaldetti M. (1980) Abnormal chromosomal marker ($D^{14}q^+$) in a patient with alpha heavy chain disease. *J. Clin. Pathol.* **33**, 136–144.

Galian A., Lecestre M.J., Scotto J., Bognel C., Matuchansky C. & Rambaud J.C. (1977) Pathological study of alpha chain disease with special emphasis on evolution. *Cancer*, **39**, 2081–2101.

Gall E.A. & Mallory T.B. (1942) Malignant lymphoma: a clinicopathology survey of 618 cases. *Amer. J. Pathol.* **18**, 381.

Gough K.R., Read A.E. & Nash J.M. (1962) Intestinal reticulosis as a complication of idiopathic steatorrhoea. *Gut*, **3**, 232–239.

Green J.A., Dawson A.A., Jones P.F. & Brunt P.W. (1979) The presentation of gastrointestinal lymphoma: study of a population. *Brit. J. Surg.* **66**, 798–801.

Gull W. (1855) Fatty stools from disease of the mesenteric glands. *Guys Hosp. Rep.*, **1**, 369.

Harris O.D., Cooke W.T., Thompson H. & Waterhouse J.A.H. (1967) Malignancy in adult coeliac disease and idiopathic steatorrhoea. *Amer. J. Med.* **42**, 899–912.

Henry K., Bird R.G. & Doe W.F. (1974) Intestinal coccidiosis in a patient with alpha-chain disease. *Brit. Med. J.* **1**, 542–543.

Henry K. & Farrer-Brown G. (1977) Primary lymphomas of the gastrointestinal tract. I Plasma cell tumours. *Histopathol.* **1**, 53−76.

Herbsman H., Wetstein L., Rosen Y., Orces H., Alfonso A.E., Iyer S.K. & Gardner B. (1980) Tumors of the small intestine. *Curr. Prob. Surg.* **17**, 121−82.

Hermans P.E., Diaz-Buxo J.A. & Stobo J.D. (1976) Idiopathic late-onset immunoglobulin deficiency. *Amer. J. Med.* **61**, 221−237.

Ho F. & Gibson J.B. (1979) Gastrointestinal lymphomas in Hong Kong Chinese. *Isr. J. Med. Sci.* **15**, 382−385.

Holmes, G.K.T., Stokes P.L., Sorahan T.M., Prior P., Waterhouse J.A.H. & Cooke, W.T. (1976) Coeliac disease, gluten-free diet and malignancy. *Gut*, **17**, 612−619.

Inunberry J., Benallegue A., Illoul G., Timsit G., Abbadi M., Benabdalla S., Boucekkine T., Ould-Aoudia J.P. & Calonna P. (1970) Trois cas de maladie des chaînes alpha observés en Algerie. *Nouv. Rev. Franc. d'Haematol.* **10**, 609−616.

Isaacson P. (1980) Malignant histiocytosis of the intestine: the early histological lesion. *Gut*, **21**, 381−386.

Isaacson P., Wright D.H., Judd M.A. & Mepham B.L. (1979) Primary gastrointestinal lymphomas: a classification of 66 cases. *Cancer*, **43**, 1805−1809.

Isaacson P. & Wright D.H. (1978) Malignant histiocytosis of the intestine — its relationship to malabsorption and ulcerative jejunitis. *Human Pathol.* **9**, 661−676.

Kahn L.B. & Novis B.H. (1974) Nodular lymphoid hyperplasia of the small bowel associated with primary small bowel reticulum cell lymphoma. *Cancer*, **33**, 837−844.

Kapadia S.B. (1979) Histiocytic lymphoma of the ileocecal region after chemotherapy for multiple myeloma. *Cancer*, **43**, 435−439.

Lamers C.B., Wagener T., Assmann K.J. & Van Tongeren J.H. (1980) Jejunal lymphoma in a patient with primary adult-onset hypogammaglobulinemia and nodular lymphoid hyperplasia of the small intestine. *Dig. Dis. Sci.* **25**, 553−557.

Laroche D., Seligmann M., Merillon H., Turpin G., Marche C., Cerf M., Lemaigre G., Forest M., & Hurez D. (1970) Nouvelle observation d'une maladie des chaines lourdes alpha au cours d'un lymphome abdominal de type Mediterranean avec tuberculose isolee des ganglions mesenteriques et pelvispondylite. *Presse Medicale*, **78**, 55−59.

Lennert K. & Stein H. (1981) *Histopathology of Non-Hodgkin's Lymphomas* (Based on the Kiel Classification). Springer-Verlag, Berlin.

Lewin K.J., Kahn L.B. & Novis B.H. (1976) Primary intestinal lymphoma of 'Western' and Mediterranean type, alpha chain disease and massive plasma cell infiltration. *Cancer*, **38**, 2511−2528.

Lightdale C.J. (1980) Classifying gastrointestinal lymphomas. *Gastroenterol.* **78**, 1641−1642.

Loehr W.J., Mujajed A., Zahn F.D., Gray G.F. & Thorbjarnarson R.D. (1969) Primary lymphoma of the gastrointestinal tract. A review of 100 cases. *Ann. Surg.* **170**, 232−238.

Magrath I., Henele W., Owor R. Olweny C. (1975) Antibodies to Epstein-Barr virus antigens before and after the development of Burkitt's lymphoma in a patient treated for Hodgkin's disease. *New Engl. J. Med.* **292**, 621−623.

Manousos O.N., Economidou J.C., Georgiadou D.E., Pratsika-Ougourloglou K.G., Hadziyannis St. J., Merikas G.E., Henry K. & Doe W.F. (1974) Alpha-chain disease with clinical, immunological and histological recovery. *Brit. Med. J.* **ii**, 397−456.

Matuchansky C., Morichau-Beauchant M., Touchard G., Lenormand Y., Bloch P., Tanzer J., Alcalay D. & Babin P. (1980) Nodular lymphoid hyperplasia of the small bowel associated with primary jejunal malignant lymphoma. Evidence favoring a cytogenetic relationship. *Gastroenterol.* **78**, 1587−1592.

Mittal V.K. & Bodzin J.H. (1980) Primary malignant tumors of the small bowel. *Amer. J. Surg.* **140**, 396−399.

Naqvi M.S., Burrows J. & Kark A.E. (1969) Lymphoma of the gastrointestinal tract. Prognostic guides based on 162 cases. *Ann. Surg.* **170**, 221−231.

Nasr K., Haghighi P., Bakhshandeh K. & Haghshenas M. (1970) Primary lymphoma of the upper small intestine. *Gut*, **11**, 673−678.

Nassar V.H., Salem P.A., Shahid M.J., Alami S.Y., Baklian J.A., Salem A.A. & Nasrallah S.M. (1978) Mediterranean abdominal lymphoma or immunoproliferative small intestinal disease. Part II. Pathological Aspects *Cancer*, **41**, 1340−1354.

Non-Hodgkin's Lymphoma Pathologic Classification Project. National Cancer Inst.-sponsored study. (1982) *Cancer* **49**, 2112−2135.

Novis B.H., Bank S. & Young G. (1973) Alpha chain disease. *Lancet*, **ii**, 498.

Novis B.H., Kahn L.B. & Bank S. (1973) Alpha-chain disease in subsaharan Africa. *Amer. J. Dig Dis.* **18**, 679−688.

Oshimura M., Freeman A.I. & Sandberg A.A. (1977) Chromosomes and causation of human cancer and leukaemia. CXVI. Banding studies in acute lymphoblastic leukaemia (ALL). *Cancer*, **40**, 1161−1172.

Penn I. (1979) Tumor incidence in human allograft recipients. *Transplant. Proceed.* **11**, 1047−1051.

Preud'homme J.L., Brouet J.C. & Seligmann M. (1979) Cellular immunoglobulins in human γ- and α-heavy chain diseases. *Clin. Exper. Immunol.* **37**, 283−291.

Rambaud J.C. & Matuchansky C. (1973) Alpha chain disease and relation to Mediterranean lymphoma. *Lancet*, **i**, 1430−1432.

Rambaud J.C., Bognel C., Prost A., Bernier J.J., LeQuintrec Y., Lanbling A., Danon F., Hurez D. & Seligmann M. (1968) Clinico-pathological study of a patient with 'Mediterranean' type of abdominal lymphoma and a new type of IgA abnormality (α chain disease). *Digestion*, **1**, 321−336.

Rambaud J.C., Galian A., Danon F. Preud'homme

J.L., Brandstaeg P., Wassef M., Le Carrer M., Mehaut M.A., Voinchet O.L., Perol R.G. & Chapman A. (1983) Alpha chain disease without qualitative serum IgA abnormality: report of two cases including a 'non-secretory' form. *Cancer.* **51**, 686–693.

Ramot B., Levanon M., Hahn Y., Lahat N. & Moroz C. (1977) The mutual clonal origin of the lymphoplasmocytic and lymphoma cell in alpha-heavy chain disease. *Clin. Exper. Immunol.* **27**, 440–445.

Ramot B., Shanin N. and Bubis J.J. (1965) Malabsorption syndrome in lymphoma of small intestine. *Isr. J. Med. Sci.* **1**, 221–226.

Ramot B. & Streifler C. (1966) Raised serum alkaline phosphatase. *Lancet,* **ii**, 587.

Rappaport H. (1966) Tumours of the haemopoietic system. In *Atlas of Tumour Pathology,* section 3, fasicle 8, US Armed Forces Institute of Pathology, Washington DC.

Robertson D.A.F., Swinson C.M., Hall R. & Losowsky M.S. (1982) Coeliac disease splenic function and malignancy. *Gut,* **23**, 666–669.

Rosenberg S.A., Diamond H.D., Jaslowitz B. & Craver L.F. (1961) Lymphosarcoma: a review of 1269 cases. *Medicine,* **40**, 31–83.

Salem P.A., Nassar V.H., Shahid M.J., Hajj A.A., Alami S.Y., Balikian J.B. & Salem A.A. (1977) Mediterranean abdominal lymphoma or immunoproliferative small intestinal disease. Part I: Clinical aspects. *Cancer,* **40**, 2941–2947.

Savilahti E., Brandtzaeg P. & Kuitenen P. (1980) Atypical intestinal alpha-chain disease evolving into selective immunoglobulin A deficiency in a Finnish boy. *Gastroenterol.* **79**, 1303–1310.

Scotto J., Stralin H. & Caroli J. (1970) Ultrastructural study of two cases of α-chain disease. *Gut,* **11**, 782–788.

Selby W.S. & Gallagher N.D. (1979) Malignancy in a 19-year experience of adult coeliac disease. *Dig. Dis. Sci.* **24**, 684–688.

Seligmann M. (1975) Alpha-chain disease. *J. Clin. Pathol.* **29**, Suppl 6, 72–76.

Seligmann M., Danon F., Hurez D., Mihaesco E. & Preud'homme J-L. (1968) Alpha chain disease: a new immunoglobulin abnormality. *Sci.* **162**, 1396–1398.

Seligmann M., Mihaesco E. & Frangione B. (1971) Studies on α chain disease. *NY Acad. Sci. Ann.* **190**, 487–500.

Seligmann M., Mihaesco E., Hurez, D., Mihaesco C., Preud'homme J.L. & Rambaud J-C. (1969) Immunochemical studies in four cases of alpha chain disease. *J. Clin. Invest.* **48**, 2374–2389.

Skinner J.M., Manousos O.N. Economidou J., Nicolau A. & Merikas G. (1976) Alpha-chain disease with localised plasmacytoma of the intestine. *Clin. Exper. Immunol.* **25**, 112–116.

Spector B., Perry G.S. & Kersey J.H. (1978) Genetically determined immunodeficiency diseases (GDID) and malignancy report from the immunodeficiency-cancer registry. *Clin. Immunol. Immunopath.* **11**, 12–29.

Stoop J.W., Ballieux R.E., Hijmans W. & Zegers B.J.M. (1971) Alpha chain disease with involvement of the respiratory tract in a Dutch child. *Clin. Exper. Immunol.* **9**, 625–635.

Sugarbaker E.D. & Craver L.F. (1940) Lymphosarcoma. *J. Amer. Med. Assoc.* **115**, 112.

Swinson C.M., Slavin G., Coles E.C. & Booth C.C. (1983a) Coeliac disease and malignancy. *Lancet,* **i**, 111–115.

Swinson C.M., Hall, P.J., Bedford P.A. & Booth C.C. (1983b) HLA antigens in coeliac disease associated with malignancy. *Gut* **24**, 925–928.

Tangun Y., Saracbasi Z., Inceman S., Danon F. & Seligmann M. (1975) IgA myeloma globulin and Bence-Jones proteinuria in a diffuse plasmacytoma of small intestine. *Ann. Intern. Med.* **83**, 673.

The Non-Hodgkin's Lymphoma Pathologic Classification Project (1982) National Cancer Institute Study Descriptions of a Working Formulation. *Cancer,* **49**, 1258–1265.

Thompson H. (1974) Necropsy studies on adult coeliac disease. *J. Clin. Path* **27** 710–721.

Treadwell I.A. & White R.R. (1975) Primary tumors of the small bowel. *Amer. J. Surg.* **130**, 749.

Weinstein, W.M., Piercey J.R.A. & Dosseter J.B. (1974) *Proceedings of the 2nd International Coeliac Symposium, Leiden,* p. 361. (Ed. by W. Hekkens & A.S. Pera). H.E. Stenfert Kroese BV, Leiden.

Whicher J.T., Ajdukiewicz A. & Davies J.D. (1977) Two cases of alpha chain disease from Nigeria. *J. Clin. Pathol.* **30**, 679–681.

Wiltshaw, E. (1976) The natural history of extramedullary plasmacytoma and its relation to solitary myeloma of bone and myelomatosis. *Medicine,* **55**, 217–238.

Wolfenstein-Todel C., Mihaesco E. & Frangione B. (1974) 'Alpha chain disease' protein Def: Internal deletion of a human immunoglobulin A$_1$ heavy chain. *Proc. Nat. Acad. Sci. USA* **71**, 974–978.

World Health Organization (1976) Alpha-chain disease and related small-intestinal lymphoma: a memorandum. *WHO Bulletin,* **54**, 615–624.

Zulman J. Jaffe R. & Talal N. (1978) Evidence that the malignant lymphoma of Sjögren's syndrome is a monoclonal B-cell neoplasm. *New Engl. J. Med.* **299**, 1215–1210.

Chapter 11
Crohn's Disease (Regional Enteritis)

D.P. JEWELL

Introduction 195
Epidemiology 195
Aetiology 196
Pathology 198
Clinical features 199
Complications 200
Diagnosis 201
Assessment of disease activity 203
Treatment 204
Prognosis 206

Introduction

The classical description by Crohn and his colleagues in 1932 was the first account of the clinical and pathological features of 'regional enteritis'. They described a condition of ileal stricture which was not due to tuberculosis, for chest X-rays were normal and Mantoux tests were negative. Nevertheless, the nineteenth century literature contains descriptions of conditions which in retrospect may have been the same disease. The clearest description before Crohn's account was given by Dalziel (1913) who recognized the clinical features of the disease, the macroscopic appearances at surgery, and the submucosal nature of the typical inflammation, with infiltration with mononuclear cells and the occasional giant cell. These early accounts described mainly ileal disease. Ileocolic disease became recognized in the late 1930s and primary Crohn's disease of the colon was described by Lockhart-Mummery and Morson in 1960.

The disease has been called terminal ileitis, regional enteritis, and granulomatous enteritis or colitis, but the eponymous term 'Crohn's disease' is preferable as it implies neither a specific anatomical location within the gastrointestinal tract nor the presence of granulomata.

There is no universally accepted definition of the disease. It is a chronic inflammatory disorder which most commonly affects the ileocaecal area, although it may involve any part of the gastrointestinal tract from mouth to anus. Characteristically, the disease is discontinuous, with abnormal segments of intestine separated by apparently normal areas. The inflammation may affect all parts of the bowel wall and consists of an infiltration with mononuclear cells and the formation of granulomata. Stricturing and fistula formation frequently occur.

Epidemiology

Crohn's disease has shown a four- to tenfold increase in incidence during the last 30 years. This has been documented in Britain, Scandinavia and Israel (Gilat & Rozen 1981). The considerable increase in Aberdeen (Kyle & Stark 1980) and Stockholm County (Hellers 1981) has occurred since the 1950s and now appears to have reached a plateau and may even be decreasing. Some of this increase is due to greater diagnostic awareness and to more accurate diagnosis but all observers agree that much of the apparent increase is real. Crohn's disease is also becoming increasingly recognized in parts of the world where it was previously thought to be very rare, such as Brazil and Japan. Ileal Crohn's disease in Japan is particularly interesting, since it is often associated with extensive longitudinal ulcers (Japanese Research Committee 1981). The disease has also become increasingly frequent in young children.

Since the incidence of the disease appears to be changing, it is difficult to know the precise frequency with which new cases occur. For the UK, the annual incidence rate is probably 2.0−3.0/1,000,000 of the population. Most studies have shown that Crohn's disease is more common in Jews.

Aetiology

The aetiology of the disease remains unknown. Genetic influences are probably of only minor importance. There is an increased incidence of Crohn's disease in the first-degree relatives of patients with the disease, but identical-twin studies show discordance in many instances. Ulcerative colitis may also occur more frequently in these families but it is exceptionally rare for husband and wife to be both affected. So far, no firm association with a histocompatibility antigen has been found, although patients with associated ankylosing spondylitis are frequently positive for HLA B27. Most recent work has concentrated on the search for an infective agent and on the role of immunological effector mechanisms in the pathogenesis of chronic inflammation.

Infective agents

In 1970, Mitchell and Rees reported that the disease could be transmitted to mice by injecting extracts of Crohn's tissue into their foot pads. Subsequently, Cave et al. (1975) claimed that granulomata appeared in the bowel wall of a proportion of rabbits injected with an ultra-filtered extract of Crohn's tissue into the subserosa of the small intestine. It took many months for the granulomata to develop but the effect could be obtained by extracts of affected intestine passaged through several generations of rabbits. As the tissue extracts had been passed through a 20-mm filter, the transmissible agent could well have been a virus although transmissibility does not prove a viral aetiology. Other workers, however, have failed to confirm these findings and a recent independent review of the original rabbit histology has suggested that the presence of foreign body material may have induced the granulomatous changes (Yardley 1981).

These studies were followed by a series of experiments in which filtrates of tissue homogenates were inoculated into cell lines in culture. When filtrates of tissue from patients with Crohn's disease were used, cytopathic changes were seen in 80–90% of filtrates which was significantly higher than occurred with control tissue filtrates (Aronson et al. 1975, Gitnick et al. 1976). Some evidence suggested that the cytopathic effect could be due to an RNA virus (Aronson et al. 1975, Gitnick et al. 1976, Whorwell et al. 1977). A recent study, however, has failed to confirm this (Phillpotts et al. 1980). The failure to find any host immune responses to chick embryo cell cultures showing cytopathic changes following inoculation of filtrates from Crohn's disease tissue is also evidence against the presence of a virus (Chiba et al. 1982). Subsequently, it has been shown that the cytopathic effect induced by filtrates of tissue homogenates may be mediated by soluble proteins (Phillpotts et al. 1981, McLaren & Gitnick 1982). Precise characterization of these proteins is awaited.

The search for a bacterial aetiology has been equally unrewarding, although there is an unconfirmed report of a cell-wall-deficient pseudomonad being isolated from the intestinal tissue of some patients with Crohn's disease (Parent & Mitchell 1978). Atypical acid-fast organisms can be grown from mesenteric lymph nodes taken from patients with Crohn's disease or ulcerative colitis (Stanford 1981) but only in one patient has the organism been identified, in that case as *Mycobacterium kansassii* (Burnham et al. 1978). A preliminary report suggests that patients with Crohn's disease have antibodies to *Mycobacterium paratuberculosis* (Thayer et al. 1983) but the identity of other isolates containing acid-fast material remains unknown.

There is therefore no convincing evidence yet available that Crohn's disease is caused by a specific infective agent.

Immunological mechanisms

The immunological phenomena associated with Crohn's disease have been reviewed by Thomas & Jewell (1979), Kirsner & Shorter (1982) and Strickland & Jewell (1983).

Patients with Crohn's disease have normal or raised serum immunoglobulin concentrations while the disease is active and abnormalities of complement components suggest that there may be an acute phase reaction. Whether there is impairment of cellular immunity is less clear-cut. Many patients show diminished delayed hypersensitivity on skin testing, there may be reduced numbers or proportions of circulating T cells and responses to non-specific mitogens are often depressed. There is much variability between different reports, however, and it is possible that these changes are secondary to nutritional deficiency or to the side-effects of therapy. Immunoregulatory mechanisms have been studied more recently. There may be reduced suppressor cell function, especially during active disease, and reduced NK activity in the mononuclear cell populations of peripheral blood. Studies on mononuclear cell populations isolated from the intestine have generally shown an increase in 'activated' T cells and greater increase in the proliferative responses to bacterial antigens. The proportions of helper to suppressor-cytotoxic cells within the mucosa, as defined by monoclonal antibodies to surface antigens, does not differ from proportions found in peripheral blood but functional assays for suppressor activity have given widely different results.

Within the inflamed mucosa there is a considerable increase in immunoglobulin-containing cells, particularly IgG-containing cells, but the antigen specificity of locally synthesized immunoglobulin has not yet been determined. During periods of active disease, patients may have circulating immune complexes in the serum but this is less frequently seen in those with ileal than in colonic Crohn's disease. The possibility that antigen–antibody reactions occurring within the mucosa may contribute to the pathogenesis of the inflammation has been strengthened by the observation that there is an increased metabolism of complement and increased titres of antibodies to complement degradation products in peripheral blood.

Finally, peripheral blood lymphocytes from patients with Crohn's disease are cytotoxic to colonic epithelial cells, even if the overt disease is confined to the ileum. However, the pathogenetic significance of this cytotoxicity is uncertain since the lymphocytes kill colonic cells specifically and do not kill ileal epithelial cells.

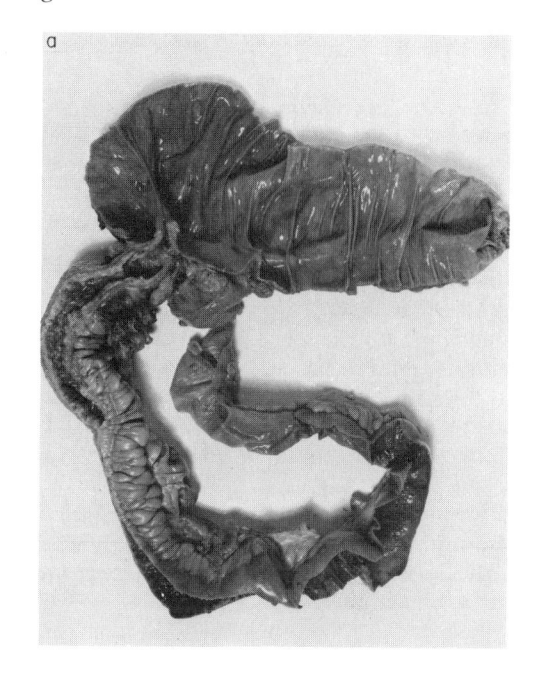

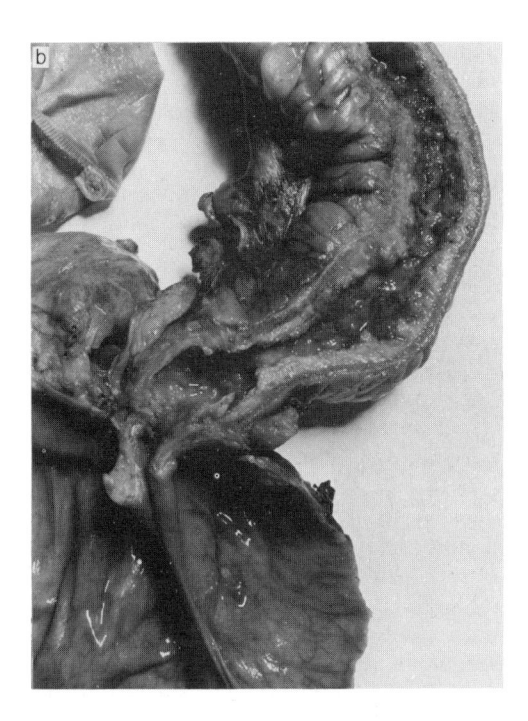

Fig. 11.1. (a) and (b) Resected specimen of ileum and colon showing classical 'hose-pipe' appearance of the terminal ileum up to the ileocaecal valve. (Courtesy of Dr A.B. Price.)

Pathology

The terminal ileum is most frequently affected by Crohn's disease, often in association with disease in the right side of the colon. Disease confined to the duodenum or the proximal intestine is rare and is more frequently seen in association with ileal disease.

Macroscopically, the affected segment of intestine is thickened, often with stricturing, and the mucosa has a 'cobble-stone' appearance caused by the combination of fissuring ulcers and submucosal oedema (Fig. 11.1). Early lesions consist of discrete shallow ulcers (aphthoid ulcers).

Histologically, the major features are a transmural inflammation of mononuclear cells, lymphoid aggregates, fissure ulcers and granulomata. Other features are pyloric metaplasia, hypertrophy of the muscle coat and neural hyperplasia. The latter consists predominantly of nerve endings which stain for VIP but whether this is specific for Crohn's disease or simply a feature of the neural hyperplasia associated with obstructive lesions is not known (Bishop et al. 1980).

Granulomata

Granulomata (Fig. 11.2) are composed of epitheloid cells. They may form a rather loose aggregate but may be more compact and contain a multinucleate giant cell. There is often a lymphocyte reaction around the granuloma. Granulomata are common in the early aphthoid ulcers and are often associated with blood vessels or lymphatics in more advanced disease. Fewer granulomata occur in ileum affected by Crohn's disease than in affected colon; in fact there appears to be a progressive increase in the number of granulomata from the ileum to a maximum in the rectal area (Chambers & Morson 1979). It has been suggested that the presence of granulomata may indicate a better prognosis than if they are absent, although this may be less true in the small intestine than in the colon (Glass & Baker 1976, Chambers & Morson 1979).

There have been few electron microscopic studies of Crohn's disease (Aluwihare 1971, Tijtgat et al. 1981). A variety of microorganisms have been observed but they probably represent secondary invasion of the damaged mucosa. Alteration of the tight junctions or of the desmosomes of the epithelial cells has not been seen (Tijtgat et al. 1981). Gebbers & Otto (1981) have shown that one of the earliest abnormalities to occur is micro-ulceration of the epithelium overlying Peyer's patches. This is accompanied by the presence of mononuclear cells associated with the M cells and by hyperplasia of the Peyer's patch. Hypothetically, antigen entry into these specialized lymphoid areas, which are known to process antigen, could be facilitated and the intestine might therefore become populated with antigen-sensitive lymphocytes (Craig & Cebra 1971).

Crohn's disease was initially thought to be a segmental, discontinuous disease which could affect any part of the gastrointestinal tract. Evidence is now accumulating that most of the intestine may be abnormal even though only a limited segment may be

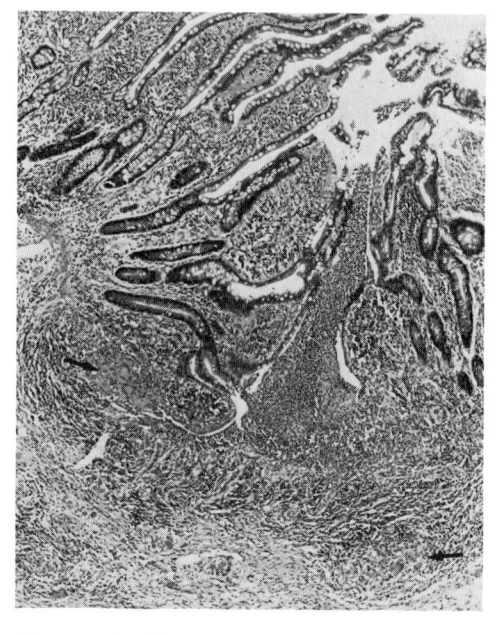

Fig. 11.2. Small intestinal mucosa showing two granulomata (arrowed) at the edge of a small apthoid ulcer in Crohn's disease (H & E × 60). (Courtesy of Dr A.B. Price.)

Crohn's Disease (Regional Enteritis)

overtly involved. For example, as many as 30% of patients with ileal disease may have a proctitis and granulomata may be found if an apparently normal rectum is biopsied (Surawicz et al. 1981). Quantitative histological observations have shown an increase in plasma cells, mast cells and macrophages in the apparently normal duodenum or proximal small intestine in patients with ileal or colonic disease (Ferguson et al. 1975, Sommers & Korelitz 1981). Furthermore, glucosamine synthetase and the disaccharidases are frequently depressed in uninvolved, proximal small intestine (Dunne et al. 1977, Goodman et al. 1976).

Clinical features

Symptoms

The commonest symptoms of small intestinal Crohn's disease are diarrhoea, abdominal pain and weight loss. The diarrhoea is usually loose and watery and the patient often has nocturnal diarrhoea. Rectal bleeding, however, is rarely seen. About 30% of patients have some degree of proctitis and this may cause some bleeding. Occasionally, patients may present with steatorrhoea.

The pain is usually colicky in nature and is centrally sited. Systemic symptoms such as nausea, vomiting, general malaise and fever are common. Some patients present with general symptoms of vague ill health, when the presence of intestinal disease may be overlooked in the absence of abdominal symptoms.

In children or in adolescents, the disorder may present with failure to thrive and growth failure. This is particularly associated with disease of the jejunum (Farmer & Michener 1979).

Clinical examination

Signs of anaemia, particularly due to iron deficiency, may be present; there may be evidence of weight loss and oedema, due to hypoalbuminaemia, may occur. Thickened loops of ileum are often palpable as a tender mass in the right iliac fossa. Perianal

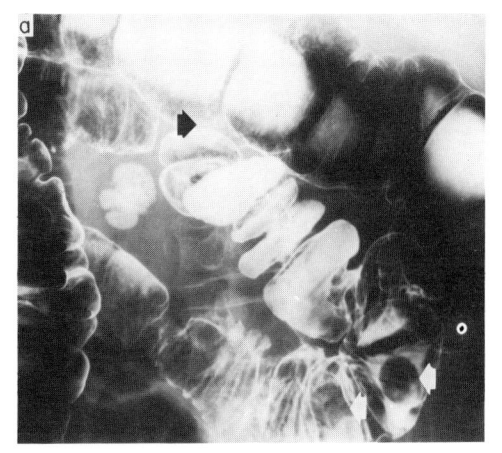

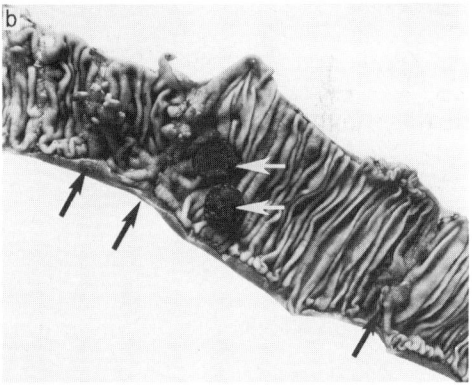

Fig. 11.3. Radiograph (a) and operative specimen (b) from a man aged 64 with recurrent Crohn's disease in whom ileotranverse colonic anastomosis had been performed at the age of 25.
(a) Radiograph showing ileal strictures proximal to the anastomosis (black arrow) and two radiolucent enteroliths outlined by contrast medium (white arrows). (b) Resected small intestine showing the site of strictures due to Crohn's disease (black arrows) and the two enteroliths in the gut lumen (white arrows).

disease in the form of fleshy skin tags, fissures and fistulae occur in some 14% of patients (Farmer et al. 1975).

In contrast with Crohn's colitis, ileal disease is associated with less rectal bleeding, less perianal disease, more abdominal pain, and the frequent occurrence of an abdominal mass. A further major difference, however, is in the frequency of the systemic manifestations such as an acute arthropathy, uveitis, and erythema nodosum, which occur in no more than 1% of patients with ileal disease alone, compared with a frequency of 20% in patients with colonic Crohn's disease.

Complications

Local complications

Perforation, acute dilatation and massive haemorrhage may all complicate Crohn's disease of the small intestine but they are rare. Fistulae to neighbouring loops of ileum or colon, or to other structures such as bladder (causing pneumaturia) or vagina, occur in about 10–17% of patients (Farmer et al. 1975). Intestinal obstruction is a frequent complication (35%).

Enterolithiasis (Fig. 11.3) may be associated with stasis, particularly of the distal small intestine, and may also be a factor causing intestinal obstruction (Atwell & Pollock 1960) and rarely perforation (Zeit 1979, Walker & Ellis 1984).

Hypolactasia

This may be secondary to diffuse involvement of proximal small intestine and the patient may therefore be intolerant of milk.

Renal

In patients with malabsorption, there may be hyperoxaluria leading to the development of renal oxalate stones, as also occurs after small intestinal resection or bypass (cf. Chapter 6). Renal stones are therefore not uncommon in Crohn's disease of the small intestine, particularly when resection has also been carried out.

Less commonly, the inflammatory tissue in the ileum or ileocolic region may involve the right ureter, causing a right hydronephrosis.

Amyloid

This is a rare but well recognized complication of Crohn's disease and may be found in kidneys, liver, spleen and intestine. Amyloid may regress following surgical resection of the intestinal disease, as illustrated by the following case history.

A 46-year-old woman was referred for management of Crohn's disease and nephrotic syndrome. She had an 8-year history of ileocolitis which responded poorly to corticosteroids. For 5 years, she had suffered from perianal fistulae. During the 6 months before referral she had developed gross ankle oedema and subsequently generalized oedema. Examination showed considerable facial, finger and dependant oedema. She was anaemic and had severe perianal disease. Investigations revealed an iron deficiency anaemia, ESR 86 mm/h, normal urea, creatinine and electrolytes. The serum albumin was 19 g/l and the urinary protein output was markedly elevated at 12 g/day. Radiologically, there was Crohn's disease of the ileum and the colon. Colonoscopic biopsies confirmed a granulomatous inflammation but also showed amyloid. A renal biopsy demonstrated amyloid deposits on the glomerular membrane with some interstitial infiltration with lymphocytes and plasma cells.

An intravenous regimen of parenteral nutrition and corticosteroids was begun but the patient deteriorated. The major part of her diseased intestine was therefore resected. An ileostomy was formed and the upper part of the rectum was brought out as a mucous fistula. Postoperative progress was excellent and during the next 3 months her oedema disappeared. The serum albumin rose to 38 g/l and the urinary protein excretion fell to less than 2 g/24 h. A repeat renal biopsy was not performed but further rectal biopsies showed no amyloid.

Joints

The incidence of arthropathy varies considerably in different reported series but joint involvement was found in one centre to occur in as many as 20% of patients with Crohn's disease, whatever its location (Haslock & Wright 1973). The attacks of acute inflammatory arthritis usually occur in large rather than small joints, and there is a suggestion that lesions are more common in legs than in arms. Severe disability, such as may occur in rheumatoid disease, is rare. Aspiration of synovial fluid may show inflammatory cells but the fluid is sterile on culture. Rose–Waaler test is negative. Arthritis usually occurs in association with exacerbations of Crohn's disease. Treatment is symptomatic in most instances but it may be necessary to consider the use of corticosteroids intra-articularly if symptoms persist.

Ankylosing spondylitis

Ankylosing spondylitis occurs almost exclusively in patients who are HLA B27 positive. It may occur long before bowel symptoms appear. Alternatively it may develop during the course of Crohn's disease. It may complicate Crohn's disease of the small intestine alone, although it is more frequent in those with colonic involvement. In many instances there is sacroileitis, sometimes only recognizable on radiological examination. In others, however, there may be progressive stiffness leading to the rigid spine characteristic of the condition.

Malnutrition

Malabsorption of vitamin B_{12} is common in patients with ileal Crohn's disease but this infrequently leads to symptoms or a frank megaloblastic anaemia. Malabsorption of bile salts may also occur which probably accounts for the high incidence of gallstones in these patients (Heaton et al. 1969, Cohen et al. 1971). Steatorrhoea usually results from bacterial overgrowth secondary to narrowing of the bowel with subsequent stasis. If prolonged, this may lead to deficiencies of the fat-soluble vitamins and rarely to osteomalacia and impaired haemostasis due to vitamin K deficiency. Nutritional deficiencies of other vitamins such as folic acid may also be present but are more commonly due to a poor dietary intake than to frank malabsorption. Deficiencies of potassium are frequently the result of severe diarrhoea. Deficiencies of magnesium and zinc have also been described.

Hepatobiliary system

Liver disease may be associated with Crohn's disease. Fatty liver may be found in any patient who is severely ill and isolated granulomata are common. Other histological abnormalities on liver biopsy range from a classical periductular fibrosis to a chronic portal inflammation with piecemeal necrosis resembling chronic active hepatitis (Chapman et al. 1980, Ludwig et al. 1981). Cirrhosis of the liver, however, is rare (Perrett et al. 1971).

The use of endoscopic retrograde cholangiopancreatography has enabled the diagnosis of sclerosing cholangitis to be made with accuracy. There are few well-documented cases of sclerosing cholangitis and Crohn's disease and only one reported case of a bile duct carcinoma (Berman et al. 1980). It appears that these forms of hepatobiliary disease complicate Crohn's disease less commonly than ulcerative colitis.

Malignancy

Adenocarcinoma of the small intestine complicating Crohn's disease was first described by Ginzburg et al. (1956). Subsequent studies have shown that carcinoma is a rare complication of small intestinal Crohn's disease. Hawker et al. (1982) were able to identify only three patients with this complication in their own clinical experience between 1968 and 1980 and they reviewed fifty-eight cases culled from the world literature. Forty-one of the tumours occurred in the ileum, eighteen in the jejunum, one in the duodenum and one in the ileum and colon. Eighteen occurred in bypassed intestinal loops. The prognosis was grave despite resection. Many patients died within a year of diagnosis.

Diagnosis

The diagnosis is confirmed by radiological studies and the small bowel enema is the procedure which provides maximal information (Nolan & Gourtsoyiannis 1980). This technique allows visualization of the early aphthoid ulcers which cannot be shown on conventional barium meal and follow-through. The characteristic radiological signs at the earliest stage are shallow aphthous ulcers (Fig. 11.4). Thereafter there are fissure-ulcers, mucosal oedema producing a

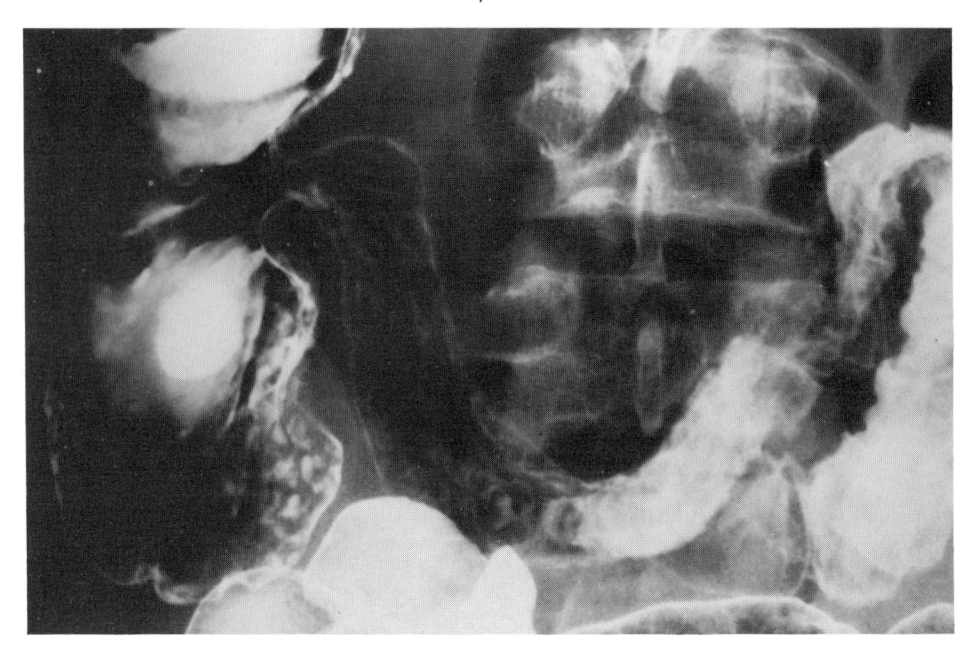

Fig. 11.4. Shallow aphthous ulcers in the terminal ileum of a patient with early Crohn's disease. (Courtesy of Dr R.A. Wilkins.)

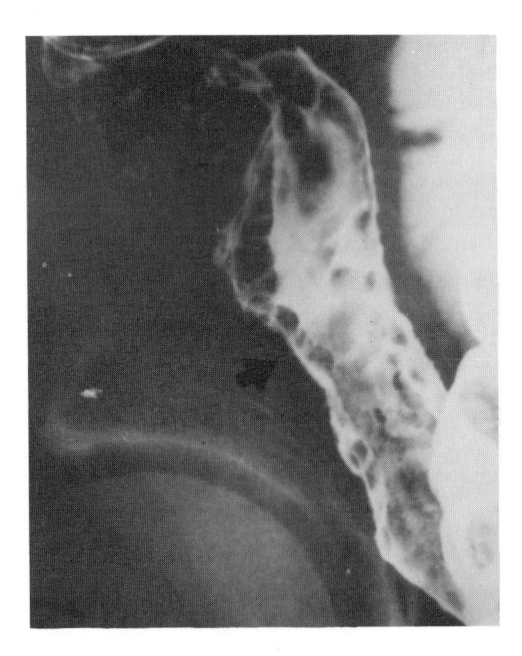

Fig. 11.5. Terminal ileitis with penetrating ulcers in Crohn's disease. (Courtesy of Dr R.A. Wilkins.)

'cobble-stone' appearance and narrowing of the intestinal lumen (Figs 11.5, 11.6 and 11.7). A barium enema should always be performed to document the presence and extent of co-existent colonic disease. Sigmoidoscopy may reveal a proctitis. A rectal biopsy specimen should be obtained even if the mucosa appears normal since granulomata may be found in up to 25–30% on histological examination (Surawicz *et al.* 1981). If the radiological appearances are not certainly diagnostic, it may be necessary to perform colonoscopy with multiple biopsies from the colon and from the terminal ileum if it can be entered.

Differential diagnosis

Crohn's disease must be differentiated from tuberculosis, yersinia, lymphoma and Behçet's syndrome. An acute presentation mimicking an acute appendicitis is characteristic of an acute ileitis but few such patients have Crohn's disease. Some cases may be due to *Yersinia enterocolitica* or *Yersinia pseudotuberculosis*. These organisms may be grown from the stool but a rise

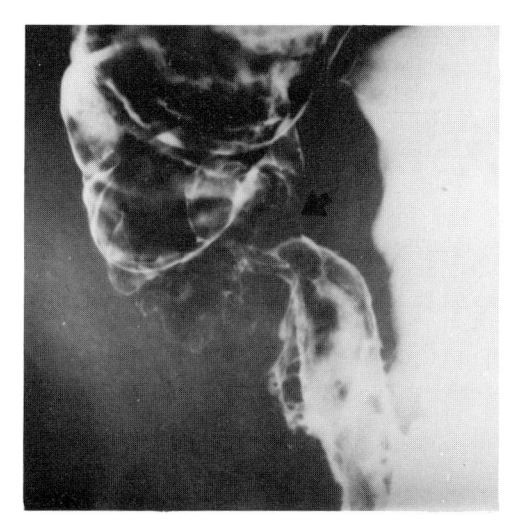

Fig. 11.6. Fistula formation (arrowed) between caecum and terminal ileum in Crohn's disease. (Courtesy of Dr R.A. Wilkins.)

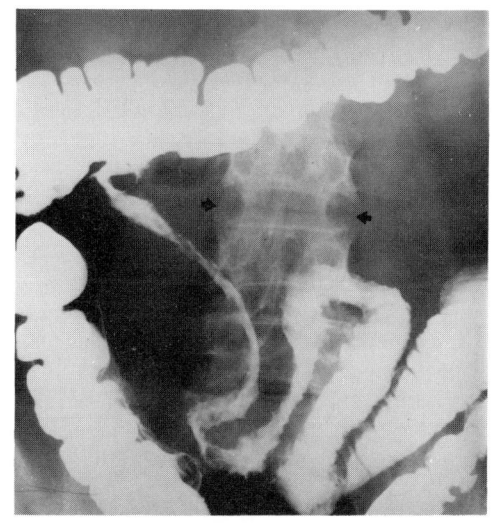

Fig. 11.7. Recurrent Crohn's disease in the ileum after right hemicolectoy and terminal ileectomy. Note calcification in the spinal ligaments (arrowed) in this patient who had ankylosing spondylitis. (Courtesy of Dr R.A. Wilkins.)

in serum antibody titres provides the most reliable diagnosis. Behçet's disease of the intestine is almost always associated with the other features of the syndrome, such as oral and genital ulceration, or ocular abnormalities, and intestinal perforation is common (Kasahara *et al.* 1981) (see Chapter 12). Actinomycosis is rarely a problem in differential diagnosis. Intestinal lymphoma may be difficult to differentiate and laparotomy may be necessary.

The most difficult diagnostic problem is tuberculosis (Marks 1983), especially when Crohn's disease occurs in Asian patients. Stool culture or serum antibody titres to mycobacteria are unhelpful. Laparoscopy is frequently useful in cases where serosal tubercles are present which can be biopsied and cultured. Radiologically, 'skip areas', so commonly seen in Crohn's disease, are unusual in tuberculosis. Other radiological features which favour tuberculosis rather than Crohn's disease are a short segment of ileum involved and the absence of cobblestoning and asymmetry (Nolan 1983). Nevertheless, it is frequently impossible to differentiate the two diseases on radiological criteria. Colonoscopy and biopsy have been used in an attempt to make a positive diagnosis of tuberculosis. If an acid-fast bacillus is found or a caseating granuloma is seen in the rectal biopsy, the diagnosis is clear, but the distinction from Crohn's disease is not usually so simple.

Assessment of disease activity

Active, extensive disease of the ileum may not be associated with clinical symptoms. In contrast, symptoms of diarrhoea, pain and weight loss may be due to fibrous strictures or bacterial overgrowth, or may be secondary to previous surgical resection. Clinical assessment of disease activity may therefore frequently be misleading. Laboratory data such as haemoglobin, albumin and erythrocyte sedimentation rate, may be useful but may also be misleading. The acute phase reactants, C-reactive protein and orosomucoid, are probably the most sensitive indicators (André *et al.* 1981). Attempts have been made to devise an activity index by Best *et al.* (1976) and by van Hees *et al.* (1980). These set out to achieve a standard method of assessment which can be applied universally but neither is simple to use in everyday practice. The assessment of disease activity is therefore not yet satisfactorily established.

Treatment

At present Crohn's disease cannot be cured. The clinician must attempt to ameliorate the inflammatory process, to correct nutritional deficiencies and to control symptoms. Most patients will require lifelong supervision even though the disease process may remit for long periods leaving the patient apparently symptom-free. Disease limited to the small intestine is less troublesome than ileocolic disease in which there is a higher incidence of internal fistulae, perianal disease and systemic complications.

Mild to moderate disease

Initially it is reasonable to give patients with a mild attack of Crohn's disease who are well enough to be treated on an out-patient basis, a trial of sulphasalazine (2−4 g/day for 1 month). During this period, the inflammatory process may remit, although data from the National Co-operative Crohn's Disease Study in the USA (N.C.C.D.S.) (Summers et al. 1979) indicates that the drug may be effective only in patients with colonic involvement. Metronidazole 800 mg/day is an alternative treatment which has been shown to be slightly more effective than sulphasalazine in double-blind cross-over trial in seventy-five Swedish patients (Ursing et al. 1982).

Steroids are used for patients with more obvious evidence of ongoing inflammation and for those who have not responded to an initial period of treatment with other medications. The recommended dose of prednisone starts at 30−60 mg/day and is tapered down as the condition improves (Summers et al. 1979). It is unwise to continue with a high dose of prednisone for more than 3 or 4 weeks. In the N.C.C.D.S. the response was essentially complete at 6−7 weeks. Moreover, there was no evidence that sulphasalazine and prednisone together conferred any additional benefit; in fact the combination appeared to be less effective than prednisone alone. Recently it has been shown that Crohn's disease of moderate severity remits if the patient is given an elemental diet and that this treatment is as effective as the use of corticosteroids (O'Morain et al. 1982).

Patients in remission should not be given maintenance treatment with either steroids or sulphasalazine. Neither treatment is effective. The role of diet in the long-term management of Crohn's disease remains uncertain. On the basis of retrospective studies it has been suggested that a fibre-rich unrefined carbohydrate diet taken by patients with Crohn's disease in remission is associated with less severe relapse (Heaton et al. 1979). A prospective trial in the UK is currently being undertaken. Evidence in favour of other forms of dietary manipulation is anecdotal.

Severe disease

Patients with severe symptomatic Crohn's disease require admission to hospital. They are usually febrile and often there is evidence of an inflammatory mass with or without sinuses or fistulae. If an abscess can be demonstrated, for example, using scanning techniques, it should be drained and the patient given broad spectrum antibiotics including metronidazole to cover anaerobic organisms. It may be necessary to defunction intestine adjacent to the abscess cavity.

If localized bacterial infection cannot be demonstrated and repeated blood cultures are sterile, the clinician should feed the patient by the parenteral route and give a high dose of prednisone. In addition, broad spectrum antibiotics should be used if an infective component is suspected. In most cases the disease remits. If it does not, then surgery is usually indicated. Azathioprine does not help in this situation (Summers et al. 1979 reporting on N.C.C.D.S.) and should not be used alone in acute Crohn's disease, although it may have a steroid-sparing effect. Patients with perianal disease or with fistulae should be treated with metronidazole (800−1200 mg/day) (Brandt et al. 1982). Losses from enterocutaneous fistulae diminish on treatment with an elemental diet and fistulae may even appear to heal.

Nevertheless, if long-standing, they rarely remain closed and are an indication for surgical resection.

Crohn's disease in remission

In the N.C.C.D.S. approximately 40% of patients studied achieved a good remission and stopped taking anti-inflammatory drugs (especially steroids). Sulphasalazine did not help in the withdrawal of prednisone (Singleton et al. 1979) and in two controlled trials it had no prophylactic value in preventing exacerbation of Crohn's disease. In addition, prednisone has no prophylactic effect against recurrence after surgery (Summers et al. 1979). The finding that azathioprine inhibits relapse (O'Donaghue 1978) needs confirmation. It is not supported by the results of a differently structured trial in the N.C.C.D.S. (Summers et al. 1979). The clinician must balance the risks of using azathioprine, for example bone marrow toxicity and increased incidence of malignant disease, against its possible prophylactic benefit.

Chronic active Crohn's disease

The majority of patients with Crohn's disease are at least mildly symptomatic most of the time. Many patients (50% in some series) continue to take steroids to suppress chronic disease and most clinicians report that symptoms recur as the dose of prednisone is reduced to 10 mg/day (Lennard-Jones 1983). It may be possible to reduce the side-effects of steroids by giving treatment as a single dose on alternate days or by using small doses of a cytotoxic drug for its steroid-sparing effects. More studies are needed to resolve these issues. Similarly there are no reports of controlled trials of the benefit of using metronidazole or broad spectrum antibiotics in the long-term control of the inflammatory process. Preparations such as codeine phosphate, loperamide or diphenoxylate are often useful for treating diarrhoea in patients with persistently active Crohn's disease. In addition, the clinician must maintain the patient's nutritional status.

Surgical management

The main indications for surgical treatment are:
1 Failure of medical therapy, either because the disease is not controlled by corticosteroids or the patient has repeated relapses once steroids are withdrawn;
2 The presence of complications such as strictures causing intestinal obstruction or fistulae.

If patients have had good medical management, they should come to surgery in a good state of nutrition and with the active inflammation under control with corticosteroids. The surgical procedure should aim to be a resection of the grossly diseased segment with an end-to-end anastomosis. Bypass operations should be avoided as they may be associated with persistent active disease, bacterial overgrowth and malabsorption, and carcinoma can occur in the bypassed segment (Greenstein et al. 1978). Wide resection is unnecessary as the presence of microscopic inflammation at the resected margins does not influence the subsequent prognosis (Papaioannou et al. 1979, Pennington et al. 1980). For the patient with diffuse small intestinal disease who has multiple strictures, minimal procedures such as a 'plasty', a localized bypass or mini-resections can be performed (Lee 1981). It is advisable to cover all surgical procedures with corticosteroids. These drugs do not seriously impair healing or predispose the patient to infective complications and they serve to suppress the disease. Postoperative fistulae are rarely seen if corticosteroids are used.

Considerable debate continues about the surgical management of patients who present as an 'acute appendicitis' and are then found to have a terminal ileitis. Only a minority will eventually prove to have Crohn's disease (de Dombal et al. 1971). If the base of the appendix is free of obvious disease, many surgeons will remove it. If, however, the base of the appendix is involved, then surgical interference is best avoided.

Prognosis

Patients are never cured of Crohn's disease. They are subject to relapse of their disease and recurrences after surgical resection. Nevertheless, with regular follow-up, maintenance of a good nutritional state and judicious medical and surgical treatment, the majority of patients lead full and active lives (Gazzard et al. 1978, Meyers et al. 1980) Following a surgical resection, about 45% of patients will have recurrent disease within 5 years (de Dombal et al. 1971, Hellers 1979), but the course of small intestinal disease following surgery appears to be more favourable than ileocolonic disease (Lock et al. 1981). A few patients will need a second or even a third resection but whether the risk of needing further surgery increases with each operation is debatable (Lee & Papaioannou 1981). The factors predisposing to recurrence are not known. Age and sex have no influence. The suggestion that diets rich in fibre but low in refined sugar may favourably influence the course of the disease (Heaton et al. 1979) is interesting and needs further study.

Mortality from Crohn's disease has been studied using actuarial methods. When survival curves have been plotted, these have progressively diverged from the expected survival curve (Truelove & Pena 1976, Weterman 1976, Hellers 1979). In other words, Crohn's disease is a disease which becomes more dangerous with the passage of time. Recent data from Birmingham, England, conflicts with these results and suggests that the highest mortality is seen in young patients in the early stages of their disease (Cooke et al. 1980). However, the majority of patients will have a good prognosis, despite considerable morbidity, and the mortality will only be about twice that expected.

References

Aluwihare A.P.R. (1971) Electron microscopy in Crohn's disease. *Gut,* **12**, 509.

André C., Descos L., Landais P. & Fermanian J. (1981) Assessment of appropriate laboratory measurements to supplement the Crohn's disease activity index. *Gut,* **22**, 571.

Aronson M.D., Phillips C.A., Beeken W.L. & Forsyth B.R. (1975) Isolation and characterisation of a viral agent from intestinal tissue of patients with Crohn's disease and other intestinal disorders. *Prog. Med. Virol.* **21**, 165.

Atwell J.A. & Pollock A.V. (1960) Intestinal calculi. *Brit. J. Surg.* **47**, 367–374.

Berman M.D., Falchuk K.R. & Trey C. (1980) Carcinoma of the biliary tree complicating Crohn's disease. *Dig. Dis. Sci.* **25**, 795.

Best W.R., Becktel J.M., Singleton J.W. & Kern F. (1976) Development of a Crohn's disease activity index. *Gastroenterol.* **70**, 439.

Bishop A.E., Polak J.M., Bryant M.G., Bloom S.R. & Hamilton S. (1980) Abnormalities of vasoactive intestinal polypeptide-containing nerves in Crohn's disease. *Gastroenterol.* **79**, 853.

Brandt L.J., Bernstein L.H., Boley S.J. & Frank M.S. (1982) Metronidazole therapy for perineal Crohn's disease: A follow-up study. *Gastroenterol.* **83**, 383.

Burnham W.R., Lennard-Jones J.E., Stanford J.L. & Bird R.G. (1978) Mycobacteria as a possible cause of inflammatory bowel disease. *Lancet,* **ii**, 693.

Cave D.R., Mitchell D.N. & Brooke B.N. (1975) Experimental animal studies of the aetiology and pathogenesis of Crohn's disease. *Gastroenterol.* **69**, 618.

Chambers T.J. & Morson B.C. (1979) The granuloma in Crohn's disease. *Gut,* **20**, 269.

Chapman R.W.G., Arborgh B.A.M., Rhodes J.M., Summerfield J.A., Dick R., Schener P.J. & Sherlock S. (1980) Primary sclerosing cholangitis: a review of its clinical features, cholangiography, and hepatic histology. *Gut,* **21**, 870.

Chiba M., McLaren L.C. & Strickland R.G. (1982) Immunity to cytopathic agents associated with Crohn's disease: a negative study. *Gut,* **23**, 333.

Cohen S., Kaplan M., Gottlieb L. & Patterson J. (1971) Liver disease and gallstones in regional enteritis. *Gastroenterol.* **60**, 237.

Cooke W.T., Mallas E., Prior P. & Allan R.N. (1980) Crohn's disease: course, treatment and long-term prognosis. *Quart. J. Med.* **49**, 363.

Craig S.W. & Cebra J.J. (1971) Peyer's patches: an enriched source of precursors for IgA-producing immunocytes in the rabbit. *J. Exp. Med.* **134**, 188.

Crohn B.B., Ginzburg L. & Oppenheimer G.D. (1932) Regional ileitis. A pathologic and clinical entity. Description of 14 cases. *J. Amer. Med. Assoc.* **99**, 1323.

Dalziel T. (1913) Chronic interstitial enteritis. *Brit. Med. J.* **2**, 1068.

De dombal F.T., Burton I.L. & Goligher J.C. (1971) Recurrence of Crohn's disease after primary excisonal surgery. *Gut,* **12**, 519.

Dunne W.T., Cooke W.T. & Allan R.N. (1977) Enzymatic and morphometric evidence for Crohn's disease as a diffuse lesion of the gastrointestinal tract. *Gut,* **18**, 290.

Farmer R.G., Hawk W.A. & Turnbull R.B. (1975)

Clinical patterns in Crohn's disease. A statistical study of 615 cases. *Gastroenterol.* **68**, 727.

Farmer R.G. & Michener W.M. (1979) Prognosis of Crohn's disease in childhood and adolescence. *Dig. Dis. Sci.* **24**, 752.

Ferguson R., Allan R.N. & Cooke W.T. (1975) A study of the cellular infiltrate of the proximal jejunal mucosa in ulcerative colitis and Crohn's disease. *Gut,* **16**, 205.

Gazzard B.G., Price H.L., Libby G.W. & Dawson A.M. (1978) The social toll of Crohn's disease. *Brit. Med. J.* **2**, 1117.

Gebbers J.-O. & Otto H.F. (1981) Immunohisto and ultracytochemical observations in Crohn's disease. In *Recent Advances in Crohn's Disease,* p. 136. (Ed. by A.S. Pena, I.T. Weterman, C.C. Booth & W. Strober). Martinus Nijhoff Publishers, The Hague.

Gilat T. & Rozen P. (1981) The épidemiology of Crohn's disease, trends and clues. In *Recent Advances in Crohn's disease,* p. 153. (Ed. by A.S. Pena, I.T. Weterman, C.C. Booth & W. Strober.) Martinus Nijhoff Publishers, The Hague.

Ginzburg L., Schneider K.M., Dreizin D.H. & Levinson C. (1956) Carcinoma of the jejunum occurring in a case of regional enteritis. *Surgery,* **39**, 347−351.

Gitnick G.L., Arthur M.H. & Shibata I. (1976) Cultivation of viral agents from Crohn's disease. A new sensitive system. *Lancet,* **ii**, 215.

Gitnick G.L. & Rosen V.J. (1976) Electron microscopic studies of viral agents in Crohn's disease. *Lancet,* **ii**, 217.

Glass R.E. & Baker W.N.W. (1976) Role of the granuloma in recurrent Crohn's disease. *Gut,* **17**, 75.

Goodman M.J., Skinner J.M. & Truelove S.C. (1976) Abnormalities in apparently normal bowel mucosa in Crohn's disease. *Lancet,* **i**, 275.

Greenstein A.J., Sachar D. & Pucillo A. (1978) Cancer in Crohn's disease after diversionary surgery. *Ann. J. Surg.* **135**, 86.

Gyde S.N., Prior P., Macartney J.C., Thompson H., Waterhouse J.A.H. & Allan R.N. (1980) Malignancy and Crohn's disease. *Gut,* **21**, 1024.

Haslock I. & Wright V. (1973) The musculo-skeletal complications of Crohn's disease. *Medicine,* **52**, 217−225.

Hawker P.C., Gyde S.N., Thompson H. & Allan R.N. (1982) Adenocarcinoma of the small intestine complicating Crohn's disease. *Gut,* **23**, 188.

Heaton K.W. & Read A.E. (1969) Gallstones in patients with disorders of the terminal ileum and disturbed bile salt metabolism. *Brit. Med. J.* **3**, 494.

Heaton K.W., Thornton J.R. & Emmett P.M. (1979) Treatment of Crohn's disease with an unrefined-carbohydrate, fibre-rich diet. *Brit. Med. J.* **2**, 764.

Hellers G. (1979) Crohn's disease in Stockholm County 1955-1974. A study of epidemiology, results of surgical treatment and long-term prognosis. *Acta Chirugica Scand. Supp,* 490.

Hellers G. (1981) Epidemiology of Crohn's disease. In *Topics in Gastroenterology,* vol. 9, p. 13. (Ed. by D.P. Jewell & Emanoel Lee). Blackwell Scientific Publications, Oxford.

Japanese Research Committee for Crohn's disease (1981) Crohn's disease in Japan. In *A Global Assessment of Crohn's Disease,* p. 136. (Ed. by E.C.G. Lee). HM & M Publishers, London.

Kasahara Y., Tanaka S., Nishino M., Umemura H., Shiraha S. & Kuyama T. (1981) Intestinal involvement in Behçet's disease. *Dis. Colon Rectum,* **24**, 103.

Kirsner J.B. & Shorter R.G. (1982) Recent developments in 'non-specific' inflammatory bowel disease. *New Engl. J. Med.* **306**,837.

Kyle J. & Stark G. (1980) Fall in the incidence of Crohn's disease. *Gut,* **21**, 340.

Lee E.C.G. (1981) Surgery in Crohn's disease. in *Recent Advances in Crohn's disease,* p. 522. (Ed. by A.S. Pena, I.T. Weterman, C.C. Booth & W. Strober). Martinus Nijhoff Publishers, The Hague.

Lee E.C.G. & Papaioannou N. (1981) Recurrences following surgery for Crohn's disease. In *Clinics in Gastroenterology,* p. 419. (Ed. by R. Farmer) W.B. Saunders Co Ltd, London.

Lennard-Jones J.E. (1983) Towards optimal use of conticosteroids in ulcerative colitis and Crohn's disease. *Gut,* **24**, 177−181.

Lock M.R., Farmer R.G., & Fazio V.W., Jagleman D.G., Lavery I.C. & Weakley F.L. (1981) Recurrence and reoperation for Crohn's disease. *New Engl. J. Med.* **304**, 1586.

Lockhart-Mummery H.E. & Morson B.C. (1960) Crohn's disease (regional enteritis) of the large intestine and its distinction from ulcerative colitis. *Gut,* **1**, 87.

Ludwig J., Barham S.S., La Ruiso N.F., Elveback L.R., Wiemer R.H. & McCall J.T. (1981) Morphologic features of chronic hepatitis associated with primary sclerosing cholangitis and chronic ulerative colitis. *Hepatol.* **1**, 632.

McLaren L.C. & Gitnick G. (1982) Ulcerative colitis and Crohn's disease tissue cytotoxins. *Gastroenterol.* **82**, 1381.

Marks I.N. (1983) Intestinal tuberculosis. In *Topics in Gastroenterology,* vol. 11. (Ed. by D.P. Jewell & H.A. Shepherd). Blackwell Scientific Publications, Oxford.

Meyers S., Walfish J.S., Sachar D.B., Greenstein A.J., Hill A.G. & Janowitz H.D. (1980) Quality of life after surgery for Crohn's disease: a psychosocial survey. *Gastroenterol.* **78**, 1.

Mitchell D.N. & Rees R.J.W. (1970) Agent transmissible from Crohn's disease tissue. *Lancet,* **11**, 168.

Nolan D.J. (1983) *Radiological Atlas of Gastrointestinal Disease.* John Wiley and Sons, Chichester.

Nolan D.J. & Gourtsoyiannis N.C. (1980) Crohn's disease of the small intestine: a review of the radiological appearances in 100 consecutive patients examined by a barium infusion tech-

nique. *Clin. Radiol.* **31**, 597.
O'Donoghue D.P., Dawson A.M., Powell-Tuck J., Baum R.L. & Lennard-Jones J.E. (1978) Double-blind withdrawal trial of azathioprine as maintenance treatment for Crohn's disease. *Lancet*, **2**, 955.
O'Morain C. & Levi A.J. (1981) Elemental diets in the treatment of acute Crohn's disease. In *Recent Advances in Crohn's disease* (Ed. by A.S. Pena, I.T. Weterman, C.C. Booth & W. Strober). Martinus Nijhoff Publishers, The Hague.
O'Morain C.A., Segal A.W. & Levi A.J. (1982) Elemental diets in the treatment of Crohn's disease: a controlled study. *Gut*, **23**, A891.
Papaioannou N., Piris J., Lee E.C.G. & Kettlewell M.G.W. (1979) The relationship between histological inflammation in the cut ends after Crohn's disease and recurrence. *Gut*, **20**, A916.
Parent K. & Mitchell P. (1978) Cell-wall defective variants of pseudomonas-like (group Va) bacteria in Crohn's disease. *Gastroenterol.* **75**, 368.
Pennington L., Hamilton S.R., Bayless T.M. & Cameron J.L. (1980) Surgical management of Crohn's disease: influence of disease at margin of resection. *Ann. Surg.* **192**, 311.
Perrett A.D., Higgins G., Johnston H.H., Massarella G.R., Truelove S.C. & Wright R. (1971) The liver in Crohn's disease. *Quart. J. Med.* **40**, 187.
Phillpotts R.J., Hermon-Taylor J., Teich N.M. & Brooke B.N. (1980) A search for persistent virus infection in Crohn's disease. *Gut*, **21**, 202.
Phillpotts R.J., Hermon-Taylor J. & Brooke B.N. (1981) Evidence against the involvement of conventional viruses in Crohn's disease. In *Recent Advances in Crohn's Disease*, p. 252. (Ed. by A.S. Pena, I.T. Weterman, C.C. Booth & W. Strober). Martinus Nijhoff Publishers, The Hague.
Rozen P., Zonis J., Yekutiel P. & Gilat T. (1979) Crohn's disease in the Jewish population of Tel-Aviv-Yafo. *Gastroenterol.* **76**, 25.
Singleton J.W., Summers R.W., Kern F.J., Becktel J.M., Best W.R., Hansen R.N., Winship D.H. (1979) A trial of sulfasalazine as adjunctive therapy in Crohn's disease. *Gastroenterol.* **77**, 887-897.
Sommers S.C. & Korelitz B.I. (1981) Duodenal biopsy cell counts and histopathology in Crohn's disease. In *Recent Advances in Crohn's Disease*, p. 47. (Ed. by A.S. Pena, I.T. Weterman, C.C. Booth & W. Strober). Martinus Nijhoff Publishers, The Hague.
Stanford J.L. (1981) Acid-fast organisms in Crohn's disease and ulcerative colitis. In *Recent Advances in Crohn's Disease*, p. 274. (Ed. by A.S. Pena, I.T. Weterman, C.C. Booth & W. Strober.) Martinus Nijhoff Publishers, The Hague.
Strickland R.G. & Jewell D.P. (1983) Immunoregulatory mechanisms in non-specific inflammatory bowel disease. *Ann. Rev. Med.* **34**, 195–204.

Summers R.W., Switz D.M., Sessions J.T., Becktel J.M., Best W.L., Kern F. & Singleton J.W. (1979) National co-operative Crohn's disease study: results of drug treatment. *Gastroenterol.* **77**, 847.
Surawicz C.M., Meisel J.L., Ylvisaker T., Saunders D.R. & Rubin C.E. (1981) Rectal biopsy in the diagnosis of Crohn's disease: value of multiple biopsies and serial sectioning. *Gastroenterol.* **80**, 66.
Thayer W.R., Coutu J.A., Chiodini R.J., Van Kruiningen H.J., & Merkol R.S. (1983) Mycobacterium paratuberculosis antibodies in Crohn's disease. *Gastroenterol.* **84**, 1334.
Thomas H.C. & Jewell D.P. (1979) *Clinical Gastrointestinal Immunology*. Blackwell Scientific Publications, Oxford.
Tijtgat G., Van Minnen A. & Verhoeven T. (1981) Electronmicroscopy in Crohn's disease. In *Recent Advances in Crohn's Disease*, p. 110. (Ed. by A.S. Pena, I.T. Weterman, C.C. Booth & W. Strober). Martinus Nijhoff Publishers, The Hague.
Truelove S.C. & Pena A.S. (1976) Course and prognosis of Crohn's disease. *Gut*, **17**, 192.
Ursing B., Alm T., Barany F., Bergelin I., Ganrot-Norlin K., Hoevels J., Huitfeldt B., Jarnerot G., Krause U., Krook A., Lindstrom B., Nordle O. & Rosen A. (1982) A comparative study of metronidazole and sulphasalazine for active Crohn's disease: The Co-operative Crohn's Disease Study in Sweden. II. Result. *Gastroenterol.* **83**, 550.
van Hees P.A.M., van Elteren P.H., van Lier H.J.J. & van Tongeren J.H.M. (1980) An index of inflammatory activity in patients with Crohn's disease. *Gut*, **21**, 279.
van Hees P.A.M., van Lier H.J.J., van Elteren P.H., Driessen W.M.M., van Hogezand R.A., Ten Velde G.P.M., Bakker J.H. & van Tongeren J.H.M. (1981) Effect of sulphasalazine in patients with active Crohn's disease: a controlled double-blind study. *Gut*, **22**, 404.
Walker J. & Ellis I.O. (1984) Cuboidal calcium enterolith causing obstruction and perforation of the small intestine. *Brit. Med. J.* **i**, 532.
Weterman I.T. (1976) Retrospective study of 226 patients with Crohn's disease. In *The Management of Crohn's Disease*. (Ed. by I.T. Weterman, A.S. Pena & C.C. Booth). Excerpta Medica, Amsterdam.
Whorwell P.J., Phillips C.A., Beeken W.L., Little P.K. & Roessner K.D. (1977) Isolation of reovirus-like agents from patients with Crohn's disease. *Lancet*, **i**, 1169.
Yardley J. (1981) In *Recent Advances in Crohn's Disease*, p. 272. (Ed. by A.S. Pena, I.T. Weterman, C.C. Booth & W. Strober). Martinus Nijhoff Publishers, The Hague.
Zeit R.M. (1979) Enterolithiasis associated with ileal perforation in Crohn's disease. *Amer. J. Gastroenterol.* **72**, 662–664.

Chapter 12
Ulcerative Lesions

CHRISTOPHER C. BOOTH AND GRAHAM NEALE

Ulceration due to known causes 209
Behçet's syndrome 209
Primary ulcer 212
Acute jejunitis 212
Idiopathic mucosal enteropathy (Syn.
   Idiopathic chronic ulcerative enteritis,
   chronic ulcerative non-granulomatous
   jejunoileitis, non-responsive coeliac
   disease, unclassified sprue) 213
Pre-stomal ileitis 216

Ulceration of the small intestine may be due to causes which are well defined. There are, however, a variety of disorders, such as Behçet's syndrome, primary ulcer of the small intestine and other conditions where the cause of intestinal ulceration remains uncertain.

Ulceration due to known causes

Ulceration of the small intestine is usually due to one or other of the disorders described in other chapters in this book. Table 12.1 lists the major causes of small intestinal ulceration. Infections such as tuberculosis and typhoid, and the inflammatory lesions of Crohn's disease are particularly associated with ulceration. Ulceration leading to perforation is a frequent presenting feature of malignant conditions of the small intestine, such as lymphoma or malignant histiocytosis. Obstructive vascular lesions leading to ischaemia often cause ulceration. Ulceration of the upper jejunum should always raise the suspicion that there is hyperacidity due to the Zollinger–Ellison syndrome, and drugs or other toxic substances should always be suspected if intestinal ulceration is found unassociated with a known aetiology. Ulceration with stricture formation may occur in coeliac disease and is presumably the result of the mucosal lesion.

The clinical features in patients with ulceration due to such lesions are those of the causative disorder. Ulceration may itself cause central abdominal pain, frequently postprandially. The major clinical complication, however, is perforation, which requires immediate surgical correction. Haemorrhage causing melaena is often seen, particularly if there is ulceration within a Meckel's diverticulum. Stricture formation may also be a sequel to long-standing ulceration.

Behçet's syndrome

Hippocrates appears to have been the first physician to describe the characteristic clinical syndrome of oral and genital ulcer-

Table 12.1. Causes of intestinal ulceration.

Infection	Bacterial (tuberculosis, typhoid), parasites
Inflammatory lesions	Acute jejunitis Crohn's disease
Mucosal lesions	Coeliac disease
Malignant tumours	Primary — lymphoma, malignant histiocytosis Secondary
Vascular abnormalities	Mesenteric vascular insufficiency, arteritis
Hyperacidity	Zollinger–Ellison syndrome, stomal ulcer, Meckel's diverticulum
Toxins	Endogenous — uraemia Exogenous — arsenic, gold, mercury, drugs such as potassium chloride or corticosteroids
Radiation	
Unknown aetiology	Behçet's syndrome Primary ulcer Idiopathic mucosal enteropathy

ation, together with chronic inflammation of the eye (Feigenbaum 1956). References to the condition up to the mid-1950s, however, are sparse. Bluthe wrote a thesis on the subject in 1908 but there appear to be few further reports until 1937 when Hulusi Behçet, Professor of Dermatology in the University of Istanbul, produced a series of important papers (Müftüoglu 1980).

The aetiology and pathogenesis of Behçet's syndrome remain obscure although recent evidence has implicated the herpes simplex virus (Denman et al. 1980, Eglin et al. 1982).

Prevalence

The prevalence of Behçet's syndrome appears to be approximately 10/100,000 in Japan (Aoki et al. 1971) and is probably similar in Turkey. The condition is relatively common in Israel and Middle Eastern countries (Chajek & Fainaru 1975) but it is much rarer in the UK where a prevalence of approximately 0.6/100,000 has been reported (Chamberlain 1980). The condition is rarer still in Minnesota (O'Duffy 1981).

HLA antigens

The relationship of the syndrome to HLA antigens remains uncertain. In Japan, Turkey and Israel HLA B5 is associated with a significantly increased relative risk. This increase is associated with Bw 51 (relative risk × 13) and not the Bw 52 split of the HLA B5 locus antigen (Yazici et al. 1980). In the USA this relationship appears not to hold true. It has been suggested that HLA B5 predisposes to ocular manifestations, B12 to the mucocutaneous syndrome and B27 to arthritic disease (Lehner & Batchelor 1979).

Clinical features

Behçet's syndrome is a multi-system disorder which commonly affects the skin, joints and vascular system and much less commonly the heart, lungs, central nervous system and gut. Characteristically the condition runs a chronic but intermittent course and there is no rational treatment.

The classical triad of oral and genital ulceration, with inflammatory lesions of the eye, presents no diagnostic problem. In many cases, however, characteristic physical signs may be transient and the clinical picture may be dominated by atypical manifestations such as ileocolitis, or thrombophlebitis migrans. Moreover, there is an obvious overlap between Behçet's disease and other multi-systemic disorders such as erythema multiforme with systemic involvement. It is often difficult to make clear-cut clinical distinctions (Bøe et al 1958).

In the Western world and the Mediterranean area, gastrointestinal involvement is a rare manifestation of Behçet's syndrome. By contrast a nationwide survey in Japan revealed that more than 10% of nearly 3000 patients registered with Behçet's disease had gastrointestinal lesions (Baba et al. 1976), particularly ulceration of the ileocaecal region (Kasahara et al. 1981). In a detailed study of a group of patients with Behçet's syndrome studied in London, nineteen out of sixty-nine patients had gastrointestinal symptoms but there was no abnormal pathology (Sladen & Lehner 1979). In many published reports it is difficult to distinguish the clinical manifestations of Behçet's enteritis from those of other forms of inflammatory bowel disease.

Diagnosis is therefore not easy. Although there is no specific diagnostic test, skin hyper-reactivity to needle prick or to the injection of saline is a useful procedure. The skin should be inspected 12–48 h after a sterile prick. In positive tests there is induration and the formation of sterile pus. This is associated with perivascular round cell infiltration and a scattering of mast cells; deposits of immunoglobulin and complement have not been demonstrated (Haim et al. 1976). In Turkey 88% of patients with clinically defined Behçet's disease had a positive skin prick test compared to only 7% of 122 healthy and diseased controls (Tüzün et al. 1980) but in the USA this test has not been found useful (O'Duffy 1974).

Intestinal manifestations

In Western medical literature most patients suffering from Behçet's syndrome with gastrointestinal involvement had a left-sided colitis. In many of these the histological features were indistinguishable from ulcerative colitis; in others the clinical and histological findings resembled a granulomatous colitis (Nilsen et al. 1977).

In Japan, however, as many as 50% of patients with Behçet's syndrome suffer from attacks of anorexia, nausea and vomiting, abdominal pain and distension and associated diarrhoea. Radiological examination of the small intestine (Fig. 12.1) shows dilated loops of intestine, excess gas and liquid, and flocculation of barium (Oshima et al. 1963). In four of fifteen patients subjected to jejunal biopsy abnormal distended lymphatic channels were found and, although there was no evidence of protein-losing enteropathy (Asakura et al. 1973), fat absorption might be impaired (Oshima et al. 1963).

Kasahara et al. (1981) have reviewed over 100 cases of Behçet's disease with localized ulceration of the gastrointestinal tract treated surgically. The distribution of ulcers was as follows: stomach 1%, duodenum 2%, small intestine (excluding terminal ileum) 4%, terminal ileum 45%, ileocaecal region 35%, caecum 10%, colon 3%. In a further twenty cases ulceration occurred in multiple sites from oesophagus to colon. In the more common localized variety there was more than one ulcer in 75% of reported cases and perforation or deep penetration of the intestinal wall occurred in more than 50%. The prognosis was not always favourable. Thirteen of 108 patients died after resection of affected intestine.

Pathology of intestinal ulcers

The pathology shows no specific features. There may be irregular undermining and swelling of the ulcer margin. The inflammation is transmural and may extend to the serosa. Granulomata are not seen, and the surrounding intestinal mucosa is usually normal. Internal thickening and thrombosis are seen in vessels around the ulcer, together with perivascular infiltration, but these changes may well be secondary to the inflammatory process.

Ulcers are usually multiple and may per-

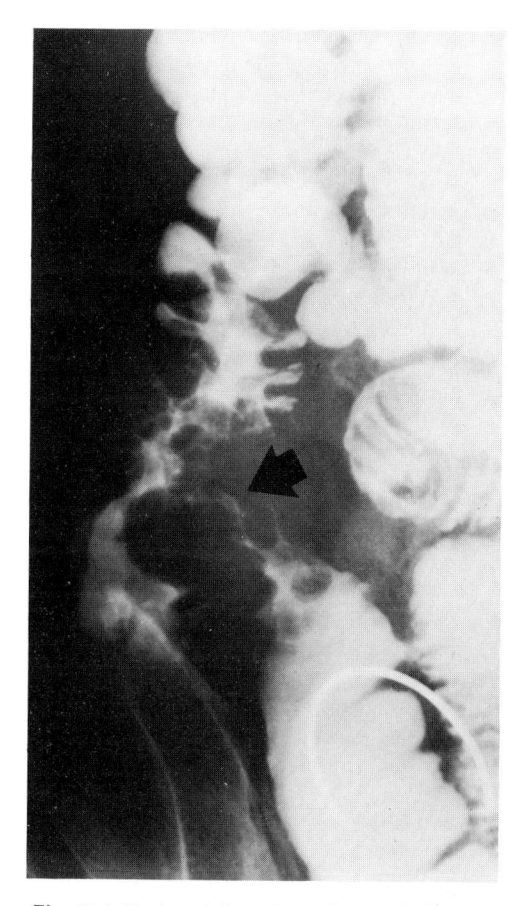

Fig. 12.1. Barium follow-through examination showing ileal involvement in Behçet's syndrome.

forate in more than one site. It has been suggested that at least 100 cm of intestine should be resected to try to prevent recurrence, but postoperative recurrence rates of 65% in 6 months have been described (Kasahara et al. 1981).

An example of Behçet's syndrome with apparent total recovery is illustrated by the following case history.

> A 10-year-old girl developed a mild generalized arthritis and vulval ulcers. Soon she had a low grade iritis and superficial punctate keratitis. The symptoms persisted for 4 years and the course of the illness was interrupted by an attack of acute appendicitis. At laparotomy the terminal ileum was noted to be thickened.

By the age of 16 years she was symptom-free but she then developed erythema nodosum and colicky abdominal pain. Examination of the small intestine by barium follow-through showed a spastic small intestine but at laparotomy no macroscopic abnormality was found. The patient was treated with corticosteroids for 4 years in order to control the erythema nodosum. She was now suffering from recurrent aphthous ulceration of the mouth. Two years after stopping steroids she presented with episodic bleeding per rectum. Barium follow-through again showed an irregular terminal ileum. This was resected at Hammersmith Hospital and found to contain one large and two small punched-out ulcers. Histologically there was dense lymphocytic infiltration of the ulcerated area. Lymphatics were dilated and there were focal collections of lymphocytes just outside the muscularis. There was no evidence of a primary vasculitis. Since the operation she has remained well. She has been asymptomatic for 10 years, has married and is the mother of two children.

Primary ulcer

The term 'primary ulcer' is used to describe a benign ulcer occurring in the small intestine distal to the duodenum for which no cause is found. Ulcers may be single, more rarely multiple, and are located in either jejunum or ileum, with a slight preponderance for the ileum. Primary ulceration may occur at any age but is more common in males (Keen 1958). Pathologically there are no specific features, although the lesion resembles that of a peptic ulcer. The size usually ranges from 0.5–4.0 cm (Morlock et al. 1956). Many ulcers perforate and stricture formation may also occur, leading to chronic obstruction. No known cause has yet been established. There is no evidence of ectopic gastric or pancreatic mucosa, no suggestion of obstructive vascular lesions and no indication that trauma is involved.

Clinical features

Many patients with primary ulcer of the small intestine are first seen with complications such as perforation, obstruction or haemorrhage (Berry & Dailey 1940). There may, however, be preceding symptoms of postprandial central, low grade abdominal pain, sometimes associated with vomiting. The diagnosis is often difficult. In the absence of complications, it is unusual to recognize a primary ulcer by standard clinical or radiological techniques. More frequently, the diagnosis is only made at laparotomy, carried out on account of complications.

Treatment

The treatment of primary ulcer of the small intestine is usually surgical (Morlock et al. 1956). The segment of small intestine containing the ulcer should be resected since it is not usually possible immediately to determine whether or not the lesion is malignant. The prognosis is usually good.

Acute jejunitis (Hertzberg 1954)

Acute jejunitis is a rare but serious disease. It has been described particularly in Norway and in Germany during the Second World War but sporadic cases have been described elsewhere. There is inflammation of the entire circumference of the jejunum. The serosa is red, congested and has a fibrin coating, so that at laparotomy the upper intestine appears thickened and plum-coloured. Segments of the intestinal wall may become necrotic. Histologically there is acute inflammation, most pronounced in the submucosa, with infiltration of the mucosa, submucosa and muscularis with polymorphonuclear leucocytes. Although clostridium infection has been postulated as a cause of the condition, bacteriological findings have been inconstant. The cause of the condition remains unknown.

Clinical features

Patients may complain of previous dyspepsia, and there may be diarrhoea. Pain is constant, occurring in the epigastrium and more generally all over the abdomen. There is frequent nausea and vomiting with both haematemesis and melaena. Diarrhoea occurs in 50% of cases. The abdomen is tender and there may be signs suggesting peritonitis. Blood can always be demonstrated in the faeces. Radiological examination reveals thickening of the intestinal wall but there is usually no obstruction. Laparotomy is indicated to establish the diagnosis and limited resection should be undertaken if there is gangrene or severe ulceration with intestinal haemorrhage. The prognosis is serious, mortality rates of 50% being reported. The condition appears to be quite distinct from Crohn's disease. If recovery occurs, it is complete.

Idiopathic mucosal enteropathy (Syn. Idiopathic chronic ulcerative enteritis, chronic ulcerative non-granulomatous jejunoileitis, non-responsive coeliac disease, unclassified sprue)

Nomenclature

Non-specific small bowel ulceration associated with malabsorption has been described since 1949 (Nyman 1947, Goulston et al. 1965, Jefferies et al. 1968, Mills et al. 1980, Baer et al. 1980). The disorder is rare. It occurs in middle age and at presentation frequently mimics adult coeliac disease since the jejunal biopsy usually reveals severe mucosal atrophy and there is malabsorption. The patients do not usually improve, except partially, with treatment with a gluten-free diet and their condition may deteriorate inexorably until death, which is frequently the result of progressive and extensive small intestinal ulceration. Since coeliac disease, by definition, improves on treatment with a gluten-free diet (see Chapter 9), the term 'non-responsive coeliac disease' is inappropriate to describe this condition.

The intestinal mucosal lesion is also different from that of coeliac disease in other ways. It may be patchy, with normal areas of intestine being found. In contrast to the predominantly jejunal lesion in coeliac disease, in which there is primary damage to the enterocytes with a compensatory hyperplasia of crypt cells, a situation analogous to that in haemolytic anaemia, in these patients there is some evidence to suggest that there is hypoplasia of the crypts of Lieberkühn, analogous to the situation in aplastic anaemia. Furthermore, the lesion is not confined to the jejunum, as is usually the case in coeliac disease, since there are frequently abnormalities in the ileum and in some instances also in the colon.

Intestinal ulceration is a frequent feature and usually involves both jejunum and ileum. Ulceration of the intestine, however, is not specific for this condition because it may also occur in coeliac disease, although here it is usually the jejunum that is involved (Bayless et al. 1977, Baer et al. 1980). Strictures may also develop, presumably as a result of fibrosis around areas of ulceration. The observation that strictures in the small intestine may occur in both coeliac disease and in non-coeliacs suggests that ulceration and stricture are secondary to mucosal damage, whatever the primary cause.

A subepithelial layer of collagen in the intestinal mucosa which may be marked in severe cases is a further feature of this condition (Neale 1968, Weinstein et al. 1970). Again the presence of subepithelial collagen is non-specific, because it is described in patients with untreated coeliac disease, in whom it may disappear following successful treatment with a gluten-free diet (Bossart et al. 1975, Cluysenar & van Tongeren 1977). Subepithelial collagen is simply a marker of an inflammatory process, whatever its cause.

The nomenclature used to describe this condition is controversial. Many writers have concentrated on the ulceration of the intestine that so frequently occurs in patients with jejunal mucosal atrophy not responding to a gluten-free diet who also develop intestinal ulceration, and have therefore used terms such as 'idiopathic chronic ulcerative enteritis' or 'chronic ulcerative non-granulomatous jejunoileitis' to describe the

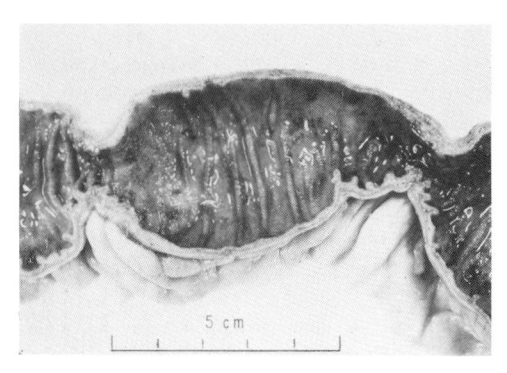

Fig. 12.2. Autopsy specimen of multiple stricutres of the jejunum in a patient with a flat jejunal mucosa and malabsorption, unresponsive to treatment with a gluten-free diet, after an operation to close a perforated ulcer of the jejunum (Neale 1970).

condition. This is probably an incorrect emphasis since there is little evidence of inflammation, except in the immediate vicinity of the ulcers. Furthermore, it seems likely that the ulceration is secondary to primary intestinal mucosal damage. We believe that it is more appropriate at this time to use a term which emphasizes the primary mucosal abnormality. In the absence of any real knowledge of aetiology we suggest 'idiopathic mucosal enteropathy (IME)' to describe the condition from which these unfortunate patients suffer. This is not intended to imply that there is always a diffuse mucosal abnormality in every patient, since it is evident that sometimes the mucosal abnormality may be patchy.

Aetiology

There is no known aetiology and the pathogenesis is uncertain. There have, however, been rare reports of individuals with apparent coeliac disease who have responded partially to treatment with a gluten-free diet initially but who have then undergone severe unremitting relapse on exposure to even small amounts of gluten (Neale 1968). In other patients, careful pathological examination of the ulcerated areas may reveal evidence of malignant histiocytosis (Isaacson & Wright 1978). Robertson et al. (1983) suggest that diffuse small intestinal ulceration with malabsorption represents a 'spectrum of disorders with an inconsistent relationship to gluten sensitivity and small intestinal lymphoma'.

Clinical findings

Patients with IME usually present with severe diarrhoea and steatorrhoea. The diarrhoea becomes chronic and continuous. The patient loses weight and becomes progressively malnourished. There is usually an anaemia, due to both iron and folate deficiency. The serum albumin falls and oedema may develop. If steatorrhoea is severe, hypocalcaemia and hypomagnasaemia may cause tetany. Zinc deficiency has also been described in such patients and in a single instance a remarkable response to treatment with zinc supplements has been recorded (Elmes et al. 1976). As the disorder progresses, evidence of intestinal ulceration may become apparent. There may be abdominal distension and severe episodes of abdominal pain. Intestinal perforation and melaena due to ulceration may occur, necessitating laparotomy and removal of ulcerated segments of small intestine. Strictures also develop (Fig. 12.2) causing symptoms of chronic intestinal obstruction. The disease progresses over a period of 1–5 years and most patients die in a state of chronic inanition or malnutrition, frequently following surgical intervention for intestinal perforation, stricture or haemorrhage.

Radiology

Ulcerated small intestine is rarely demonstrated by routine radiological studies in these patients. More frequently, barium follow-through examination reveals a featureless small intestine, the usually feathery pattern being lost and replaced by a 'hosepipe' appearance (Pink & Creamer 1967). Strictures are sometimes demonstrated.

Intestinal mucosa

Jejunal biopsies usually show a severe degree of villous atrophy and the surface enterocytes are markedly flattened and in some instances scarcely seen. Subepithelial collagen may be dense. Crypts may be reduced in number and mitotic figures absent. On the other hand there are also patients in whom only partial villous atrophy is found (Robertson et al. 1983). The mucosal lesion may also be patchy, since normal villi may be found in areas of the intestine distant from the ulcerated areas (Modigliani et al. 1979). Studies of the ileum in such patients, either at laparotomy or at autopsy, often show changes as severe as in the jejunum and in some instances a virtual absence of crypts has been described (Hourihane 1963, Cluysenar & van Tongeren 1977), suggesting that in contrast to the hyper-regenerative mucosa of coeliac disease, the mucosa in IME is hypoplastic. Further evidence that the mucosa is not regenerating normally is provided from studies, using intubation techniques, of the loss into the gut lumen of DNA derived from the normal turnover of cells in the intestinal epithelium. Whereas the loss of DNA into the gut is increased in coeliac disease, Barry et al. (1970) showed a reduced DNA loss in a single patient with IME. Furthermore, Jones & Peters (1977) have shown that in five patients with 'unresponsive coeliac disease' the incorporation of a radioactive precursor into DNA by jejunal biopsies kept in tissue culture is markedly reduced. By contrast, coeliac biopsies demonstrate, as would be expected of a regenerating mucosa, an enhanced turnover as evidenced by incorporation of increased amounts of labelled DNA precursor.

There is, therefore, evidence to suggest that hypoplasia of the enteroblasts is the basic abnormality in at least some patients. This leads to a markedly reduced production of enterocytes, often to a severely flattened mucosa, and there may be total loss of villi. Under such circumstances, ulceration of the small intestine follows.

The cause of the reduced enteropoiesis remains uncertain. It is unknown whether there is inhibition of the response of intestinal regulatory peptides such as enteroglucagon which are markedly enhanced in coeliac disease (Chapter 9). In some cases, retrospective histological examination has revealed atypical histiocytic cells in the ulcerated areas of intestine, as well as in other tissues (Isaacson & Wright 1978). In such patients the diagnosis of IME may readily be confused with that of malignant histiocytosis. It is therefore important that the pathologist seek assiduously for evidence of malignancy in tissue obtained from these patients. In the eight patients with small intestinal ulceration reported by Robertson et al. (1983), three had coeliac disease, two had malabsorption unresponsive to treatment with a gluten-free diet, but the remaining three had malignant histiocytosis.

Treatment and progress

As already indicated, exclusion of gluten from the diet is ineffective, though a gluten-free diet must be instituted at the outset since the failure to respond often establishes the diagnosis. Corticosteroids (prednisone or prednisolone in initial dosage of 40–80 mg/day reducing gradually to a maintenance dose of 10–20 mg/day) have usually proved only temporarily helpful. An indication of the progressive and intractable nature of this disorder is given by the following account of a patient with malabsorption who had apparently been in good health on a gluten-free diet but who relapsed after inadvertent gluten ingestion, developing severe and progressive villous atrophy and malabsorption that led to his death. He also had a cutaneous vasculitis.

> At the age of 36, H.S. had presented with malabsorption and a mild megaloblastic anaemia. He was treated with a gluten-free diet for a 10-year period but at the end of this time a jejunal biopsy still showed partial villous atrophy. A year later he developed epigastric discomfort for which he was treated with Nulacin, an antacid with a flour base. He then had a severe relapse, with marked steatorrhoea, diarrhoea and loss of weight. Despite treatment with a strict gluten-free diet within a metabolic unit, his condition deteriorated and steatorrhoea became so severe that he was excreting as much as 70 g of fat daily. His jejunal biopsy is shown in Fig. 12.3.

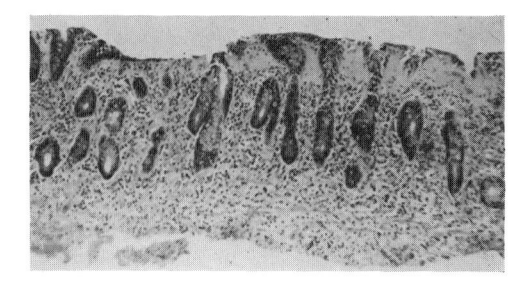

Fig. 12.3. Severe villous atrophy in a patient with malabsorption unresponsive to treatment with a gluten-free diet. There is dense collagen beneath the grossly abnormal enterocytes (Neale 1968).

There was a dense layer of collagen beneath the enterocytes and severe villous atrophy. Despite a milk-free diet, prednisone and a period on a total protein-free diet, his condition steadily deteriorated over the next 12 months. He was then intermittently fed intravenously and for the last 3 months of his life received total parenteral nutrition. Despite all these measures, his condition inexorably progressed until his death of septicaemia after 18 months. During the last 6 months of his life he developed a cutaneous arteritis and evidence of cryoglobulinaemia. Autopsy revealed marked thinning of the small intestine and there was extensive superficial ulceration of the jejunum. Arteritis was restricted to the skin, no vascular lesions being present in the gastrointestinal tract (Neale 1968).

This report illustrates the serious problems which may develop during the treatment of these patients. Nevertheless, continued parenteral feeding must clearly offer patients with this often fatal condition some hope and it is worth trying if all else fails. Early resection of ulcerated lesions has also been claimed to be beneficial.

Pre-stomal ileitis

In patients with prolonged and chronic obstruction at an ileostomy opening, ulceration of the terminal ileum may develop. Morson & Dawson (1979) have described linear, deep and clear-cut ulcers in the ileum but the intervening mucosa is histologically normal. There may be a variable degree of granulomatous reaction but the lesions are not thought to be typical of Crohn's disease. The condition should be suspected in patients with ileostomy dysfunction who have excessive loss of ileostomy effluent. Thayer & Spiro (1962) demonstrated that prestomal ileitis is characterized by the development of profuse watery discharge days or years after an ileostomy has been constructed. There may also be a systemic reaction with pyrexia, tachycardia and anaemia. Perforation may occur, but is rare. The clinical and pathological findings have been reviewed by Knill-Jones *et al.* (1970).

References

Aoki K., Fujioka K. & Katsumata H. (1971) 100 cases of Behçet's disease in Hokkaido *Jap. J. Clin. Ophthalmol.* **25**, 1751–1754.

Asakura H., Morita A., Morishita T., Tsuchiya M., Watanabe Y. & Enomoto Y. (1973) Histopathological and electron microscopic studies of lymphangiectasia of the small intestine in Behçet's disease. *Gut*, **14**, 196–201.

Baba S., Maruta M., Ando K., Tatsuo T. & Endo I. (1976) Intestinal Behçet's disease: report of five cases. *Dis. Colon Rectum*, **19**, 428–440.

Baer A.N., Bayless T.M. & Yardley J.H. (1980) Intestinal ulceration and malabsorption syndromes. *Gastroenterol.* **79**, 754–765.

Barry R.E., Morris J.S. & Read A.E.A. (1970) A case of small intestinal mucosal atrophy. *Gut*, **11**, 743–747.

Bayless T.M., Baer A., Yardley J.H. & Hendrix T.R. (1977) Intestinal ulceration, flat mucosa and malabsorption. Report of registry of 33 patients. In *Perspectives in Coeliac Disease,* (Ed. by B. McNicholl, C.F. McCarthy & P.F. Fottrell) pp. 311–312. M.T.P. Press, Lancaster.

Berry L.H. & Dailey U.G. (1940) Primary ulcer of the jejunum. *Amer. J. Digest. Dis.* **7**, 63–65.

Bøe J., Dalgaard J.B. & Scott D. (1958) Mucocutaneous-ocular syndrome with intestinal involvement. *Amer. J. Med.* **25**, 857-867.

Bossart R., Henry K., Booth C.C. & Doe W.F. (1975) Subepithelial collagen in intestinal malabsorption. *Gut*, **16**, 18–22.

Chajek T. & Fainaru M. (1975) Behçet's disease: report of 41 cases and a review of the literature. *Medicine*, **54**, 179–196.

Chamberlain M.A. (1980) Behçet's syndrome as seen in England. *Haematologica*, **65**, 384–389.

Cluysenar O.J.J. & van Tongeren J.H.M. (1977) *Malabsorption in Coeliac Sprue,* p. 228. Martinus Nijhoff, The Hague.

Denman A.M., Fralkow P.J., Pelton B.K., Salo, A.C., Appleford D.J. & Gilchrist C. (1980) Lymphocyte abnormalities in Behçet's syndrome. *Clin. Exp. Immunol.* **42**, 175–185.

Eglin R.P., Lehner T. & Subak-Sharpe J.H. (1982) Detection of RNA complementary to herpes-simplex virus in mononuclear cells from patients with Behçet's syndrome and recurrent oral ulcers. *Lancet*, **ii**, 1356–1361.

Elmes M., Golden M.K. & Love A.H.G. (1976) Unresponsive coeliac disease. *Quart. J. Med.* **45**, 696–697.

Feigenbaum A. (1956) Description of Behçet's syndrome in the Hippocratic third book of endemic diseases. *Brit. J. Ophthalmol.* **40**, 355–357.

Goulston S.J., Skyring A.P. & McGovern V.J. (1965) Ulcerative jejunitis associated with malabsorption. *Aust. Ann. Med.* **14**, 57–64.

Haim S., Sobel J.D., Friedmann-Birnbaum R. & Lichtig C. (1976) Histological and direct immunofluorescence study of cutaneous hyperreactivity in Behçet's disease. *Brit. J. Dermatol.* **95**, 631–636.

Hertzberg J. (1954) Jejunitis acuta. *Acta Chir. Scand.* **194**, Suppl., 1–151.

Hourihane D. O'B. (1963) The histology of intestinal biopsies. *Proc. Roy. Soc. Med.* **56**, 1073–1077.

Isaacson P. & Wright D.M. (1978) Malignant histiocytosis of the intestine. Its relationship to malabsorption and ulcerative jejunitis. *Hum. Pathol.* **9**, 661–677.

Jefferies G.H., Steinberg H. & Sleisenger M.H. (1968) Chronic ulcerative (nongranulomatous) jejunitis. *Amer. J. Med.* **44**, 47–59.

Jones P.E. & Peters T.J. (1977) DNA synthesis by jejunal mucosa in responsive and non-responsive coeliac disease. *Brit. Med. J.* **i**, 1130–1131.

Kasahara Y., Tanaka S., Nishino M., Umemura H., Shiraha S. & Kuyama T. (1981) Intestinal involvement in Behçet's disease. *Dis. Colon Rectum*, **24**, 103–106.

Keen G. (1958) Simple ulcer of the small intestine. *Brit. J. Surg.* **45**, 652–655.

Knill-Jones R.P., Morson B. & Williams R. (1970) Prestomal ileitis: clinical and pathological findings in five cases. *Quart. J. Med. N.S.*, **39**, 287–297.

Lehner T. & Batchelor J.R. (1979) Classification and an immunogenetic basis of Behçet's syndrome. In *Behçet's Syndrome: Clinical and Immunological Features*, pp. 13–32. (Ed. by T. Lehner & C.C. Barnes) Academic Press, London.

Mills P.R., Brown I.L. & Watkinson G. (1980) Idiopathic chronic ulcerative enteritis. *Quart. J. Med.* **49**, 133–149.

Modigliani R., Poitras P., Galian A., Messing B., Guyet-Rousset P., Libeskind M., Piel-Desruisseaux J.L. & Rambaud J.C. (1979) Chronic non-specific ulcerative duodenojejunoileitis: report of four cases. *Gut*, **20**, 318–328.

Morlock C.G., Goehrs H.R. & Dockerty M.B. (1956) Primary non-specific ulcers of the small intestine: a clinicopathologic study of 18 cases with follow-up of 14 previously reported cases. *Gastroenterol.* **31**, 667–680.

Morson B.C. & Dawson I.M.P. (1979) *Ileostomy Dysfunction.* In *Gastrointestinal Pathology* 2nd ed., pp. 318–319 Blackwell Scientific Publications, Oxford.

Müftüoglu A.Ü. (1980) Symposium on the haematological and immunological aspects of Behçet's disease. *Haematologica*, **65**, 374–380.

Nilsen K.H., Jones S.M. & Shorey B.A. (1977) Behçet's syndrome with perforation of the colon. *Postgrad. Med. J.* **53**, 108–110.

Neale G. (1970) A case of malabsorption, intestinal mucosal atrophy and ulceration, cirrhosis and emphysema. *Brit. Med. J.* **3**, 207–212.

Neale G. (1968) A case of coeliac disease resistant to treatment. *Brit. Med. J.* **ii**, 678–684.

Nyman E. (1947) Ulcerative jejuno-ileitis with symptomatic sprue. *Acta Med. Scand.* **134**, 275–283.

O'Duffy J.D. (1974) Suggested criteria for the diagnosis of Behçet's disease. *Proc. 6th Pan American Congress on Rheumatic Disease.* J. Rheumatol, 1, Suppl. 1, p.18.

O'Duffy J.D. (1981) Behçet's disease. In *Textbook of Rheumatology*, Chapter 74 (Ed. by W.N. Kelley, E.D. Harris, Jr, S. Ruddy & C.B. Sledge). W.B. Saunders Co., Philadelphia.

Oshima Y., Shimizu T., Yokohari R., Matsumoto T., Kano K., Kagami T., & Nagayan H. (1963) Clinical studies on Behçet's syndrome. *Ann. Rheum. Dis.* **22**, 36–45.

Pink I.J. & Creamer B. (1967) Response to a gluten-free diet in the coeliac syndrome. *Lancet*, **i**, 300–304.

Robertson, D.A.F., Dixon M.F., Scott, B.B., Simpson F.G. & Losowsky, M.S. (1983) Small intestinal ulceration: diagnostic difficulties in relation to coeliac disease. *Gut*, **24**, 565–574.

Sladen G.E. & Lehner T. (1979) Gastrointestinal disorders in Behçet's syndrome. In *Behçet's Syndrome: Clinical and Immunological Features*, pp. 151–158. (Ed. by T. Lehner & C.C. Barnes) Academic Press, London.

Thayer W.R. & Spiro H.M. (1962) Ileitis after ileostomy: prestomal ileitis. *Gastroenterol.* **42**, 547–554.

Tüzün Y., Altaç M., Yazici H., Basöz A., Yurdakul S., Pazarli H., Yalcin B. & Müftüoglu A. (1980) Non-specific skin reactivity in Behçet's disease. *Haematologica*, **65**, 395–398.

Weinstein W.M., Saunders D.R., Tytgat G.N. & Rubin C.E. (1970) Collagenous sprue — an unrecognised type of malabsorption. *New Engl. J. Med.* **283**, 1297–1301.

Yazici H., Chamberlain M.A., Schreuder I., D'Amara J. & Müftüoglu M. (1980) HLA antigens in Behçet's disease: a reappraisal by a comparative study of Turkish and British patients. *Ann. Rheum. Dis.* **39**, 344–348.

Chapter 13
Infiltrative Lesions

GRAHAM NEALE AND CHRISTOPHER C. BOOTH

Amyloidosis	218
Systemic sclerosis	221
Eosinophilic gastroenteritis	222
Systemic mastocytosis	225
Malignant infiltration	226
Lipid storage disease	226
Pneumatosis cystoides intestinalis	227

There are a number of generalized systemic disorders associated with infiltration of many organs in the body with abnormal cells or material and in many of these conditions the small intestine may be involved. In most instances the intestinal lesion is part of a generalized abnormality, other organs being involved to a varying degree. In rare instances, however, the small intestine may be the main if not the sole organ involved, in which case the patient may present with symptoms and signs of small intestinal disease without other evidence of the primary pathological abnormality. Such a presentation of amyloidosis or systemic sclerosis, for example, may cause considerable difficulty in diagnosis.

Amyloidosis

Amyloidosis commonly affects the small intestine, often without producing symptoms but sometimes severely affecting absorptive function. The deposition of amyloid is unpredictable. It may be primarily perivascular causing patchy ischaemic damage, perforation (Griffel et al. 1975), bleeding (Levy et al. 1982) or protein-losing enteropathy (Jarnum 1965). It may damage the neuromuscular components, thereby affecting motility (Gilat & Spiro 1968), or it may be largely submucosal with associated malabsorption (Kyle & Bayrd 1975). It may also be deposited in sufficiently large quantities to obstruct the intestine or to simulate malignancy (Johnson et al. 1982).

The nature of amyloid

Amyloid is an extracellular scleroprotein. Under the light microscope it is amorphous, eosinophilic and hyaline. With polarized light it shows a characteristic green birefringence and electron micrography reveals a specific fibrillar structure. There are two basic components. The fibrils consist of twisted anti-parallel β-pleated polypeptide chains, the components of which vary with the cause. In multiple myeloma the polypeptide structure is closely akin to that of immunoglobulin light chains. In the familial varieties of amyloid it is one of a number of variants of pre-albumin, and in amyloidosis secondary to inflammatory disease (including familial Mediterranean fever) it is amyloid A substance.

The fibrils are associated with a glycoprotein, an α_1-globulin designated amyloid P substance. This component is probably derived from a circulating polypeptide, serum amyloid P (SAP), which in turn is structurally related to C-reactive protein. SAP, however, is not an acute phase reactant (Pepys 1982, Falck et al. 1983).

Classification

Amyloidosis has been classified as primary, secondary, heredofamilial, senile, and that related to multiple myeloma. It also occurs locally in some endocrine tumours.

Primary amyloidosis

In the Western world generalized amyloidosis is a rare disease. If there is no apparent underlying cause, the patient is said to have primary amyloidosis and the distribution of amyloid deposits often follows a characteristic pattern involving heart, kidney, gastrointestinal tract, liver and spleen. It is almost certainly due to a pathological process associated with a plasma cell dyscrasia in which the clone of abnormal cells lacks the malignant behaviour of multiple myeloma (Isobe & Osserman 1974, Kyle 1984). Amyloid is deposited principally in the outer coats of small- and medium-sized blood vessels and in the muscle layers of the intestine in both primary amyloidosis and in amyloidosis associated with multiple myeloma (Gilat *et al.* 1969).

Secondary amyloidosis

Inflammatory disorders of prolonged duration, including familial Mediterranean fever and Crohn's disease, have long been recognized as causes of generalized amyloidosis. In the small intestine the deposits of amyloid are found especially within the inner coat of small blood vessels and in the mucosa.

Heredofamilial amyloidosis

Several distinct entities of hereditary generalized amyloidosis have been described (Mahloudji *et al.* 1969). In two of these, type I (Andrade or Portuguese variety) and type III (van Allen or Iowa variety), the small intestine is frequently involved. At autopsy amyloid has been found distributed throughout the muscularis mucosae and the muscular layers with involvement of enteric nerve plexuses (Ikeda *et al.* 1982).

Localized amyloidosis

In the aged, local deposition of amyloid is common. Brain, heart, aorta and pancreas are the organs most frequently affected (Wright *et al.* 1969) and the small intestine is spared. Localized amyloid may also occur in association with endocrine tumours such as medullary carcinoma of the thyroid. Very rarely amyloid appears in single organs of apparently healthy subjects. Such a condition has been found in the small intestine (Long *et al.* 1965, Berardi *et al.* 1973, Griffel *et al.* 1975).

Diagnosis

The diagnosis of amyloidosis depends on histological examination of involved tissue. With generalized disease rectal biopsy is the procedure of choice (Kyle & Bayrd 1975). Occasionally however it may be necessary to examine aspirates from the spleen or biopsies from other organs, including the jejunum (Green *et al.* 1961).

Radiology

The extent and location of involvement of the small intestine in generalized amyloidosis is variable. Thickening of the valvulae conniventes giving the whole small intestine a uniform appearance is said to be the characteristic radiological feature of diffuse submucosal deposits (Marshak & Lindner 1976). On the other hand barium studies of the small intestine may appear normal even when there is extensive involvement with amyloid.

Clinical features

Most patients with generalized amyloidosis do not have prominent gastrointestinal disease even though post-mortem studies usually show some deposits of amyloid in the gut, particularly around blood vessels. There may, however, be wide-ranging effects on structure and function (Brody *et al.* 1984). In the patient presenting with gastrointestinal symptoms but without obvious signs of amyloidosis, the recognition of other features of amyloid disease may be useful in alerting the clinician to the diagnosis. In the nervous system, for example, the patient may complain of symptoms of the carpal tunnel syndrome due to amyloid deposition under the flexor retinaculum or of a peripheral neuropathy secondary to involvement of the vasa nervorum.

Disorders of motility

In the Andrade type of hereditary amyloidosis, there is often progressive peripheral and autonomic neuropathy, and this may involve the small intestine. Several hundred kindreds have been reported especially from

Portugal, Japan and Sweden. The condition has also been described in other countries including Britain. The relentless course of the illness is illustrated by the following case history:

> L.P., an English woman, presented at the age of 25 years with intermittent vomiting and diarrhoea. She had a peripheral neuropathy affecting the lower more than the upper limbs and she later developed an autonomic neuropathy causing marked postural hypotension. Barium follow-through showed mild dilatation of the small intestine. Faecal weight varied between 200−500 g/day but there was no steatorrhoea. Jejunal biopsy was normal. Biopsy of the rectal mucosa revealed amyloidosis for which there was no obvious cause. Concentrations of circulating immunoglobulins were normal and there was no evidence of myeloma. The pattern of illness and subsequent course was typical of type I heredofamilial amyloidosis (Andrade or Portuguese variety). There was no obvious family history of the condition although the patient's father had died suddenly in middle age with a cardiac dysrhythmia, raising the possibility of amyloid heart disease.

The course of the illness was relentlessly progressive. The gastrointestinal symptoms were exacerbated by incontinence. No treatment was of any avail and the patient died after 5 years of unremitting disease. At autopsy there was diffuse organ involvement with amyloidosis including perivascular and perineural deposits in the small intestine (Fig. 13.1) (courtesy of Professor L.A. Turnberg).

Malabsorption

Five to ten per cent of patients with diffuse amyloidosis are reported to have malabsorption (Kyle & Bayrd 1975). Digestive function may be impaired as a result of amyloid infiltration of stomach and pancreas. Disordered motility may lead to bacterial overgrowth in the small intestine and amyloid infiltration of the submucosa of the small intestine may itself hinder absorption. No correlation has been demonstrated between the degree of amyloidosis in biopsies of jejunal mucosa and the impairment of fat absorption (Green et al. 1961). It has been reported that disaccharidase deficiency may occur in association with secondary amyloidosis (Petterson & Wegelius 1972).

Bleeding and protein loss into the small intestine

Gastrointestinal bleeding may occur as a result of ulceration of a localized plaque of amyloid or from small areas of infarction caused by vascular insufficiency. Protein-losing enteropathy has been ascribed to the same mechanisms (Jarnum 1965, Gilat et al. 1969).

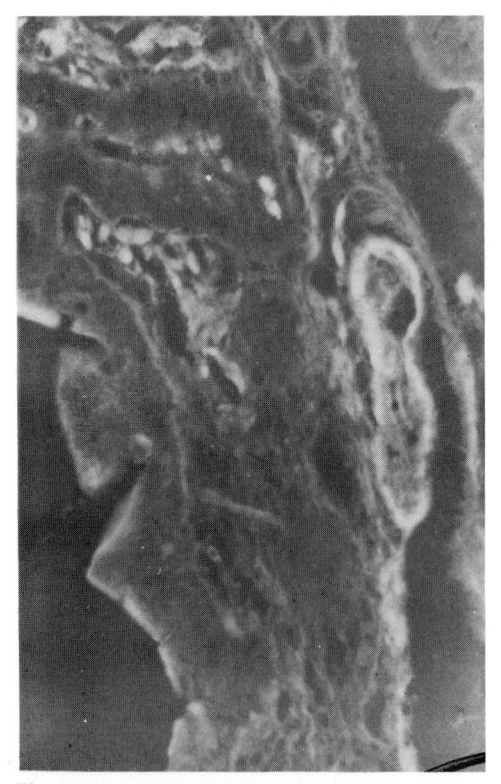

Fig. 13.1. Small intestinal mucosa in amyloidosis. Staining with Thioflavin T showing amyloid deposition around blood vessels and within enterocytes (× 200). (Courtesy of Dr A.W. Jones.)

Intestinal ischaemia and perforation of the small intestine

Amyloid infiltration of the walls of small mesenteric vessel leads to progressive ischaemia and may cause segmental bowel infarction with or without perforation (Gilat et al. 1969). Rupture of the fragile rigid wall of a small intestine which has been largely replaced with amyloid has also been described (Griffel et al. 1975).

Prognosis

The mean survival of patients with generalized amyloidosis is usually less than 2 years. Cardiac or renal failure account for half the mortality. Prognosis may improve as a result of the more vigorous treatment of multiple myeloma and of primary amyloidosis with cytotoxic drugs. Early treatment of the causative disorder in patients with secondary amyloidosis may also improve prognosis. There are occasional reports of regression of amyloid deposits in patients treated successfully (Grigor et al. 1974, Kyle & Bayrd 1975).

Systemic sclerosis

Systemic sclerosis (scleroderma) is a generalized disorder of unknown aetiology involving many organs and characterized by a proliferation of fibrous tissue. It may also be associated with a widespread vasculitis. Whereas the disorder characteristically involves the skin, visceral abnormalities may occur in the absence of skin changes, particularly in the gastrointestinal tract. Oesophageal involvement is a predominant feature of systemic sclerosis, occurring in as many as 80% of patients when the diagnosis is established by sensitive manometric techniques (Neschis et al. 1970). Detailed radiological and functional studies have shown that the small intestine is involved in up to 60% of patients (Bluestone et al. 1969). As with amyloidosis, diffuse small bowel disease causing malabsorption has been described in the absence of involvement of other organs (Leneman et al. 1962).

Pathology

There is diffuse infiltration of the muscle layers of the small intestine with sheets of fibrous tissue, leading to muscular atrophy. The mucosa is usually normal, but occasionally there may be oedema and cellular infiltration of the submucosa and serosa, with eventual fibrosis. Jejunal biopsy, however, is usually normal. The pathological changes result in disordered motility of the small intestine, with dilatation and atony due to failure of peristalsis. Infarction of the ileum and colon have been reported and pneumatosis cystoides intestinalis is a rare complication.

Clinical features

Patients with dermatological lesions may show the characteristic features of Raynaud's syndrome, with tight, shiny, atrophic skin over the fingers and in the face around the mouth and nose. There is often telangiectasia involving the face and hands, and the finger tips may be atrophic with palpable deposits of calcification.

Radiologically the duodenum is almost always dilated, often grossly, and there may be stasis within the intestinal lumen as a result of peristaltic failure. The small intestine may also be diffusely dilated but the lesion is most frequently maximal in the jejunum. There is reduced peristalsis, dilatation and often a characteristic 'spiculation' of the mucosa (Fig. 13.2). Pseudo-diverticula may also be seen. Clinical symptoms do not always correlate well with the severity of radiological changes, extensive dilatation being found in individuals without gastrointestinal symptoms.

There may be bloating, abdominal distension and excessive borborygmi after meals. Most patients with small intestinal involvement develop diarrhoea, but diarrhoea may alternate with constipation. In other patients, obstinate constipation alone may be the major symptom. There is often nausea but rarely vomiting.

Absorption

Malabsorption with steatorrhoea occurs in as

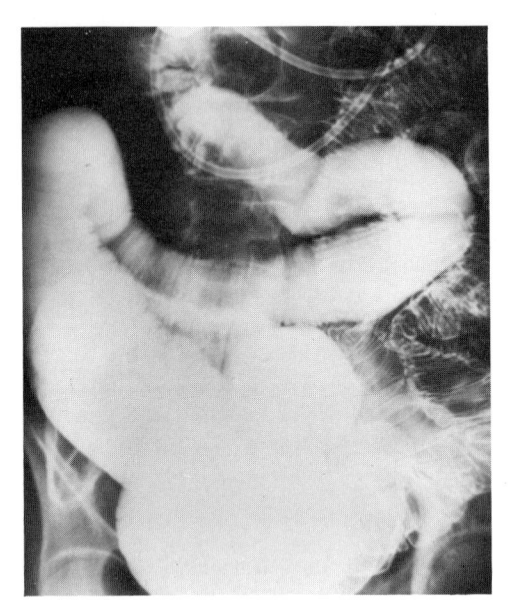

Fig. 13.2. Enteroclysis in systemic sclerosis with small intestinal involvement. There is widespread dilatation. The arrows indicate areas of 'spiculation'. (Courtesy of Dr Sue Barter.)

many as 80% of patients with small bowel involvement. Faecal fat is increased and the absorption of both xylose and vitamin B_{12} (given with intrinsic factor) impaired. In many cases, malabsorption is caused by bacterial overgrowth as a result of intestinal stasis due to the abnormal motility of the small intestine (Chapter 15, Kahn et al. 1966).

Treatment

In patients with documented bacterial overgrowth, treatment with oral broad spectrum antibiotics (tetracycline 1–2 g daily or ampicillin 2 g daily) may rapidly relieve diarrhoea. Faecal fat and vitamin B_{12} absorption may return to normal within a few days. Surgical intervention should be avoided at all costs.

Eosinophilic gastroenteritis

Eosinophilic infiltration of the intestine occurs rarely and usually without apparent cause. In some cases there is evidence of an allergic response either to parasites (Greenberger & Gryboski 1978) or to food antigens (Caldwell et al. 1975, Cello 1979) but more often this is not so.

Aetiology

From the time of the earliest report (Kaijser 1937) many attempts have been made to demonstrate that the eosinophilic infiltration represents an allergic response. In many instances there may be excess circulating eosinophils and atopic disorders such as seasonal rhinitis, asthma, eczema and urticaria may be associated with this condition. An intolerance of specific foodstuffs has been postulated but in general the putative antigen is presumptive and unspecified. Positive skin-prick tests to allergens have been described but the results are usually variable. There is usually a good response to treatment with corticosteroids. In most reported cases the evidence for an allergic cause is weak and contradictory, and some form of allergy has only been adequately demonstrated in less than a quarter of reported cases (Johnstone & Morson 1978a). The direct effect of putative antigens on the small intestinal mucosa has been rarely reported. An increase in tissue eosinophils after meat challenge has been described (Klein et al. 1970) but in the most complete study of a single patient in whom oral challenges with steak or soyabean produced symptoms, significant changes were not found either in villous architecture or in the degree of eosinophilic infiltration. This study was performed meticulously over 2½ years and involved the examination of 303 per-oral biopsies of jejunal mucosa. The evidence suggests that eosinophilic gastroenteritis is usually not a simple allergic process (Leinbach & Rubin 1970).

Pathology

Eosinophilic gastroenteritis occurs mainly in young adults. It causes diffuse thickening of one or more segments of the gut and is characterized by oedematous swelling of the gut wall associated with eosinophilic infiltration. It appears in the medical literature under various pseudonyms including pyloric hypertrophy with eosinophilic infiltration,

Loeffler's syndrome of the gastrointestinal tract, eosinophilic granuloma of the gut, infiltrative eosinophilic gastroenteritis and allergic gastroenteritis. Organs other than the gut may be infiltrated with eosinophils including the prostate, the bladder and the gall bladder (Johnstone & Morson 1978a). The disorder is rare but occurs world-wide.

Differential diagnosis

In appropriate areas it is important to exclude rare parasitic disorders such as *Angiostrongyloidiasis* (Morera 1973), *Anisakiasis* (Marsden 1978) and *Macracanthorhynchus hirudinaceus* (Hemsrichart et al. 1983). On the other hand doubt has been cast on data implicating the larva of *Eustoma rotandatum* (carried in slightly salted raw herring) in eosinophilic disease of the small intestine (Kuipers et al. 1960, Ashby et al. 1964, Williams 1965). Some nematodes present as tumour-like granuloma formations. These are easily recognized in segments of small intestine resected at surgery or during postmortem examination.

It is also important to exclude eosinophil proliferation associated with Crohn's disease, the presence of foreign bodies and malignant conditions such as primary intestinal lymphoma and Hodgkin's disease. Multi-focal eosinophilic granulomata (histiocytosis X) appears not to involve the small intestine although the common bile duct may be affected (Jones et al. 1981). On the other hand 50% of patients with the hyper-eosinophilic syndrome have gastrointestinal symptoms and the pathology of the small intestine may be similar to that of eosinophilic gastritis. This is a multi-system disease and the principal features are endomyocardial fibrosis and thromboembolic disease (Spry et al. 1983).

The putative diagnosis of eosinophilic gastroenteritis is often supported by the finding of elevated levels of circulating eosinophils and confirmed by histological examination of multiple biopsies of jejunal mucosa. The initial findings, however, are not specific. It is usually easy to exclude coeliac disease, radiation enteritis and ischaemic disease but it may be much more difficult to eliminate the possibility of polyarteritis, early Crohn's disease and visceral lymphoma. It is important to remember that the changes in villous architecture and the degree of mucosal eosinophilia vary greatly even in an individual biopsy. Many histological sections should be examined before coming to a conclusion (Leinbach & Rubin 1970).

Clinical features

The clinical manifestations of eosinophilic gastroenteritis are variable. For descriptive purposes it is useful to recognize three forms: mucosal disease, muscle layer disease, and predominantly subserosal disease (Klein et al. 1970).

Mucosal involvement

The mucosa is involved in about 25% of patients with eosinophilic gastroenteritis. Nausea, vomiting and abdominal pain may be presenting symptoms. There is often diarrhoea and loss of weight. Radiology of the small intestine may show non-specific signs such as coarsening and nodularity of mucosal folds and occasionally this is sufficiently marked to give a saw-tooth appearance (Fig. 13.3).

Tests of absorptive function are usually mildly abnormal with some steatorrhoea and frequently evidence of protein-losing enteropathy. In the mucosal form of eosinophilic gastroenteritis there may be evidence of atopic disease. Nevertheless in only occasional cases has it been possible to control the disease solely by use of an elimination diet. Acute exacerbations usually respond well to short periods of corticosteroids (prednisolone 20–40 mg/day for 10 days) and some patients are best maintained on small doses for prolonged periods. Most patients become asymptomatic and the mucosal pattern reverts to normal. Rarely the disease is progressive and fatal.

Muscle involvement

In 50% of patients with eosinophilic gastroenteritis the gut wall is diffusely involved.

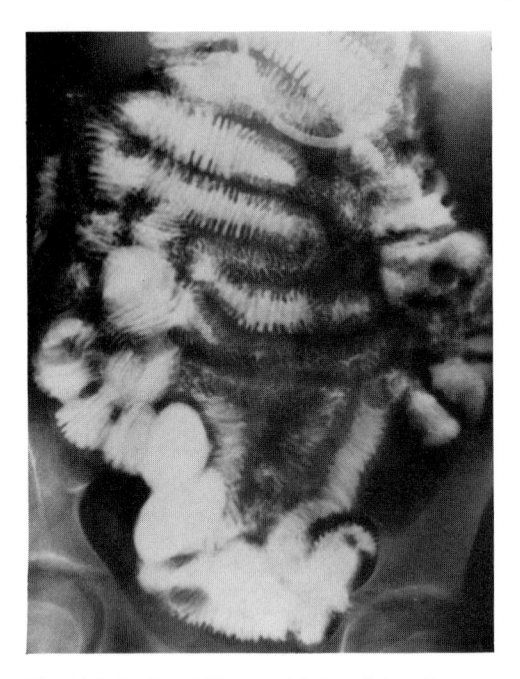

Fig. 13.3. Eosinophilic enteritis involving the small intestine showing 'saw-tooth' appearance. (Courtesy of Dr Sue Barter.)

Patients in this group present in early adult life with nausea, vomiting and abdominal pain.

There is usually a peripheral eosinophilia but the radiological appearances are different from those seen in the mucosal disorder. There is marked rigidity of the affected gut wall often with polypoid filling defects. The gastric antrum is most commonly affected. It is irregularly narrowed with decreased peristalsis and the appearances may simulate those of carcinoma. The lesions in the small intestine may be localized or diffuse. There is extensive thickening and induration of the wall. Some parts may even feel cartilagenous. The mesenteric nodes are hyperplastic and infiltrated with diffuse sheets of mature eosinophilic leucocytes. In approximately two-thirds of cases the changes are limited to antrum and pylorus; in the remaining one-third the small intestine is involved, usually in association with a gastric lesion. Laparotomy is necessary for a firm diagnosis. The symptoms are usually readily controlled with corticosteroids.

Serosal involvement

Less than one in four patients with eosinophilic gastroenteritis have significant involvement of the serosal surface of the small intestine. The serosa is markedly thickened and patients present with ascites. The ascitic fluid contains large numbers of eosinophil leucocytes and clears promptly on treatment with corticosteroids (Klein *et al.* 1970). Eosinophils and mast cells may also infiltrate the lamina propria of the small intestine in patients with collagen-vascular disorders. This infiltrate may be a cause of intestinal dysfunction (De Schryver-Kecskemeti & Clouse 1984).

Eosinophilic pseudo-tumoral enterocolitis

Enterocolitis with a massive infiltration of eosinophils has been recently described in a young woman from the Antilles. The course of the illness was dominated by the formation of tumour-like granulomata in both the large and small intestine associated with bleeding and protein-losing enteropathy. This may be a florid form of eosinophilic gastroenteritis but the disease was totally unresponsive to treatment with corticosteroids. The patient was well for a year after colectomy but then developed ulcerating tumours in the ileostomy and died after an illness which lasted 6 years (Malè *et al.* 1983).

Localized eosinophilic granuloma (inflammatory fibroid polyp)

Infiltration with eosinophils is often a prominent feature of inflammatory fibroid polyps of the gastrointestinal tract. The original report described 'circumscribed granuloma with eosinophilic infiltration' (Vanek 1949). The condition has been confused with eosinophilic gastroenteritis but should be regarded as a separate entity (Johnstone & Morson 1978b). It affects both sexes in the age range 40–60 years. Usually there is no peripheral eosinophilia and no evidence of allergy. The lesions are firm and well circumscribed. They occur most commonly in the stomach close to the pylorus and less often in the small and large intestine. In the small intestine they may cause obstructive symptoms often with a tendency to intussusception. Ileal lesions may mimic acute appendicitis (Salmon & Paulley 1967). The condition is cured by surgical resection.

Systemic mastocytosis

Gastrointestinal symptoms occur in 50% of patients with systemic mastocytosis. Proliferation of mast cells occurs most frequently in skin (as urticaria pigmentosa), bones and lymph nodes, but also may affect any parenchymatous organ including the small intestine. Mast cells produce, store and liberate histamine, heparin, kinins and serotonin. These may act locally in the intestine (paracrine effect) or by an endocrine process. Dyspepsia due to peptic ulceration and diarrhoea are the major gastroenterological problems.

Involvement of the small intestine may be suspected radiologically. Characteristically there is increased rugosity of the gastric

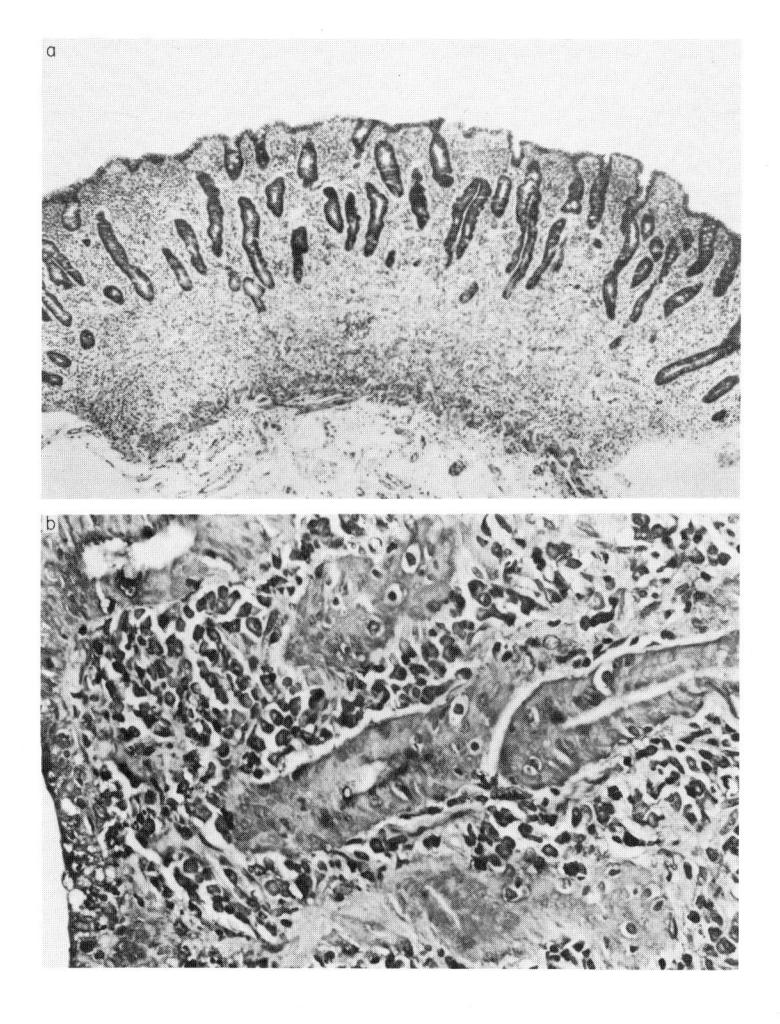

Fig. 13.4. Small intestine in mast cell disease. (a) Jejunal biopsy showing subtotal villous atrophy and cellular infiltration (H & E × 10). (b) Mast cells (darkly stained) (Toluidine Blue × 160). (Courtesy of Professor M.S. Losowsky.)

mucosa associated with nodular filling defects in the small intestine (especially the duodenum) (Clemett *et al.* 1968). The infiltration with mast cells may be seen in biopsies of the jejunal mucosa (Fig. 13.4). Usually there is marked submucosal oedema (Scott *et al.* 1975).

The diarrhoea of systemic mastocytosis is usually copious and watery. More rarely there is intestinal malabsorption with steatorrhoea (Broitman *et al.* 1970). In some cases it has been related to gastric hypersecretion as in the Zollinger−Ellison syndrome; but it may also be due to the direct secretory effects of other mast cell products including prostaglandin D2 (Poynard *et al.* 1982).

Treatment with oral disodium cromoglycate is moderately effective in controlling symptoms (Soter *et al.* 1979). The prognosis is variable. In children the mastocytosis frequently disappears at puberty; in adults the disease may become extremely long-standing with persistent diarrhoea for 40 years or more (Mahood *et al.* 1982). A proportion of patients develop a rapidly progressive lymphoma or myeloproliferative disorder with fatal consequences.

Malignant infiltration

Lymphoma, α-chain disease and tumours of the small intestine are described in Chapters 10 and 22.

Leukaemia

Leukaemia not infrequently involves the gastrointestinal tract especially in the later stages of the disease. The infiltrating cells may form nodules, plaques or polyps with or without diffuse infiltration. The stomach, ileum and colon are most frequently affected. With ileocolonic involvement secondary bacterial or fungal infection is common. It may be associated with local ulceration of deposits or a more diffuse leukaemic ileocolitis. Bleeding, perforation and intussusception of the small intestine are complications of involvement of the small intestine by leukaemic cells (Sherman *et al.* 1973).

Vigorously treated leukaemia is now recognized as the commonest cause of neutropenic enterocolitis, a condition which also occurs in cyclic neutropenia (Wright *et al.* 1981) and drug-induced agranulocytosis (Braye *et al.* 1982). Recent evidence implicates infection with *Clostridium septicum* in the pathogenesis of neutropenic ileocolitis. In patients at risk active immunization may be justified (King *et al.* 1984).

Waldenström's macroglobulinaemia

In this condition, which is due to an IgM monoclonal gammopathy, proteinaceous material may accumulate in lacteals and in the lamina propria of the villi of the small intestine (Fig. 13.5).

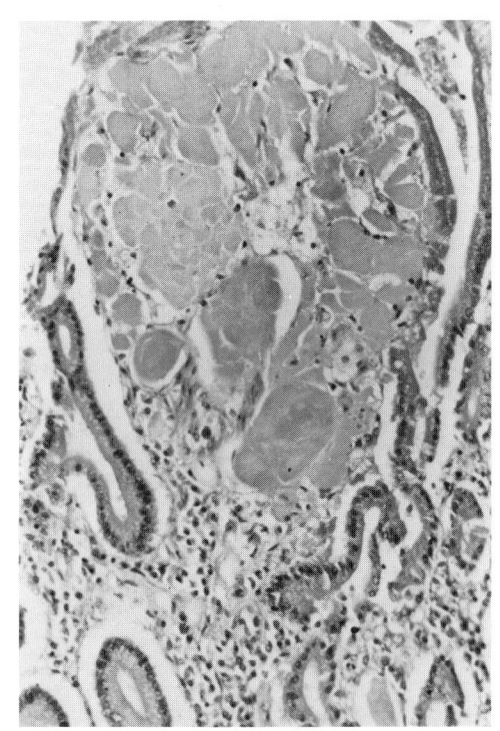

Fig. 13.5. Waldenström's macroglobulinaemia showing the distended villi filled with amorphous eosinophilic material representing deposition of immunoglobulin (H & E × 315). (Courtesy of Dr. A.B. Price.)

Lipid storage disease

Three familial lipid storage diseases (Tangier

disease, Wolman's disease and cholesterol ester storage disease) are characterized by accumulation of cholesterol ester and carotenes in parenchymatous organs. The liver and spleen are predominantly affected.

In Tangier disease (circulating alpha-lipoprotein deficiency) the intestinal mucosa appears normal under the light microscope and there are no gastrointestinal symptoms. Peripheral neuropathy is the major feature of the disease.

In Wolman's disease (lysosomal acid esterase deficiency) the intestinal mucosa is infiltrated with fat-laden histocytes. Affected infants have persistent diarrhoea and rarely survive for more than a year.

Cholesterol ester storage disease is also associated with a deficiency of lysozymal acid esterase but is a much more benign condition. The lamina propria of the small intestine is infiltrated with cholesterol ester and carotenes giving the mucosal surface a distinct orange tinge. Lipid droplets accumulate alongside the endothelium of lacteals, in mucosal smooth muscle and in vascular pericytes. It is postulated that there is a block in the transport of cholesterol into lacteals independent of the plasma lipoprotein system (Partin & Schubert 1969). The condition is extremely rare and although affected subjects have hepatosplenomegaly they are usually healthy and do not have steatorrhoea (Schiff et al. 1968).

Pneumatosis cystoides intestinalis

This is a benign rare condition affecting the small intestine, mesentery and omentum and sometimes the colon. Gas appears to infiltrate along tissue planes and accumulates in cysts which are usually lined by endothelial cells. These cells aggregate and they may form giant cells. The surrounding connective tissue is inflamed and accumulates lymphocytes, plasma cells, eosinophils and occasionally epithelioid cells which form into granulomata. Disappearance of cysts may be preceded by a progressive fibrotic reaction.

Aetiology

The cause is unknown. It occurs at any age and more frequently in males than females. About two-thirds of reported cases have co-existent gastrointestinal disease of which peptic ulceration is the most common. It has been described with most inflammatory diseases of the small intestine, with intestinal ischaemia and after bowel anastomosis (Table 13.1) (Ghahremani et al. 1974). Acute or chronic obstructive airways disease is associated with most of the cases without gastrointestinal pathology.

Table 13.1. Conditions associated with pneumatosis cystoides intestinalis.

Gastric	Peptic ulcer
	Ingestion of caustic agents
Small intestine	Crohn's disease
	Whipple's disease
	Jejunal diverticulosis
	Systemic sclerosis
	Idiopathic mucosal enteropathy
	Acute necrotizing enterocolitis
	Parasitic disease
	Lymphoreticular neoplastic disease
	Catheter jejunostomy feeding
Large intestine	Diverticular disease (perforated)
	Ulcerative colitis
	Post sigmoidoscopy (with biopsy)
General	Intestinal obstruction
	Post-intestinal anastomosis
	Mesenteric vascular occlusion
	Abdominal trauma
	Lung disease

Gas is probably forced into tissue spaces in the gut either by peristaltic pressure or by the effort of vomiting. In cases associated with lung disease (Klausen et al. 1982) it is thought that air from emphysematous bullae infiltrates into the mediastinum and dissects along fascial planes or along the course of blood vessels to reach the subserosa of the gut. The condition is nearly always benign and rupture of cysts does not cause peritonitis. The gas is predominantly nitrogen with up to 20% oxygen and 10% carbon dioxide. Very rarely, death from gas embolism associated with pneumatosis has been described (Bonnell & French 1982).

Pneumatosis occurring in association with ischaemic bowel disease is a more serious event. The cysts may contain gas-forming bacteria and gas may enter the portal venous system, usually with fatal consequences (Chapter 20) (Scott et al. 1971).

Clinical features

In most cases symptoms are non-specific. Patients complain of cramping abdominal pain, recurrent diarrhoea and the passage of mucus. Rarely the intestine obstructs. The diagnosis is usually made on the appearances of a simple radiograph of the abdomen. Occasionally there is free gas under the diaphragm, indicating cyst rupture. If the lower colon is involved a characteristic appearance may be seen at sigmoidoscopy. Pale rounded soft masses, often with a bluish tinge, are seen. They may be mistaken for polyps but their structure collapses after biopsy.

A single patient with fatal malabsorption syndrome secondary to pneumatosis cystoides has been described (Yunich & Fradkin 1958).

Treatment

The majority of patients require no specific treatment. Diagnosis is important to prevent unnecessary surgery and to direct the attention of the clinician to finding an underlying cause. The cysts may persist, in which case it is worth trying oxygen therapy. The patient is given oxygen over several days (24 h a day) to raise the partial pressure of the gas in the circulation to 300 mmHg. This reduces the partial pressure of nitrogen in the circulation and promotes diffusion of nitrogen into the surrounding tissue (Down & Castleden 1975 Miralbés et al. 1983). Occasionally surgery may be necessary for obstructive symptoms. Unfortunately pneumatosis has a tendency to recur after resection of involved proximal segments (Witkowski et al. 1955).

References

Abrams G.D., Bauer H. & Sprinz H. (1963) Influence of the normal flora on mucosal morphology and cellular renewal in the ileum. A comparison of germ-free and conventional mice. *Lab. Invest.* **12**, 355–364.

Ashby R.S., Appleton P.J. & Dawson I. (1964) Eosinophilic granuloma of the gastro-intestinal tract caused by herring parasite, Eustoma rotundatum. *Brit. Med. J.* **i**, 1141–1145.

Berardi R.S. & Malette W.G. (1973) Focal amyloidosis of the small bowel mesentery. *Int. Surg.* **58**, 491–494.

Bluestone R., MacMahon M. & Dawson J.M. (1969) Systemic sclerosis and small bowel involvement. *Gut*, **10**, 185–193.

Bonnell H. & French S.W. (1982) Fatal air embolus associated with pneumatosis cystoides intestinales. *Amer. J. Forensic Med. Pathol.* **3**, 69–72.

Braye S.G., Copplestone J.A. & Garrell P.C. (1982) Neutropenic enterocolitis during mianserin-induced agranulocytosis. *Brit. Med. J.* **285**, 1117–1118.

Brody, I.A. Wertlake P.T. & Laster L. (1984) Causes of symptoms in intestinal amyloidosis. *Arch. Int. Med.* **113**, 512–518.

Broitman S.A., McCray R.S., May J.C., Deren J.J., Ackroyd F., Gottlieb L.S., McDermott W. & Zamcheck N. (1970) Mastocytosis and intestinal malabsorption. *Amer. J. Med.* **48**, 382–389.

Caldwell J.H., Tennenbaum J.I. & Brostein H.A. (1975) Serum IgE in eosinophilic gastroenteritis. Response to intestinal challenge in two cases. *New Engl. J. Med.* **292**, 1388–1390.

Cello J.P. (1979). Eosinophilic gastroenteritis — a complex disease entity. *Amer. J. Med.* **67**, 1097–1104.

Clemett A.R., Fishbone G., Levine J., Everette-James A. & Janower M. (1968) Gastrointestinal lesions in mastocytosis. *Amer. J. Roentgenol.* **103**, 405–409.

de Castro C.A., Dockerty M.B. & Mayo C.W. (1957). Metastatic tumours of the small intestine. *Surg. Gynec. Obstet.* **105**, 159–164.

De Schryver-Kecskemeti, K. & Clouse, R.E. (1984) A previously unrecognized subgroup of eosinophilic gastroenteritis. Association with connective tissue diseases. *Amer. J. Surg. Pathol.* **8**, 171–180.

Down R.H.L. & Castleden W.M. (1975). Oxygen therapy for pneumatosis coli. *Brit. Med. J.* **i**, 493–495.

Falck H.M., Maury C.P.J., Teppo A.-M. & Wegelius O. (1983) Correlation of persistently high serum amyloid A protein and C-reative protein. Concentrations with rapid progression of secondary amyloidosis. *Brit. Med. J.* **286**, 1391–1393.

Ghahremani G.G., Port R.B. & Beachley M.C. (1974) Pneumatosis coli in Crohn's disease. *Dig. Dis.* **19**, 315–320.

Gilat T. & Spiro H.M. (1968) Amyloidosis and the gut. *Amer. J. Dig. Dis.* **13**, 619–625.

Gilat T., Revach M. & Sohar E. (1969) Deposition of amyloid in the gastro-intestinal tract. *Gut*, **10**, 98–104.

Goldstein W.B. Poker N. (1966) Multiple myeloma involving the gastrointestinal tract. *Gastro-*

enterol. **51**, 87–93.

Gordon H.A. & Pesti L. (1971) The gnotobiotic animal as a tool in the study of host-microbial relationships. *Bacteriol. Rev.* **35**, 390–429.

Green P.A., Higgins T.A., Brown Jr A.L. & Hoffman H.N. (1961) Appraisal of infiltration biopsy of the small intestine in diagnosis. *Gastroenterol.* **41**, 452–457.

Greenberger N. & Gryboski J.D. (1978) Allergic disorders of the intestine and eosinophilic gastroenteritis. In *Gastrointestinal Disease* (Ed. by Sleisenger M.V. & Fordtran J.S.), p. 1228. W.B. Saunders Co., Philadelphia.

Griffel B., Man B. & Kraus L. (1975). Selective amyloidosis of the small intestine. *Arch. Surg.* **110**, 215–217.

Grigor R.R., Lang W.R. & Nicholson G. (1974) Gut amyloidosis in lepromatous leprosy regressing with therapy. *Lepr. Rev.* **45**, 313–320.

Hemsrichart V., Pichyangkura C., Chitchang S., Yuti Chamnong U. (1983) Eosinophilic enteritis due to Macra-canthorhynchus hirudinaceus infection: report of 3 cases. *J. Med. Assoc. Thai*, **66**, 303–310.

Heneghan J.B. (1963) Influence of microbial flora on xylose absorption in rats and mice. *Amer. J. Physiol.* **205**, 417–420.

Ikeda S.-I., Makishita H., Oguchi K., Yanagisawa N. & Nagata T. (1982) Gastro-intestinal amyloid deposition in familial amyloid polyneuropathy. *Neurol. (NY)* **32**, 1364–1368.

Ingelfinger F.J., Lowell F.C. & Franklin W. (1949) Gastro-intestinal allergy. *New Engl. J. Med.* **241**, 303–308; 337–340.

Leneman F., Fierst S., Gabriel J.B. & Ingegno A.P. (1962) Progressive systemic sclerosis of the intestine presenting as malabsorption syndrome. *Gastroenterol.* **42**, 175–180.

Isobe T. & Osserman E.F. (1974) Patterns of amyloidosis and their association with plasma cell dyscrasia, monoclonal immunoglobulins and Bence-Jones proteins. *New Engl. J. Med.* **290**, 473–477.

Jarnum S. (1965) Gastrointestinal hemorrhage and protein loss in primary amyloidosis. *Gut*, **6**, 14–18.

Johnson D.H., Guthrie T.H., Tedesco F.J., Griffin J.W. & Anthony Jr H.F. (1982) Amyloidosis masquerading as inflammatory bowel disease with a mass lesion simulating a malignancy. *Amer. J. Gastroenterol.* **77**, 141–145.

Johnstone J.M. & Morson B.C. (1978a) Eosinophilic gastroenteritis. *Histopathol.* **2**, 335–348.

Johnstone J.M. & Morson B.C. (1978b) Inflammatory fibroid polyp of the gastro-intestinal tract. *Histopathol.* **2**, 349–361.

Jones M.B., Voet R., Pagani J., Lotysch M., O'Connell T. & Koretz R.L. (1981) Multifocal eosinophilic granuloma involving the common bile duct: histologic and cholangiographic findings. *Gastroenterol.* **80**, 384–389.

Kahn I.J., Jefferies G.H. & Sleisenger M.H. (1966) Malabsorption in intestinal scleroderma. Correction by antibiotics. *New. Engl. J. Med.*, **274**, 1339–1344.

Kaijser R. (1937) Zür kenntnis der allergischen Affektionen des Verdauungs-kanals von Standpumkt des Chirurgen aus. *Archiv. für Klin. Chir.* **188**, 36–64.

King A., Rampling A., Wight D.G.D & Warren R.F. (1984) Neutropenic enterocolitis due to Clostridium septicum infection. *J. Clin. Path.* **37**, 335–343.

Klausen N.O., Agner E., Tongaard L. & Sørensen B. (1982) Pneumatosis cystoides coli in chronic respiratory failure. *Brit. Med. J. (Clin. Res.)* **284**, 1834–1835.

Klein N.C., Hargrove R.I., Sleisenger M.H. & Jefferies G.H. (1970) Eosinophilic gastroenteritis. *Medicine*, **49**, 299–319.

Kuipers F.C., van Thiel P.H., Rodenburg W., Wielinga W.J. & Roskam R.T.H. (1960) Eosinophilic phlegmon of the alimentary tract caused by a worm. *Lancet*, **ii**, 1171–1173.

Kyle R.A. (1984) 'Benign' monoclonal gammopathy. A misnomer? *J.A.M.A.* **251**, 1849–1854.

Kyle R.A. & Bayrd E.D. (1975) Amyloidosis: review of 236 cases. *Medicine*, **54**, 271–299.

Leinbach G.E. & Rubin C.E. (1970) Eosinophilic gastroenteritis: A simple reaction to food allergens? *Gastroenterol.* **59**, 874–889.

Leneman F., Fierst S., Gabriel J.B. & Ingegno A.P. (1962) Progressive systemic sclerosis of the intestine presenting as malabsorption syndrome. *Gastroenterol.* **42**, 175–180.

Levy D.J., Franklin G.O. & Rosenthal W.S. (1982) Gastro-intestinal bleeding and amyloidosis. *Amer. J. Gastroenterol.* **77**, 422–426.

Long L., Mahoney T.D. & Newell W.R. (1965) Selective amyloidosis of the jejunum: case report of a rare cause for gastro-intestinal bleeding. *Amer. J. Surg.* **109**, 217–220.

Mahloudji M., Teasdell R.D., Adamkiewicz J.J., Hartmann W.H., Lambird P.A., & McKusick V.A. (1969) The genetic amyloidoses. *Medicine*, **48**, 1–37.

Mahood J.M., Harrington C.L., Slater D.N. & Corbett C.L. (1982) Forty years of diarrhoea in a patient with urticaria pigmentosa. *Acta Dermatol.-Venereol.* **62**, 264–265.

Malè P.J., de Toledo F., Widgren S., de Peyer R. & Berthoud S. (1983) Pseudo tumoral enterocolitis and massive eosinophilia. *Gut*, **24**, 345–350.

Marsden P.D. (1978) Other nematodes. *Clin. Gastroenterol.* **7**, 219–229.

Marshak R.H. & Lindner A.E. (1976) Amyloidosis. In *Radiology of the Small Intestine*, 2nd ed, p. 62. W.B. Saunders Co., Philadelphia.

Miralbés M., Hinojosa J., Alonso J., Berenguer J. (1983) Oxygen therapy in pneumatosis coli. What is the minimum oxygen requirement? *Dis. Colon Rectum* **26**, 458–60.

Morera P. (1973) The history and redescription of angiostrongylus costaricensis morera and cespedes. *J. Trop. Med. Hyg.* **22**, 613–621.

Neschis M., Siegelman S.S. & Rotstein J. (1970) The oesophagus in progressive systemic sclerosis: a manometric and radiographic correlation. *Amer. J. digest. Dis.* **15**, 443–447.

Partin J.C. & Schubert W.K. (1969) Small intestinal mucosa in cholesterol ester storage disease. *Gastroenterol.* **57**, 542–558.

Patterson T. & Wegelius O. (1972) Biopsy diagnosis of amyloidosis in rheumatoid arthritis. *Gastroenterol.* **62**, 22–27.

Pepys M.B. (1982) Biology of serum amyloid P component. *Ann. N.Y. Acad. Sci.* **389**, 286–298.

Perla D. & Gross H. (1935) Atypical amyloid disease. *Amer. J. Path.* **11**, 93–112.

Poynard T., Natal C., Messing B., Modigliani R. Lecompte T., Nicholas P., Dray F. & Ferme C. (1982) Secretory diarrhoea and prostaglandin D2 overproduction in secretory diarrhoea. *New Engl. J. Med.* **307**, 186.

Salmon P.R. & Paulley J.W. (1967) Eosinophilic granuloma of the gastrointestinal tract. *Gut*, **8**, 8–13.

Schiff L., Schubert W.K., McAdams A.J., Spiegel E.L. & O'Donnell J.F. (1968) Hepatic cholesterol ester storage disease. A familial disorder. *Amer. J. Med.* **44**, 538–546.

Scott B.B., Hardy G.J. & Losowsky M.S. (1975) Involvement of the small intestine in systemic mast cell disease. *Gut*, **16**, 918–924.

Scott J.R., Miller W.T., Urso M. & Stadalnik R.C. (1971) Acute mesenteric infarction. *Amer. J. Roent. Radium Ther. Nuc. Med.* **113**, 269–272.

Sherman N.J., Williams K. & Woolley M.M. (1973) Surgical complications of leukemia. *J. Pediat. Surg.* **8**, 235–239.

Soter N.A., Austen K.F. & Wassermann S.I. (1979) Oral disodium cromoglycate in the treatment of systemic mastocytosis. *New Engl. J. Med.* **301**, 465–468.

Spry C.J.F., Davies J., Tai P.C., Olsen E.G.J., Oakley C.M. & Goodwin J.F. (1983) Clinical features of fifteen patients with the hypereosinophilic syndrome. *Quart. J. Med.* **52**, 1–22.

Vanek T. (1949) Gastric submucosal granuloma with eosinophilic infiltration. *Amer. J. Path.* **25**, 397–411.

Williams H.H. (1965) Roundworms in fishes and so-called 'Herring worm disease'. *Brit. Med. J.* **1**, 964–967.

Witkowski L.J., Pontius G.V. & Anderson R.E. (1955) Gas cysts of the intestine. *Surgery*, **37**, 959–963.

Wright D.G., Dale D.C., Fauci A.S. & Wolff S.M. (1981) Human cyclic neutropenia. Clinical review and long-term follow-up of patients. *Medicine (Balt.)* **60**, 1–13.

Wright J.R., Calkins E., Breen W.J., Stolte G. & Schultz R.T. (1969). Relationship of amyloid to aging. *Medicine (Balt.)* **48**, 39–60.

Yunich A.M. & Fradkin N.F. (1958) Fatal sprue (malabsorption) syndrome secondary to extensive pneumatosis cystoides intestinalis. *Gastroenterol.* **35**, 212–217.

Chapter 14
Infections

SHERWOOD L. GORBACH

Control mechanisms 231
Bacterial diarrhoea 232
Toxigenic infections 232
Invasive infections 236
Viral diarrhoea 240
Tuberculosis 243
Diagnostic features of diarrhoeal disease 245

The small bowel is exposed to a wide range of pathogenic micro-organisms in the environment. Considering the many bacteria, viruses, parasites, and fungi that contaminate food and drink, it is remarkable that the gut is able to sustain an effective 'Pax intestinum'.

Control mechanisms

Gastric acidity

Acid production in the stomach acts as a defence mechanism against exogenous pathogenic micro-organisms, as well as suppressing colonization of the small bowel by the normal flora from the oropharynx (Drasar et al. 1969, Gray & Shiner 1967). Increased susceptibility to cholera and salmonellosis is associated with hypochlorhydria due to atrophic gastritis, after gastric surgery, or the use of blockers of hydrogen-ion secretion such as cimetidine (Gitelson 1971). Administration of such pathogenic organisms with sodium bicarbonate dramatically reduces the infectious inoculum in volunteers by as much as 100,000-fold (Hornick et al. 1971).

Motility

Intestinal motility is an important host defence mechanism that limits the proliferation of organisms in the small bowel, both those from the normal flora and exogenous pathogens (Dixon 1960). Impaired peristalsis increases bacterial overgrowth of the upper gut and facilitates implantation of pathogens. Bile has antibacterial properties, and this may be another factor in controlling the microbial milieu of the small bowel.

Receptors

Protection against random infection by the numerous organisms in nature is dependent, to some extent, on the specific configuration of receptors on the intestinal cells of the host (Keusch 1979). Adherence and colonization by pathogenic micro-organisms are determined by specific recognition between surface structures on the micro-organisms and the mucosal cell. In some instances this involves recognition between sugar-binding proteins (lectins) and characteristic oligosaccharides on the interacting membrane. Another adherence mechanism, found in strains of E. coli that infect piglets, involves the presence of protein structures known as pili on the bacterial cell wall (Fig. 14.1). The specific pili for piglets, K-88, recognizes glycoconjugates containing terminal Ga1NAc or G1cNAc on the mucosal cells of the pig intestine (Anderson et al. 1980). Strains of E. coli infecting humans have different pili structures; the specific receptor in the human intestine has not yet been identified. Thus, site colonization and host specificity are based on biochemical determinants both in the bacteria and on the surface of epithelial cells of the host.

Immunity

Immune mechanisms in the small intestine play a major role in protection from invasion by pathogens (McNabb & Tomasi 1981).

Bacterial diarrhoea

The acute bacterial diarrhoeas can be classified into *toxigenic* forms in which an enterotoxin is the major, if not exclusive, pathogenic mechanism, and *invasive* forms, in which the organism penetrates the intestinal mucosa, causing disruption of the epithelial architecture (Keusch & Donta 1975). (Some invasive bacteria produce an enterotoxin as well.) In general, the toxigenic bacteria, such as *Vibrio cholerae*, involve the small intestine while the highly invasive organisms, such as Shigella, involve the large intestine.

Enterotoxins may be demonstrated in the laboratory by the rabbit ileal loop model and the suckling mouse model, or by *in vitro* tests involving a tissue culture line such as Y-1 adrenal cells or Chinese hamster ovary cells. These toxins are broadly grouped into two categories: *cytotonic* — producing fluid secretion by activation of intracellular enzymes, e.g. adenylate cyclase, without any damage to the epithelial surface; and *cytotoxic* — causing injury to the mucosal cell, as well as inducing fluid secretion, but not primarily by activating cyclic nucleotides (Table 14.1).

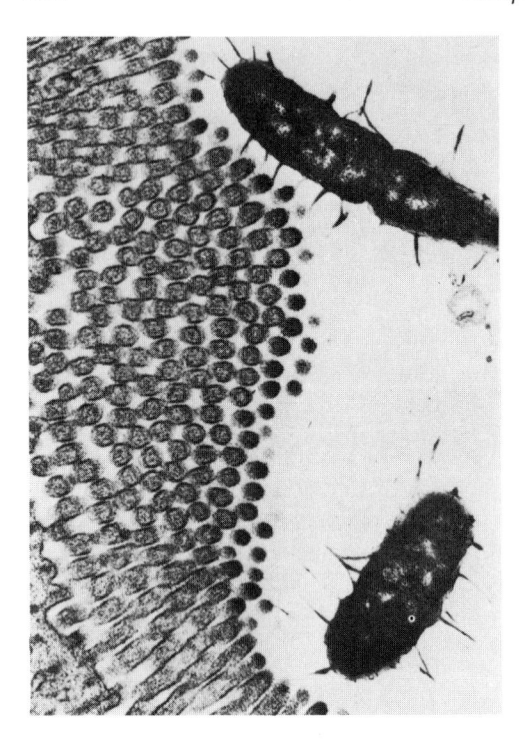

Fig. 14.1. Electron micrograph of two cells of *Escherichia coli* strain 74-5208 carrying several large appendages that contact epithelial microvilli (seen on left of picture) (Moon *et al.* 1977).

Secretory immunoglobulin A (S-IgA) can prevent adherence of micro-organisms to epithelial cells (Gibbons 1974). Some bacteria have developed a defensive weapon in the form of IgA proteases (Plaut 1978). This enzyme has specificity for the IgA-1 immunoglobulin subtype found in humans. Cleavage occurs in the hinge region, and involves either a prolyl-threonyl or a prolyl-seryl peptide bond, depending on the bacterial species of origin. Bacterial hydrolysis of IgA yields intact Fab_a or Fc_a, with a sharp reduction in antibody activity. IgA protease is made by several pathogens that colonize mucosal surfaces, including *Neisseria gonorrhoeae, N. meningiditus, Streptococcus pneumoniae* and *Haemophilus influenzae* (Kornfeld & Plaut 1981). Similar proteases have not yet been identified in bacteria associated with small bowel infection.

Toxigenic infections

Vibrio cholerae and enterotoxigenic *E. coli* are the major organisms in this category. Both produce enterotoxins of the cytotonic type. The clinical disease has the following characteristics:

1 The entire disease consists of intestinal fluid loss which is related to the action of the enterotoxin on the small bowel epithelial cell.

2 The organism itself does not invade the mucosal surface; rather, it colonizes the upper small bowel, 'sticking' to the epithelial cells and elaborating an enterotoxin. The mucosal architecture remains intact, with no evidence of cellular destruction. Bacteraemia does not occur.

3 The faecal effluent is watery and often voluminous, producing clinical features of dehydration. The fluid comes from the upper small bowel, where the enterotoxin has its

Table 14.1. Classification of bacterial toxins associated with diarrhoea.

Cytotonic	Cytotoxic
Vibrio cholerae	Shigella
Escherichia coli (LT & ST)	Clostridium perfringens (Types A & C)
Bacillus cereus	Clostridium difficile
? Aeromonas	Staphylococcus aureus
? Coliforms	? Yersinia
? Yersinia	? Campylobacter

greatest activity.

Cholera

Cholera is a severe dehydrating diarrhoea that can produce massive intestinal purging and death within 3–4 h of onset. Faecal output can exceed 1 litre/hour at the height of disease, and daily outputs of 15–20 litres can be observed when adequate replacement of fluids is given.

Since the 1960s cholera has been a major stimulus to studies of acute diarrhoea and intestinal physiology. On a world-wide scale cholera is not a major problem, since it tends to occur in epidemics and in relatively localized areas but it is important as the prototype of toxigenic diarrhoea. The pathophysiology has been defined; the enterotoxin has been purified; the epidemiology has been elucidated; new forms of treatment such as oral rehydration, have been devised; and means of immunologic protection, especially by the use of vaccines, have been developed. The lessons of cholera have direct application to other forms of diarrhoea. Whatever successes or failures have been achieved with cholera, their counterparts have been realized with the other diarrhoeal diseases.

Vibrio cholerae

The organism is a short, Gram-negative curved rod that looks like a comma (Finkelstein 1973). It is strongly aerobic and prefers an alkaline and salty environment, characteristics that play a role in the epidemiology of the disease. Two major biotypes are recognized, *classic* and *El Tor*. The current pandemic of cholera, dating since the 1960s, has been caused by the El Tor biotype. Although the two biotypes cause similar clinical manifestations, El Tor produces a milder disease. Inaba and Ogawa are the two major antigenic types. In individual areas a specific biotype and serotype usually dominates but over a period of years this may change as the inhabitants develop immunity.

All wild strains of *V. cholerae* elaborate the same enterotoxin, a protein molecule with a molecular weight of 84,000 daltons. Like the diphtheria toxin, it is composed of two subunits. Each toxin molecule has five 'B' subunits that encircle a single 'A' subunit (Gill 1977). The B subunit is responsible for binding to the receptor on the mucosal cell membrane, identified as a GM_1 ganglioside. The A subunit is responsible for binding and activation of adenylate cyclase located on the inner cellular membrane.

Epidemiology

The epidemiology of cholera has been studied since the mid-nineteenth century when the first pandemics were recorded. The current pandemic is the seventh, an outbreak that started in 1961 in Indonesia and made its way across Asia, into the Middle East, and finally into Africa, with occasional forays into Southern Europe. Contaminated water and food are the major vehicles for the spread of cholera. This observation is based in part on the relatively large inoculum required to cause disease, which is approximately 10^9 organisms. Person-to-person spread is relatively uncommon. Health workers are generally spared the disease, even when working closely with cholera patients. Gastric acid is an important barrier to infection. It is extremely difficult to infect healthy people with normal acid production, unless a buffering solution is given simultaneously with the inoculum of vibrios.

Pathogenesis and clinical features

The clinical picture of cholera with massive

loss of fluid is caused by the action of toxin on the upper intestine (Carpenter 1982). This is a form of 'overflow' diarrhoea: the large volume of fluid produced in the upper intestine overwhelms the absorptive capacity of the lower small bowel and colon. Cholera toxin increases adenylate cyclase activity, resulting in elevated levels of cyclic AMP in the intestinal mucosa. There appear to be differential actions on the mucosal cells, in that there is a direct secretory effect on the crypt cells and an anti-absorptive effect on the villous cells.

Cholera stools resemble 'rice water'; the stool has lost all pigment and becomes a clear fluid with small flecks of mucus. The electrolyte composition is isotonic with plasma, and the effluent has a low protein concentration. There is a characteristic pattern of electrolytes in the stool; sodium, 126 ± 9 mEq/1; potassium, $19 \pm$ mEq/1; bicarbonate, 47 ± 10 mEq/1; and chloride, 94 ± 9 mEq/1. On microscopic examination, there are no inflammatory cells in the faecal effluent; all that can be seen are small numbers of shed mucosal cells.

The clinical spectrum extends from the subject who is an asymptomatic carrier to the patient with severe purging. The extreme end of this spectrum is characterized by profound dehydration and hypovolaemic shock progressing to renal failure. Mild fever may be present, but there are no signs of sepsis.

Immunologic responses are registered by two serum components, vibriocidal antibody directed against the somatic antigens of the organism, and anti-toxin antibody against the enterotoxin (Mosley 1969). Relative protection is correlated with the height of antibody response, although this may be variable. In areas of endemicity such as the Indian subcontinent, the titre of vibriocidal antibody rises with age. Thus, the disease in these areas is confined largely to young children who have not yet developed antibody. Epidemics in previously virgin territories for cholera are characterized by infection in all ages.

Treatment

This is largely concerned with replacement of fluid and electrolytes, based on physiological principles. The severely ill need rapid administration of an isotonic fluid containing electrolytes in similar concentrations to those found in the stool. Particular attention should be paid to the replacement of the excessive losses of potassium and bicarbonate. In the less severely ill, rehydration can be effected orally (Hirschhorn *et al.* 1973).

Antimicrobial agents are important ancillary measures since they reduce the amount of fluid loss and shorten the carrier phase. For example, tetracycline shortens the duration of diarrhoea by 60% and decreases the duration of positive stool cultures by 80% or more (Carpenter *et al.* 1964, Greenough *et al.* 1964). Alternative agents are chloramphenicol and trimethoprim/sulfamethoxazole.

There has been a remarkable reduction in mortality by the use of simple fluid replacement and antibiotics. Up to 1960, mortalities of 50% or more were recorded whereas today the mortality rate in well-functioning units is approximately 1% in adults and 3–5% in children (Glass *et al.* 1983).

Prevention

A vaccine is available for parenteral administration. Unfortunately, it is not uniformly effective, not more than 50% of immunized individuals being protected. This is probably because the parenteral vaccine is relatively ineffective in stimulating the production of secretory IgA in the intestine.

Escherichia coli

Outbreaks of severe, often fatal diarrhoea in new-born nurseries have been ascribed to *E. coli*. This connection was made in the 1920s, but it was not until the availability of serotyping in the late 1930s that certain antigenic types, known as enteropathogenic *E. coli* (EPEC), were related epidemiologically to neonatal diarrhoea. With the tremendous strides in cholera research, there followed a renaissance of interest in *E. coli* as an intestinal pathogen. Originally in India, and thereafter in many parts of the world,

Table 14.2. Types of *E. coli* intestinal pathogens.

Common name	Toxin	Mechanism
Enteropathogenic (EPEC)	—	Not known; associated by serotype
Enterotoxigenic (ETEC)	LT	Activates adenylate cyclase
	ST	Activates guanylate cyclase
Invasive	—	Penetrates colonic epithelium
RDEC-1	—	Adheres to brush border, destroys microvilli; no invasion

strains of *E. coli* causing diarrhoea in humans were found to produce an enterotoxin similar to that of choleratoxin. These toxigenic strains have become known as enterotoxigenic *E. coli* (ETEC). Subsequently, other forms of *E. coli* intestinal pathogens have been discovered (Table 14.2).

Enteropathogenic E. coli (EPEC)

Among the more than 150 somatic antigens used in the typing schema for *E. coli*, approximately fifteen have been designated as EPEC. In neonates an association has been established between a specific *E. coli* serotype and diarrhoea, but this does not appear to be relevant to cases of sporadic diarrhoea in older children or adults. Indeed, the isolation of EPEC serotypes in the faeces of older children with diarrhoea (about 5%) is similar to or only slightly more frequent than findings in the stools of healthy children.

Laboratory investigations have failed to reveal the pathogenic mechanisms in EPEC. They do not seem to produce enterotoxin, nor do they invade the mucosal wall. There is no doubt, however, that EPEC cause intestinal infection, since administration of these strains to volunteers produces acute diarrhoea (Levine *et al.* 1978).

Certain *E. coli* strains designated RDEC produce diarrhoea in rabbits (Cantey & Blake 1977). These organisms adhere avidly to the intestinal mucosa, particularly in the ileum (Inman *et al.* 1983). A similar type of organism has been associated with diarrhoea in children (Ulshen & Rollo 1980). Again, the organisms stick to the microvilli of the small intestine, extensively colonizing its surface. By electron microscopy, the *E. coli* bacteria can be seen adherent to the brush border. Although there is no invasion of the mucosal cell, the microvilli are extensively disrupted. Children develop chronic diarrhoea lasting several months, which seems to respond to antibiotic treatment, although the result of such therapy is certainly not dramatic.

Enterotoxigenic E. coli (ETEC)

While not belonging to the specific serotypes known as EPEC, the toxin-producing strains associated with human diarrhoea (ETEC) do have certain serotype preferences, for example 06, 078, 0148. Infection by ETEC occurs mostly in children, principally in the developing countries (Sack 1980). Adult travellers to these regions can also become infected (Gorbach & Hoskins 1980).

Two pathogenic mechanisms are required for ETEC to cause diarrhoea. The first requirement is colonization of the upper small intestine. These pathogens adhere to the epithelial cell by means of specific protein antigens known as pili. The antigenic structure of adherence pili determines the host specificity of the ETEC strains. Several types of pili have been associated with infection in humans, but these pili are clearly different from those associated with infections in piglets or calves (Evans *et al.* 1975, Deneke *et al.* 1981).

Enterotoxin production is the other pathogenic determinant in ETEC (Sack 1975). Two such toxins can be produced by ETEC: a heat-labile toxin (LT) which is a protein with a molecular weight of approximately 80,000; and a heat-stable toxin (ST) with a relatively small molecular weight of 4,500. The LT resembles choleratoxin in its biochemical features, immunologic reactivity, and pathophysiology (adenylate cyclase activation). ST, however, seems to activate guanylate cyclase and has an entirely different chemical structure (Hughes *et al.* 1978, Field *et al.* 1978 Moseley *et al.* 1983). Strains of ETEC can elaborate either LT or ST alone,

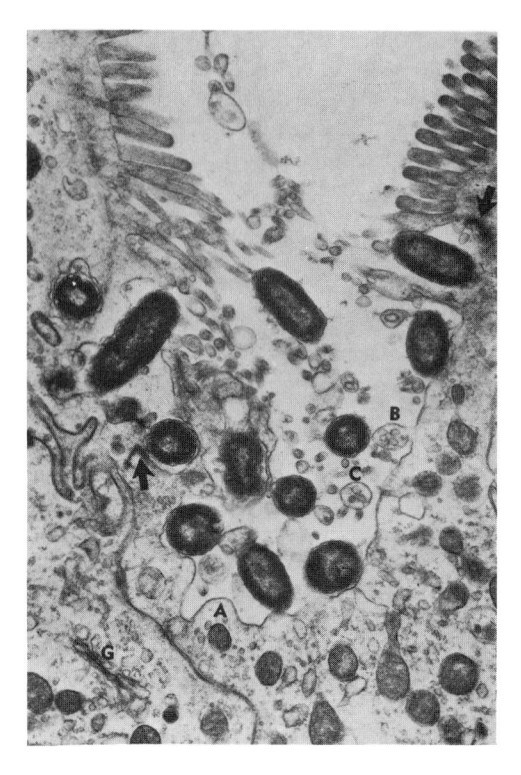

Fig. 14.2. Electron micrograph of *S. typhimurium* invading ileal epithelium of a guinea-pig. The microvilli, terminal web, and apical cytoplasm are replaced by a cavity lined with bleb-like projections (A), some of which contain small vesicles (B) and (C). An intercellular junctional complex is laterally displaced (arrows) while the bacteria are being internalized. (Courtesy of A. Takeuchi.)

or both toxins.

A mild case of traveller's diarrhoea can be caused by ETEC, resulting in a brief interruption of a holiday. On the other end of the spectrum, a severe form of dehydrating diarrhoea, recognized in Calcutta as 'acute undifferentiated diarrhoea', is caused by ETEC (Gorbach et al. 1971). In general, ETEC diarrhoea is less voluminous than cholera, although the two diseases may be difficult to distinguish at the onset. ST-only strains generally produce a milder form of diarrhoea with vomiting and intestinal cramps (Merson et al. 1980).

The epidemiology of ETEC is similar to cholera with transmission by contaminated food and water, mediated by a human carrier. ETEC is more cosmopolitan than cholera, causing diarrhoea in virtually every area, with a pattern of mostly endemic disease and occasional small-scale epidemics. The reservoirs of ETEC in animals are probably not important since these organisms lack the specific pili for infecting the human small intestine.

Protection from reinfection is associated with the presence of serum and intestinal antibodies against either the toxin or the specific adherence pili. People residing in areas of high risk for ETEC are relatively protected from new infection. Studies of individuals attending international meetings in Tehran and Mexico City showed that Europeans and North Americans experienced assorted intestinal agonies, whereas Asians, Africans and South Americans were relatively unscathed.

The treatment of ETEC diarrhoea is based on providing symptomatic relief with attention to fluid and electrolyte replacement. Antibiotics such as doxycycline and trimethoprim/sulfamethoxazole seem to shorten the duration of purging by a few hours, but this small benefit must be weighed against the risk of side-effects from the antibiotic itself (Merson et al. 1980).

Invasive infections

Salmonellosis

Non-typhoidal salmonellosis can be caused by many of the 1700 Salmonella serotypes found in animals and birds. Approximately twenty serotypes are responsible for 85% of human Salmonella infections, the most common being *S. typhimurium*. Regional patterns of serotypes are determined by local epidemiologic circumstances.

Pathogenesis

The main portal of entry for Salmonella is the gastrointestinal tract (Takeuchi 1966, Takeuchi & Sprinz 1967). These organisms are unique in attacking mainly the ileum (Fig. 14.2) and to a lesser extent the colon. They cause mild epithelial ulceration and rapidly make their way through the mucosa to the lamina propria, thence to the lymphatics and bloodstream. Histologic sections of ileum show oedematous, shortened villi and numerous polymorphonuclear leucocytes in the lamina propria. The organisms are spread to other organs by haematogenous dissemination.

The exact mechanisms responsible for diarrhoea are not clear, although penetration of the mucosa and inflammation appear to be the important components. Two virulence factors must be present in order that a specific Salmonella strain is pathogenic: a factor that causes mucosal invasion, and another that causes secretion of fluid and electrolytes into the lumen (Giannella *et al.* 1973). Cyclic AMP is stimulated by some strains that produce fluid accumulation. Indomethacin, which blocks prostaglandin synthesis, inhibits intestinal secretion in experimental Salmonella infections (Giannella *et al.* 1975).

A high degree of intrinsic pathogenicity is possessed by certain strains, and this feature is related to the inoculum size required to initiate disease. For example, 10^5 *S. newport* produced disease in volunteers, whereas 10^9 *S. pullorum* was ineffective (McCullough & Eisele 1951a, McCullough & Eisele 1951b). In experimental situations the inoculum size can be reduced when animals are pre-treated with antibiotics. Blocking gastric acid production also increases the susceptibility to infection.

Clinical features

Five clinical syndromes are seen with Salmonellosis: (i) gastroenteritis, noted in 70% of infections; (ii) bacteraemia, with or without gastrointestinal involvement, seen in approximately 10%; (iii) typhoidal or 'enteric fever' seen with all typhoid strains and in approximately 5% of other Salmonella infections; (iv) localized infections, i.e. bones, joints, and meninges, seen in approximately 5%; and (v) a carrier state in asymptomatic individuals. The organism is usually harboured in the gall bladder (Saphra & Winter 1957, Rubin & Weinstein 1977).

The most common syndrome is gastroenteritis. The usual incubation period is 6–48 h, although latency can last as long as 7–12 days. The initial symptoms are nausea and vomiting, followed by abdominal cramps and diarrhoea. The diarrhoea usually lasts 3–4 days, and is accompanied by fever in about 50% of cases. In general, the pain of Salmonella gastroenteritis is located in the peri-umbilical area or the right lower quadrant. The diarrhoea is variable. It may be no more than a few loose stools; a dysenteric picture with grossly bloody and purulent faeces; or a cholera-like syndrome. The latter condition with massive purging has been described in patients who are achlorhydric (Gray & Trueman 1971).

Salmonella bacteraemia is similar to sepsis caused by any other Gram-negative bacterium, although there is an impression that it is less severe. Once the organism has disseminated it can produce meningitis, arteritis, endocarditis, osteomyelitis, wound infection, septic arthritis, and focal abscesses (Black *et al.* 1960).

A number of associated conditions seem to increase the risk of salmonellosis (Table 14.3). Haemolytic anaemias, such as occur with sickle-cell disease and with malaria, predispose to Salmonella infection (Black *et al.* 1960, Hook 1961). This increased susceptibility may be due to blockage of the reticuloendothelial system by the breakdown products of red blood cells (Kaye *et al.* 1967). A defect in opsonization of Salmonella has been described among patients with sickle-cell anaemia, based on defective activation of the alternative complement pathway (Hand & King 1977).

Table 14.3. Predisposing conditions in Salmonella infection.

Haemolytic anaemia	Achlorhydria
Sickle-cell disease	Gastro-duodenal
Malaria	surgery
Bartonellosis	Idiopathic
Malignancy	Ulcerative colitis
Lymphoma	
Leukaemia	Schistosomiasis
Disseminated	
carcinoma	
Immunosuppression	
Steroid therapy	
Chemotherapy	
Radiation	

Treatment

Although many antibiotics have been used to treat non-typhoidal Salmonella gastroenteritis, all have failed to alter the rate of clinical recovery when compared to untreated controls (Rosenstein 1967, Kazemi *et al.* 1973). Indeed, antibiotic therapy increases the incidence and duration of intestinal carriage of the organism (Askerkoff & Bennett 1969). For these reasons, antimicrobial therapy is not generally employed in Salmonella gastroenteritis. Some clinical situations, however, dictate that antibiotics be used (Rubin & Weinstein 1977). Therapy should be given when Salmonella infection occurs in the presence of a lymphoproliferative disorder; prosthetic heart valves; vascular grafts; aneurysms; foreign bodies implanted in the skeletal system; and in patients with haemolytic anaemia; or at the extreme ages of life. Signs of sepsis, i.e. high fever, rigors, hypotension, decreased renal function, and systemic toxicity, would provide a sound rationale for therapy.

Resistance to one or more antimicrobial agents is almost universal among salmonellae, probably related to the use of antibiotics in animal feed. Ampicillin (or amoxicillin) or trimethoprim/sulfamethoxazole are the preferred agents, unless resistance is high in the local area.

Typhoid fever

Typhoid fever is more a systemic illness than a gastroenteritis, although the portal of entry is the GI tract. *Salmonella typhi* is the main cause of typhoid fever, but other Salmonella serotypes occasionally produce the same clinical features, known variously as typhoidal disease, enteric fever, or paratyphoid fever. *Salmonella typhi* is remarkably adapted to humans who represent the only natural reservoir, whereas the other salmonellae are widely dispersed in nature.

Pathogenesis

Following ingestion, the organism penetrates the small bowel mucosa, sparing the stomach, and makes its way rapidly to the lymphatics, the mesenteric nodes, and within minutes to the bloodstream (Hornick *et al.* 1970). There is little inflammation, which explains the lack of intestinal symptoms at this initial stage. This sequence of events contrasts with with other forms of salmonellosis in which the intestinal findings are prominent at the onset. Following the initial bacteraemia, the organism is sequestered in macrophages and monocytic cells of the reticuloendothelial system in the liver and spleen. After multiplying for approximately 7–10 days, it emerges in recurrent waves of bacteraemia, an event that initiates the symptomatic phase of infection. The intestinal tract is seeded by direct bacteraemic spread, especially to Peyer's patches in the terminal ileum. Alternatively, the gut may be infected by passage of bacilli down the biliary tree from the gall bladder.

Hyperplasia of the reticuloendothelial system, including lymph nodes, liver and spleen is characteristic of typhoid fever (Stuart & Pullen 1946, Walker 1965, Hoffman *et al.* 1975). Inflammation of the gall bladder is common and may lead to acute cholecystitis. Lymphoid follicles in the gut (Peyer's patches) become hyperplastic with the infiltration of macrophages, lymphocytes and red blood cells. Subsequently, the epithelium over a follicle may ulcerate. The lymphoid tissue penetrates through the submucosa to the intestinal lumen, discharging in its wake large numbers of typhoid bacilli. As the bowel wall is progressively involved, it becomes paper-thin and is susceptible to transmural perforation into the peritoneal cavity. This sequence of events accounts for the dreaded complications of typhoid fever, intestinal bleeding and perforation, which occur in the second and third week of illness (Woodward & Smadel 1964).

Clinical features

Typhoid fever has an insidious onset after an incubation period of 10–14 days. The patient usually complains of general malaise, dull headache, aches and pains, chills and often a cough. His appetite is poor and often he is constipated. Atypical presentations include septicaemic collapse or signs of focal infection such as meningitis, lobar pneumonia or cholecystitis. Mental disturbances are common, occasionally to the point of an acute psychosis.

The clinician is rarely able to document the classical step-like rise in fever but characteristically at the end of the first week of illness the patient has a temperature of 102–104°F (38.8–40°C). He is tired and toxic, the headache persists and the abdomen is slightly tender. Now the tip of the spleen becomes palpable and rose spots may be detected on the lower chest and abdomen. Commonly there are only four or five macules 1–2 mm in diameter; two dozen would be diagnostic luxury.

From this stage onwards signs of small intestinal disease become increasingly common. Diarrhoea is usual. It has a pea-soup appearance because of pus and necrotic material shed from the ulcerating Peyer's patches. Before the days of chloramphenicol 10–20% of patients bled from these ulcers; in more recent series the incidence is only 1–3%. Intestinal perforation has a similar incidence and is the more serious complication. It occurs silently in the patient treated late who is already very sick and who has a distended, vaguely tender abdomen. But it also occurs in the treated patient who seems to have entered the convalescent phase of his illness. In such cases diagnosis is rarely difficult.

Today most patients escape the many complications of typhoid fever caused either by Salmonella localizing in a specific organ (e.g. cholecystitis, osteomyelitis) or as a consequence of severe illness (e.g. hypostatic pneumonia, thrombophlebitis). But many still suffer relapse despite effective treatment with chloramphenicol. Salmonella organisms are unusually tenacious and may be carried by humans for years.

Diagnosis

The initial diagnosis of typhoid fever depends on culturing *S. typhi* especially from blood. Repeated samples should be taken and culture may be positive into the third week of illness, but the number of organisms is often small and prolonged culture (10–12 days) may be necessary especially if treatment with antibiotics has been started. There is a high rate of positive cultures of bone marrow aspirates, even when patients are being treated with antibiotics, and this is a useful diagnostic technique in the difficult case.

Culture of faeces is also helpful, even in the first week of illness when by careful subculturing techniques the organism can be isolated from 50% of samples. By the third week the organism should be found without difficulty.

Agglutinating antibodies in serum (Widal test) may be expected to aid diagnosis. A positive reaction merely indicates contact with an organism, dead or alive, recently or not so recently, Salmonella or other, that possesses the relevant antigens. In an uninoculated patient, recently exposed, a titre of 1/40 for O and H antibodies in the first week of a febrile illness is suggestive of enteric infection; at 1/80 the diagnosis is almost certain. A rising titre over 4 or 5 days is also very good evidence but in some patients the expected increase does not occur.

In inoculated patients, however, no titre is diagnostic and even a rise after a few days may be misleading. In areas where enteric infection is common it is essential to know the average level of antibodies in the normal healthy population. In such an area a high O titre is of more significance than a high H titre and second tests are necessary if one is to make a useful deduction. It is often stated that a rise in H antibody may be provoked by a non-specific stimulus; this is true but under the right circumstances increasing titres are much more likely to be due to enteric fever. Antibiotics appear to delay but not to affect the final level of antibody titres.

In temperate climates the Widal test is particularly helpful in diagnosing a cryptic case of fever in a returning traveller or even in the rare autochthonous case.

Paratyphoid

Salmonella paratyphi usually causes a mild typhoid-like disease. Not infrequently, however, it produces an acute enteritis similar to that caused by *S. typhimirium* and sometimes one type of illness is followed by the other. *Salmonella paratyphi* A and C are more likely to cause an invasive fever than *S. paratyphi* B. With all three organisms symptomless excretors are much more common than with *S. typhi*.

Treatment

All patients with typhoid fever should receive antimicrobial drugs. Chloramphenicol remains the treatment of choice for most cases. Resistance to this organism has been relatively uncommon. Alternative agents are ampicillin, amoxacillin, and trimethoprim/sulfamethoxazole.

Yersinia enterocolitica

This organism is a non-lactose-fermenting, Gram-negative rod that causes a spectrum of illness from simple gastroenteritis to invasive ileitis and colitis (Morris & Feeley 1976, Bottone 1977). The organism is widely dispersed in nature, it infects many animals, especially cows and chickens. It is an important pathogen in Scandinavia, other European countries, and in Canada, although found rather infrequently in the USA.

Clinical features

The clinical syndrome tends to vary with the age of the patient and the underlying disease state (Bottone 1977, Ahvonen 1972). Acute diarrhoea is the most frequent presentation, occurring in two-thirds of reported cases. Children less than 5 years of age are most commonly afflicted with this non-specific diarrhoeal disease, which usually lasts 1–3 weeks (Marks *et al.* 1980). Older children and young adults have mesenteric adenitis and associated ileitis. Exploratory laparotomy may be mistakenly performed for the presumptive diagnosis of appendicitis. Enlarged mesenteric nodes and ulcerative ileitis are encountered at surgery. Yersiniosis is less common in adults; when present, it causes acute diarrhoea which may be followed by joint symptoms and rash (erythema nodosum or erythema multiforme) (Winblad 1975). This symptom complex is usually associated with HLA-B27. Immunosuppressed hosts may suffer a severe, and often fatal, Yersinia bacteraemia.

Although the organism is sensitive to many antibiotics, there is no evidence that therapy alters the course of the disease. Indeed, the diagnosis is often established in retrospect by positive culture or serology.

Viral diarrhoea

Most acute gastrointestinal infections are caused by viruses. It is particularly frustrating for physicians and laboratory workers alike to be unable to culture or to even define the majority of responsible viral agents. Even using the best techniques of electron microscopy and immunochemistry, only one-third of cases can be assigned to a specific viral agent. The remaining two thirds are implicated by epidemiologic and clinical data, but the viral agents are as yet undiscovered. Two groups of viruses have received most attention: the rotaviruses, which cause endemic diarrhoea in children, and the Norwalk viruses, which appear in epidemics and attack all age groups (Table 14.4) (Cukor & Blacklow 1984).

Rotaviruses

Originally discovered in Australia during the 1970s, these viruses are cosmopolitan in distribution. They measure 70 nm in diameter, and contain a double-walled outer capsid (Flewett & Woode 1978). They are RNA viruses that are extremely stable to heat and environmental pressures, and can be maintained in storage for long periods of time. The agent is visualized in faecal specimens by electron microscopy (Fig. 14.3), and it can be identified by various immunological techniques. Propagation in tissue

Table 14.4. Clinical and laboratory characteristics of human gastroenteritis viruses of medical importance.

Feature	Norwalk virus	Rotavirus
Biologic characteristics		
Diameter, shape	27 nm, round	70 nm, with double-shelled capsid
Nucleic acid	Not known	Double-stranded, segmented RNA
Density (cesium chloride)	1.36–1.41 g/cm^3	1.35–1.37 g/cm^3
Number of serotypes	At least 3	At least 2
Replication in cell culture	No	Incomplete for wild strains
Clinical characteristics		
Epidemiology	Family and community epidemics, often in winter	Sporadic cases, usually in winter, occasionally epidemic
Age primarily affected	Older children, adults	Infants, young children
Method of transmission	Faecal-oral, contaminated water and shellfish	Faecal-oral
Incubation period	1–2 days	1–3 days
Duration of illness	Usually 1–2 days	Usually 5–8 days
Pathogenetic characteristics		
Attack rate in adult volunteers	About 50%	Low
Site of human infection	Small bowel	Small bowel
Mechanisms of immunity	? Non-immune genetic factors; not local or systemic antibody	Local intestinal IgA antibody, not systemic antibody
Disease production in animals	No	Yes, particularly young animals
Major diagnostic tests	Immune electron microscopy, radioimmunoassay; serologic adaptation of above tests	Electron microscopy, radioimmunoassay, enzyme-linked immunosorbent assay, counterimmuno-electrophoresis, cell-culture antigen production; serologic adaptation of some of the above tests

From Blacklow & Cukor (1981).

cultures has been extremely difficult, and simple animal models have not been developed. At least three, and possibly as many as five, serotypes of human rotavirus have been discovered, each with its own immunologic specificity. For this reason children have multiple attacks until they have developed protective antibodies to all serotypes.

Pathology

Intestinal biopsy in young children infected with rotavirus has shown a patchy abnormality, confined mostly to the epithelial cells of the upper intestine (Bishop et al. 1973, Davidson & Barnes 1979). In its severe form, gross destruction of the villous architecture and flattening of the epithelial surface are observed. These changes may persist for 3–8 weeks and are associated with reduced levels of disaccharidase enzymes. In addition, the absorption of xylose is decreased.

Clinical features

The disease is mostly confined to children aged 6–24 months (Tallett et al. 1977, Rodriguez et al. 1977). Older siblings and adults may be excreting the virus, but they seldom develop clinical illness. Vomiting often heralds the disease, and is usually followed by watery diarrhoea which lasts for 3–5 days. Some instances of chronic diarrhoea have been reported.

Antibodies to the rotavirus can be demonstrated in serum and in intestinal secretions (Kapikian et al. 1976). Secretory

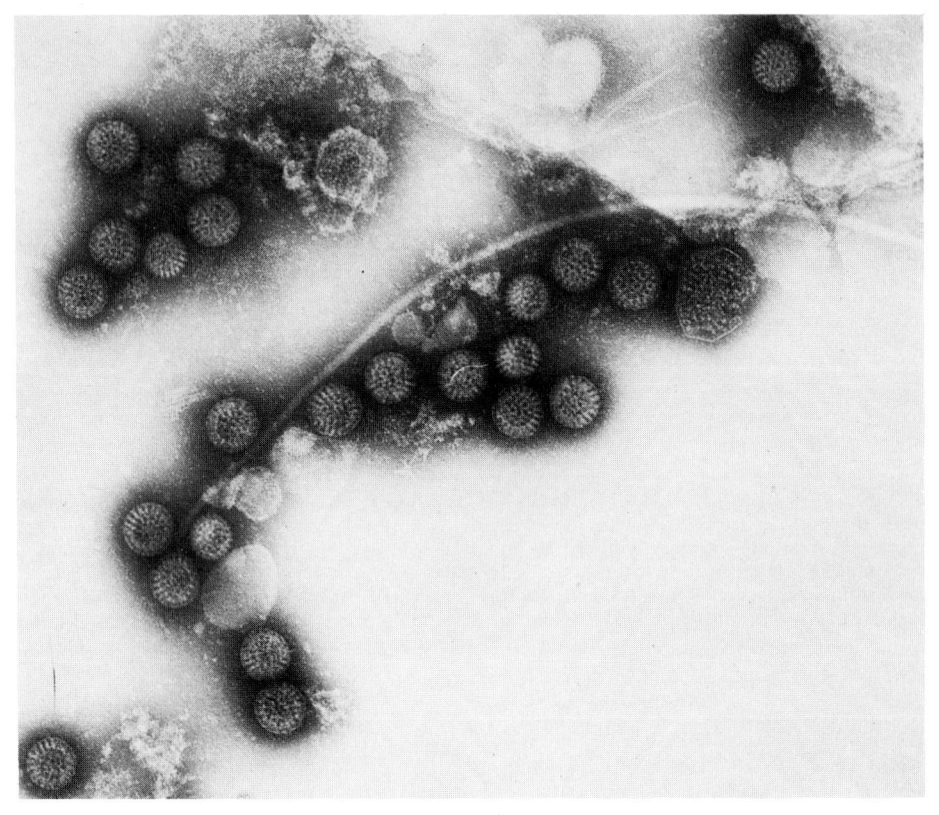

Fig. 14.3. Rotavirus demonstrated by electron microscopy in faeces of child with neonatal diarrhoea (× 40,000). (Courtesy of Professor Raymond Heath.)

antibody of the IgA type provides protection, and breast-feeding may offer some benefit against this infection (Totterdell et al. 1980).

Fluid and electrolyte replacement is the mainstay of therapy and, as in mild cholera, oral rehydration is usually sufficient (Nalin et al. 1979).

Norwalk virus

This virus is also cosmopolitan in distribution, having been isolated in the USA, Hawaii, UK, Australia and Japan (Cukor & Blacklow 1984). It is a very small agent with a diameter of 27 nm. Most evidence suggests that it is a DNA-containing virus, although its exact place in taxonomy has not been determined. Because of the problems in identifying the virus in faecal effluent and the lack of suitable tissue culture sytems or animal models, our knowledge of this agent is limited. Most information has come from epidemiologic observations and experimental infections in volunteers.

Clinical features

Vomiting and diarrhoea can occur together or independently. The disease is often epidemic in nature, with an attack rate of 70% or more. In community outbreaks, a broad spectrum of illness is observed, ranging from mild anorexia and malaise, to severe diarrhoea, vomiting, myalgias and fever. The illness usually lasts for no longer than 24−48 h (Blacklow et al. 1972, Wyatt et al. 1974).

Intestinal biopsies reveal that the upper small bowel is the main focus of attack, with sparing of the stomach and colon (Schreiber et al. 1973). Patchy mucosal lesions are noted in symptomatic individuals, and such lesions have also been found in asymptomatic volunteers receiving the virus. Since the virus particles are extremely small, they cannot be seen on electron microscopy, in contrast to the rotavirus. Several physiologic abnormalities have been observed during the course of Norwalk infection, including malabsorption of fat and xylose, reduced disaccharidase activity, and delayed gastric emptying; these abnormalities are reversed within 1–2 weeks.

The disease is spread mainly by person-to-person contact (Greenberg et al. 1979), although some infections have been traced to foods, especially shellfish and oysters. There is no respect for age, since all age groups are infected. This age distribution reflects unusual immunologic events, best demonstrated in volunteer studies (Parrino et al. 1977). Volunteers who became sick during the initial challenge became ill when re-challenged 24–40 months later. Those who resisted an initial challenge also resisted subsequent challenge. Antibody in serum and intestinal juice showed higher titres in the volunteers who became ill, both on the initial and subsequent challenge. Nevertheless, the antibody offers some short-lived protection. Early rechallenge at 6–14 weeks did not produce disease. Yet the same group with antibody became ill when rechallenged several months later. It is postulated that non-immune mechanisms in the intestine are responsible for resistance to infection by this virus. Antibody provides only transient protection. For these reasons some people experience repeated infection with this virus.

Miscellaneous viral agents

The medical literature is replete with reports of viruses associated with gastroenteritis in humans. Unfortunately, it is not clear whether these viruses are truly infectious agents or merely innocent bystanders. New viral pathogens undoubtedly will be described in the future, since two-thirds of what are presumably viral infections of the gastrointestinal tract are undiagnosed by the available techniques. The burden of proof rests with showing that the specific virus is not part of the normal viral flora, nor even a transient passenger in the gut, but an aetiologic agent.

The classic enteroviruses — echovirus and coxsackievirus — are rare causes of simple gastroenteritis. They tend to cause diarrhoea in association with involvement of other organs such as the lungs, the central nervous system and the heart. Cytomegaloviruses (CMV) have been recognized as the cause of diarrhoea in some patients. Intestinal X-rays have shown punctate ulcerations in the stomach and small intestine, especially the ileum. Adenoviruses have been identified by culture and direct electron microscopy in patients with diarrhoea; some of the viruses observed by electron microscopy cannot be cultivated, suggesting that they may not be conventional members of the adenovirus group. Since this group of viruses is ubiquitous in our environment and is a common cause of respiratory illness, its relative importance in diarrhoeal disease is unclear.

Calicivirus has been identified by electron microscopy in several outbreaks of gastroenteritis among children. Certain structural features bear resemblances to the Norwalk agent, although this point remains disputed.

There have been reports of astrovirus and coronavirus causing infections in humans, but since these viruses cannot be propagated in tissue culture or in experimental animals — a feature common to many of the viral pathogens in diarrhoeal disease — a paucity of information on their overall significance exists.

Tuberculosis

Before the availability of chemotherapy intestinal involvement was noted at autopsy in 55–90% of patients with pulmonary tuberculosis (Jordan & DeBakey 1954). Gastrointestinal involvement was related to the severity of pulmonary infection, and was most common in patients with lung cavitation and positive sputum smears (Mitchell & Bristol 1954). In more recent series, however, the chest X-ray has appeared completely normal in the majority of patients with intestinal tuberculosis (Abrams & Holden 1964, Bentley & Webster 1967, Schulze et al.

1977). *Mycobacterium tuberculosis* is the major pathogen in the industrialized countries. An organism found in dairy products, *M. bovis*, is still encountered in developing countries, but it is now rarely found in areas where milk products are pasteurized. Swallowed organisms present either in sputum or in food products remain the major vehicle of infection of the gut.

Clinical features

The ileocaecal region is the most frequently infected, being involved in about 90% of patients. Other locations, in order of incidence, are ascending colon, jejunum, appendix, duodenum, stomach, sigmoid colon and rectum. The ileocaecal valve is often incompetent in tuberculosis, a finding which may distinguish this process from Crohn's disease. Indeed, much of the older literature confused intestinal tuberculosis with Crohn's disease, so one cannot rely on data published more than 40 years ago.

Classically, three forms of intestinal tuberculosis are recognized: (i) ulcerative, in 60% of patients. Multiple, superficial ulcers are present on the epithelial surface of the bowel. This is a virulent process with a high mortality; (ii) hypertrophic, occurring in 10% of patients. Scarring, fibrosis and heaped-up mass lesions are characteristic of this condition; and (iii) ulcerohypertrophic, in 30% (Hoon *et al.* 1950).

At surgery, the bowel wall is thickened with an inflammatory mass surrounding the ileocaecal region. Active inflammation, along with strictures and fistulae, are present. The serosal surface is covered by multiple tubercles. The regional mesenteric nodes are enlarged and thickened with caseous necrosis. In contrast to Crohn's disease, the superficial ulcers tend to be circumferential, with the long axis perpendicular to the lumen. When these ulcers heal, the associated fibrosis causes strictures and stenosis of the lumen.

Chronic abdominal pain, non-specific in nature, is the most common complaint reported by 80−90% of patients. Non-specific symptoms such as fever, weight loss and malaise are also frequent problems.

Complications of intestinal tuberculosis include haemorrhage, perforation, obstruction, fistula formation and malabsorption syndrome (Sherman *et al.* 1980). Intestinal obstruction is a common occurrence. It forms in a segmental, stenotic fashion, and may require surgical intervention for relief, even with appropriate drug therapy. Malabsorption can be caused by bacterial overgrowth in the dilated, proximal loops or by obstruction of the mesenteric lymphatic system.

Roentgenographic examination of the bowel reveals a thickened mucosa with distortion of the mucosal folds, ulcerations, various degrees of thickening and stenosis of the bowel, and pseudo-polyp formation (Werbeloff *et al.* 1973, Kolawole & Lewis 1975). The caecum is contracted, with disease on both sides of the valve, and the valve itself is often distorted and incompetent. Tuberculosis tends to involve small segments of the intestine with stenosis and fistula formation. In the hypertrophic form a mass can be mistaken for caecal carcinoma. Calcified mesenteric lymph nodes and an abnormal chest X-ray when present, are helpful signs.

Treatment

Standard anti-tuberculous treatment gives a high cure in what was formerly a severe, often fatal disease. While there are no control studies to determine optimal therapy, it seems reasonable to use three active drugs (isoniazid, ethambutol and rifampicin) for a period of 12−18 months. It may occasionally be necessary to intervene surgically, especially in cases involving the ileum. Obstruction and fistula formation are the major indications for surgery, although mass lesions may require laparotomy for definitive diagnosis (Bentley & Webster 1967). In many cases tuberculosis is diagnosed at operation, which was undertaken for other presumed pathology such as carcinoma or Crohn's disease. Minimal resection is recommended since much of the disease will yield to medical therapy.

Table 14.5. Faecal leucocytes in intestinal infections.

Present	Variable	Absent
Shigella	Salmonella	V. cholerae
Campylobacter	Yersinia	Toxigenic E. coli (ETEC)

Invasive E. coli	V. parahaemolyticus
	Clostridium difficile
	(antibiotic-associated colitis)
		Enteropathogenic E. coli (EPEC)
		Rotavirus
		Norwalk virus
		Giardia lamblia
		Entamoeba histolytica
		Food-poisoning
		    Staphylococcus aureus
		    Clostridium perfringens
		    Bacillus cerus

Diagnostic features of diarrhoeal disease

A presumptive diagnosis of the aetiologic agent can be made by considering the clinical features and pathogenic mechanisms (DuPont & Pickering 1980). A number of agents involve the upper small intestine, including toxigenic bacteria (E. coli, V. cholerae), viruses, and the parasite Giardia. These organisms produce watery diarrhoea, which may lead to dehydration. Abdominal pain, although often diffuse and poorly defined, is generally peri-umbilical in location. Organisms attacking the large bowel, such as Shigella and Campylobacter, are invasive and produce the clinical syndrome of dysentery. Characteristic rectal pain, known as tenesmus, indicates colonic involvement. Although initially the faecal effluent may be watery, by the second or third day of dysentery there is a relatively small volume stool, often bloody and mucoid. Certain pathogens invade the lower small bowel, especially the ileum, but also the colon; Salmonella and Yersinia are in this category. Whereas watery diarrhoea is the usual presentation, depending on the focus of infection the spectrum of disease extends from dehydrating diarrhoea to frank colitis.

Microscopic examination of the stool is a useful technique in establishing a presumptive diagnosis in infectious diarrhoea (Harris et al. 1972, Pickering et al. 1977) (Table 14.5). Using two drops of Loeffler's methylene blue mixed with a small amount of stool on a slide, a search for leucocytes and erythrocytes is undertaken. (An experienced observer can do the examination without the stain, thereby looking for protozoa and other parasites on the same slide). Invasive pathogens, such as Shigella and Campylobacter, produce many polymorphonuclear leucocytes ('a sea of polys') easily visible on every coverslip, as well as red blood cells. The toxigenic organisms, viruses, Giardia, and food-poisoning bacteria cause a watery stool that harbours very few cellular elements.

Several organisms produce variable findings on microscopic stool examination, depending on the invasive properties of the strain and the degree of colonic involvement. This category includes Salmonella, Yersinia, and V. parahaemolyticus. Pseudomembranous colitis and antibiotic-associated diarrhoea, caused by Clostridium difficile, have unpredictable findings with regard to cellular elements in the stool. Most cases show a profusion of sloughed epithelial cells and red blood cells, but only rare polymorphonuclear leucocytes. An acute exacerbation of ulcerative colitis can produce a great discharge of leucocytes and erythrocytes into the stool, resulting in an exudative microscopic appearance that resembles bacillary dysentery.

Although the faecal microscopic examination is neither infallible nor even helpful in all cases, it is inexpensive and yields immediate information that can guide

References

Abrams J.S. & Holden W.D. (1964) Tuberculosis of the gastrointestinal tract. *Arch. Surg.* **89**, 282–293.

Ahvonen P. (1972) Human yersiniosis in Finland. II. Clinical features. *Ann. Clin. Res.* **4**, 39–48.

Anderson M.J., Whitehead J.S. & Kim Y.S. (1980) Interaction of *Escherichia coli* K88 antigen with porcine intestinal brush border membrane. *Infect. Immun.* **29**, 897–901.

Askerkoff B. & Bennett J.V. (1969) Effect of antibiotic therapy in acute salmonellosis on the faecal excretion of salmonellae. *N. Engl. J. Med.* **281**, 636–640.

Bentley G. & Webster J.H.H. (1967) Gastrointestinal tuberculosis: A 10-year review. *Brit. J. Surg.* **54**, 90–96.

Bishop R.F., Davidson G.P., Holmes I.H. & Ruck B.J. (1973) Virus particles in epithelial cells of duodenal mucosa from children with acute non-bacterial gastroenteritis. *Lancet* **ii**, 1281–1283.

Black P.H., Kunz L.J. & Swartz M.N. (1960) Salmonellosis — a review of some unusual aspects. *N. Engl. J. Med.* **262**, 811–817.

Blacklow N.R. & Cukor G. (1981) Viral gastroenteritis. *N. Engl. J. Med.* **304**, 397–407.

Blacklow N.R., Dolin R., Fedson D.S., DuPont H., Northrup R.S., Hornick R.B. & Chanock R.M. (1972) Acute infectious nonbacterial gastroenteritis: etiology and pathogenesis. *Ann. Intern. Med.* **76**, 993–1008.

Bottone E.J. (1977) *Yersinia enterocolitica*: A panoramic view of a charismatic microorganism. *CRC Crit. Rev. Microbiol.* **5**, 211–241.

Cantey J.R. & Blake R.K. (1977) Diarrhoea due to *Escherichia coli* in the rabbit: A novel mechanism. *J. Infect. Dis.* **35**, 454–462.

Carpenter C.C.J. (1982). The pathophysiology of secretory diarrheas. *Med. Clin. N. Amer.* **66**, 597–610.

Carpenter C.C.J., Sack R.B., Mondal A. & Mitra P.P. (1964) Tetracycline therapy in cholera. *J. Ind. Med. Assoc.* **43**, 309–312.

Cukor G. & Blacklow N.R. (1984). Human viral gastroenteritis. *Microbiol. Rev.* **48**, 157–179.

Davidson G.P. & Barnes G.L. (1979) Structural and functional abnormalities of the small intestine in infants and young children with rotavirus enteritis. *Acta Paediatr, Scand.* **68**, 181–186.

Deneke C.F., Thorne G.M. & Gorbach S.L. (1981) Serotypes of attachment pili of enterotoxigenic *Escherichia coli* isolated from humans. *Infect. Immun.* **32**, 1254–1260.

Dixon J.M.S. (1960) The fate of bacteria in the small intestine. *J. Path. Bact.* **79**, 131–140.

Drasar B.S., Shiner M. & McLeod G.M. (1969) Studies on the intestinal flora. I. The bacterial flora of the gastrointestinal tract in healthy and achlorhydric persons. *Gastroenterol.* **56**, 71–79.

DuPont H.L. & Pickering L.K. (1980) *Infections of the Gastrointestinal Tract: Microbiology, Pathophysiology, and Clinical Features*. Plenum Medical Books, New York.

Evans D.G., Silver R.P., Evans D.J., Chase D.G. & Gorbach S.L. (1975) Plasmid-controlled colonization factor associated with virulence in *Escherichia coli* enterotoxigenic for humans. *Infect. Immun.* **12**, 656–667.

Field M., Graf L.H. Jr., Laird W.J. & Smith P.L. (1978) Heat-stable enterotoxin of *Escherichia coli: In vitro* effects on guanylate cyclase activity, cyclic GMO concentration, and ion transport in small intestine. *Proc. Natl. Acad. Sci. USA*, **75**, 2800–2804.

Finkelstein R.A. (1973) Cholera. *CRC Crit. Rev. Microbiol.* **2**, 553–623.

Flewett T.H. & Woode G.N. (1978) The rotaviruses: Brief review. *Arch. Virol.* **57**, 1–23.

Giannella R.A., Formal S.B., Dammin G.J. & Collins H. (1973) Pathogenesis of salmonellosis. *J. Clin. Invest.* **52**, 441–453.

Giannella R.A., Gots R.E., Charney A.N., Greenhough III W.B. & Formal S.B., (1975) Pathogenesis of salmonella-mediated intestinal fluid secretion: activation of adeylate cyclase and inhibition by indomethacin. *Gastroenterol.* **69**, 1238–1245.

Gibbons R.J. (1974) Bacterial adherence to mucosal surfaces and its inhibition by secretory antibiotics. In *The Immunoglobulin A System*, pp. 315–325. (Ed. by J. Meslecky & A.R. Lawton) Plenum Press, New York.

Gill D.M. (1977) The mechanisms of action of cholera toxin. *Advan. Cyclic Nucleotide Res.* **8**, 85–118.

Gitelson S. (1971) Gastrectomy, achlorhydria and cholera. *Isr. J. Med. Sci.* **7**, 663–667.

Glass R.I., Svennerholm A.M., Stoll B.J., Khan M.R., Hossain K.M.B., Hug M.I. & Holmgren J. (1983). Protection against cholera in breast-fed children by antibodies in breast milk. *New Engl. J. Med.* **308**, 1389–1392.

Gorbach S.L., Banwell J.G., Chatterjee B.D., Jacobs B. & Sack R.B. (1971) Acute undifferentiated human diarrhoea in the tropics. I. Alterations in intestinal microflora. *J. Clin. Invest.* **50**, 881–889.

Gorbach S.L. & Hoskins D.W. (1980) Traveller's diarrhoea. *Disease-a-Month* **27**. 1–44.

Gray J.D.A. & Shiner M. (1967) Influence of gastric pH on gastric and jejunal flora. *Gut*, **8**, 574–581.

Gray J.A. & Trueman A.M. (1971) Severe salmonella gastroenteritis associated with hypochlorhydria. *Scot. Med. J.* **16**, 255–258.

Greenberg H.B., Valdesuso J., Yolken R.H., Gangarosa E., Gary W., Wyatt R.G., Konzo T., Suzuki H., Chanock R.M. & Kapikian A.Z. (1979) Role of Norwalk virus in outbreaks of nonbacterial gastroenteritis. *J. Infect. Dis.* **139**,

564–568.

Greenough W.B., Gordon R.S., Rosenberg I.S., Davies B.I. & Benseson A.S. (1964) Tetracycline in the treatment of cholera. *Lancet*, **i**, 355–357.

Hand W.L. & King N.L. (1977) Serum opsonization of salmonella in sickle-cell anaemia. *Amer. J. Med.* **64**, 388–395.

Harris J.C., DuPont H.L. & Hornick R.B. (1972) Fecal leucocytes in diarrheal illness. *Ann. Intern. Med.* **76**, 697–703.

Hirschhorn N., McCarthy B.J., Ranney B., Hirschhorn M.A., Woodward S.T., Lacapa A., Cash R.A. & Woodward W.E. (1973) Ad libitum oral glucose-electrolyte therapy for acute diarrhea in Apache children. *J. Pediatr.* **83**, 562–571.

Hoffman T.A., Ruiz C.J., Counts G.W., Sachs J.M. & Nitzkin J.L. (1975) Waterborne typhoid fever in Dade County, Florida: clinical and therapeutic evaluations of 105 bacteremic patients. *Amer. J. Med.* **59**, 481–487.

Hook E.W. (1961) Salmonellosis: Certain factors influencing the interaction of salmonella and the human host. *Bull. N.Y. Acad. Med.* **37**, 499–512.

Hoon J., Dockerty M. & Pemberton J. (1950) Collective review: Ileocaecal tuberculosis including comparison of this disease with nonspecific regional enterocolitis and noncaseous tuberculated enterocolitis. *Int. Abstr. Surg.* **91**, 417–440.

Hornick R.B., Greisman S.E., Woodward T.E., DuPont H.L., Dawkins A.T. & Snyder M.J. (1970) Typhoid fever: pathogenesis and immunologic control. *N. Engl. J. Med*, **283**, 739–746.

Hornick R.B., Music S.I., Wenzel R., Caseh R., Libonati J.P., Snyder M.J. & Woodward T.E. (1971) The Broad Street pump revisited: Response of volunteers to ingested cholera vibrios. *Bull. N.Y. Acad. Med.* **47**, 1181–1191.

Hughes J.M., Murad F., Chang B. & Guerrant R.L. (1978) Role of cyclic GMP in the action of heat-stable enterotoxin of *Escherichia coli*. *Nature*, **271**, 755–756.

Inman L.R. & Cantey J.R. (1983). Specific adherence of *Escherichia coli* (strain RDEC-1) to membranous (M) cells of Peyer's patch in *Escherichia coli* diarrhea in the rabbit. *J. clin. Invest.* **71**, 1–8.

Jordan Jr G., DeBakey M. (1954) Complication of tuberculous enteritis occurring during antimicrobial therapy. *Arch. Surg.* **69**, 688–693.

Kapikian A.Z., Kim H.W., Wyatt R.G., Cline W.L. Arrobio J.O., Brandt C.D., Rodriguez W.J., Sack D.A., Chanock R.M. & Parrott R.H. (1976) Human reovirus-like agent as the major pathogen associated with 'winter' gastroenteritis in hospitalized infants and young children. *N. Engl. J. Med.* **294**, 965–972.

Kaye D., Gill F.A. & Hook E.W. (1967) Factors influencing host resistance to salmonella infections: The effects of hemolysis and erythrophagocytosis. *Amer. J. Med. Sci.* **254**, 205–215.

Kazemi M., Gumpert T.G. & Marks M.I. (1973) A controlled trial comparing sulphamethoxazole-trimethoprim, ampicillin, and no therapy in the treatment of Salmonella gastroenteritis in children. *J. Pediatr.* **83**, 646–650.

Keusch G.T. & Donta S.T. (1975) Classification of enterotoxins on the basis of activity in cell culture. *J. Infect. Dis.* **131**, 58–63.

Keusch G.T. (1979) Specific membrane receptors: Pathogenic and therapeutic implications in infectious diseases. *Rev. Infect. Dis.* **1**, 517–529.

Kolawole T.W. & Lewis E.A. (1975) A radiologic study of tuberculosis of the abdomen (gastrointestinal tract). *Amer. J. Roentgenol. Radium Ther. Nucl. Med.* **123**, 348–358.

Kornfeld S.J. & Plaut A.G. (1981) Secretory immunity and bacterial IgA proteases. *Rev. Infect. Dis.* **3**, 521–534.

Levine M.M., Nalin D.R., Hornick R.B., Berquist E.J., Waterman D.H., Young C.R. & Sotman S. (1978) *Escherichia coli* strains that cause diarrhoea but do not produce heat-labile or heat-stable enterotoxins and are noninvasive. *Lancet*, **i**, 1119–1122.

Marks M.I., Pai C.H., Lafleur L., Lackman L. & Hammerberg O. (1980) *Yersinia enterocolitica* gastroenteritis: A prospective study of clinical, bacteriologic, and epidemiologic features. *J. Pediatr.* **96**, 26–31.

McCullough N.B. & Eisele C.W. (1951) Experimental human salmonellosis. IV. Pathogenicity of strains of *Salmonella pullorum* obtained from spray-dried whole egg. *J. Infect. Dis.* **88**, 278–289.

McCullough N.B. & Eisele C.W. (1951) Experimental salmonellosis. III. Pathogenicity of strains of *Salmonella newport*, *Salmonella derby*, and *Salmonella bareilly* obtained from spray-dried whole egg. *J. Infect. Dis.* **89**, 209–213.

McNabb P.C. & Tomasi T.B. (1981) Host defense mechanism at mucosal surfaces. *Ann. Rev. Microbiol.* **35**, 477–496.

Merson M.H., Sack, R.B., Islam S., Saklayen G., Huda N., Hug I., Zulich A.W., Yolken R.H. & Kapikian A.Z. (1980) Disease due to enterotoxigenic *Escherichia coli* in Bangladeshi adults: Clinical aspects and a controlled trial of tetracycline. *J. Infect. Dis.* **141**, 702–711.

Mitchell R. & Bristol L. (1954) Intestinal tuberculosis: analysis of 346 cases diagnosed by routine intestinal radiography on 5529 admissions for pulmonary tuberculosis, 1924–49. *Amer. J. Med. Sci.* **227**, 241–249.

Morris G.K. & Feeley J.C. (1976) *Yersinia enterocolitica*: A review of its role in food hygiene. *Bull. WHO*, **54**, 79–85.

Moon H.W., Nagy B. & Issacson R.E. (1977) Intestinal colonization and adhesion by enterotoxigenic *Escherichia coli*: ultrastructural observations on adherence to ileal epithelium of the pig. *J. Infect. Dis.* **136**, Suppl., S124–S129.

Mosley W.H. (1969) The role of immunity in

cholera. A review of epidemiological and serological studies. *Texas Report Biol. Med.* **27**, Suppl. 1, 227–241.

Moseley S.L., Samadpour-Motalebi M. & Falkow S. (1983). Plasmid association and nucleotide sequence relationship of two genes encoding heat-stable enterotoxin production in *Escherichia coli* H-10407. *J. Bacteriol.* **156**, 441–443.

Nalin D.R., Levine M.M. & Mata L. (1979) Oral rehydration and maintenance of children with rotavirus and bacterial diarrhoeas. *Bull. WHO* **57**, 453–459.

Parrino T.A., Schreiber D.S., Trier J.S., Kapikian A.Z. & Blacklow N.R. (1977) Clinical immunity in acute gastroenteritis caused by Norwalk agent. *N. Engl. J. Med.* **297**, 86–89.

Pickering L.K., DuPont H.L., Olarte J., Conklin R. & Ericsson C. (1977) Fecal leucocytes in enteric infections. *Amer. J. Clin. Path.* **68**, 562–565.

Plaut A.G. (1978) Microbial IgG proteases. *N. Engl. J. Med.* **298**, 1459–1463.

Rodriguez W.J., Kim H.W., Arrobio J.O., Brandt C.D., Chanock R.M., Kapikian A.Z., Wyatt R.B. & Parrott R.H. (1977) Clinical features of acute gastroenteritis associated with human reovirus-like agent in infants and young children. *J. Pediatr.* **91**, 188–193.

Rosenstein B.J. (1967) Salmonellosis in infants and children: epidemiologic and therapeutic considerations. *J. Pediatr.* **70**, 1–7.

Rubin H.R. & Weinstein L. (1977) *Salmonellosis: Microbiologic, Pathologic and Clinical Features.* Stratton Intercontinental Medical Book Corporation, New York.

Sack R.B. (1980) Enterotoxigenic *Escherichia coli*: identification and characterization. *J. Infect. Dis.* **142**, 279–286.

Sack R.B. (1975) Human diarrheal disease caused by enterotoxigenic *Escherichia coli*. Ann. Rev. Microbiol. **29**, 333.

Saphra I. & Winter J.W. (1957) Clinical manifestations of salmonellosis in man. *N. Engl. J. Med.* **256**, 1128–1134.

Schreiber D.S., Blacklow N.R. & Trier J.S. (1973) The mucosal lesion of the proximal small intestine in acute infectious nonbacterial gastroenteritis. *N. Engl. J. Med.* **288**, 1318–1323.

Schulze K., Warner H.A. & Murray D. (1977) Intestinal tuberculosis: experience at a Canadian teaching institution. *Amer. J. Med.* **63**, 735–745.

Sherman S., Rohwedder J.J., Ravikrishnan K.P. & Weg J.G. (1980) Tuberculous enteritis and peritonitis: Report of 36 general hospital cases. *Arch. Intern. Med.* **140**, 506–508.

Stuart B.M. & Pullen R.L. (1946) Typhoid: Clinical analysis of three hundred and sixty cases. *Arch. Intern. Med.* **78**, 629–661.

Takeuchi A. (1966) Electron microscope studies of experimental salmonella infection. I. Penetration into the intestinal epithelium by *S. typhimurium*. *Amer. J. Pathol.* **50**, 109–136.

Takeuchi A. & Sprinz H. (1967) Electron microscope studies of experimental salmonella infection in the preconditioned guinea pig. II. Response of the intestinal mucosa to the invasion by *S. typhimurium*. *Amer. J. Pathol.* **51**, 137–161.

Tallett S., MacKenzie C., Middleton P., Kerzner B. & Hamilton R. (1977) Clinical, laboratory and epidemiological features of a viral gastroenteritis in infants and children. *Pediat.* **60**, 217–222.

Totterdell B.M., Chrystie I.L. & Banetvola J.E. (1980) Cord blood and breast milk antibodies in neonatal rotavirus infection. *Brit. Med. J.*, **200**, 828–830.

Ulshen M.H. & Rollo J.L. (1980) Pathogenesis of *Escherichia coli* enteritis in man — another mechanism. *New Engl. J. Med.*, **302**, 99–101.

Walker W. (1965) The Aberdeen typhoid outbreak of 1964. *Scot. Med. J.*, **10**, 466.

Weberloff L., Novis B.H., Bank S. & Marks I.N. (1973) The radiology of tuberculosis of the gastrointestinal tract. *Brit. J. Radiol.* **46**, 329–336.

Winblad S. (1975) Arthritis associated with *Yersinia enterocolitica* infections. *Scand. J. Infect. Dis.*, **7**, 191–195.

Woodward T.E. & Smadel J.E. (1964) Management of typhoid fever and its complications. *Ann. Intern. Med.*, **60**, 144–157.

Wyatt R.G., Dolin R. Thornhill T.S., Blacklow N.R. Dupont H.L., Buscho R.F., Kapikian A.Z. & Chanock R.M. (1974) Comparison of three agents of acute infectious non-bacterial gastroenteritis by cross-challenge in volunteers. *J. Infect. Dis.*, **129**, 709–714.

Chapter 15
Bacterial Overgrowth

SOAD TABAQCHALI AND CHRISTOPHER C. BOOTH

Introduction 249
Normal bacterial flora 249
Factors encouraging an abnormal bacterial flora 250
Micro-organisms isolated under abnormal circumstances 251
Deleterious effects of bacterial overgrowth .. 252
Clinical assessment of bacterial overgrowth 260
Clinical conditions associated with an abnormal bacterial flora 261
Treatment 266

Introduction

In 1890, White drew attention to patients with changes in the small intestine who died with pernicious anaemia. This observation, together with other reports of macrocytic or megaloblastic anaemia in patients with lesions of the distal small intestine causing stasis (Faber 1895), suggested that bacteria within the intestine might elaborate toxins which caused megaloblastic change in the bone marrow. It was not until the discovery of the efficacy of liver treatment for Addisonian pernicious anaemia in the 1920s, and subsequently the isolation of vitamin B_{12} in 1948, that the megaloblastic anaemia associated with what became known as the 'stagnant loop syndrome' was shown to be due to vitamin B_{12} deficiency and that this was caused by malabsorption of vitamin B_{12}. The recognition that the physiological absorption of vitamin B_{12} takes place in the ileum explained why patients with lesions of the distal small intestine, such as those originally described by Faber (1895), were particularly vulnerable to the development of megaloblastic anaemia, a frequent feature of the stagnant loop syndrome.

In recent years, microbiologists have been involved in the dramatic renaissance that has characterized studies of the small intestine. The microbiology of this region of the alimentary tract has been extensively investigated and considerable progress has been made towards establishing the nature of the bacterial populations of proximal and distal small intestine in health and disease. At the same time, modern biochemical techniques, microbiological assay methods, and the use of isotopically labelled substances have made it possible to unravel some of the complex metabolic effects of bacteria in the small intestine. Detailed studies, both in man and in experimental animals, have shown how bacteria within the small intestine may interfere with the digestion and absorption of nutrients, particularly of fat and vitamin B_{12}, as well as producing localized damage to the intestinal mucosa (Donaldson 1970, Tabaqchali 1970, King & Toskes 1979).

Normal bacterial flora

The bacterial flora of the gastrointestinal tract is derived from the oropharynx, saliva and food. There are two types of flora, the resident indigenous flora which varies little under constant conditions, and a transient flora which is introduced with meals and causes a wave of increase in the microbial population postprandially.

The normal fasting proximal small intestine usually harbours a sparse microflora, but in the distal small bowel there is a characteristic indigenous flora (Gorbach et al. 1967). The numbers of bacteria in the upper intestine rarely exceed $10^3 - 10^4$/ml. They are composed predominantly of Gram-positive organisms, including streptococci, staphylococci, lactobacilli and fungi. The numbers of bacteria present in the upper intestine tend to reflect social and environmental conditions since individuals studied in developing countries have higher bacterial counts than those in the Western world.

The microbial flora of the ileum is different and may represent a transitional zone between the upper intestinal flora and that found in the colon, where facultative Gram-negative enterobacteria and enterococci are present (10^8-10^9 organisms/g) and where anaerobes such as bacteroides and bifidobacteria are found in high concentrations ($10^{10}-10^{11}$ organisms/g). The ileum contains a similar flora to that of the jejunum, but in addition there are coliforms, bacteroides, anaerobic lactobacilli and faecal streptococci. The concentrations are usually higher than those in the jejunum, reaching 10^6-10^7/ml.

The bacterial flora in the small intestine is closely associated with the mucus layer covering the mucosa and cannot be dislodged by repeated washing (Fig. 15.1). Frozen sections of intestinal mucosa obtained from both experimental animals and man show large numbers of rods and cocci within the intestinal mucus. Culture of mucosal biopsy specimens reveals similar micro-organisms to those found in the lumen of the small bowel.

The role of the indigenous flora

Studies in animals raised in germ-free conditions suggest that the establishment of the bacterial flora within the small intestine, presumably during the neonatal period, plays an important part in inducing the development of the immunocytes of the lamina propria. This may be important in the development of protective mechanisms against ingested pathogens (Mackowiak 1982). In the germ-free state, the lamina propria of the small intestinal mucosa is poorly developed and there is a striking reduction in the cellular infiltrate, plasma cells being conspicuously absent. The mucosa of the small intestine of the neonate appears similar (Perkkio & Savilahti 1980). Furthermore, there is a reduction in the mucosal thickness of the small intestine. The villi are slender and the crypts are shallow as compared with the deep crypts and numerous mitotic figures of the conventional animal. There is also an overall reduction in the turnover of intestinal epithelial cells in the germ-free state. These observations suggest that the bacterial flora may also play a role in controlling the growth of the small intestinal mucosa, in addition to the nutritional and hormonal factors already described in Chapter 6.

Factors encouraging an abnormal bacterial flora

Three types of gastrointestinal abnormality encourage bacterial growth in the small intestine (Table 15.1). Since gastric acidity is important in controlling the entry of micro-organisms into the small intestine (Chapter 14), the first group includes abnormalities of the stomach such as gastric atrophy due to Addisonian pernicious anaemia, partial gastrectomy and vagotomy with pyloroplasty or gastroenterostomy.

Secondly, there may be areas of stasis within the small intestine, as in diverticulosis of duodenum and jejunum, or surgically created blind loops due to entero-anastomosis and strictures. If normal peristalsis is inhibited, as in scleroderma, diabetic neuropathy or after treatment with ganglion-blocking agents, a profuse bacterial flora may also develop in the areas of stasis. It has further been claimed that bacterial

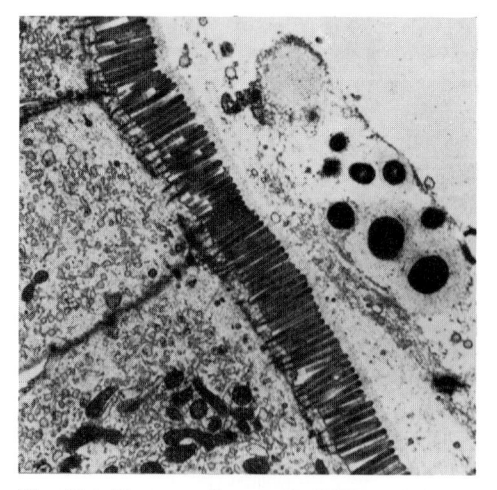

Fig. 15.1. Electron micrograph of the enterocyte showing the microvilli and glycocalyx with a mucus layer overlying the mucosa containing micro-organisms ($\times$ 11,000).

Table 15.1. Conditions associated with an abnormal flora.

Abnormalities of gastric function	Pernicious anaemia Polya partial gastrectomy — afferent loop syndrome Malfunctioning gastrojejunostomy

Conditions causing stasis	Surgical blind loops
	Entero-anastomosis
	Strictures
	  Congenital
	  Crohn's disease
	  Tuberculosis
	Adhesions
	  X-ray irradiation
	Small intestinal diverticulosis
	Abnormal motility
	  Scleroderma
	  Diabetic neuropathy
	  Vagotomy
	  Ganglion-blocking agents
	Partial biliary obstruction with cholangitis
	? Ageing

Free communications between large and small bowel	Gastrocolic fistula Enterocolic fistula Massive intestinal resection

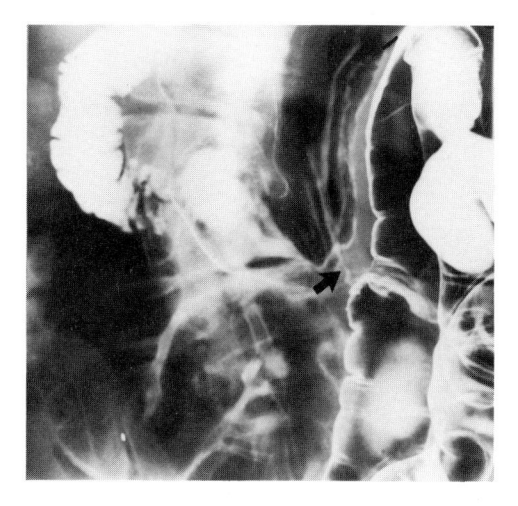

Fig. 15.2. Gastrocolic fistula revealed by barium enema. The barium can be seen passing through the fistula (arrowed) into the stomach and duodenal loop on the left.

overgrowth may occur in the small intestine in old age without demonstrable intestinal lesions (McEvoy *et al.* 1983). Whether this is due to an undiscovered and occult lesion, or possibly a motility disorder due to ageing, or to hypochlorhydria, is at present uncertain.

Thirdly, there may be a free communication between the small intestine and colon through a fistula, as in gastrocolic or enterocolic fistulae (Fig. 15.2), or following surgical anastomoses between the large and small bowel. Under these circumstances, the small intestine is exposed to the high concentration of bacteria in the colon, which have unimpeded entry as a result of the higher pressure present in the colon than in the small intestine. This may also occur after resection of the small intestine with the loss of the ileocaecal valve.

Micro-organisms isolated under abnormal circumstances
(Simon & Gorbach 1984)

When there is bacterial overgrowth in the small intestine, the abnormal bacterial flora appears to develop within the lumen of the gut, and in close association with the mucosa (Fig. 15.3). Unless there is ulceration, as may occur in an infected diverticulum or blind loop, the organisms do not invade the jejunal mucosa, in contrast to some of the pathogens described in Chapter 14. Whether the small intestinal micro-organisms in the stagnant loop syndrome adhere to the mucosa, as in the case of enterotoxic *E. coli* or cholera, is uncertain. Multiple O and H serotypes and biotypes of *E. coli* are represented along the entire length of the intestine, although usually a single serotype predominates in each patient. The serotypes isolated from the stomach and small intestine are represented in the faeces (Tabaqchali *et al.* 1977). This indicates a stable ecosystem in each patient and may require specific oral antibiotics to alter it.

A wide variety of micro-organisms has been cultured from the intestinal lumen in patients with the stagnant loop syndrome. The bacterial flora, however, may vary at

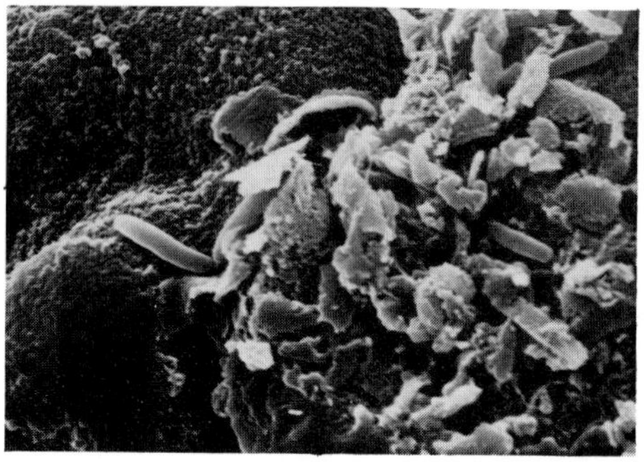

Fig. 15.3. Scanning electron micrograph of jejunal biopsy from a patient with intestinal stasis due to intestinal pseudo-obstruction showing bacteria enmeshed in surface mucus (× 3500). (Courtesy of Dr David Levinson and Mr Peter Crocker.)

different levels of the intestine. In general, the development of an abnormal small intestinal microflora is related to the site and the extent of the causative abnormality (Gorbach & Tabaqchali 1969). In a patient with multiple jejunal diverticulosis, for example, there may be a diffuse and generalized bacterial proliferation throughout the small intestine, and the same situation may develop in a generalized disorder of motility, such as scleroderma. On the other hand, a single duodenal diverticulum may be associated with a significant bacterial flora which is limited to the upper intestine, and conversely a distal intestinal stricture, involving the terminal ileum, for example, may encourage bacterial proliferation only in the ileum.

The bacterial counts in intestinal fluid from patients with conditions favouring stasis are usually markedly increased, ranging from 10^6 to as high as 10^9 organisms/ml. Coliforms and other aerobic organisms are invariably present, but there are also high counts of anaerobic organisms such as bacteroides, anaerobic lactobacilli and clostridia. These anaerobic organisms are of particular importance since it is the anaerobic flora that is responsible for the majority of the deleterious effects of bacteria in the small intestine.

Figure 15.4 illustrates the bacterial flora at different levels of the gastrointestinal tract of a patient with severe malabsorption due to multiple small intestinal diverticulosis. The numbers of coliforms, bacteroides and streptococci range from 10^6-10^9/ml throughout the small intestine. Other organisms were present in lower concentrations. In this patient, therefore, the bacterial populations throughout the small bowel were relatively uniform.

By contrast, there are other intestinal abnormalities which involve specific areas of the small intestine, in which the bacterial flora at different levels of the bowel may vary. Figure 15.5 illustrates the distribution of two micro-organisms at different levels of the small intestine in three other examples of gastrointestinal disorders. The two micro-organisms are *E. coli*, to represent the aerobic flora, and bacteroides, a fastidious anaerobe whose distribution in the small intestine appears to be particularly related to stasis. In the first patient who had a Polya partial gastrectomy without evidence of stasis, coliforms were present throughout the small intestine in concentrations of 10^6-10^9/ml. Bacteroides, however, were not detected at any level, although present in normal concentrations in stool. In the second and third patients, coliforms were also present at all levels, but bacteroides were only present in the areas of stasis, proximally in the patient with a single duodenal diverticulum, and only in the area of stasis in the distal small intestine in the patient who had an ileal stricture. These observations indicate that the nature of the abnormal bacterial flora may be determined by the presence or absence of stasis, and that the development of the anaerobic flora is particularly correlated with areas of stasis. As is the case after small intestinal resection, the site and extent of the causative lesion may therefore be of great importance in determining the severity of malabsorption and malnutrition that may result.

Deleterious effects of bacterial overgrowth

Mucosal injury

In experimental animals, there is abundant

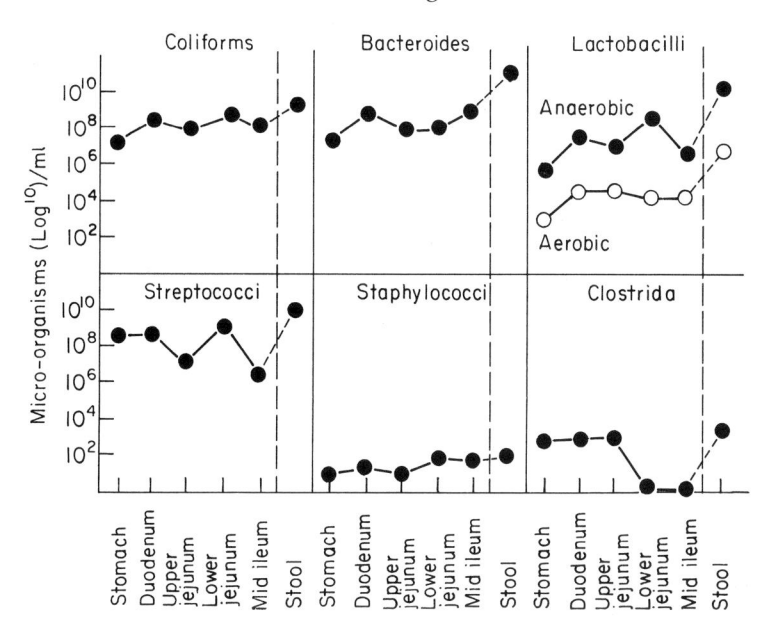

Fig. 15.4. Bacterial flora at different levels of the gastrointestinal tract from a patient with multiple small intestinal diverticulosis. There is marked bacterial overgrowth of both aerobic and anaerobic bacteria throughout the small intestine. Bile salt deconjugation was present in all samples from duodenum to mid-ileum (Gorbach & Tabaqchali 1969).

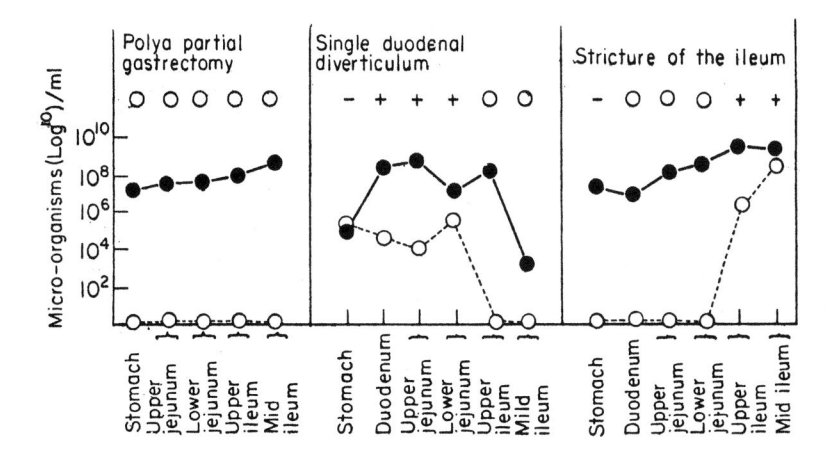

Fig. 15.5. Distribution of E. coli (●——●) and Bacteroides (○——○) at different levels of the gastrointestinal tract in Polya partial gastrectomy, a single duodenal diverticulum and stricture of the ileum. The presence (+) or absence (○) of bile salt deconjugation is also shown (Gorbach & Tabaqchali, 1969).

evidence that bacterial overgrowth within the small intestine is associated with abnormalities of the mucosa (King & Toskes 1979). Histochemical and biochemical studies have shown reduction of enzyme activities in brush border membranes, mitochondria and endoplasmic reticulum (Riepe et al. 1980). There may also be reduced transport of substances such as sugars (Gracey et al. 1971) and amino acids, and on light and electron microscopy abnormalities of enterocytes and of villi have been shown (Gracey et al. 1974).

In man, the evidence is less clear-cut. Patients with bacterial overgrowth have been described in whom there was no abnormality of the small intestine on light or electron microscopy, but other reports have documented significant abnormalities (Ament et al. 1972). It seems likely that the mucosal lesion if present in the stagnant loop syndrome is patchy and that a diffuse abnormality, such as is seen in the jejunum of coeliac disease, does not occur unless there is severe nutritional deficiency, in which case the mucosal abnormality may be the result of malnutrition rather than bacterial overgrowth. Unquestionably, the mucosa may become ulcerated, as in the areas of stasis proximal to a stricture or within a diverticulum or blind loop. Ulceration may be particularly important in such patients (Fig. 15.6) for they may develop signs of iron deficiency due to chronic blood loss (Tabaqchali 1970), or in some cases, acute haemorrhage causing severe melaena.

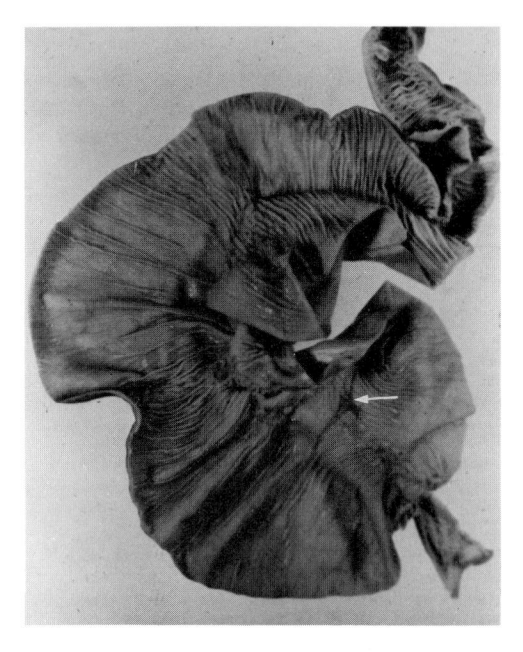

Fig. 15.6. Ulceration of the small intestinal mucosa with a stagnant area proximal to a congenital ileal stricture.

Bacteria and absorption

Carbohydrates

After oral administration of a test dose of xylose, diminished urinary excretion has been described both in the experimental and human blind loop syndrome. The cause of this reduced urinary xylose excretion appears to be predominantly bacterial catabolism of xylose by bacteria in the upper small intestine (Goldstein et al. 1970). There may be an element of xylose malabsorption due to mucosal damage, particularly in experimental animals, but direct studies of ^{14}C-xylose metabolism in animals with experimental blind loops or patients with bacterial overgrowth have shown a significant catabolism of xylose by small intestinal bacteria. Further evidence of intraluminal bacterial metabolism of carbohydrates in the stagnant loop syndrome is provided by the demonstration of elevated levels of volatile fatty acids produced from carbohydrate by bacteria within the small intestine in experimental animals and in man (Chernov et al. 1972).

In addition to these bacterial reactions within the small intestine, there is experimental evidence for diminished mucosal uptake of monosaccharides. Malabsorption of disaccharides may also be associated with the abnormalities of brush border enzymes caused by damage to the brush border of the enterocyte. Carbohydrate malabsorption is therefore a multi-factorial process, involving predominantly bacterial catabolism within the intestinal lumen but there may in addition be an element of mucosal malabsorption (King & Toskes 1979).

Fat

Steatorrhoea is not universally present in patients with the stagnant loop syndrome. The degree of steatorrhoea depends on two main factors: first, the site and extent of the lesion, and second, the degree of bacterial overgrowth present. A patient with a terminal ileal stricture, with bacterial overgrowth limited to the terminal ileum, may have no steatorrhoea, a situation comparable to that described after distal intestinal resection in Chapter 6. On the other hand, a diffuse and generalized bacterial overgrowth in the small intestine, as occurs in massive jejunal diverticulosis, may be associated with severe steatorrhoea. By contrast, however, there may be only mild bacterial overgrowth in massive jejunal diverticulosis and in such patients there may also be no significant steatorrhoea (Tabaqchali et al. 1968).

When there is steatorrhoea, it is predominantly due to malabsorption of dietary fat and not to bacterial synthesis of fatty acids. There are occasional reports of patients with small intestinal bacterial overgrowth who excrete more fat in the stools than taken in the diet, but evidence for this is scanty. There is little doubt that bacteria are capable of metabolizing dietary fat, at least to a certain extent. In vitro incubation of fatty acids with bacteria leads to the production of hydroxyacids and these may be increased in the stools of patients with bacterial overgrowth in the small intestine, as well as those with distal small intestinal resection (Webb et al. 1963). Their presence acts as a stimulus to intestinal secretion (Ammon et al. 1974) which in turn may cause the diarrhoea which occurs in some patients with the stagnant loop syndrome.

Bile acids

The major abnormality produced in the small intestine by bacteria is deconjugation and dehydroxylation of the bile salts. The intestinal flora contains micro-organisms capable of transforming bile acids into a variety of metabolites (Fig. 15.7). These reactions occur in the colon under normal circumstances, but also take place in the small intestine if there is significant bacterial overgrowth. The main reaction is the splitting of the conjugated bile salts by hydrolysing the peptide bond linking the bile acids to taurine or glycine, thus forming free bile acids. The next reaction is the elimination of the hydroxyl group at C-7 to form the secondary bile acids, deoxycholic acid from cholic acid and lithocholic acid from chenodeoxycholic acid. Some micro-organisms can further oxidase the hydroxyl groups to form keto acids or reduce them to α or β epimers. Pure cultures of some strains of enterococci and clostridia are capable of in vitro hydrolysis of the conjugated bile salts and deoxycholic acid and lithocholic acid are also produced.

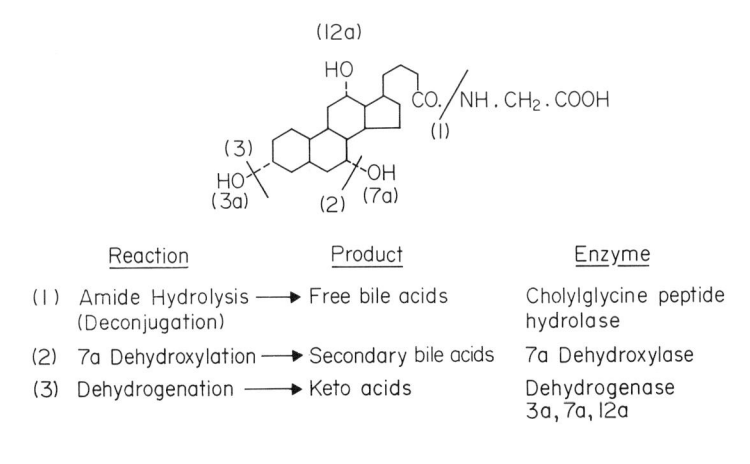

Reaction	Product	Enzyme
(1) Amide Hydrolysis (Deconjugation) →	Free bile acids	Cholylglycine peptide hydrolase
(2) 7α Dehydroxylation →	Secondary bile acids	7α Dehydroxylase
(3) Dehydrogenation →	Keto acids	Dehydrogenase 3α, 7α, 12α

Fig. 15.7. Effects of intestinal bacteria on bile acids.

Although it has been well established that the bulk of the normal intestinal flora in man consists of micro-organisms belonging within the families Lactobacilliaceae and Bacteroidaceae, the ability of these micro-organisms to transform bile acids was not investigated until Drasar et al. (1966) demonstrated that some strains of the anaerobic micro-organism bacteroides were capable of this reaction. The ability to deconjugate and dehydroxylate the conjugated bile salts is not possessed by all micro-organisms but is present in the strictly anaerobic micro-organisms such as bacteroides, veillonella, clostridia, and bifidobacteria (anaerobic lactobacilli). Some strains of *Streptococcus faecalis* and *Staph. aureus* also possess this activity. However, *E. coli*, non-faecal streptococci, aerobic lactobacilli, and the yeasts are incapable of this reaction, although some strains of *Pseudomonas aerigunosa* are capable of dehydroxylation. The enzymes taurocholate amidase and cholate dehydroxylase which carry out these reactions have been shown to be present in these micro-organisms and have a pH optimum of 6.0–7.0. Since bacteroides and bifidobacteria are often the most numerous of the small intestinal bacteria in lesions associated with the stagnant loop syndrome, these micro-organisms may play a major role in altering bile salt metabolism and thus contributing to steatorrhea. Deconjugation of bile salts only occurs in areas of stasis where conditions favour the growth of the anaerobic flora and it is likely that bacteroides is the bacterial species responsible for deconjugation *in vivo* (Gorbach & Tabaqchali 1969). Figures 15.3 and 15.4 illustrate the relationship between bile salt deconjugation and the presence of coliforms or bacteroides at different levels of the small intestine. Free bile acids were only present in the areas where bacteroides were isolated in the areas of stasis.

The evidence for incriminating bacteroides in deconjugation of bile salts *in vivo* is largely circumstantial, however, and it is possible that this micro-organism may only be serving as a marker for the physico-chemical environment of a stagnant area which allows the deconjugation reaction to proceed.

Bile acids and steatorrhoea

The deconjugation of bile acids by bacteria in the small intestine results in a reduction in the levels of the conjugated bile salts, predominantly involving the taurine conjugates, and a marked increase in the free bile acids. The reduction in the intraluminal concentration of the conjugated bile salts, which may occur at all levels of the small intestine if there is diffuse bacterial overgrowth, is important in causing steatorrhoea, since conjugated bile salts are necessary for normal micelle formation and fat absorption (Tabaqchali et al. 1968). However, free bile acids, particularly deoxycholic acid, may under certain circumstances be toxic to the small intestinal mucosa and there is evidence that this toxicity may contribute to the inhibition of fat absorption when there is significant bacterial overgrowth. It is likely, however, that the reduction in the conjugated bile salts is of greater importance in the majority of patients, for studies in both experimental animals and in man have demonstrated that the feeding of conjugated bile salts will improve fat absorption in the stagnant loop syndrome. Furthermore, the improvement in fat absorption that occurs after antibiotic therapy may occur remarkably rapidly, suggesting that the deleterious effects of bacteria on fat absorption are readily reversible. Precipitation of bile acids around an organic nucleus such as a fruit pip may produce enteroliths which may develop within duodenal or jejunal diverticula and may be associated with chronic small bowel obstruction (Shockett & Simon 1982).

Serum bile acids

Using either thin layer chromatography (Panveliwalla et al. 1970) or mass spectrometry (Setchell et al. 1982), it may be shown that the changes in the bile acid pattern in the intestine in the stagnant loop syndrome are reflected in the serum. Patients with bacterial overgrowth and significant bile salt deconjugation in the small intestine have markedly elevated levels of total bile salt concentration in the serum and this increase is almost entirely due to the presence of excessive amounts of free bile acids, cholic, chenodeoxycholic and deoxycholic acids. The serum conjugated bile acids are either normal or only slightly elevated. The pattern of conjugated bile acids, however, is abnormal in that there is a reduction in the taurine conjugates, a reflection of the reduced taurine conjugates in the intestinal bile acids of such patients. As noted in Chapter 6, the presence of excessive amounts of free bile acids in the serum is not specific to small intestinal bacterial overgrowth since similar abnormalities are seen in patients with ileal resection who have malabsorption of the conjugated bile salts.

Fat-soluble vitamins

Malabsorption of fat in the stagnant loop syndrome may be associated with malabsorption of fat-soluble vitamins such as vitamins A and D. Vitamin K, however, does not appear to cause significant problems in patients with bacterial overgrowth, probably because this vitamin may be synthesized by intestinal bacteria.

Protein

Bacteria within the small intestine are able to catabolize protein in the same way that they catabolize carbohydrate. This may lead to effective protein deprivation by diversion of dietary protein from the host by bacterial metabolism (Jones et al. 1968, Varcoe et al. 1974). The metabolites of bacterial activity on protein may be excreted in the urine as indolic substances (derived from trytophan) or phenols (derived from tyrosine), and indicanuria has therefore been used as an indicator of small intestinal bacterial overgrowth. Unfortunately, it is not possible to separate catabolism of the substrates for indican by small intestinal bacteria from those in the colon, and indicanuria correlates more closely with the degree of malabsorption than with small intestinal bacterial overgrowth. Studies of protein and ammonia metabolism in the stagnant loop syndrome, however, have provided elegant evidence of bacterial catabolism of protein in the gut lumen and this has also been shown experimentally in rats with surgically created blind loops (King et al. 1976). Although it is not possible for these studies to quantitate precisely the amount of dietary protein deaminated by bacteria, it is evident that a large proportion of dietary protein may be metabolized in this way if there is a heavy overgrowth of bacteria in the proximal small intestine. In such patients, there is usually severe malabsorption and the faecal nitrogen excretion is often grossly increased.

Bacteria may also inhibit protein digestion and absorption. Diminished levels of enterokinase and brush border peptidase have been demonstrated in the experimental blind loop syndrome. Furthermore, disordered absorption of amino acids, both *in vitro* and *in vivo*, has also been shown.

Protein-losing enteropathy, causing a loss of serum proteins across the intestinal mucosa, has been demonstrated in the experimental blind loop syndrome of the rat, but appears to be less frequent in man. Jeejeebhoy & Coghill (1961), however, demonstrated severe gastrointestinal protein loss in a patient with multiple tuberculous strictures of the ileum, which was corrected by resection of the affected area. In patients with protein-losing enteropathy, hypoproteinaemia is due to increased catabolism of serum proteins which leak out into the intestinal lumen and the products of catabolism are reabsorbed. There is therefore no true malabsorption of protein and in contrast to patients with bacterial catabolism of dietary protein due to severe bacterial overgrowth, the excretion of faecal nitrogen in protein-losing enteropathy is usually normal.

Vitamin B_{12} and folic acid

Megaloblastic anaemia is frequently associated with bacterial overgowth in the small intestine. Using radiolabelled vitamin B_{12}, it has been shown that there may be malabsorption of vitamin B_{12} and, unlike Addisonian pernicious anaemia, this is not corrected by administration of intrinsic factor (IF). If the ileum is present and not short-circuited, however, absorption frequently improves to normal after treatment with oral broad spectrum antibiotics.

The bacteria responsible for malabsorption of intrinsic factor-bound vitamin B_{12} appear to be predominantly the anaerobic flora, which are capable of binding B_{12}, even when it is bound to IF (Schjønsby 1973, 1974; Schjønsby et al. 1973). Furthermore experimental studies have shown that antimicrobial therapy with metronidazole alone, a specifically anti-anaerobe agent, corrects the B_{12} malabsorption of the experimental blind loop model (King & Toskes 1979). There appears to be no direct effect of bacteria on either intrinsic factor or brush border uptake in the ileum, and malabsorption appears to be predominantly associated with bacterial binding of the B_{12}–IF complex (Schjønsby et al. 1973). It is possible that bacterial production of B_{12} analogues such as cobamides may also contribute to B_{12} malabsorption since such analogues may compete for the ileal B_{12} receptor. This has not hitherto been demonstrated in man.

As with substances such as fat, the site and extent of the causative lesion determines whether there is B_{12} malabsorption. A localized lesion of the ileum, for example, is likely to cause B_{12} malabsorption. By contrast, a proximal small intestinal lesion may cause no malabsorption of vitamin B_{12} even in the presence of bacterial overgrowth and bile salt deconjugation in the jejunum.

The absorption of folic acid in patients with bacterial overgrowth in the small intestine is usually normal.

Nutritional deficiency

Vitamin B_{12} and folic acid

Megaloblastic anaemia due to B_{12} deficiency which responds fully to treatment with parenteral B_{12}, is frequently associated with the stagnant loop syndrome. The anaemia is usually more severe than that seen after distal intestinal resection. Subacute combined degeneration of the cord, similar to that seen in Addisonian pernicious anaemia, also occurs (Richmond & Davidson 1958), but rarely. Vitamin B_{12} deficiency in patients with bacterial overgrowth may also be associated with sterility.

When an intestinal abnormality is created surgically, resulting in bacterial overgrowth and the stagnant loop syndrome, it may be several years before B_{12} deficiency develops for, as after total gastrectomy or resection of the ileum, this will only occur when the hepatic stores of B_{12} have been exhausted. Megaloblastic anaemia may therefore be an incident occurring during the course of prolonged and irreparable disease, associated with obvious symptoms and steatorrhoea. By contrast, patients with a lesion of the ileum, in which there may only be malabsorption of B_{12}, may have no intestinal symptoms and it is the anaemia that draws attention to a surgically correctable lesion. A similar megaloblastic anaemia due to B_{12} deficiency may also occur without intestinal symptoms in patients with widespread lesions of the small intestine such as massive jejunal diverticulosis, who have bacterial overgrowth sufficient to inhibit B_{12} absorption but not to cause steatorrhoea.

Folic acid deficiency is exceptionally rare in the stagnant loop syndrome. More frequently, there are high levels of serum folate as a result of folate synthesis by intestinal bacteria (Hoffbrand et al. 1971). The type of folic acid present is 5-methyl tetrahydrofolate, as in control subjects. The highest levels of serum folic acid occur in patients with jejunal lesions which encourage bacterial overgrowth. Patients with ileal lesions do not usually have a high serum folate level, probably because folic acid is predominantly absorbed in the proximal small intestine in man and is only poorly absorbed from the ileum (Hepner et al. 1968). Megaloblastic anaemia in patients with bacterial overgrowth may occasionally fail to respond to treatment with physiological amounts of both B_{12} and folic acid. The anaemia may then respond after treatment with oral broad spectrum antibiotics. It is possible that in such cases bacteria may have in some way inhibited the bone marrow,

Bacterial Overgrowth

possible by synthesis of such substances as B_{12} analogues which could inhibit the action of vitamin B_{12}.

Iron

Iron deficiency may sometimes be the predominant cause of anaemia in patients with the stagnant loop syndrome (Rampal et al. 1981). This is usually due to occult bleeding from ulcerated mucosa in stagnant areas of small intestine. In patients with blind loops, however, haemorrhage may sometimes be so severe as to produce melaena.

Protein

Serum proteins may be reduced in patients who have protein-losing enteropathy. This commonly occurs in patients with inflammatory lesions of the small intestine such as Crohn's disease or radiation enteritis. In such patients, oedema may develop as a result of hypoproteinaemia but, as in the nephrotic syndrome, there is no overall body protein deficiency. Oedema is therefore the main clinical feature of serum protein deficiency due to protein-losing enteropathy.

By contrast, in patients with severe malabsorption due to massive bacterial overgrowth in the small intestine, so great may be the bacterial metabolism of dietary protein that severe protein deficiency may develop. Under these circumstances, there may be not only reduced serum proteins due to reduced synthesis, but also protein deficiency affecting many other organs in the body. In some cases, protein-calorie malnutrition may be so severe as to resemble kwashiorkor (Neale et al. 1967).

Intestinal infantilism in the stagnant loop syndrome

In children with long-continued caloric undernutrition due to the stagnant loop syndrome, there may be failure of growth and sexual development. These findings are demonstrated in the following case report.

> A boy of 18 years had undergone repeated operations on the distal small intestine for a congenital ileal stricture. He was dwarfed and there had been no development of secondary sex characteristics. Height was 1.35 m, and weight 30 kg. Bone age was 10 years. Barium meal showed grossly dilated distal small intestine. Cultures of intestinal fluid produced a profuse growth of coliforms and bacteroides. There was marked steatorrhoea (faecal fat 20 g/day), creatorrhoea (faecal nitrogen 3.4/day), subnormal vitamin B_{12} absorption and

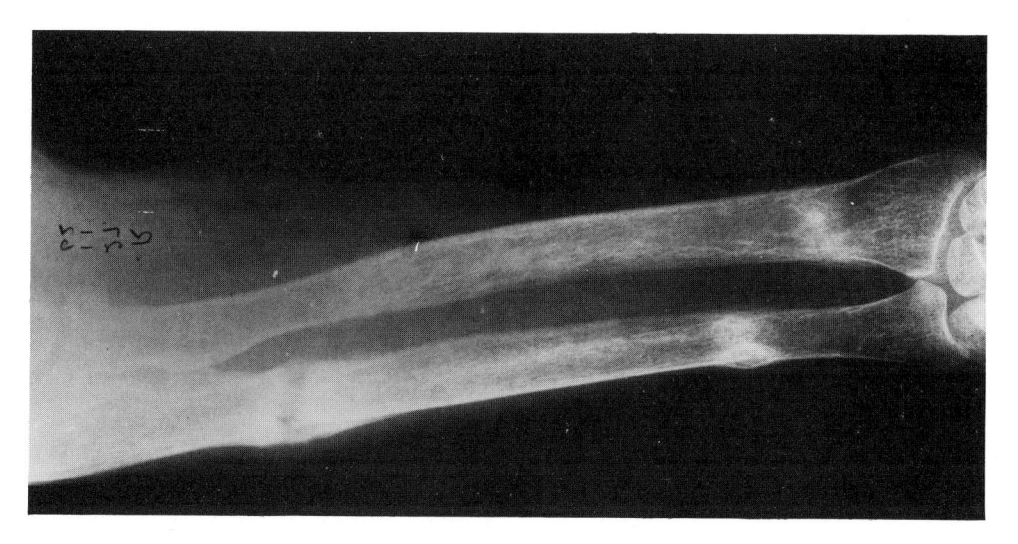

Fig. 15.8. Forearm fractures and osteomalacia in a patient with malabsorption and bacterial overgrowth due to a chronic stricture of the ileum.

indicanuria. Endocrine function was normal for a boy of 10 years (Tabaqchali & Booth 1970).

Vitamin D

Osteoporosis may occur in patients with long-standing and surgically uncorrectable lesions of the small intestine causing bacterial overgrowth. Deficiency of vitamin D, sufficient to cause osteomalacia, is rare and there are few reports of metabolic bone disease with pseudo-fractures and the radiological signs of osteomalacia (Schjønsby 1977). A rare example of severe osteomalacia causing bone fractures in an elderly patient with a stricture of the ileum is shown in Fig. 15.8.

Other substances

Decreased serum levels of vitamin A and its precursor β-carotene are frequently found in patients with malabsorption secondary to bacterial overgrowth. Ocular abnormalities have been recorded but are unusual (Levy & Toskes 1974). In a single patient with jejunal diverticulosis and severe malabsorption, an encephalopathic syndrome resembling that of nicotinic acid deficiency has been described. The patient had stupor and marked generalized rigidity with bilateral grasp reflexes. The electroencephalogram was grossly abnormal. With 3h of a single intravenous injection of 100 mg nicotinic acid, the patient had fully recovered (Tabaqchali & Pallis 1970).

Clinical assessment of bacterial overgrowth

It is first necessary, by appropriate radiological techniques, to establish that the patient has a lesion of the small intestine which might be associated with bacterial overgrowth. The most satisfactory and direct method of establishing that there is significant bacterial overgrowth is by collecting from the small intestine an aspirate which is cultured both under aerobic and anaerobic conditions. Collection of such aspirates may be carried out using a non-sterile polyvinyl tube. Air should not be injected at any time and the initial aspirate of a volume at least equal to that of the collecting tube, should be discarded. Sampling under nitrogen has been advocated when stricter methods of quantitative anaerobic bacteriology have been employed.

Since bacterial culture methods are not always available, indirect methods of detecting bile-salt-hydrolysing bacteria have been introduced, such as mixing intestinal aspirates with conjugated bile salts and testing for the presence of free bile acids after incubation. The most widely used indirect test, however, has been the bile acid breath test (Fromm & Hofmann 1971). A ^{14}C-labelled conjugated bile acid is given by mouth and the amount of $^{14}CO_2$ appearing in the breath provides a measure of bacterial deconjugation and further metabolism of the labelled bile acid. This test is particularly useful in the diagnosis of bacterial overgrowth (Lauterberg et al. 1978) but it has the disadvantage that it is also abnormal in patients with disease or resection of the ileum (James et al. 1973, Hepner 1978) and only detects the presence of organisms capable of degrading bile acids.

A ^{14}C-xylose breath test has also been developed, a test dose of xylose labelled with 10 μc of ^{14}C being given by mouth. Providing that the amount of xylose given is small (1 g), this test appears to be a particularly sensitive screening test for bacterial overgrowth (King et al. 1980). Breath hydrogen measurements after oral administration of glucose have also been useful in detecting bacterial overgrowth, and the hydrogen breath test appears to be more sensitive than the bile acid breath test (Metz et al. 1976). This is because it also detects the presence of facultative anaerobic bacteria, such as *Enterobacteriaceae*. All these tests are indirect measurements of bacterial enzymic activity, and wide variations in the results occur regularly.

Absorption tests carried out before and after the administration of oral broad spectrum antibiotics may also provide good evidence of bacterial overgrowth. Faecal fat excretion, if abnormal, may be restored to normal. The B_{12} absorption test before and after antibiotics is also a sensitive indicator of the presence in the small intestine of micro-organisms which interfere with B_{12} absorption.

Clinical conditions associated with an abnormal bacterial flora

These conditions are listed in Table 15.1. It is, however, essential to recognize that the presence of an abnormal bacterial flora in the small intestine does not necessarily have deleterious effects. It is only a relatively small proportion of patients who develop the full picture of the stagnant loop syndrome, with steatorrhoea and megaloblastic anaemia. Furthermore, in conditions such as biliary obstruction, the presence of bacterial overgrowth is of more theoretical than practical importance.

Gastric abnormalities

Although the contents of the normal fasting stomach are usually sterile or have low counts of oral flora because of the bactericidal effect of gastric acid (Garrod 1939), it is well documented that in patients with hypochlorhydria or pernicious anaemia, bacterial overgrowth occurs in the stomach (Hurst 1934, Drasar et al. 1966). Furthermore, bacterial colonization with coliforms, yeasts and increased counts of oral flora also occur in patients in whom the stomach contents are made alkaline, either by antacids or H_2 receptor antagonists (Ruddell et al. 1980, Hillman et al. 1982).

Pernicious anaemia

The microflora of the stomach and upper small intestine in such patients can occasionally be normal, but in most patients an abnormal bacterial flora with coliform organisms is present in concentrations of 10^4-10^7/ml of gastric or intestinal aspirate. In general, however, the flora has no functional significance. Malabsorption, other than of B_{12} due to gastric atrophy and intrinsic factor deficiency, does not occur in pernicious anaemia unless there is an associated intestinal lesion such as duodenal or jejunal diverticulosis.

Partial gastrectomy

Studies of the microflora of the small intestine of patients with Polya or Bilroth I partial gastrectomy have revealed an abnormal flora of colonic type. The concentrations usually range from 10^4-10^8 organisms/ml of intestinal aspirate. In many instances, the abnormal microflora appears to play little part in inducing malabsorption, steatorrhoea being more frequently associated with defects of the mixing of food with digestive enzymes. The bacterial flora, however, may play a minor role in some of these patients.

In rare patients with partial gastrectomy, a massive bacterial overgrowth occurs causing severe steatorrhoea. Such patients may develop a severe form of protein-calorie malnutrition which may be so extreme as to resemble kwashiorkor (Krikler & Schrire 1958). Neale et al. (1967) described three such patients, all of whom had extensive bacterial colonization of the small intestine. Two of these patients had stagnant and redundant duodenal loops. The third had jejunal diverticulosis, as well as a partial gastrectomy. In addition to hypoproteinaemic oedema, these patients had signs of severe protein−calorie malnutrition. The skin was abnormal, the hair dry, sparse and depigmented and in one extreme example total alopecia developed. The patients also showed the features of apathetic misery characteristic of severe malnutrition and there were abnormalities in the electroencephalogram. Electrocardiography showed low voltage complexes and periodic arrhythmias. The most striking biochemical feature involved the plasma proteins which were markedly reduced. There was also a reduction in the level of essential amino acids in the plasma as is seen in kwashiorkor. Liver function tests were abnormal and the urinary excretion of urocanic acid after histidine loading was greatly increased, an additional feature of severe protein malnutrition. A normochromic normocytic anaemia was a constant feature. All these patients had marked malabsorption and, in contrast to most patients with protein-losing enteropathy, the faecal nitrogen was grossly increased. These abnormalities were partially reversed, first by treatment with antibiotics and subsequently there was striking improvement following surgical correction of the intestinal lesions.

Vagotomy with pyloroplasty or gastrojejunostomy

Patients with vagotomy and pyloroplasty or gastrojejunostomy have minor changes in bacterial flora in the upper small intestine and the presence of these organisms does not appear to contribute to the steatorrhoea and diarrhoea that may occur. Vitamin B_{12} absorption is usually normal, although serum levels of B_{12} and folate may be slightly reduced (Tinker *et al.* 1971).

Intestinal stasis

Diverticulosis

Duodenal diverticula are increasingly frequent with increasing age. They are not usually associated with bacterial overgrowth and malabsorption unless there is significant stasis within a diverticulum and particularly if associated with achlorhydria. This can be demonstrated radiologically by carrying out a barium follow-through examination. In later films, when the barium has reached the caecum, barium seen persisting in a duodenal diverticulum may indicate stasis. Under these circumstances, an abnormal flora may develop in the upper intestine. Steatorrhoea, however, is rare in patients with single or even multiple duodenal diverticula, although malabsorption of vitamin B_{12} may occur in a small proportion of patients, particularly if there is achlorhydria. Occasionally bacterial overgrowth in a diverticulum close to the ampulla of Vater leads to ascending cholangitis and pancreatitis (Eggert *et al.* 1982).

Jejunal diverticulosis is uncommon. The autopsy incidence is approximately 0.5%. The jejunum is more frequently involved than the ileum and the number of diverticula usually diminishes distally. They are wide-mouthed and situated on the mesenteric border of the small intestine (Fig. 15.9).

Jejunal diverticula usually occur after the age of 50 and patients with symptoms are from the older age groups. They are frequently asymptomatic, the diverticula being found incidentally either on radiological examination or at autopsy. Complications may include perforation, volvulus and haemorrhage, sometimes severe enough to cause melaena. Some patients may develop colicky abdominal pain and borborygmi. The abdomen may be distended and a plain abdominal radiograph in the erect posture may show fluid levels in the diverticula (Fig. 15.10). These appearances can be mistaken for intestinal obstruction and may lead to unnecessary laparotomy. The erroneous diagnosis of intestinal obstruction in patients with jejunal diverticulosis has been emphasized by a recent report describing the frequency with which surgical exploration of the abdomen is carried out in such patients (Krishnamurthy *et al.* 1983). Eight patients with jejunal diverticulosis had undergone a total of eighteen operations. Six of these patients had ten operations for suspected small bowel obstruction although none was found.

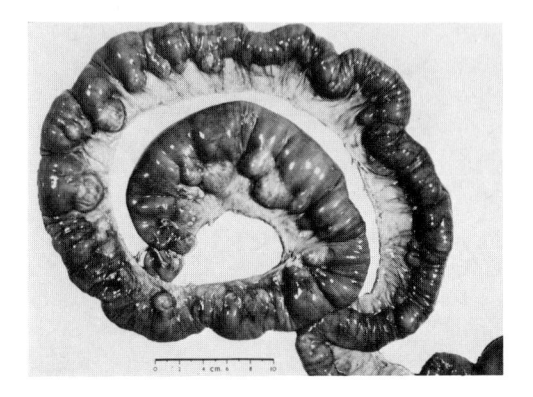

Fig. 15.9. Multiple jejunal diverticula on mesenteric border of the small intestine.

Bacterial overgrowth is variable. If only few bacteria are present, they may be insufficient to influence absorption or nutrition. Heavier bacterial overgrowth may result in deconjugation of bile acids, but if the degree of deconjugation of bile salts is low and the conjugated bile salts are maintained at a satisfactory level, there may be no steatorrhoea (Tabaqchali 1970). If there is extensive bacterial colonization of the small

production organisms such as enterotoxigenic *E. coli* or *Aeromonas* species has not yet been determined.

Although megaloblastic anaemia may occur in patients with steatorrhoea and diarrhoeal symptoms, in some cases bacterial overgrowth may be sufficient to cause malabsorption of vitamin B_{12} without causing steatorrhoea. Such patients may develop megaloblastic anaemia without intestinal symptoms and a mistaken diagnosis of Addisonian pernicious anaemia may be made. In some patients there may be little or no anaemia, yet the patient has B_{12} deficiency of sufficient severity to cause symptoms and signs of subacute combined degeneration of the spinal cord. It is tempting to speculate that bacterial synthesis of folic acid maintains the haemoglobin level but accentuates B_{12} deficiency in such patients. The diagnosis becomes apparent when normal gastric acidity is demonstrated and a barium follow-through is performed (Ward *et al.*, 1983).

Blind loops

It is only *anti-peristaltic* loops of intestine that act as blind loops and become colonized by bacteria. *Isoperistaltic* loops of intestine are capable of emptying themselves and therefore do not encourage bacterial overgrowth except in some which are particularly long as may occur with the operation of jejunoileal bypass for obesity (Powell-Jackson *et al.* 1979). The duodenal stump after partial gastrectomy is an example of a self-emptying isoperistaltic loop and for this reason it rarely acts as a blind loop. Blind loops develop when the intestine is anastomosed side-to-side, and the end of the proximal portion of the small intestine dilates to form a blind loop. Blind loops are now rarely seen since end-to-end or end-to-side anastomoses are preferred by gastrointestinal surgeons. The location of the blind loop in the intestine determines the degree of malabsorption likely to occur, a proximal loop being more likely to be associated with severe malabsorption than a distal lesion, in which nutritional effects may be limited to inhibition of vitamin B_{12} absorption. Blind loops are parti-

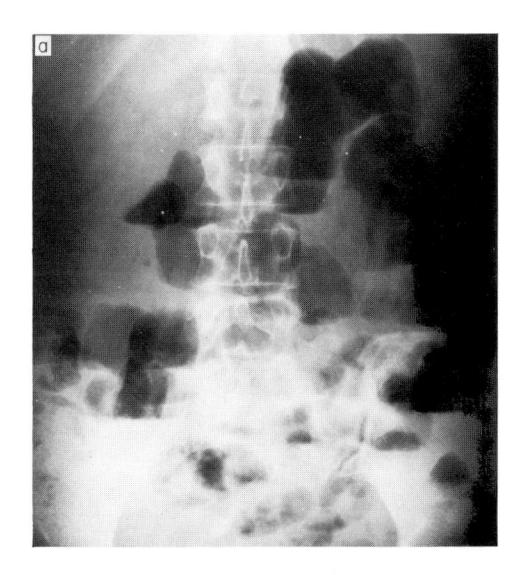

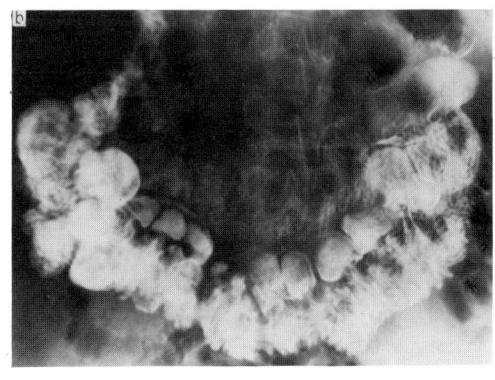

Fig. 15.10. Jejunal diverticulosis. (a) Plain abdominal radiograph in the erect posture showing fluid levels in the diverticula which are not due to obstruction. (b) Barium follow-through showing multiple jejunal diverticula.

intestine, however, as shown in Fig. 15.4, there may be extensive deconjugation of bile salts and large amounts of free bile acids are present. Under these circumstances, there may be marked steatorrhoea and the patient frequently has severe diarrhoea. There is loss of weight and megaloblastic anaemia due to B_{12} deficiency is frequently present. The diarrhoea may be mistaken for an infective diarrhoea, since if treatment with broad spectrum antibiotics is given, symptoms may be temporarily relieved. Periodic explosive episodes of diarrhoea occur in these patients. Whether these episodes are associated with the new acquisition of toxin-

cularly likely to bleed, causing both iron deficiency, anaemia and, on occasions, severe melaena. Rampal and colleagues (1981) studied sixteen patients with stagnant loops and demonstrated that ileocolic anastomoses, with blind loops, were more frequently complicated by intestinal haemorrhage and iron deficiency than by B_{12} deficiency. They also showed that treatment with antibiotics was not usually effective in controlling anaemia in these patients and that surgical correction of the blind loop was invariably required.

Strictures

Although tuberculosis is still an important cause of ileal stricture in the developing world, Crohn's disease is now the commonest cause of stricture in western Europe and the USA. Other causes include congenital strictures or bands. Strictures frequently involve the distal small intestine, and may therefore cause B_{12} deficiency. Rarely, there may be no intestinal symptoms and the recognition of B_{12} deficiency may lead to the discovery of the causative lesion, as illustrated by the following patient:

> A married woman aged 36 presented with symptoms of anaemia. She had been married for 10 years but had failed to become pregnant. The haemoglobin was 9.6 g/dl and stained blood films showed macrocytes and signs of iron deficiency. Sternal marrow was megaloblastic and her serum B_{12} concentration was subnormal (45 pg/ml). She had occult blood in her stools. Since she had free acid in the gastric juice, it was unlikely that she had Addisonian pernicious anaemia and a barium follow-through revealed gross dilatation of the terminal ileum indicating chronic intestinal obstruction. After treatment with iron, vitamin B_{12} and antibiotics, laparotomy was performed by Mr R.H. Franklin, who discovered a grossly dilated segment of terminal ileum, obstructed by a congenital band a few inches proximal to the ileocaecal valve. When the intestine was opened, a large ulcerated area was seen in the stagnant and dilated segment of intestine (Fig. 15.6). Resection of the stricture and end-to-end anastomosis was performed and the result was excellent. After the operation the patient had two uneventful and successful pregnancies.

Abnormal motility

The most frequent causes of bacterial overgrowth due to abnormal motility are scleroderma, intestinal pseudo-obstruction and, in some instances, the autonomic neuropathy of diabetes mellitus. Patients with these disorders may have steatorrhoea, but anaemia due to vitamin B_{12} deficiency is unusual. Severe watery diarrhoea is more frequently present in these patients. The mechanism of this diarrhoea has not been established but the role of bacterial toxins has not been excluded. Surgical correction is not possible in these patients but intermittent courses of oral broad spectrum antibiotics may be helpful.

Free communication between large and small bowel

Where there is a fistula between the small and large intestine, a barium follow-through frequently fails to reveal the lesion. This is because the pressure in the colon is higher than that in the small intestine and the flow of intestinal contents is therefore from large to small intestine. A barium enema is the radiological investigation of choice to reveal a fistula.

Gastrocolic fistula

This may occur when a stomal ulcer following gastroenterostomy erodes into the colon. It is an unusual cause of bacterial overgrowth since gastroenterostomy is now rarely performed. Gastrocolic fistula may also occur from cancer of either stomach or transverse colon if the tumour erodes its way into adjacent organs. Patients with gastrocolic fistula usually develop severe diarrhoea and steatorrhoea quite suddenly, with marked loss of weight associated with hypoalbuminaemia. There is usually no evidence of vitamin B_{12} deficiency since the onset is so acute that there is little time for hepatic stores of vitamin B_{12} to be exhausted.

Duodenocolic fistula

Duodenocolic fistula is a rare complication of duodenal ulcer. It may occur as a result of tumours eroding the duodenum from the colon. There are also cases of benign duodenocolic fistula in which no cause has been found (Chandler & Longmore 1960). Malabsorption and diarrhoea may occur depending on the degree of bacterial contamination, but unlike gastrocolic fistula, symptoms of duodenocolic fistula may be remarkably mild. The patient sometimes only presents with megaloblastic anaemia due to B_{12} deficiency, suggesting that symptomless malabsorption of vitamin B_{12} may have been present for a considerable time. This is illustrated by the following case report:

> A widowed seamstress aged 67 years was admitted to Hammersmith Hospital with symptoms of anaemia of 1 year's duration. Investigations revealed a megaloblastic anaemia (Hb 10 g/dl; serum B_{12} 45 pg/ml). There was no steatorrhoea and xylose absorption was normal. Absorption of vitamin B_{12}, measured by Schilling test, was grossly reduced, both without and with the addition of intrinsic factor, indicating an intestinal absorptive defect. Gastric acid secretion was normal. A barium meal examination showed some slight dilatation of the small intestine, but it was on barium enema that a fistula between the transverse colon and the duodenum was revealed. This was successfully closed surgically by Mr R.H. Franklin. There were a few diverticula in the sigmoid colon but none were found in the transverse colon or at the area where the fistula had formed. The cause of the fistula is unknown but it is tempting to speculate that in a seamstress such a lesion may have been produced by a needle, inadvertently swallowed.

Enterocolic fistula

The commonest cause of enterocolic fistula is Crohn's disease. It may also be due to diverticulitis of the colon if an inflamed diverticulum erodes into the small intestine. The symptoms of enterocolic fistula are related to the causative lesion and, as with blind loops, the degree of malabsorption and diarrhoea usually depends on the site of the lesion.

Massive small intestinal resection

The small intestinal flora after intestinal resection appears to be controlled by the extent of intestinal resection and the presence or absence of the ileocaecal valve. Gastric acid secretion in these patients is usually normal or sometimes increased, which may limit the entry of microorganisms into the small bowel. In distal small intestinal resections, with the loss of the ileocaecal valve, the situation may be similar to that of an ileocolic fistula with backwash into the distal part of the intestine from the colon, whereas the proximal bowel may remain normal. If the resection is extensive, however, there may be a profuse microbial flora in the small intestinal remnant, simulating a proximal stagnant loop syndrome and bacterial colonization, with bile salt deconjugation, may exacerbate the already existing malabsorption. This is illustrated by the following case report:

> W.D. had only 35 cm of jejunum remaining anastomosed end-to-end to the transverse colon, resection having been carried out for infarction following mesenteric vascular occlusion. Bacterial counts were made of stomach, duodenum and jejunal contents in the fasting state and after a meal. During fasting there were low counts of coliforms and other organisms, but anaerobic bacteroides were not isolated and there was no bile salt deconjugation. After a meal, however, there must

have been regurgitation of colonic contents into the residual small intestine for the bacterial counts were as high as 10^8-10^9 organisms/ml with the appearance of bacteroides and anaerobic lactobacilli. At the same time, there was evidence of extensive bile salt deconjugation in samples from duodenum and jejunum. In the fasting state, there were only conjugated bile salts present in the duodenum, the concentration being 7.4 mM. After a meal, bile salt deconjugation occurred, with the appearance of free cholic acid and chenodeoxycholic acid, the total free bile acids being 6.9 mM. There was a reduction in the conjugated bile salts to 2.7 mM. Subsequent antibiotic therapy was followed by a slight but significant fall in steatorrhea which deteriorated after cessation of therapy. The bile acid pattern in the intestine was reflected by the serum bile acids, elevated levels of both cholic and chenodeoxycholic acid being present. The secondary bile acid, deoxycholic acid, however, was not present in samples either from the intestine or the serum (Tabaqchali 1970). The absence of the secondary bile acid deoxycholic acid was not due to lack of organisms capable of dehydroxylating bile acids, since *in vitro* incubation of the bacteroides species from this patient with bile salts produced deoxycholic acid.

By contrast, studies in a second patient with a similar amount of small intestine remaining but an intact ileocaecal valve and a short segment of ileum, showed a different bacterial flora. Although there were coliforms, streptococci and lactobacilli present, there were no bacteroides and there was no deconjugation or dehydroxylation of bile acids within the small intestine. Furthermore, the patient's malabsorption did not improve with antibiotic therapy.

Treatment

If there is a surgically correctable lesion present, such as a fistula, stricture or blind loop, the treatment of choice is surgery and the results may be excellent. The correction of nutritional deficiencies (Gracey 1979) and treatment with oral broad spectrum antibiotics are necessary preliminaries to operation.

There may, however, be other lesions such as diverticulosis of the small intestine or scleroderma where surgical correction of the causative lesion is not feasible. Under these circumstances, correction of nutritional deficiencies is the first step in treatment. Thereafter, the potential value of oral broad spectrum antibiotics must be considered. In many patients with only mild intestinal symptoms, no antibiotic treatment may be necessary. If there is significant diarrhoea and steatorrhoea, however, antibiotics may dramatically relieve both symptoms and malabsorption. Figure 15.11 illustrates the use of oral tetracycline in a patient with jejunal diverticulosis and malabsorption. There was a dramatic restoration of normal small intestinal function, together with a striking fall in indicanuria following treatment. This was associated with marked symptomatic improvement.

The correct antibiotic to be used in these circumstances should theoretically be one which has anti-anaerobic activity, such as lincomycin or metronidazole given orally (Joiner & Gorbach 1979). Neomycin (2.0 g daily) given orally has also been shown to be effective and leads to a reduction in the anaerobic bacterial counts in the small intestine despite its known inactivity against these organisms by *in vitro* testing (Schjønsby et al 1973). Tetracycline is a useful antibiotic when given in a dose of 2.0 g daily in divided dosage, but recent surveys have shown that a high percentage of bacteroides species and *E. coli* are resistant to this antibiotic. Treatment, continued for 1 week or more, frequently corrects symptoms and, despite cessation of therapy, there may be no relapse. If symptoms persist, however, it is possible to consider the use of tetracycline, neomycin, or cotrimoxazole over a prolonged period to control symptoms of bacterial overgrowth. If possible, however, antibiotic sensitivity testing of the organisms should be carried out before initiating such therapy. In some patients, such as those with strictures caused by chronic adhesive tuberculous

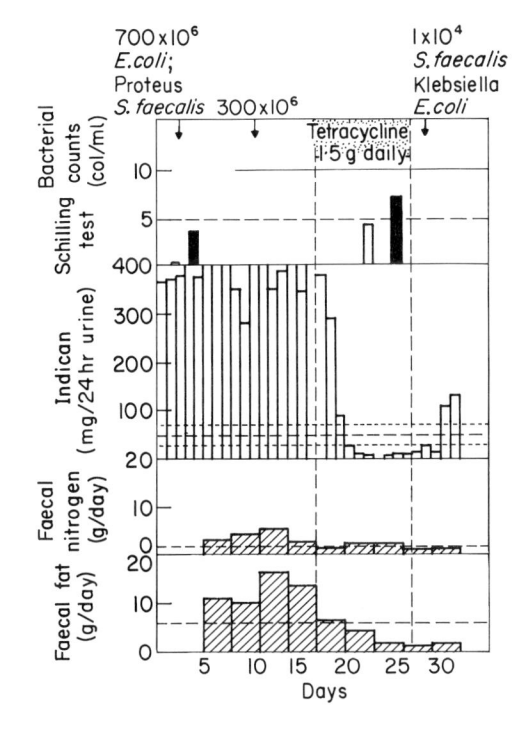

Fig. 15.11. Antibiotic response in jejunal diverticulosis in a patient treated with oral broad-spectrum antibiotic. The figure shows: bacteria count in jejunal fluid, vitamin B12 absorption (normal value > 5%), urinary indicans, faecal nitrogen and faecal fat. Upper limit of normal range for these last three measurements are indicated by the interrupted lines.

peritonitis, surgical correction may not be technically possible and yet steatorrhoea may persist. Continued antibiotic treatment may be not only impracticable but unnecessary, as shown by the following case report:

> A young woman 25 years of age first presented at Hammersmith Hospital in 1943 with tuberculous peritonitis. In 1944 and 1946 recurrent bouts of intestinal obstruction necessitated entero-entero anastomoses as life-saving procedures. Following these operations, which created blind loops, she had diarrhoea and 4 years later in 1950 developed a megaloblastic anaemia. This was associated with a subnormal serum B$_{12}$ concentration (70 pg/ml.) There was also significant steatorrhoea. She was treated by Professor D.L. Mollin first with a single injection of 20 µg of vitamin B$_{12}$ and there was an excellent reticulocyte response and rise in her red cell count. She continued to receive 40 µg B$_{12}$ monthly until 1954, since when 200 µg have been given by injection monthly. Apart from a recurrence of her intestinal tuberculosis in 1957, she has remained well without other treatment. The presence of large amounts of free bile acids in the serum, together with an improvement in vitamin B$_{12}$ absorption following short-term treatment with oral broad spectrum antibiotics, provides evidence for extensive small intestinal bacterial overgrowth in this patient which has been present for nearly 40 years. Her diarrhoea has been controlled by a low fat diet and in recent years has caused no symptoms. In 1980 she developed a carcinoma of the tonsillar fossa which was successfully treated by radiotherapy (Dr Mary Catterall). Subsequently she has unfortunately developed a carcinoma of the oesophagus.

Such observations illustrate that despite the remarkable range of potentially harmful effects of bacterial overgrowth described in this chapter, man can co-exist in remarkable symbiosis with an abnormal and profuse bacterial flora in the small intestine for a prolonged period of time without overt harmful effect.

References

Ament M.E., Shimoda S.S., Saunders D.R. and Rubin, C.E. (1972) Pathogenesis of steatorrhea in three cases of small intestinal stasis syndrome. *Gastroenterol.* 63, 728–747.

Ammon H.V., Thomas P.H. & Phillips S.F. (1974) Effects of oleic and ricinoleic acid on net jejunal water and electrolyte movement. *J. Clin. Invest.* 53, 374–379.

Chernov A.J., Doe W.F. & Gompertz D (1972) Intrajejunal volatile fatty acids in the stagnant loop syndrome. *Gut,* 13, 103–106.

Chandler G.N. & Longmore A.J. (1960) Benign duodeno-colic fistula. *Gut,* 1, 253–257.

Donaldson Jr R.M. (1970) Small bowel bacterial overgrowth. *Adv. Intern. Med.* 16, 191–212.

Drasar B.S., Hill M.J. & Shiner M. (1966) The deconjugation of bile salts by human intestinal bacteria. *Lancet,* **i,** 1237–1238.

Eggert A., Teichmann W. & Wittman D.H. (1982) The pathological implications of duodenal diverticula. *Surg. Gynae. Obst.* **152,** 62–64.

Faber K. (1895) Perniciøs Anaemia som Føe af Tarmlidelse Hosp. *Tid. Kjøbenh.* **4,** 601–615.

Fromm H. & Hofmann A.F. (1971) Breath test for altered bile acid metabolism. *Lancet,* **ii,** 621–625.

Garrod I.P. (1939) A study of the bactericidal power of hydrochloric acid and of gastric juice. *St. Bart. Hosp. Rep.* **75,** 145–150.

Goldstein F., Karacadag S., Wirts C.W. and Kowlessar O.D. (1970) Intraluminal small-intestinal utilization of d-xylose by bacteria. A limitation of the d-xylose absorption test. *Gastroenterol.* **59,** 380–386.

Gorbach S.L., Plaut A.G., Nahas L. Weinstein L., Spanknebel G. and Levitan, R. (1967) Studies of intestinal microflora. II. Micro-organisms of the small intestine and their relations to oral and fecal flora. *Gastroenterol.* **53,** 856–867.

Gorbach S.L. & Tabaqchali S. (1969) Bacteria, bile, and the small bowel. *Gut,* **10,** 963–972.

Gracey M.J. (1979) The contaminated small bowel syndrome: pathogenesis diagnosis and treatment. *Ann. J. Clin. Nut.* **32,** 234–243.

Gracey M., Burke V., Oshin A. Barker J. & Glasgow E.F. (1971) Bacteria, bile salts, and intestinal monosaccharide malabsorption. *Gut,* **12,** 683–692.

Gracey M.J., Papadimitrious J. & Bower G. (1974) Ultrastructural changes in the small intestines of rats with self-filling blind loops. *Gastroenterol.* **67,** 646–651.

Hepner G.W. (1978) Breath tests in gastroenterology. *Adv. Intern. Med.* **23,** 25–45.

Hepner G.W., Booth C.C., Cowan J. Hoffbrand A.V. and Mollin D.L. (1968) Absorption of crystalline folic acid in man. *Lancet,* **ii,** 302–306.

Hillman K.M., Riordan T., O'Farrell S.M. & Tabaqchali S. (1982) Colonisation of gastric contents in critically ill patients. *Crit. Care Med.* **10,** 444–447.

Hoffbrand A.V., Tabaqchali S., Booth C.C. and Mollin D.L. (1971) Small intestinal bacterial flora and folate status in gastrointestinal disease. *Gut,* **12,** 27–33.

Hurst A.F. (1934) The clinical importance of achlorhydria. *Br. Med. J.* **ii,** 665–670.

James O.F.W., Agnew J.E. & Bouchier I.A.D. (1973) Assessment of the ^{14}C-glycocholic acid breath test. *Br. Med. J.* **3,** 191–195.

Jeejeebhoy K.N. & Coghill N.F. (1961) The measurement of gastrointestinal protein loss by a new method. *Gut,* **2,** 123–130.

Joiner K.A. & Gorbach S.L. (1979) Antimicrobial therapy of digestive disorders. *Clin. in Gastroenterol.* **8,** 3–35.

Jones E.A., Craigie A., Tavill A.S. Franglen G. and Rosenoes V.M. (1968) Protein metabolism in the intestinal stagnant loop syndrome. *Gut,* **9,** 466–469.

King C.E. & Toskes P.P. (1979) Small intestinal bacterial overgrowth. *Gastroenterol.* **76,** 1035–1055.

King C.E., Lorenz E. & Toskes P. (1976) The pathogenesis of decreased serum protein levels in the blind loop syndrome: evaluation including a newly-developed ^{14}C-amino acid breath test (abstr.) *Gastroenterol.* **70,** 901.

King C.E., Toskes P.P., Guilarte R.R., Lorenz E. & Welkos S.L. (1980) Comparison of the one-gram d-^{14}C xylose breath test to the ^{14}C bile acid breath test in patients with small intestine bacterial overgrowth. *Dig. Dis. Sci.* **25,** 53–58.

Krikler D.M. & Shrire V. (1958) Kwashiorkor in an adult due to an intestinal blind loop. *Lancet,* **i,** 510-511.

Krishnamurthy S., Kelly M.M., Rohrmann C.A. & Schuffler M.D. (1983) Jejunal diverticulosis. A heterogenous disorder caused by a variety of abnormalities of smooth muscle or myenteric plexus. *Gastroenterol.* **85,** 538–547.

Lauterburg B.H., Newcomer A.D., & Hofmann A.F. (1978) Clinical value of the bile acid breath test: evaluation of the Mayo Clinic experience. *Mayo Clin. Proc.* **53,** 227–233.

Levy N.S., Toskes P.P. (1974) Fundus albipunctatus and vitamin A deficiency. *Amer. J. Ophthalmol.* **78,** 926–929.

Mackowiak P.A. (1982) The normal bacterial flora. *New Engl. J. Med.* **307,** 83–93.

Metz G., Gassull M.A., Drasar B.S. Jenkins D.J.A. and Blendis L.M. (1976) Breath-hydrogen test for small intestinal bacterial colonization. *Lancet,* **i,** 668–669.

McEvoy A., Dutton J. & James O.F.W. (1983) Bacterial contamination of the small intestine is an important cause of occult malabsorption in the elderly. *Brit. Med. J.* **ii,** 789–793.

Neale G., Antcliff A., Welbourn R. Mollin D.L. and Booth, C.C. (1967) Protein malnutrition after partial gastrectomy. *Quart. J. Med.* **36,** 469–494.

Panveliwalla D., Lewis B., Wootton I.D.P. & Tabaqchali S. (1970) Determination of individual bile acids in biological fluids by thin layer chromatography and fluorimetry. *J. Clin. Path.* **23,** 309–314.

Perkkio M. & Savilahti E. (1980) Time of appearance of immunoglobulin-containing cells in the mucosa of the neonatal intestine. *Pediatr. Res.* **14,** 953–955.

Powell-Jackson P.R., Maudgal D.P., Sharp D., Goldie A. & Maxwell J.O. (1979) Intestinal bacterial metabolism of protein and bile acids: role in pathogenesis of hepatic disease after jejunoileal surgery. *Brit. J. Surg.* **66,** 772–775.

Rampal P., Karsenty C., Faure X., Math M. & Delmont J. (1981) Les anemies au cours du syndrome de l'anse borgne. *Gastroenterol. Clin. Biol.* **5,** 156A.

Richmond J. & Davidson S. (1958) Subacute combined degeneration of the spinal cord in non-Addisonian megaloblastic anaemia. *Quart. J. Med.* **27,** 517–531.

Riepe S.P., Goldstein J. & Alpes D.H. (1980) Effect of secreted Bacteroides proteases on human intestinal brush border hydrolases. *J. clin. Invest.* **66**, 314–322.

Ruddell W.S.J., Axon A.T.R., Findlay J.M. Bartholemeco B.A. and Hill M.J. (1980) Effect of cimetidine on the gastric bacterial flora. *Lancet*, **i**, 672–674.

Schjønsby H. (1973) Studies on vitamin B_{12} absorption in the blind loop syndrome. MD Thesis, University of Bergen.

Schjønsby H. (1974) The absorption of vitamin B_{12} in the blind loop syndrome. *Scand. J. Gastroenterol.* **29**, Suppl., 65.

Schjønsby H. (1977) Osteomalacia in the stagnant loop syndrome. *Acta Medica Scandinavica* **603**, Suppl., 39–41.

Schjønsby H., Drasar D.S., Tabaqchali S. & Booth C.C. (1973) Uptake of vitamin B_{12} by intestinal bacteria in the stagnant loop syndrome. *Scand. J. Gastroenterol.* **8**, 41–47.

Setchell K.D.R., Worthington J., Smith S.M. & Murphy G.M. (1982) Diurnal pattern of unconjugated bile acid concentrations in the peripheral circulation of patients with ileal resection. *Falk Symposium No. 33. 'Bile acids and cholesterol in health and disease'.* Int. Bile Acid Meeting, Basle. Lancaster, MTP Press.

Shockett E. & Simon S.D. (1982) Small bowel obstruction due to an enterolith formed in a duodenal diverticulum. A case report and review of the literature. *Amer. J. Gastroenterol.* **77**, 621–624.

Simon G.L. & Gorbach S.L. (1984) Intestinal flora in health and disease. *Gastroenterlogy* **86**, 174–193.

Tabaqchali S. (1970) Case study of a patient with massive intestinal resection. *7 Int. Congr. Clin. Chem, Geneva, 1969. Digestion and Intestinal Absorption.* pp. 119–123. Karger, Basle.

Tabaqchali S. (1970) The pathophysiological role of small intestinal bacterial flora. *Scand. J. Gastroenterol.* **6**, Suppl., 139–163.

Tabaqchali S., Hatzioannou J. & Booth C.C. (1968) Bile salt deconjugation and steatorrhea in patients with the stagnant loop syndrome. *Lancet*, **ii**, 12–16.

Tabaqchali S. & Booth C.C. (1970) Bacteria and the small intestine. In *Modern Trends in Gastroenterology*, vol. 4, pp. 143–179. (Ed. by W.I. Card & B. Creamer). Butterworth, London.

Tabaqchali S., Howard A., Teoh-Chan C.H., Bettelheim K.A. & Gorbach S.L. (1977) *Escherichia coli* serotypes throughout the gastrointestinal tract of patients with intestinal disorders. *Gut*, **18**, 351–355.

Tabaqchali S. & Pallis C. (1970) Reversible nicotinamide deficiency encephalopathy in a patient with jejunal diverticulosis. *Gut*, **11**, 1024–1028.

Tinker J., Hoffbrand A.V., Mitchison R.S., Tabaqchali S. & Cox A.G. (1971) Gastrointestinal flora and diarrhoea after vagotomy. *S. Afr. Med. J.* **45**, 1258–1262.

Varcoe R., Holliday D. & Tavill A. (1974) Utilization of urea nitrogen for albumin synthesis in the stagnant loop syndrome. *Gut*, **15**, 898–902.

Ward K., Robinson A., McMurray M. & Weir D.G. (1983) Massive jejunal diverticulosis and subacute combined degeneration of the cord. *Ir. J. Med. Sci.* **152**, 289–291.

Webb J.P.W., James A.T. & Kellock T.D. (1963) The influence of diet on the quality of faecal fat in patients with and without steatorrhoea. *Gut*, **4**, 37–41.

White W.H. (1890) On the pathology and prognosis of pernicious anaemia. *Guy's Hosp., Rep.* **47**, 149–194.

Chapter 16
Whipple's Disease (Intestinal Lipodystrophy)

H.J.F. HODGSON

Introduction 270
Pathology 270
Clinical features 274
Investigations 276
Treatment 277
Aetiology 277
Conclusion 280

Introduction

In 1899 a young medical missionary arrived in Constantinople and almost immediately developed a transient arthritis, the first indication of the condition that led to his death; he died in Baltimore in 1907. G.H. Whipple, future Nobel laureate, performed the autopsy and reported 'a hitherto undescribed disease, characterized anatomically by deposits of fat and fatty acids in the intestinal and mesenteric lymphatic tissues'. He suggested the term 'intestinal lipodystrophy' for the condition, but the name 'Whipple's disease' has become the accepted usage.

There is an interesting footnote to this story. Morgan (1961) stained some material preserved in the Westminster Hospital Pathology Department since 1894 and demonstrated the characteristic pathological findings of Whipple's disease in tissue from a London policeman who died 12 years before Whipple's patient of 'diarrhoea and wasting'. This case was reported to the Pathological Society of London as a case of 'lymphangiectasis intestini' (Allchin & Hebb 1895).

The study of Whipple's disease developed with the description of the dramatic staining properties of the affected tissues (Black-Schaffer 1949), the description of the clinical response to antibiotics (Paulley 1952) and the description of bacillary bodies in affected tissues in 1961 (Yardley & Hendrix 1961, Chears & Ashworth 1961). Despite this finding, the disease has not been universally recognized as an infectious process. This arises from the difficulties in characterizing and culturing the bacteria, and other evidence suggesting an underlying immuno-deficiency in the host.

The initial clinical description of G.H. Whipple's patient illustrates that, whilst Whipple's disease often presents with intestinal symptoms, and is usually classified as a gastroenterological disorder, it is a multi-system disease. Symptoms referable to other organ systems may be present for many years before gastrointestinal involvement becomes manifest.

Pathology

The term intestinal lipodystrophy was suggested by Whipple to describe the most dramatic autopsy finding, widespread fat deposits in the intestinal mucosa and intraabdominal lymph nodes. It is now apparent that such deposits are a secondary manifestation of the disease, and reflect lymphatic obstruction and extravasation of fat from lymphatics (Enzinger & Helwig 1963, Trier et al. 1965). The characteristic histopathological feature of untreated Whipple's disease is the finding in small intestine and lymph nodes of large numbers of 'foamy' macrophage cells 20–30μ across with pale vesicular nuclei and vacuolated cytoplasm (Fig. 16.1). Periodic acid Schiff reagent (PAS) stains these cells a brilliant and startling magenta, and this reaction is diastase-resistant (Fig. 16.2). The PAS stains a glycoprotein, which is apparently a product of the bacteria also found in affected tissues. Isolated PAS-positive macrophages may occasionally be found in small intestinal tissue from normal individuals, and more commonly in colonic tissue, but such cells are normally distinguishable from Whipple's disease on light-microscopic grounds; fur-

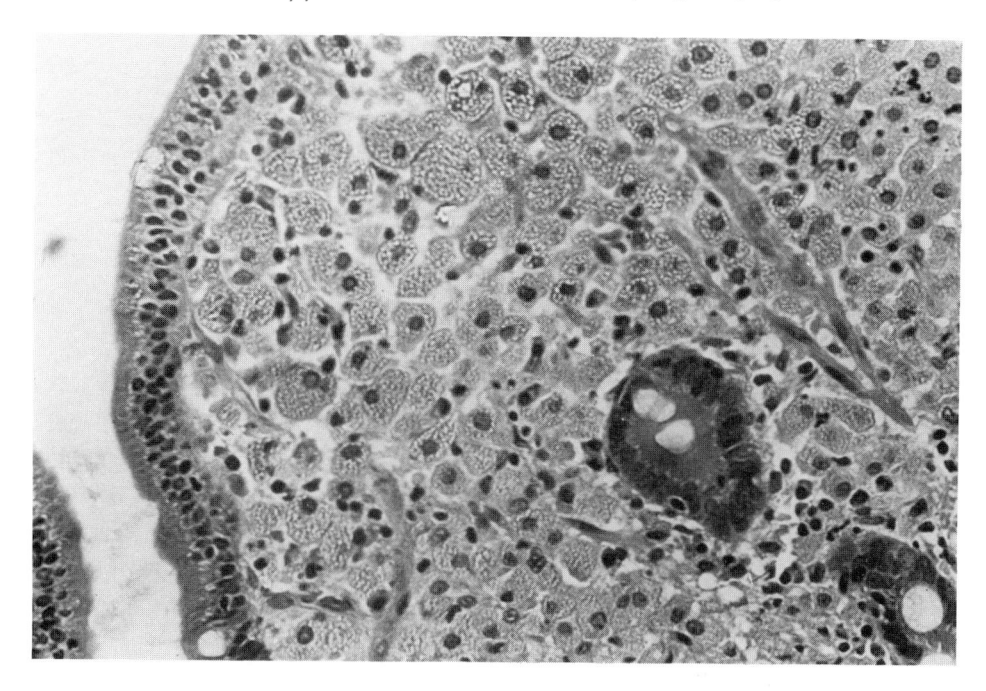

Fig. 16.1. Foamy macrophages in jejunal mucosa in a patient with Whipple's disease (H & E × 400).

thermore, in almost all cases of untreated Whipple's disease, PAS-positive macrophages are present in large numbers.

Subsequently these foamy macrophages were detected not only in the small intestine and abdominal lymph nodes, but in every system of the body. Sieracki (1958) commented that the PAS-positive material within the cells assumed shapes reminiscent of sickled erythrocytes, and suggested the cumbersome term 'sickle-form-particle containing cell' (SPC cell) for the pathognomomic cell of Whipple's disease. In a survey of autopsy cases, SPC-cells were found in the heart, lungs, spleen, pancreas, throughout the intestine, lymph nodes, bone marrow, central nervous system and retroperitoneal tissues, and even scantily in the genito-urinary system (Sieracki & Fine 1959). Cells other than macrophages, for example, fibrocytes, smooth muscle and endothelial cells, can also contain PAS-positive material, but in far less dramatic amounts (Enzinger & Helwig 1963).

Whipple had described a 'rod-shaped organism' present in considerable numbers in affected lymph nodes and suggested that it might be the causative agent. Electron microscopic reports have subsequently shown bacillary bodies in small intestinal mucosa, as well as in other organs throughout the body, such as heart, brain, lung, liver and joints. The bacteria stain the same brilliant magenta with PAS, and it is the presence of whole and degenerating bacteria, together with granules of membranous material within the macrophages, that explains the staining properties and the sickle-form particles of that cell.

Small intestinal involvement

In the past, it was thought that the small intestine is always involved in the disease process in patients with untreated Whipple's disease. Recent reports, however, have described patients in whom small gut involvement has been absent or minimal (Romanul et al. 1977, Mansbach et al. 1978), and relapses in previously treated Whipple's disease may also occur in the absence of small intestinal involvement (Feurle et al. 1979). In over 98% of reported cases of Whipple's disease, however, diffuse small intestinal abnormalities are present. The mucosal surface is oedematous, either with total loss of

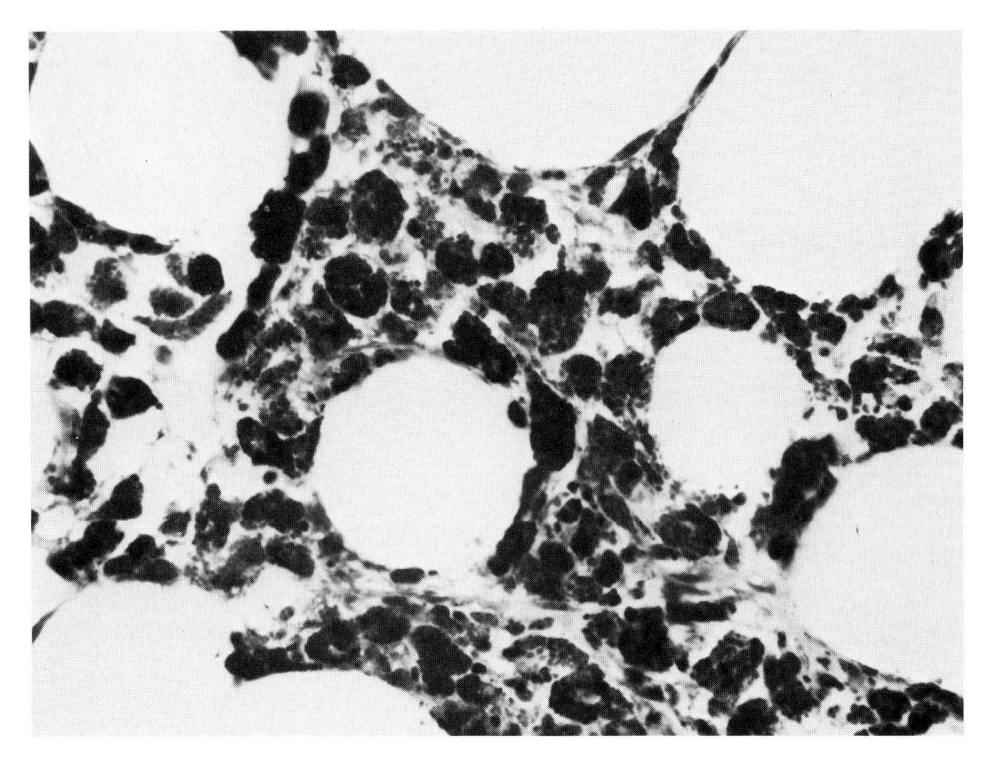

Fig. 16.2. Dark (magenta) staining macrophages in jejunal mucosa in a patient with Whipple's disease. Similar staining material is also seen extracellularly (PAS × 400).

villous pattern or more often with clubbed, flattened villi giving a coarse granular appearance (Fig. 16.3). The intestinal wall becomes thickened and doughy, and yellow lipid deposits may occur in all layers beneath the epithelium; ulceration of the mucosa is not a characteristic feature but has been reported. Whereas jejunal and ileal involvement almost invariably occur, the duodenum is less commonly abnormal (Maizel et al. 1970, Enzinger & Helwig 1963).

Histologically the villi are distorted by the characteristic foam-laden macrophages (Figs 16.1 and 16.2); they are most densely packed, and stain most brilliantly, near the luminal surface (Trier et al. 1965). Fat-filled spaces are often though not invariably present. In contrast to many other diffuse small intestinal diseases, the enterocyte layer is relatively normal, though there may be patchy areas where the cells are cuboidal and vacuolated. Intraepithelial lymphocytes are not present in increased numbers but, unlike the normal state, a few polymorphonuclear leucocytes, eosinophils and macrophages lie within the epithelial cell layer (Austin & Dobbins 1982). The bacterial bodies (Fig. 16.4) within and between the macrophages are more abundant just beneath the epithelial basement membrane; some are also seen between enterocytes (Trier et al. 1965, Dobbins & Kawanishi 1981).

Mesenteric lymphatic nodes

Mesenteric and retroperitoneal nodes are greatly enlarged — in advanced cases up to 3–4 cm across — and are often filled with irregular fat-filled cystic spaces. In the intersitium of such nodes foamy macrophages and areas of fibrosis occur, and granulomas may be seen fairly frequently (Maizel et al. 1970) in contrast with the small intestine where granulomata are rare (Babaryka et al. 1979). Bacilli are also demonstrable in the nodes (Whipple 1907, Kojecky et al. 1964).

Other abdominal findings

Peritoneal adhesions and thickening of the capsule of the liver and spleen are commonly seen at autopsy, and almost one third of patients develop ascites, which is often chylous. PAS-positive macrophages and granulomas (Saint-Marc girardin et al. 1984) are identifiable in the liver (mainly in Kuppfer cells) spleen and pancreas, but only rarely in organs of the genito-urinary system (Sieracki & Fine 1959, Viteri et al. 1979).

Heart

Valvular endocarditis was found in thirty-two out of ninety-five autopsies with a distribution of lesions similar to that of rheumatic heart disease, commonly involving mitral, mixed mitral and aortic, or aortic valves (Enzinger & Helwig 1963). PAS-positive cells and bacilli were identified in the vegetations. Fibrinous pericarditis has been reported in up to two thirds of cases coming to autopsy, and myocarditis and coronary arteritis have also been reported (James & Haubrich 1975, Lie & Davis 1976, Vliestra et al. 1978).

Pulmonary involvement

Pleural adhesions have been found in 60% of autopsied cases, usually in those with pericardial disease, and effusions are about half as frequent. Nodular involvement of the lung parenchyma with peribronchial and perivascular inflammation containing PAS-positive histiocytes has also been described (Winberg et al. 1978).

Central nervous system

Involvement of the central nervous system occurs in about 10% of autopsied cases, even in patients in whom there had been no clinical evidence of brain involvement (Romanul et al. 1977). The gross pathological appearances include cortical atrophy, ventricular dilatation, patches of spongy degeneration and areas of infarction. PAS-positive

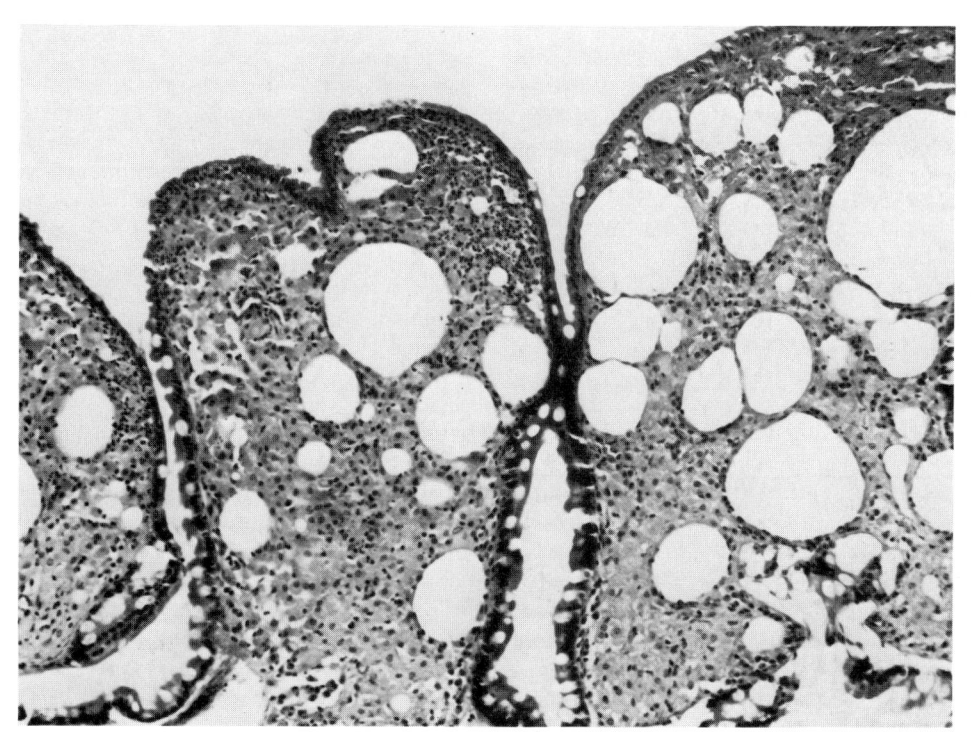

Fig. 16.3. Clubbed villi of jejunal mucosa in Whipple's disease. The lamina propria is full of foamy macrophages, and fat-filled spaces are prominent (H & E × 150).

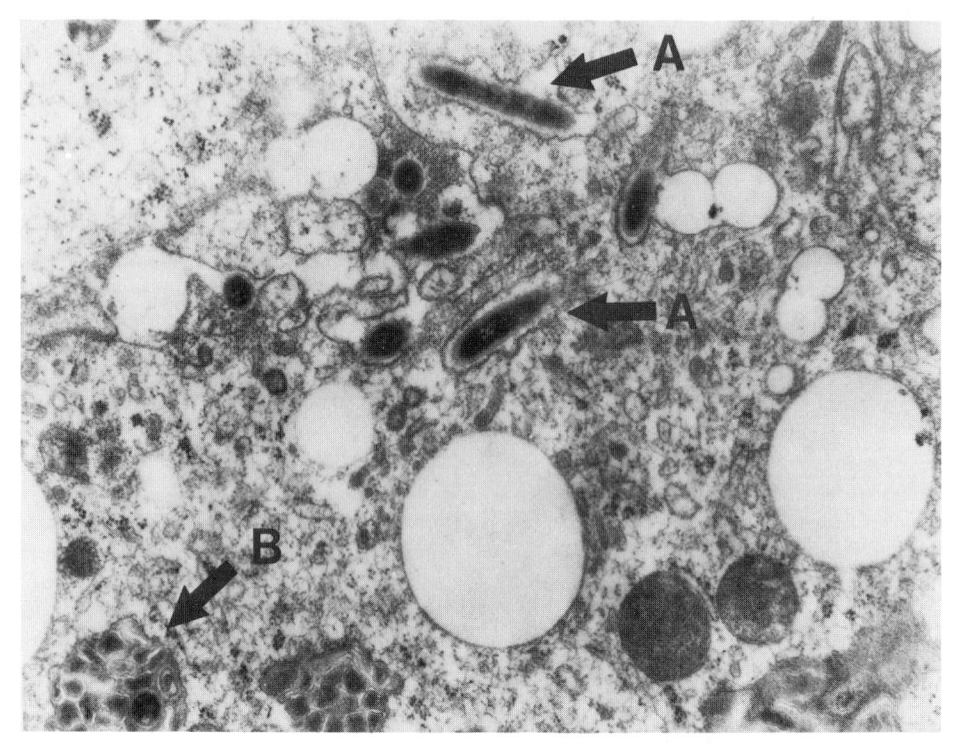

Fig. 16.4. Electron micrograph showing foamy macrophages within jejunal mucosa. Whole bacilli (A) with typical membranes are seen, as well as the characteristic intracellular granules (B) containing disintegrating membranous material (× 20,000).

inclusions are found in both glial cells and neurones and PAS-positive macrophages may appear in the cerebrospinal fluid (Feurle et al. 1979).

Amyloidosis

This has been described in Whipple's disease (Farr et al. 1983).

Clinical features

Eighty to ninety per cent of affected individuals are male and middle-aged, mostly presenting between the ages of 30 and 70 (Kelly & Weisiger 1963, Maizel et al. 1970). Nevertheless, cases have been reported in teenagers, and even in infants. The majority of patients are Caucasian but Negroes and Indians have also been affected.

The disease is systemic, and symptoms and signs of involvement of almost any organ system may occur. The commonest early symptoms, however, presenting from 1–10 years or more before symptoms of intestinal disease occur, are arthritis, fever, malaise and pulmonary complaints.

Cutaneous manifestations

One half to one-third of patients are pigmented especially in areas of exposed skin. A variety of other non-specific skin manifestations occur, including petechiae, ecchymoses, follicular hyperkeratosis and subcutaneous nodules (Whipple 1907, Enzinger & Helwig 1963). The diagnosis may be made by examining a biopsy of a skin nodule (Good et al. 1980). Finger clubbing, although reported, occurs in only a minority of patients.

Arthritis

Joint complaints are recorded in 60–90% of patients, especially in those with pulmonary involvement (Kelly & Weisiger 1963). The arthritis mainly affects peripheral joints, usually causing swelling, redness and other signs of synovial inflammation, but occasionally presenting only with pain. Symptoms are usually episodic, lasting from only a few hours to several weeks. Virtually every joint may be affected, but knees, ankles, fingers, hips, wrists, elbows and hands are most commonly affected. Involvement may be unilateral or bilateral, symmetrical or asymmetrical. There is virtually no tendency to develop deformity, and radiological changes are rare. Tests for rheumatoid factor are negative. Back pain is relatively common, but sacroiliitis or spondylitis are present in only 6–8% respectively (Canoso et al. 1978).

Investigations of the arthritis by biopsy or synovial fluid analysis have not been often reported, but a pleocytic synovial fluid, with a protein content of 3–4 g/100 ml, and biopsy appearances of synovial hyperplasia with increased vascularity and a perivascular infiltrate are recorded (Caughey & Bywaters 1963). An arthritis in combination with a chronic infection may reflect either joint infection or an antigen–antibody complex-mediated immune response. The findings in the synovium of PAS-positive macrophages and electron microscopic descriptions of bacilli similar to those found elsewhere (Hawkins et al. 1976) suggest that direct infection causes the arthritis. Dobbins & Kawanishi (1981) have, however, suggested that these particular electron micrographs may be illustrating Weibel–Palade bodies, a normal finding in capillary endothelia.

Cardiac abnormalities

The commonest cardiac problem is pericarditis, detectable by a pericardial friction rub and ECG changes in about 10% of patients (McAllister & Fenoglio 1975). Constrictive pericarditis has also been described (Vliestra et al. 1978, Crake et al. 1983). Myocarditis is rarely clinically manifest, but heart failure may occur due both to this and to valvular disease; conduction defects occur and may return to normal after treatment. The endocarditis of Whipple's disease may be further complicated by a more conventional bacterial endocarditis. Occasionally valvular involvement in Whipple's disease has necessitated valve replacement (Wright et al. 1978).

Pulmonary involvement

In addition to pleurisy, cough is a common early manifestation of Whipple's disease, occurring in approximately half the reported cases. Radiographs of the chest may reveal transient infiltrates, increased perivascular markings, or pleural effusions. (Winberg et al. 1978).

Reticuloendothelial system

Peripheral lymphadenopathy is an important clinical sign in Whipple's disease, occurring in approximately 50% of patients, and biopsy of axillary, inguinal or cervical nodes may be diagnostic (Maizel et al. 1970). There is a well-documented case of axillary node biopsy leading to a diagnosis in a patient in whom the histology of repeated small intestinal biopsies was apparently normal (Mansbach et al. 1978). Hepatomegaly and splenomegaly occur, but in less than 5% of cases. The liver involvement leads to no clinical symptoms (Viteri et al. 1979).

Central nervous system

Central system involvement occurs in less than 5% of patients and usually follows the initial systemic manifestations by some years (Knox et al. 1976, Maizel et al. 1970). There are occasional reports of symptoms of involvement of the central nervous system providing the presenting features of the disease in patients with minimal or even absent intestinal changes (Moorthy et al. 1977, Romanul et al. 1977). The manifestations are again non-specific, ranging from depression or apathy, to mild progressive dementia, fits, myoclonus, dizziness and deafness. Ocular manifestations include supranuclear ophthalmoplegia, papilloedema, optic atrophy and scotomata, vitreous opacities and haemorrhages (Leland & Chambers 1978). Uveitis has also been reported in association with spondylitis (Canoso et al. 1978).

Meningitis with PAS-positive cells in the CSF has occurred (Thompson et al. 1978). Central nervous system manifestations may also complicate the course of patients whose intestinal Whipple's disease has been successfully treated in the past with antibiotics, or even during remission with continuing antibiotic therapy. In some of these patients symptoms have suggested hypothalamic involvement, with symptoms either of insomnia or excessive somnolence and of hyperphagia and polydypsia (Knox et al. 1976, Feurle et al. 1979). At the time of central nervous system relapse, the jejunal histology may show no evidence of Whipple's disease.

The diagnosis of Whipple's disease affecting the brain may clearly present difficulties, particularly in view of the protean clinical manifestations. Although cerebrospinal fluid examination may reveal PAS-containing cells, the CSF may be of normal protein content, at normal pressure and free of cells, or be non-specifically abnormal with increased numbers of lymphocytes and elevated protein concentration (Romanul et al. 1977). Whilst brain biopsy has been used to confirm the diagnosis (Johnson & Diamond 1980), a therapeutic trial of antibiotics is preferable if the diagnosis is considered.

Intestinal disease

Despite the belief that the gut is the portal of entry of the bacillus, the clinical manifestations of gut disease are late. Furthermore, there is nothing specific in the clinical features when they occur. They consist of diarrhoea, weight loss, abdominal pain and distension. Diarrhoea reflects steatorrhoea, weight loss reflects malabsorption and anorexia, and is usually associated with anaemia and often oedema, especially in association with protein-losing enteropathy. Abdominal distension may reflect gas, ascitic fluid or mesenteric and retroperitoneal node enlargement. Occasionally bleeding from the gastrointestinal tract occurs, rarely as melaena, more often as occult blood loss. Investigation may reveal sigmoidoscopic appearances suggestive of ulcerative colitis (Hendrix et al. 1950, Enzinger & Helwig 1963, Maizel et al. 1970).

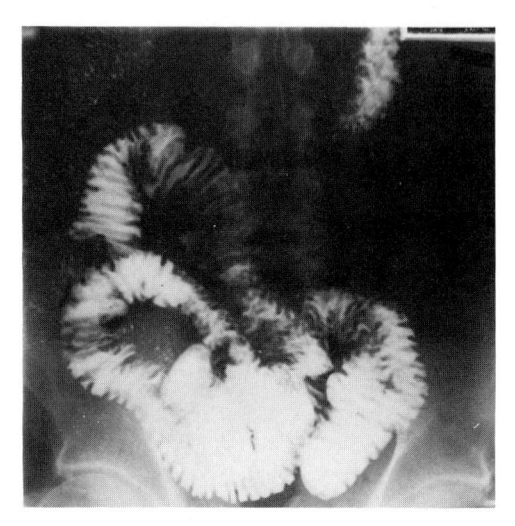

Fig. 16.5. Dilated oedematous small bowel radiograph, typical but not diagnostic of Whipple's disease.

Investigations

The diagnosis of Whipple's disease depends on the demonstration of the characteristic pathological findings, most commonly in the jejunal mucosa on biopsy, but also in lymph nodes and other tissues. The demonstration of PAS-positive staining material in rectum only is not diagnostic.

Routine haematological tests show an elevated erythrocyte sedimentation rate, and an anaemia which is either hypochromic or normochromic and normocytic, and reflects iron deficiency, folic acid deficiency and the effects of chronic inflammation. B_{12} levels are usually normal, with B_{12} absorption tests abnormal in only a minority (Maizel et al. 1970). Leucocytosis, occasionally eosinophilia and thrombocytosis are reported in untreated cases (Nuzum et al. 1981).

Serum albumin is usually low, reflecting in large part a protein-losing enteropathy associated with the lymphatic abnormalities. Despite this protein loss, globulin levels are usually normal or may even be elevated as a response to chronic infection. Hypocalcaemia and hypokalaemia are common. The steatorrhoea in patients with frank clinical involvement of the intestine usually ranges from 20–30 g daily.

In virtually every untreated case, the small

intestinal appearances are abnormal. Endoscopy may show obvious abnormalities, with thickened folds and yellow-white areas representing enlarged villi (Volpicelli et al. 1976). Small intestinal biopsies taken from the jejunum usually show diffuse abnormalities, although occasionally they may be patchy. Despite the prominence given to the rare exceptions, small intestinal biopsy remains the most important single investigation in Whipple's disease. The radiological investigation of the small intestine is normal in about 15% of cases (Maizel et al. 1970), but frequently shows varying degrees of dilatation and oedema (Fig. 16.5).

Other radiological investigations may show inflammatory colonic disease, lymphadenopathy, and minor changes in joints such as narrowing of the joint space. Computerized axial tomography (Rijke et al. 1983) would be expected to show retroperitoneal lymphadenopathy and in the brain has shown patchy areas of abnormal density.

Treatment

Paulley (1952) reported a dramatic and sustained clinical improvement in a patient with Whipple's disease, after treatment with chloramphenicol. This initial report was ignored and during the next decade corticosteroids or ACTH were used to bring about clinical improvement, although never cure (Holt et al. 1961). It was not until the 1960s, following the electron microscopic descriptions of the bacillary bodies, that antibiotics became increasingly recognized as the primary means of treatment. The use of corticosteroids is now limited to short-term supportive care in desperately sick patients.

Many antibiotics have been used with success, and no comparative trials have been performed. Penicillin, streptomycin, tetracyclines and sulphonamide-trimethoprin combinations have all been successful (Bayless 1970, Tauris & Moesner 1978) but instances of failure to respond occur. In particular, relapse during continuous tetracycline therapy has been reported and a change to another antibiotic has sometimes been effective (Trier et al. 1965, Feurle et al. 1979).

Effective treatment leads to clinical improvement within a few days with defervescence, cessation of diarrhoea and arthritis, reversal of cardiac failure and weight gain over a few weeks. Recovery of central nervous system manifestations, as would be expected, is often slow and incomplete (Knox et al. 1976). Occasionally the initiation of successful treatment has been associated with fever and exacerbation of symptoms suggestive of a Herxheimer reaction (Trier et al. 1965, Tauris & Moesner 1978).

Despite the rapid response to antibiotics, there is a high incidence of relapse after or even during continuous treatment: perhaps 20–30% of patients will relapse at some time, so life-long follow-up is indicated (Maizel et al. 1970, Knox et al. 1976). Serial histological studies show that successful treatment removes the bacteria from the intestine within a few weeks, though the PAS-positive macrophages may remain for years (Trier et al. 1965, Martin et al. 1972). Clinical relapse may be preceded and foretold by the reappearance of bacteria in the intestine, although as already mentioned, relapse may be indicated by signs in the central nervous system in the presence of a persistently normal jejunal biopsy (Feurle et al. 1979). In view of this, it seems appropriate to commence therapy with high doses of parenteral antibiotics in the hope that this will provide high enough concentrations within the central nervous system to eliminate the bacteria (Knox et al. 1976). A regime of 1.2 mega units of penicillin and 1 g streptomycin for 2 weeks, followed by long-term tetracycline, has been recommended (Maizel et al. 1970).

Aetiology

Whipple's disease results from tissue invasion by bacteria coupled with an unusual response from the macrophage cell line. Two central questions remain unanswered. Is there a specific organism, or can different types of bacteria initiate the disease? Is the response by the host a normal but rare form of immune response brought on by an unusual pathogen, or is it a primary abnormality in host defence mechanisms permitting invasion by a number of different bacteria in different individuals?

The epidemiological findings are not particularly helpful. Eighty to ninety per cent of individuals are male, and the disease is mainly reported from North America and Europe. The majority of cases occur in middle age, in Caucasian individuals, though there are scattered reports in children and in coloured races. Two sets of affected brothers have been reported (Gross et al. 1959, Puite & Tesluk 1955). Whilst the predeliction for middle-aged males has been thought to indicate a disease based on host factors, the majority of diseases particularly affecting this population (coronary artery disease, chronic bronchitis and lung cancer) have prominent environmental causes.

The bacteria

The bacillary bodies (Fig. 16.4) in the tissues in Whipple's disease appear similar in reports by many authors, and are rods, $1-1.5\mu$ long, 0.25μ across (Chears & Ashworth 1961, Yardley & Hendrix 1961). They may be seen actively dividing both freely in the tissues and in macrophages (Trier et al. 1965). There is a definite cell wall (of interest in view of some of the cultivation techniques discussed below) and there is both an inner and outer trilaminar membrane applied to the wall (Dobbins & Kawanishi 1981). Bacteria are most common just beneath the intestinal epithelial basement membrane, and decrease in numbers as the submucosa is approached, supporting the concept of invasion from the luminal side. The bacilli are also seen within and between epithelial cells, though it has been suggested that these are invaded from the lamina propria (Dobbins & Ruffin 1967). The relative abundance of bacilli in the abdomen, in small intestine and in mesenteric nodes, together with the relative difficulty initially experienced in identifying them in systemic sites, also argues in favour of the gut as the usual portal of entry. Bacilli have now been identified in heart, central nervous system, joints, lymph nodes and lung (Lie & Davis 1976), Schochet & Lampert 1969, Hawkins et al. 1976, Mansbach et al. 1978, Winberg et al. 1978, Viteri et al. 1978).

Identification of the bacteria has proved difficult despite many attempts, initially at culturing bacteria but more recently using immunological techniques for identifying surface antigens.

Culture techniques

Kjaerheim et al. (1966) isolated four different genera of bacteria from jejunal submucosa at autopsy — E. coli, Enterococci, Clostridia and Haemophilus, but such observations may be influenced by contaminating micro-organisms. Cultures of jejunal mucosa taken during life may well also be contaminated by adherent micro-organisms, which are more likely to colonize diseased mucosa: Kok et al. (1964) identified over ten different species of bacteria from repeated small bowel biopsies before and during treatment of a case of Whipple's disease. They argued on morphological grounds that the Haemophilus isolate was likely to represent the organisms responsible, resembling the Gram-negative rods seen in the jejunal tissue: the same conclusion was reached by Tytgat et al. (1977) following similar observations in another patient. Kok and others also isolated species of Corynebacterium from jejunal tissues, and a low virulence Streptococcus. Klebsiella and Nocardia have also been reported (Kok et al. 1964, Fontana et al. 1974).

In view of the difficulties in interpreting the bacteriology of intestinal tissues, the results of culture of lymph nodes seem more persuasive, particularly when there is morphological evidence of bacteria in the cultured nodes. Caroli and his colleagues (1963) isolated a Corynebacterium anaerobium from an inguinal lymph node, and isolates of similar bacteria have been made from mesenteric nodes, and axillary nodes (Greenberger et al. 1971). An anaerobic Corynebacterium, differentiatable from Caroli's isolate by fermentation reactions and identified as Corynebacterium bovis, has also been isolated from an inguinal node (Hodgson 1981). Certain of the anaerobic Corynebacterium would now be classified as Propionobacteria. These have emerged as potential pathogens in a variety of individuals, mainly in immunosuppressed hosts, but a cautionary note is sounded by their culture from lymph nodes of normal individuals (White & Stanford 1981).

More sophisticated culture techniques have been used, as well as animal innoculation studies, to provide a better milieu for this organism which is clearly visible in the tissues in large numbers but difficult to grow. Charache et al. (1966) cultured an atypical, cell-wall-deficient Enterococcus from a lymph node and blood, and under different culture conditions grew it with a cell wall. Similarly Clancy et al. (1975) grew, in a tissue culture of a patient's lymph node cells, cell-wall-deficient Streptococci (S. dysgalactiae) and showed that these bacteria could absorb out antibody from the patient's serum which reacted with intracellular material within the foamy macrophages. Yet bacteria with deficient cell walls are not found by the electron microscope and the report remains unconfirmed (Keren 1981).

Serological identification

The use of antibacterial sera offers a more direct approach to identifying bacteria in tissue, using fresh or paraffin-embedded material (Keren et al. 1976, Kirkpatrick et al. 1978, Kent & Kirkpatrick 1980). Grouping sera against bacteria, which react most strongly with polysaccharide components of bacterial cell walls, have been shown to react not only with the bacteria but also with the PAS-positive material within macrophages in the Whipple's tissue. It must be emphasized that, although similar findings have been reported in different studies, the findings are not sufficiently specific to incriminate a particular bacterial species. Unfortunately, there is cross-reactivity of the grouping antisera between both species and genera of bacteria; this probably reflects similar carbohydrate composition of the cell walls.

In all three studies reported so far no fluorescence was seen in the macrophages of tissues from controls but strong fluorescence was obtained in Whipple's disease tissue with antisera to Streptococci group A, B and G, with less strong fluorescence to Streptococci C, D and F; antisera to Shigella B also proved strongly positive, and some fluorescence was observed with an anti-Propionobacterium antiserum. No positives were noted with antisera to certain other candidate bacteria, notably Haemophilus and Klebsiella.

The sub-classes of Streptococci and Shigella B show a similar surface carbohydrate structure, and the results in Whipple's disease suggest the Whipple's bacillus is similarly endowed. The similarities in all these studies so far, taken with the uniform morphological appearances of the bacteria, suggest that a single organism or closely related group is responsible for the disease. Since this staining technique is applicable in formalin-fixed tissues, and as specific monoclonal antibodies to bacterial antigens become available, it is likely that a specific organism will soon be identified.

Immunology

The candidates for the title of Whipple's bacillus — Streptococci, Corynebacterium, Haemophilus and so on — are not notable for causing chronic infections persisting over decades. The eventual identification of a single organism might explain this conundrum — for example if it possessed a powerful method of diverting the host immune response; alternatively a basic defect in host immunity, or loss of a non-specific bacterial defence mechanism may permit the bacteria to survive.

The lack of any obvious general susceptibility to infection before the onset of disease in patients with Whipple's disease is a strong argument against defective host defences. There is, however, a large body of evidence suggesting defective immunity in patients with active Whipple's disease, both during and after treatment.

HLA typing in many diseases has implied a genetic background favouring the development of enhanced or abnormal immunity. A number of patients with Whipple's disease have been HLA-typed, and in Feurle et al.'s series (1979), four out of nine patients possessed the B27 haplotype, whereas only one would have been expected. Dobbin's survey

(1981) of studies in Whipple's disease found six out of fifteen patients B27 positive, but this small group includes those in Feurle's paper. The B27 antigen, which is strongly associated with ankylosing spondylitis, may be associated with a tendency to react to certain antigens, particularly certain intestinal bacteria, in an abnormal fashion (Ebringer et al. 1979), but whether the antigen is really commoner in Whipple's disease remains uncertain.

In untreated patients conventional assessments of immune competence, both humoral and cell-mediated, frequently show abnormalities, but this is not uncommon in ill patients. On the humoral side serum immunoglobulin levels are rarely abnormal despite protein loss into the gut (Anton 1961). In some patients, serum IgA is raised, as is often the case in diffuse mucosal disease of the gut (Hodgson & Jewell 1978). Autoantibodies are not usually found. The local gut antibody system shows some abnormalities, with reduced numbers of IgA, IgG and IgM plasma cells, but this probably simply reflects displacement of cells from the lamina propria by the abundant foamy macrophages, for the numbers of plasma cells return to normal after treatment (Keren et al. 1976).

There have been a few studies on non-specific defence mechanisms — cytotoxicity and adherence by cells of the monocyte–macrophage series, phagocytosis by leucocytes — but no consistent abnormal pattern has emerged (Clancy et al. 1977, Dobbins 1981).

The role of cell-mediated immunity has been more deeply studied, following an early demonstration of decreased *in vitro* cell-mediated immune responsiveness (Maxwell et al. 1968), and the realization that adequate macrophage function, and the ability to kill intracellular bacteria, depend upon co-operation between macrophages and T-lymphocytes. The data on *in vitro* and *in vivo* testing of cell-mediated immunity have been summarized by Dobbins (1981) and by Keren (1981). The majority of authors report diminished T-cell function, although this is most striking during active disease.

Conclusion

Whipple's disease is a chronic infection by an unidentified organism. In the future the use of more specific antibodies to stain the bacilli in tissue should identify the infectious agent. The organism may be specific, rather than the disease arising when one of a number of bacteria infect an immunodeficient host. What part, if any, abnormal host defence mechanisms play should become apparent when the bacterium is identified.

Over 80 years the disease has changed from a fatal intra-abdominal condition to a treatable multi-system disorder. It presents a diagnostic opportunity in conditions as various as seronegative arthritis, culture negative endocarditis, pre-senile dementia or ill-defined collagenosis, provided the physician is alert to the possibility.

References

Allchin W.H. & Hebb R.G. (1895) Lymphangiectasis intestini. *Trans. Path. Soc. Lond.* **46**, 221–223.

Anton A. (1961) Agammaglobulinaemia complicating Whipple's disease. *Ohio State Med. J.* **57**, 650–653.

Austin L.L. & Dobbins W.O. (1982) Intraepithelial leucocytes of the intestinal mucosa in normal man and Whipple's disease. *Dig. Dis. Sci.* **27**, 311–320.

Babaryka I., Thorn L. & Langer E. (1979) Epithelial cell granulomata in the mucosa of the small intestine in Whipple's disease. *Virchows Arch. Path.* **382**, 227–235.

Bayless T.M. (1970) Whipple's disease — newer concepts of therapy. *Adv. Int. Med.* **16**, 171–189.

Bayless T.M. & Knox D.L. (1979) Whipple's disease: a multisystem infection. *New Engl. J. Med.* **300**, 920–921.

Black-Shaffer B. (1949) Tinctorial demonstration of glycoproteins in Whipple's disease. *Proc. Soc. Exp. Biol. Med.* **72**, 225–227.

Canoso J.J., Saini M. & Hermos J.A. (1978) Whipple's disease and ankylosing spondylitis: simultaneous occurrence in HLA B27 positive males. *J. Rheumatol.* **5**, 79–84.

Caroli J., Julien C., Etévé J., Prevot A.R. & Sébald M. (1963) Trois cas de maladie de Whipple. *Sem. Hop. Paris*, **31**, 1457–1480.

Caughey D.E. & Bywaters, E.G.L. (1963). The arthritis of Whipple's syndrome. *Ann. Rheum. Dis.* **22**, 327–335.

Charache P., Bayless T.M., Shelly W.M. & Hendrix T.R. (1966) Atypical bacteria in Whipple's disease. *Trans. Assoc. Am. Phys.* **79**, 399–408.

Chears W.C. & Ashworth C.T. (1961) Electron microscopic study of the intestinal mucosa in Whipple's disease — demonstration of encapsulated bacilliform bodies in these lesions. *Gastroenterol.* **41**, 129–138.

Clancy R.L., Tomkins W.A.F., Muckle T.J., Richardson H. and Rawls W.E. (1975) Isolation and characterization of an aetiologic agent in Whipple's disease. *Brit. Med. J.* **ii**, 568–570.

Clancy R.L., Muckle T.J., de Jesus D. & Stevens D. (1977) Characteristics of the immune response in a patient with Whipple's disease. *Aust. N.Z. Med. J.* **7**, 294–298.

Crake T., Sandleg. I., Crisp A.J. & Record C.D. (1983). Constrictive pericarditis and intestinal haemorrhage in Whipple's disease. *Postgrad. Med. J.* **59**, 194–195.

Dobbins W.O. (1981) Is there an immune deficit in Whipple's disease? *Dig. Dis. Sci.* **26**, 247–252.

Dobbins W.O. & Kawanishi H. (1981) Bacillary characteristics in Whipple's disease: An electron microscopic study. *Gastroenterol.* **80**, 1468–1475.

Dobbins W.O. & Ruffin J.M. (1967) A light and electron microscopic study of bacterial invasion in Whipple's disease. *Amer. J. Path.* **51**, 225–242.

Ebringer R., Cawdwell D. & Ebringer A. (1979) *Klebsiella pneumoniae* and acute anterior uveitis in ankylosing spondylitis. *Brit. Med. J.* **i**, 382.

Enzinger F.M. & Helwig E.B. (1963) Whipple's disease — a review of the literature and report of 15 patients. *Virchows Arch. Path. Anat.* **336**, 238–269.

Farr M., Morris C., Hollywell C.A., Scott D.L., Walton K.W. & Bacon P.A. (1983). Amyloidosis in Whipple's disease. *J. Roy. Soc. Med.* **76**, 963–965.

Feurle G.E., Dörken B., Schöpf E. & Lenhard V. (1979) HLA B27 and defects in the T-cell system in Whipple's disease. *Euro. J. Clin. Invest.* **9**, 385–389.

Feurle G.E., Volk B. & Waldherr R. (1979) Cerebral Whipple with negative jejunal histology. *New Engl. J. Med.* **300**, 907–908.

Fontana G., Caletti G., Bolondi L. & Costa P. (1974) Recenti acquisizioni eziopatogenetiche sul morbo di Whipple. *Rec. Prog. Med.* **56**, 322.

Good A.E., Beals T.F., Simmons J.L. & Ibrahim M.A.H. (1980) A subcutaneous nodule with Whipple's disease — key to early diagnosis. *Arth. Rheum.* **23**, 856–858.

Greenberger N.J., Debor J., Fisher J., Perkins R.L., Murad T. & Kapral F. (1971) Whipple's disease. Characterization of anaerobic corynebacteria and demonstration of bacilli in vascular endothelium. *Dig. Dis. Sci.* **16**, 1127–1136.

Groll A., Volberg L.S., Simon J.D., Eidinger D., Wilson B. & Forschyke D.B. (1972) Immunological defect in Whipple's disease. *Gastroenterol.* **63**, 943–950.

Gross J.B., Wollaeger E.E., Sauer W.G., Huizenga K.A., Dahlin D.C. & Power M.H. (1959) Whipple's disease: report of four cases including two brothers with observations on pathologic physiology, diagnosis and treatment. *Gastroenterol.* **36**, 65–93.

Hawkins C.F., Farr M., Morris C.J., Hoare A.M. & Williamson N. (1976) Detection by electron microscopy of rod-shaped organisms in synovial membrane from a patient with the arthritis of Whipple's disease. *Ann. Rheum. Dis.* **35**, 502–509.

Hendrix J.P., Black-Shaffer B., Withers R.W. & Handler P. (1950) Whipple's intestinal lipodystrophy: Report of 4 cases and discussion of possible pathogenic factors. *Arch. Int. Med.* **85**, 91–131.

Hodgson H.J.F. (1981) Whipple's disease — any progress? In *Advanced Medicine*, p. 17. (Ed. by D.P. Jewell). Pitman Medical, London.

Hodgson H.J.F. & Jewell D.P. (1978) The humoral immune system in inflammatory bowel disease. *Amer. J. Dig. Dis.* **23**, 123–128.

Holt P.R., Isselbacher K.J. & Jones C.M. (1961) The reversibility of Whipple's disease. *New Engl. J. Med.* **264**, 1335–1337.

James T.N. & Haubrich W.S. (1975) Bacterial arteritis in Whipple's disease. *Circulation*, **52**, 722–731.

Johnson L. & Diamond I. (1980) Cerebral Whipple's. Diagnosis by brain biopsy, *Amer. J. Clin. Path.* **74**, 486–490.

Kelly J.J. & Weisiger B.B. (1963) The arthritis of Whipple's disease. *Arth. Rheum.* **6**, 615–632.

Kent S.P. & Kirkpatrick S.M. (1980) Whipple's disease. Immunological and histopathological studies of eight cases. *Arch. Path. Lab. Med.* **104**, 544–547.

Keren D.F. (1981) Whipple's disease — a review emphasising immunology and microbiology. *Crit. Rev. Clin. Lab. Sci.* **14**, 75–108.

Keren D.F., Weisburger W.R., Yardley J.H., Salyer W.R., Arthur R.R. & Charache P. (1976) Whipple's disease: demonstration by immunofluorescence of similar bacterial antigens in macrophages from three cases. *Johns Hopkins Med. J.* **139**, 51–59.

Keren D.F., Weinrieb I.J., Bertovich M.J. & Brady P.G. (1979) Whipple's disease: no consistent mitogenic or cytotoxic defect in lymphocyte function from three cases. *Gastroenterol.* **77**, 991–996.

Kirkpatrick P.M., Kent S.P., Mikas A. & Pritchett P. (1978). Whipple's disease: a case report with immunological studies. *Gastroenterol.* **75**, 297–301.

Kjaerheim A., Midtredt T., Skrede S. & Gjone E. (1966) Bacteria in Whipple's disease. Isolation of a haemophilus strain from the jejunal propria. *Arch. Path. Microbiol. Scand.* **66**, 135–142.

Knox D.L., Bayless T.M. & Pittman F.E. (1976) Neurologic disease in patients with treated Whipple's disease. *Medicine (Balt.)* **55**, 467–476.

Kojecky A., Malinsky J., Kodousek R., Marsalek E.

(1964) Frequency of occurrence of microbes in the intestinal mucosa and the lymph nodes during a long-term observation of a patient suffering from Whipple's disease. *Gastroenterol. (Basel)* **101**, 163–173.

Kok N., Dykbaer R. & Rostgaard J. (1964) Bacteria in Whipple's disease. *Acta Path. Microbiol. Scand.* **60**, 431–449.

Leland J.M. & Chambers J.K. (1978) Ocular findings in Whipple's disease. *Southern Med. J.* **71**, 335–338.

Lie T.J. & Davis J.S. (1976) Pericarditis in Whipple's disease. Electron microscopic demonstration of intra-cardiac bacillary bodies. *Amer. J. Clin. Path.* **66**, 22–32.

McAllister H.A. & Fenoglio J.J. (1975) Cardiac involvement in Whipple's disease. *Circulation*, **52**, 152–156.

Maizel H., Ruffin J.M. & Dobbins W.O. (1970) Whipple's disease. A review of 19 patients from one hospital and a review of the literature since 1950. *Medicine (Balt.)* **49**, 175–205.

Mansbach C.M., Shelbourne J.D., Stevens R.D. & Dobbins W.O. (1978) Lymph node bacilliform bodies resembling those of Whipple's disease in a patient without intestinal involvement. *Ann. Int. Med.* **89**, 64–66.

Martin F.F., Vilseck J. & Dobbins W.D. (1972) Immunologic alterations in patients with treated Whipple's disease. *Gastroenterol.* **63**, 6–18.

Maxwell J.D., Fergusson A., McKay A.M., Imrie R.C. & Watson W.C. (1968) Lymphocytes in Whipple's disease. *Lancet*, **i**, 887–889.

Moorthy S., Nolley G. & Hermos J.A. (1977) Whipple's disease with minimal intestinal involvement. *Gut*, **18**, 152–155.

Morgan A.D. (1961) The first recorded case of Whipple's disease? *Gut*, **2**, 370–372.

Nuzum C.T., Sandler R.S. & Paulk H.T. (1981) Thrombocytosis in Whipple's disease. *Gastroenterol.* **80**, 1465–1467.

Paulley J.W. (1952) A case of Whipple's disease (intestinal lipodystrophy). *Gastroenterol.* **22**, 128–133.

Puite R.H. & Tesluk H. (1955) Whipple's disease. *Amer. J. Med.* **19**, 383–400.

Rijke A.M., Falke T.H. & Vries R.R. (1983). Computed tomography in Whipple's disease *J. Compit. Assist. Tom.* **7**, 1101–1102.

Romanul F.C.A., Radvany T. & Rosales R.K. (1977) Whipple's disease confined to the brain: a case studied clinically and pathologically *J. Neurol. Neurosurg. Psych.* **40**, 901–909.

Saint-Marc Girardin M.F. Zafrani E.S. Chaumette M.T., Delcher J.C. & Métreau J.M. (1984). Hepatic granulomas in Whipple's disease. *Gastroenterol.* **86**, 753–756.

Schochet S.S. & Lampert P.W. (1969) Granulomatous encephalitis in Whipple's disease: Electron microscopic observations. *Acta Neuropathol.* **13**, 1–12.

Sieracki J.C. (1958) Whipple's disease — observations on systemic involvement 1. Cytologic observations. *AMA Arch. Path.* **66**, 464–467.

Sieracki J.C. & Fine G. (1959) Whipple's disease — observations on systemic involvement. 11. Gross and histologic observations. *Arch. Path.* **67**, 81–93.

Tauris P. & Moesner P. (1978) Whipple's disease. *Acta Med. Scand.* **204**, 423–427.

Thompson D.G., Ledingham J.M., Howard A.J. & Brown C.L. (1978) Meningitis in Whipple's disease. *Brit. Med. J.* **ii**, 14–15.

Trier J.S., Phelps J.C., Eidelman S. & Rubin C.E. (1965) Whipple's disease. Light and electron microscopic correlation of jejunal mucosal histology with antibiotic treatment and clinical status. *Gastroenterol.* **48**, 384–407.

Tytgat G.N., Hoogendijk J.L., Agenant D. & Schellekens P.T. (1977) Etiopathogenetic studies in a patient with Whipple's disease. *Digestion*, **15**, 309–321.

Viteri A.L., Stinson J.C., Barnes M.C. & Dyck W.C. (1979) Rod-shaped organism in the liver of a patient with Whipple's disease. *Dig. Dis. Sci.* **24**, 560–564.

Vliestra R.E., Lie J.T., Kuhl W.E., Danielson G.K. & Roberts M.K. (1978) Whipple's disease involving the pericardium. Pathological confirmation during life. *Aust. N.Z. J. Med.* **8**, 649–651.

Volpicelli N.A., Salyer W.R., Milligan F.D., Bayless T.M. & Yardley J.H. (1976) The endoscopic appearance of the duodenum in Whipple's disease. *Johns Hopkins Med. J.* **138**, 19–23.

Whipple G.H. (1907) A hitherto undescribed disease characterized anatomically by deposits of fat and fatty acids in the intestinal and mesenteric lymphatic tissues. *Johns Hopkins Hosp. Bull.* **198**, 382–391.

White S.A. & Stanford J.L. (1981) Investigation into the identity of acid fast organisms isolated from Crohn's disease and ulcerative colitis. In *Recent Advances in Crohn's Disease*, p. 278–282. (Ed. by A.S. Pena, I.T. Weterman, C.C. Booth and W. Strober). Martinus Nijhoff, The Hague.

Winberg C.D., Rose M.E. & Rappaport H. (1978) Whipple's disease of the lung. *Amer. J. Med.* **65**, 873–880.

Wright C.B., Hiratzka L.F., Crossland S., Isner J. & Snow J.A. (1978) Aortic insufficiency requiring valve replacement in Whipple's disease. *Ann. Thor. Surg.* **25**, 466–469.

Yardley J.H. & Hendrix T.R. (1961) Combined electron and light microscopy in Whipple's disease — demonstration of bacillary bodies in the intestine. *Bull. Johns Hopkins Hosp.* **109**, 76.

Chapter 17
Parasitic Infection

G. C. COOK

Parasites not associated with malabsorption	283
Parasites associated with malabsorption	288

The majority of mankind harbours at least one species of parasite within the lumen of the small intestine. The presence of small intestinal parasites is therefore the *normal* state for *Homo sapiens* (Anderson & May 1982, Sorvillo & Ash 1982). Clinical, parasitological (WHO 1981) and immunological (Cohen & Warren 1982) aspects of these infections have been reviewed. The majority are asymptomatic and contribute to little, if any, ill health. Some can be associated with severe disease; hookworm, for example, can produce severe anaemia and hypoalbuminaemia (Blumenthal 1977), while the protozoan, *Giardia lamblia*, can be associated with gross absorptive defects. There is good evidence that malnutrition is enhanced and pubertal development in children retarded by some parasitic infections of the small intestine (Cole et al. 1982).

Intestinal parasites are appropriately classified as those not associated with malabsorption, and those in which there is evidence that they cause malabsorption (Cook 1980).

Parasites not associated with malabsorption

Hookworm (ankylostomiasis)

A large proportion of the population of developing countries is infected with this nematode, and infections are frequently heavy. Like most intestinal parasites, the life cycle is complex (WHO 1981). Figure 17.1 illustrates the development of a larva from an ovum. Entry of larvae from moist, warm soil contaminated with human faeces, takes place through intact skin, usually the feet because they are most likely to be exposed. Local irritation ('ground-itch') may follow. Oral infection is also possible (Ray & Shrivastava 1981). Following migration through various organs and tissues of the body, during which pulmonary symptoms may be evident, the adult worms emerge in the proximal small intestine. By means of small hooks (Fig. 17.2) they anchor themselves to the small intestinal mucosa, where they produce blood loss into the intestinal lumen, the quantity of blood loss varying with the species of the parasite. Approximately 0.2 ml may be lost daily for every adult *Ankylostoma duodenale*, and 0.05 ml for a single *Necator americanus*. With loads of several hundred adult worms or more, daily blood loss is often gross and iron deficiency anaemia follows. As a consequence it is not uncommon for individuals in developing tropical countries to have haemoglobin concentrations as low as 1 g/dl. A superimposed folic acid deficiency, of dietary origin, may give rise to a 'mixed' haematological picture. Cardiac failure is frequently a complication. Similarly, protein loss may be marked and a very low serum albumin concentration results; marginal malnutrition may thus become overt. In most cases anaemia rapidly responds to oral iron supplements; blood transfusion is potentially dangerous in the presence of such a chronic anaemia. If required (in a small minority of patients) packed red blood cells should be used, and a potent intravenous diuretic given simultaneously.

Clinical features

Epigastric discomfort, a very common symptom in developing countries, can be

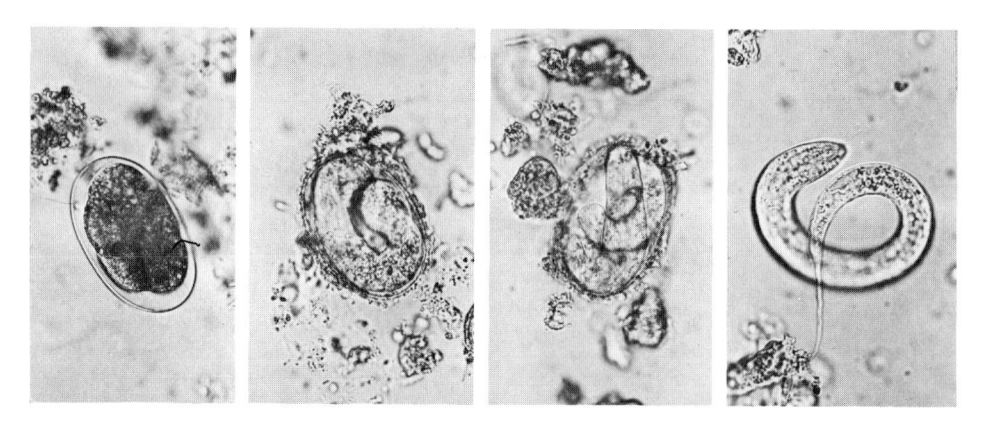

Fig. 17.1. *Ankylostoma duodenale* (hookworm). Stages in the development of the larva (right) from the ovum (left).

caused by heavy hookworm infections and a duodenitis has been described (Corachan *et al.* 1981).

Although limited evidence of malabsorption in the presence of hookworm infection has been documented in some Asian countries, this has not been confirmed by studies in Africa (Gilles *et al.* 1964, Cook 1980). If malabsorption does occur it must be unusual, and minor effects must be differentiated from the mild abnormalities in small intestinal structure (*tropical enteropathy*) and function (*sub-clinical malabsorption*) which are very common in all tropical countries and which are not associated with helminthic infections (Cook 1980).

Investigations sometimes reveal an eosinophilia, of varying degree, depending on the degree of tissue invasion. Serum IgE concentration is often elevated, but is rarely of diagnostic value (Cruickshank & Mackenzie 1981). Adult worms — approximately 1 cm in length — can be detected in duodenal and jejunal fluid, and can be seen associated with the mucosa in jejunal biopsy specimens; ova are demonstrable in faecal specimens. As the disease progresses, an iron-deficient or 'mixed' anaemia and a low serum albumin concentration can be demonstrated.

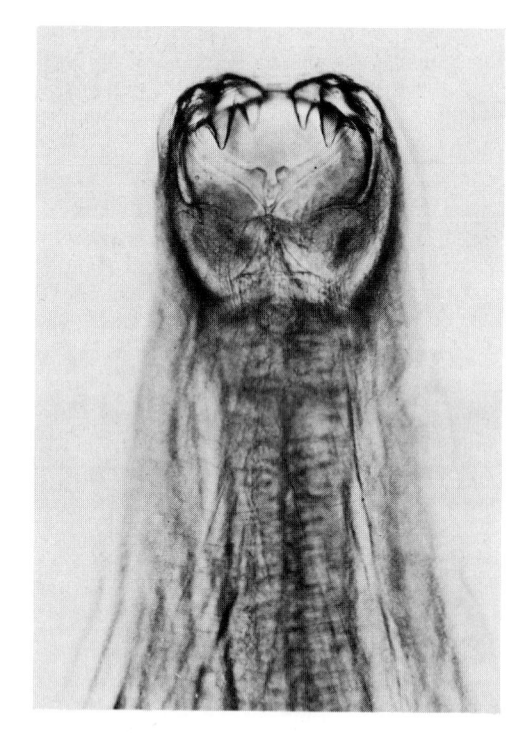

Fig. 17.2. *Ankylostoma duodenale*. Head and 'teeth' of an adult hookworm.

Treatment

Bephenium hydroxynaphthoate ('Alcopar') in an oral dose of 5 g on three consecutive mornings after overnight fasts is effective. More recently mebendazole ('Vermox') (100 mg twice daily for 3 days), pyrantel embonate ('Combantrin') (1.1 g in a single oral dose), and levamisole ('Ketrax') (150 mg in a single oral dose) have been used with a high degree of success. Cure rates (as judged by negative stool examination for ova 2 weeks after treatment) in patients with a *N. americanus* infection have been reported to be 100% after mebendazole, 73% after pyrantel embonate and 40% after bephenium hydroxynaphthoate (Griffin *et al.* 1982). Results with flubendazole are as good as those for mebendazole (Feldmeier *et al.* 1982). Albendazole, recently introduced, has also given satisfactory results (Pene *et al.* 1982; Rossignol & Maisonneuve 1983). Owing to its low cost, tetrachlorethylene (0.12 ml orally/kg body weight) is frequently used in developing countries. If a concurrent roundworm infection is demonstrated it is customary to first eradicate that parasite. Oral iron supplements and rarely transfusion with packed red blood cells may be required for the anaemia. Treatment of associated cardiac failure may also be necessary. Recent evidence suggests that after raising the serum iron concentration, other infections tend to become more common (Murray *et al.* 1978a).

Other hookworms

The monkey hookworm (*Ternidens deminutus*) occasionally infects man and may give rise to a similar clinical picture to that of *A. duodenale* and *N. americanus*.

Roundworm (ascariasis)

This is also a very common infection in people living in developing countries, as many as 70 or 80% of some population groups being affected. The parasitology has recently been reviewed (WHO 1981). Unlike the hookworm, which is dependent on warm, moist soil for survival of its larvae, the roundworm survives in the form of ova (Fig. 17.3) in soil which may be neither warm nor moist. Human infection, which is acquired by ingesting ova, is thus not confined to the tropics. After action of digestive enzymes, emergence of the rhabditiform larvae takes place; they migrate throughout the body, often producing transient pulmonary symptoms. Following migration the adult worms, which are some 10–30 cm in length, develop in the small intestine, usually the mid-jejunum; there they anchor themselves to the mucosal surface. There may be from one to several hundreds of adult worms present.

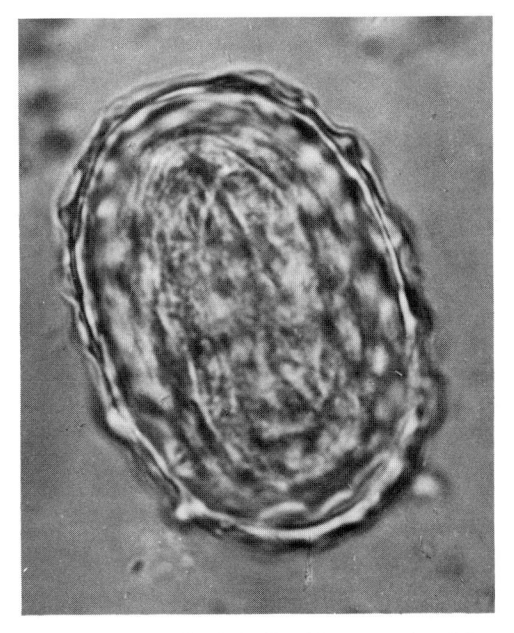

Fig. 17.3. *Ascaris lumbricoides*. Mature ovum of the roundworm, containing the developing larva.

Clinical features

Epigastric pain, which may resemble peptic ulcer disease, is sometimes a presenting symptom. A duodenitis is recorded (Corachan *et al.* 1981). Complications include: intestinal obstruction which may be caused by a ball of worms, especially in children, perforation and volvulus, which are rare, and obstruction to the common bile duct and pancreatic duct. Ascariasis must always be considered in the differential diagnosis of obstruction of the biliary passages in an individual who has undergone tropical exposure; that is, however, an unusual complication (Lloyd 1981). In a 7-year period at Kenyatta hospital, Nairobi, 624 patients (360 adults and 264 children) were treated for intestinal obstruction, and in fifty of the children the cause was *Ascaris lumbricoides* (Ochola-Abila & Barrack 1982). Constipation, abdominal pain, vomiting, distension and an abdominal mass were the major presenting symptoms. Adult worms have occasionally been detected at laparotomy within the peritoneal cavity after intestinal perforation caused by salmonella infection.

Although a minority of reports claim that malabsorption occurs occasionally with this infection, the evidence overall is unimpressive. Associated malnutrition (Jeliffe & Jeliffe 1981) seems far more likely to be due to nutrient ingestion by the parasite, and protein loss at the anchorage site; that is dependent on worm load. There is no direct relationship between infection and the presence of malnutrition (Cerf *et al.* 1981), and eradication of infection in Bangladeshi children does not enhance growth (Greenberg *et al.* 1981). An *inverse* relationship between the incidence of ascariasis and that of malaria has been documented (Murray *et al.* 1978b).

A peripheral eosinophilia of varying concentration may be present during the invasive stage. Adult worms are occasionally vomited, or 'hooked' with a jejunal biopsy capsule; more often they are passed per rectum. Ova are detected in stool specimens. Barium within the worm is sometimes demonstrated during a gastrointestinal radiological examination; alternatively the whole worm may be outlined with barium. If obstruction is present, fluid levels may be apparent on an abdominal radiograph.

Treatment

Piperazine preparations have for long been the stand-by. Piperazine phosphate ('Pripsen') 4 g is given orally with an evening meal; the adipate and citrate can also be used. Dizziness and ataxia are occasional side-effects. A possibility of carcinogenicity due to nitrosation in the stomach has been suggested (Bellander *et al.* 1981); that is only likely to occur after prolonged piperazine administration. More recently mebendazole ('Vermox') 100 mg twice daily by mouth for 3 days, pyrantel embonate ('Combantrin') 1.1 g as a single oral dose, and levamisole ('Ketrax') 150 mg as a single oral dose have also been given, with good effect. Albendazole (Rossignol & Maisonneuve 1983) and flubendazole (Kan 1983) have also proved effective. Population dynamics of *A. lumbricoides* in developing countries indicate that mass eradication is likely to be very difficult, even with the use of potent chemotherapeutic agents (Anderson & May 1982, Croll *et al.* 1982).

Other nematodes

Human trichostrongyliasis, usually due to *Trichostrongylus orientalis*, is usually asymptomatic. Ova excreted in faeces should be distinguished from those of hookworm. Bephenium and pyrantel are effective therapeutic agents. *Gnathostoma spinigerum*, which possesses an animal reservoir (in raw fish, chicken, frog or snake meat) rarely gives rise to symptoms. *Anisakis* and *Phocanema* infections, obtained from eating poorly cooked and infected fish may produce acute abdominal symptoms (Valdiserri 1981); lower abdominal pain, nausea, vomiting and fever, sometimes misdiagnosed as appendicitis or inflammatory bowel disease several days after infection, is characteristic. *Trichinella spiralis* can invade the small intestine during its migratory cycle. *Eustoma rotundum* usually involves the pyloric antrum.

Tapeworms

This group contains the longest worms to infect the human small intestine. The most common species in the Western world is the beef tapeworm, *Taenia saginata*. Organic symptoms are few, if any; more important is the psychiatric state associated with the passage of segments (proglottids) in the stool. Infection follows ingestion of infected beef. The epidemiology in the Philippines has been reviewed by Cabrera & Arambulo (1977). Segments are passed in the stool and can be easily identified; ova are detected in a faecal specimen. There may be a mild eosinophilia in the peripheral blood.

The more important species is *T. solium* (the pork tapeworm) (Fig. 17.4). Infection, which follows the eating of measly, undercooked pork has afflicted man for thousands of years and was a problem in ancient Egypt (Cockburn 1981). The intestinal stage, which is similar to that of *T. saginata*, is asympto-

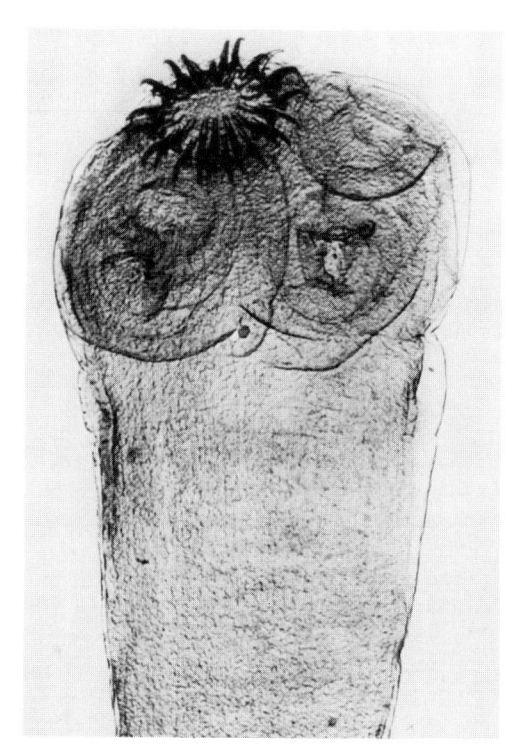

Fig. 17.4. *Taenia solium*. Head of the pork tapeworm, showing hooks and suckers.

matic and non-pathogenic. Cysticercosis, however, is a serious manifestation with a significant mortality rate. Cysts are deposited thoughout the organs of the body, and are frequently demonstrable radiologically as calcifications in skeletal muscles, especially affecting the calves and thighs. Cysts in the brain substance, which calcify much later than those in muscles, can give rise to epilepsy and other neurological and psychiatric disturbances. A large outbreak has recently been reported from Irian Jaya (Subianto *et al.* 1978, Tjahjadi *et al.* 1978).

It seems very unlikely that infection significantly impairs the host's nutritional status (Hall 1983), although growth of the parasite seems to be dependent on the protein content of the host's diet.

Serological tests are diagnostically useful. The ELISA technique is reliable (Diwan *et al.* 1982); however, cross-reaction with schistosomiasis, echinoccosis and possibly angiostrongylosis has been reported.

Treatment

Mepacrine one gram is given by a duodenal intubation technique after an overnight fast; an anti-emetic should be given, especially with *T. solium* infections, to prevent regurgitation. More recently, niclosamide ('Yomesan') and dichlorophen ('Anthiphen') have been used with good effect. Treatment for cysticercosis has formerly been unsatisfactory. Recently, praziquantel, sometimes given with prednisolone (30 mg daily) (or dexamethasone) if there is cerebral involvement, has given encouraging results in cysticercosis resulting from several tapeworm species in both animals and man (Botero & Castaño 1982, Spina-França *et al.* 1982, Thomas *et al.* 1982 Sotelo *et al.* 1984).

Less clinically important tapeworms, including *Hymenolepis nana* and *H. diminuta* are widespread in their occurrence (Kan *et al.* 1981). Although usually asymptomatic, disseminated infection can occur in immunosuppressed patients. Praziquantel and niclosamide are effective therapeutic agents.

Intestinal flukes

The major example is *Fasciolopsis buski* which is the largest fluke (trematode) to infect man. It is endemic in some areas of the tropics, e.g. South-east Asia (Hadidjaja *et al.* 1982) and Bangladesh (Gilman *et al.* 1982). Pigs form an important reservoir. Despite its size, symptoms are few; anorexia, vomiting and diarrhoea may occasionally be present. Anaemia, oedema and ascites have all been recorded and a peripheral eosinophilia may be present. Treatment is either with praziquantol, niclosamide, hexylresorcinol or tetrachlorethylene.

Other flukes

Small intestinal diarrhoea, associated with abdominal pain, malaise and dehydration, has occasionally been reported in infections with *Heterophyes heterophyes, Metagonimus yokogawai, Stellantchasmus falcatus, Pygidiopsis summa, Haplorchis tachiui, Centrocestus armatus* and *Cryptocotyle lingua*. Rarely, *Schistosoma mansoni* and *S. japonicum* can give rise to significant small intestinal involvement. Similarly, *Paragonimus westermani* can rarely involve this organ.

Eosinophilic gastroenteritis remains an enigma; various nematodes have at various times been associated with it (Cello 1979). Sarcosporidiosis, which is closely related to isosporiasis (*see below*), has been causally associated with segmental eosinophilic enteritis or necrotizing enteritis in Thailand (Bunyaratvej *et al*. 1982).

Parasites associated with malabsorption

In an extensive literature on the subject it is difficult to be certain which parasitic infections are able to impair small intestinal absorption significantly. However, *Giardia lamblia*, *Strongyloides stercoralis*, *Capillaria philippinensis* and coccidiosis (*Sarcocystis hominis*, *Isospora belli* and *Cryptosporidium*) seem beyond doubt to have a clear causative association (Cook 1980; Groupe de travail scientifique de L'OMS 1981). The underlying mechanism is, in most cases, not clear. The fresh water fish tapeworm, *Diphyllobothrium latum*, causes vitamin B_{12} deficiency on rare occasions, but that is a result of vitamin ingestion from the small intestinal lumen rather than a true malabsorption. The malaria parasite, *Plasmodium falciparum*, has been associated with intestinal abnormalities, including malabsorption, during the acute phase of the disease (Cook 1980), when severe diarrhoea may occur. In severe kala-azar (visceral leishmaniasis) the small intestine may also be heavily involved and malabsorption has been documented (Muigai *et al*. 1983).

Differential diagnosis of tropical malabsorption

Whenever overt clinical malabsorption is suspected in a tropical context (in indigenous and expatriate people in the tropics, or after tropical exposure) a number of conditions other than parasitic infection should be considered (Cook 1974, 1980). These are:

1 Chronic calcific pancreatitis.
2 Cirrhosis and other hepatic conditions.
3 Small intestinal lymphomas (including Mediterranean lymphoma).
4 Intestinal resection (following trauma, intussusception, etc.).
5 *Severe* malnutrition (Kwashiorkor).
6 Tropical sprue (Chapter 19).
7 Gluten-induced enteropathy.
8 Genetically determined hypolactasia.
9 Ileocaecal tuberculosis.

Sub-clinical malabsorption can result from systemic bacterial infections, folate deficiency and possibly *mild* malnutrition (Cook 1980).

In a developing tropical country it is frequently difficult to carry out adequate investigation of suspected malabsorption due to the paucity of laboratory amenities; the 5-h xylose excretion test, 72-h faecal fat examination and Schilling test of B_{12} absorption should, however, all be carried out if possible, as part of a basic screen.

Giardiasis

The flagellated protozoan *Giardia lamblia* is responsible for the most common human small intestinal parasitic infection in Britain. The trophozoite was first demonstrated in Delft in 1681 by van Leeuwenhoek while examining his own faeces microscopically. This organism has for long been recognized to be pathogenic to children — causing diarrhoea, failure to thrive and fretfulness. However, only recently has its importance in adult life been clearly demonstrated, despite the fact that in World War I (1914—18) good evidence was presented that it was closely associated with severe diarrhoea (Fantham 1916, Kennedy & Rosewarne 1916, Porter 1916). Historically it now seems possible that the entity described by Hillary in Barbados in 1759 (Booth 1964) was epidemic giardiasis. Similarly, hill diarrhoea (Grant 1854), a major menace in the hill stations of India, was perhaps giardiasis contracted from mountain stream water, now known to be an important source of infection.

There have been a number of major outbreaks among travellers during the past decade. In the early 1970s, 324 American tourists entered the Soviet Union and at an average of 14.5 days later, many developed acute symptoms (Brodsky et al. 1974). The untreated illness lasted a mean of 6.2 weeks. Infection was related to the drinking of tap water. There are also numerous reports from the USA. In 1965-66, 11% of skiers at Aspen, Colorado, were infected by well water (Moore et al. 1969); in 1972, 300 residents of Boulder, Colorado were infected; in 1974, 34 of 52 sociology students at Utah were infected by drinking from a contaminated stream; 6% of 1100 residents and visitors were also infected via the main water supply in New Hampshire (Brady & Wolfe 1974, Schultz 1975).

It seems to be especially common in sufferers from the acquired immunodeficiency syndrome (AIDS) (Pearce 1983), which might result from a mitogenic effect of the parasite on T-cell activity which predisposes to viral replication.

Clinical features

Classically, the disease most commonly presents acutely about 2 weeks after infection, with watery diarrhoea associated with excessive wind and passage of flatus (Wolfe 1978), followed by progressive weight loss. Growth retardation is prominent in some infected pre-school children (Gupta & Urrutia 1982). The severity of the clinical picture varies, however, from a sub-clinical one, to traveller's diarrhoea (Merson et al. 1976), to gross diarrhoea and malabsorption, followed by malnutrition and weight loss. Tiredness, lethargy and alcohol intolerance may be marked. Secondary lactose intolerance occurs. The condition is difficult to differentiate from tropical sprue, but it is more likely to be epidemic and in some cases there is very marked flatus. Giardiasis also tends to be more acute in its course and is sometimes more severe than tropical sprue. The following case history illustrates the features of giardiasis:

A 23-year-old English woman (HTD-TA 8579) presented in London, following an overland journey, from Australia, across Asia (Indonesia, Malaysia, Singapore, Thailand, Nepal, India, Pakistan and Iran). Whilst in Nepal she developed acute diarrhoea (eight stools daily) associated with excessive flatus; she was first seen 7 months later. By then she had two to eight pale, frothy, stools daily, had lost 16 kg over the previous 4 months, and was tired, clinically anaemic, and had a sore tongue. Investigations showed numerous *G. lamblia* trophozoites in the jejunal aspirate, but not in the stool. Haemoglobin was 10.2 g/dl and bone marrow showed megaloblastic erythropoiesis; serum folate was low, (1.9 ng)/ml and serum B_{12} was 165 pg/ml; whole body B_{12} absorption was less than 0.1% (normal > 20%) (Tomkins et al. 1978a). Jejunal biopsy showed an abnormal mucosa, with broad leaves and ridges; 5-h urine xylose after a 25 g load was 1.0 (normal range 8−16) mmol; stool weight ranged from 500−1500 g daily and faecal fat was 135 mmol/24 h. She was treated with oral metronidazole 2 g daily for 3 days and folic acid 5 mg three times daily for 3 months. She was also advised to avoid milk products. There was gradual improvement. Weight increased by 5 kg over the next 2 months, and diarrhoea by then had stopped. At 3 months after presentation, jejunal biopsy showed broad leaves only, and there were no *G. lamblia* trophozoites in the jejunal aspirate. Ultimate recovery was complete.

Parasitology

This has recently been reviewed by Ackers (1980), by Owen (1980a & b) and by the WHO (1981). The cysts are ingested and the trophozoites emerge in the duodenum and upper jejunum. Several members of the same household may be infected. It is more common in male homosexuals (Phillips et al 1981). It seems possible that infection may also be by inhalation (Schuman et al 1982). Infection from domestic animals is a further source, but its frequency is unknown (Lopez-Brea 1982). Following passage down the small intestine, the parasites encyst and are passed in the stool in the cystic form. Passage of cysts may be cyclical.

Trophozoites (Fig. 17.5a) can be identified in samples of jejunal fluid, jejunal biopsies or by the 'string test'. Clumps of mucus from the jejunum should be smeared on to a microscope slide and stained by the Giemsa method. Cysts (Fig. 17.5b) can easily be recognized in stool samples; cyst excretion is not a reliable indicator of the severity of infection (Olveda et al. 1982). It is important not to confuse the cysts with those of isospora and sarcocystis. A fluorescent antibody technique gives positive results *only* if malabsorption is currently present; it is positive in most patients with giardia *and* malabsorption, but negative in those without malabsorption (Moody et al. 1982). IgG antibodies to G. lamblia can be detected by an ELISA technique in a high percentage of affected individuals (Smith et al. 1981a). Morphological changes in murine giardiasis have been summarized by Ferguson et al. (1980).

Jejunal mucosa

In man, the jejunal mucosal changes vary from normality to gross villous blunting with ridging on dissecting microscopy; there is an inflammatory infiltrate with lymphocytes and plasma cells in the lamina propria. A flat mucosa, such as occurs in coeliac disease, is rare.

It seems probable that parasite rather than host factors are the major determinants of the severity of the initial mucosal damage and that host factors dominate the disease thereafter (Lancet 1982). A local antibody response to the parasite has been demonstrated (Briaud et al. 1981). An allograft type of reaction caused by hypersensitivity, in which T cells react vigorously to an antigen by releasing enteropathic lymphokines may be important (Mowat & Ferguson 1981). Abnormalities of absorption reflect the severity of the condition. Seventy-two-hour faecal weight gives a good indication of the severity of malabsorption.

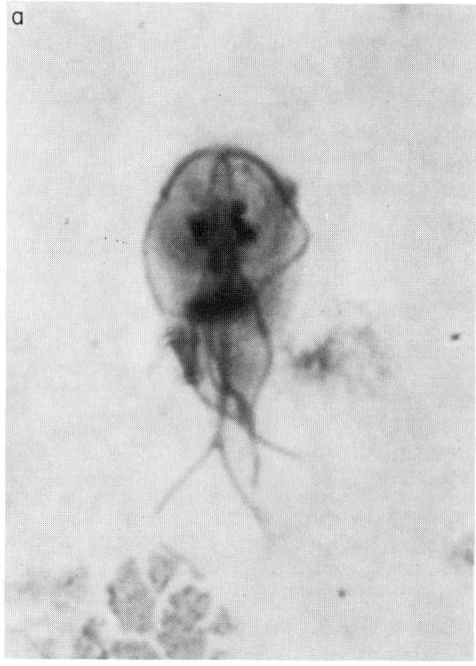

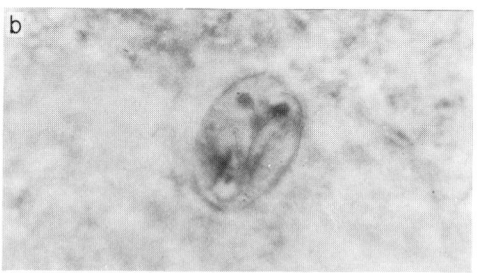

Fig. 17.5. (a) *Giardia lamblia*. Trophozoite of the flagellated protozoan in jejunal fluid. (b) *Giardia lamblia*. Cyst stage in faecal specimen.

Predisposing factors

The question as to why some infected individuals suffer *severe* symptoms and others run a sub-clinical course is unanswered; several possibilities have been advanced: the size of infecting dose, strain variability, and acquired immunity have all been suggested. There may be a genetic predisposition, for Roberts-Thomson et al. (1980) demonstrated a high frequency of infection in individuals with HLA A1 and B12. Immunosuppression may also increase the severity of infection (Nair et al. 1981), but immunological mechanisms probably play a relatively insignificant role in protection against giardiasis in man (Webster 1980). In mice, cortisone has been shown to increase the magnitude of infection and also to produce a recrudescence of an occult infection of G. muris (Nair et al. 1981). Depressed cellular immunity resulting from irradiation and thymectomy has also been shown to increase the intensity of infection with G. lamblia in mice (Vasudev et al. 1982). The only immunological abnormality in severely affected patients seems to be a low serum IgD concentration (Jokipii & Jokipii 1982a).

Treatment

Metronidazole ('Flagyl') is currently most widely used as an oral dose of 2 g daily on 3 consecutive days. Nausea and alcohol intolerance are significant side-effects; alcohol should therefore be forbidden during treatment. In chronic infections, metronidazole combined with mepacrine has given satisfactory results (Smith et al. 1982). Recently, tinidazole (2 g orally in a single dose) has given comparable results (Mendelson 1980). In a further study, tinidazole and ornidazole at a single 1.5 g dose gave an initial cure rate close to 100% in 100 infected patients (Jokipii & Jokipii 1982b). Nimorazole has also been used (WHO 1981). Alternatively, mepacrine (100 mg three times daily for 10 days by mouth) usually gives a satisfactory result.

Strongyloidiasis

There is no doubt that the nematode *Strongyloides stercoralis* can be associated with significant malabsorption, despite some conflicting reports. Invasion by larvae (Fig. 17.6a), either through intact skin or orally, initiates human infection. As with most other intestinal nematodes (see above), the life cycle is complex and pulmonary symptoms — cough, asthma, etc. may occur during migration through the lungs (Gill 1980). Adult worms are produced in the proximal small intestine where they burrow into the mucosa and submucosa, with production of an inflammatory infiltrate in the lamina propria. Ova are then produced (Fig. 17.6b). Infection can exist for 40 years or more, due to continuous auto-infection; larvae re-enter the body in the lower intestinal tract, including the anal region, thus initiating further migratory cycles which keep the infection extant. This has recently been documented in ex-prisoners of war from South-east Asia during World War II (1939—45). A high proportion (13% or more) still have an active infection (Gill & Bell 1982). Strongyloidiasis has also been shown to be a common infection in elderly men in the USA with chronic and debilitating illnesses from a low socio-economic background (Walzer et al. 1982).

Historically, a high incidence of infection was recognized in South-east Asia during the nineteenth century (Cook 1980) but its pathological significance was in doubt, largely because it was so common — involving up to 30% of the indigenous populations.

Clinical features have recently been reviewed (Milder et al. 1981). The onset of diarrhoea is insidious and much less spectacular compared with G. lamblia infections. Weight loss is also not usually so extreme. Urticaria and 'creeping eruption', with subcutaneous haemorrhage, may occur periodically during successive migratory phases. Heavy infections may also be asymptomatic and with no clinical signs (Shelhamer et al. 1982). An illustrative case history follows:

> A 71-year-old Englishman (HTD TD-4132) presented in London 2 weeks after a 35-day climbing expedition in Nepal. He had had several bouts of colic and diarrhoea which had settled on conservative treatment. For the previous week he had had severe diarrhoea — up to twelve fluid stools every 24 h — and his stools floated on water. Weight loss was approximately 9.5 kg. There had been no response to a course of metronidazole. There were no abnormalities on physical examination; he was afebrile. Investigations showed: total WBC 21.8 (16.4 eosinophils) $\times 10^9$/l; haemoglobin 14.9 g/dl; ESR 5 mm/1 h; stool-numerous larvae of strongyloides with no bacteriological abnormality; filarial serology > 1 : 512 and amoebic

serology negative. Serum B_{12} and folate normal. Five hour urinary xylose 5.0 (normal range 8.0–16.0) mmol; faecal fat 91 (normal range 11–18) mmol/24 h. He was treated with thiabendazole 1.5 g daily for 3 days; his symptoms rapidly subsided and he was symptomatically normal after a further week; 2 weeks later, body weight had increased by 3.3 kg and repeat investigations were normal.

Larvae can be demonstrated by the string test and less frequently in jejunal biopsy specimens. Ova and sometimes larvae also are found in the stool. Apart from absorption defects, there may be an eosinophilia, which is sometimes gross. Definitive diagnosis may be exceedingly difficult, in that both ova and larvae are very difficult to find. An IFAT gives a positive result in some 70% of cases; however, there is cross-reaction with all forms of filariasis. An ELISA test has given promising results (Carroll et al. 1981); a positive result was obtained in 84% of parasitologically proven cases of strongyloidiasis. In immunosuppressed patients the serological tests are often negative. In larva migrans, serology may be positive for strongyloidiasis, as well as for filariasis and toxocariasis. Recently, an immunofluorescent assay for strongyloides antibodies has also given satisfactory results (Grove & Blair 1981).

Hyperinfection syndrome

One very important complication of strongyloidiasis is disseminated or overwhelming infection in the presence of immunosuppression as associated with conditions such as renal transplantation or systemic lupus erythematosis (Hoy et al. 1981). Most organs of the body, including the lungs, may be involved and a significant mortality results. Response to treatment may be impaired and repeated courses may be necessary (Shelhamer et al. 1982).

The hyperinfection syndrome may also occur in the absence of immunosuppression. It is rare, but may affect an individual who has harboured strongyloides without any apparent ill effects for many years. The

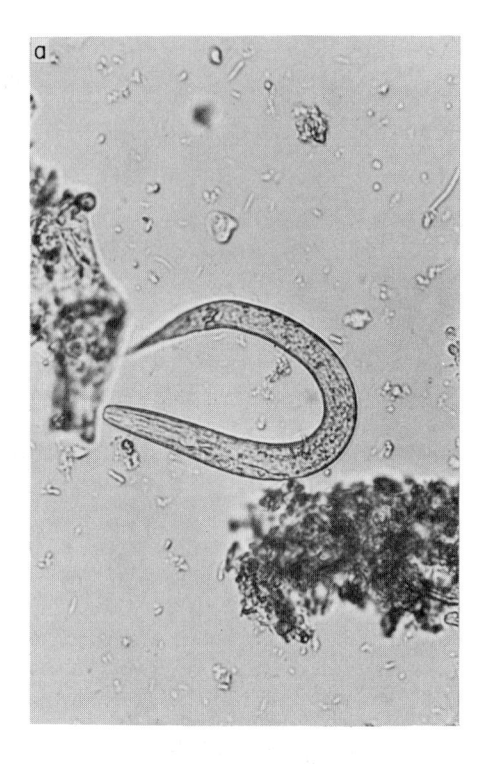

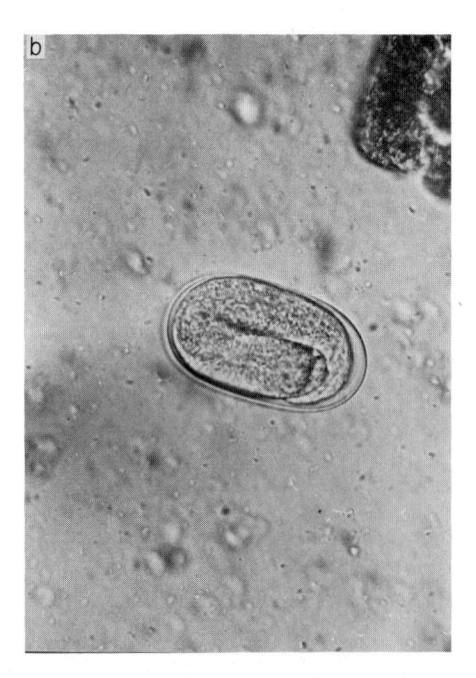

Fig. 17.6. *Strongyloides stercoralis*. Larval stage in jejunal fluid. (b) *Strongyloides stercoralis*. Mature ovum in faecal specimen.

patient may develop severe anorexia and there is frequently obstinate constipation and abdominal pain. The features at this stage may simulate subacute intestinal obstruction and such patients are frequently subjected to laparotomy with disastrous results. The diagnosis should be suspected in patients exposed to possible infection (for example, immigrants from the Caribbean living in Britain).

Diagnosis is often delayed when the presentation is not suggestive of parasitic disease. The condition may masquerade as a malabsorptive disorder associated with small intestinal obstruction (Walker-Smith et al. 1969, Toh & Chow 1969), or as an acute abdominal emergency. The migrating larvae may carry bacteria into the circulation causing septicaemia and meningitis (Brown & Perna 1958).

Strongyloides hyperinfection may be explosive in onset and can also occur many years after exposure to the parasite. If recognized, the condition usually responds well to treatment but a patient, seen at Hammersmith Hospital, recovered from hyperinfection and appeared completely well for 5 years. She then presented again with a rapidly progressive retroperitoneal (mixed histiocytic, lymphocytic) lymphoma and died within a few months. Her case history follows:

> K.T. came to London from Jamaica in 1956. In 1965 during the course of a normal pregnancy she was noted to have S. stercoralis ova in her stools. In 1973 she presented to the emergency team at Hammersmith Hospital with an acutely swollen abdomen associated with vomiting. The radiological appearances were those of a paralytic ileus. Strongyloides infection was diagnosed by biopsy of the duodenal mucosa and the patient responded dramatically to treatment with thiabendazole. On admission the circulating concentrations of proteins had been unremarkable considering the severity of the intestinal damage (Total protein 65 g/l, albumin 29, IgG 15.5, IgA 1.6 and IgM 0.4 g/l). Within 3 weeks the patient was perfectly well and there was a satisfactory rise in the protein levels. Only the concentration of IgG was increased above normal (21.5/100 ml).
> Five years later the patient returned to hospital with a history of weight loss and abdominal pain. On examination there was a mass in the left hypochondrium. At laparotomy there was diffuse retroperitoneal infiltration with a non-Hodgkin's lymphoma (histiocytic–lymphocytic). Initially the condition responded moderately well to chemotherapy but she died 6 months later.

Treatment

Treatment is with thiabendazole ('Mintezol') at a dose of 1.5 g b.d. on 3 successive days; nausea, drowsiness and vertigo may be troublesome. Clearance of infection is certainly not 100% (Grove 1982a). Repeated courses may be required, especially in the presence of an immunodeficiency state (Shelhamer et al. 1982). Mebendazole (100 mg b.d. for 4 days) is less effective; that agent has been shown to be of value in the disseminated hyperinfection syndrome, as has albendazole also (Rossignol & Maisonneuve 1983). In animal experiments, cambendazole seems to have significant advantages over thiabendazole and mebendazole (Grove 1982b). An ideal therapeutic agent is not yet available.

Other strongyloides species

In Zambia, and more recently in western Papua New Guinea, S. fuelleborni (a nematode previously thought to have originated in sub-human primates) has been implicated in a syndrome of severe malabsorption, stunting and 'pot belly' (Ashford et al. 1981); children are usually affected, and a significant mortality rate has been reported. Nippostrongylus brasiliensis infections in rats have provided a good experimental model for the study of human strongyloidiasis (Carter et al. 1981). Infections have been shown to be especially persistent in the presence of malnutrition (Tomkins et al. 1978b).

Capillaria philippinensis

Outbreaks of infection with this parasite have been recorded in the Luzon region of the northern Philippines and Thailand. It is common in areas where the human population eats raw freshwater fish (Cross & Basaca-Sevilla 1983); a fish−bird cycle is though to form an important reservoir for human infection. Onset is acute, with severe malabsorption, and significant mortality may occur. There may be an associated protein-losing enteropathy. Treatment is difficult but some success has been achieved with mebendazole, even in short-course regimes (Singson et al. 1975; 1977).

Cryptosporidiosis

Cryptosporidium is a coccidian parasite which infects many species of mammals, birds and reptiles; the disease is a zoonosis (Angus 1983). Although it has been known since 1970 that diarrhoea in calves (and less commonly lambs and piglets) can result from infection, awareness of its importance in man has lagged behind that amongst veterinarians. Experimental infection of lambs with human cryptosporidium has been reported; there was resultant diarrhoea (Tzipori et al. 1982). The life cycle is direct with faecal−oral transmission; it is probable that parasites infecting different animals belong to a single species. The organism attaches to the microvillous border of the enterocyte and colonocyte. Diagnosis is by demonstration in a faecal specimen — stained with Giemsa, modified Ziehl−Neelsen or dilute carbol fuchsin — or by a flotation technique; however, more sensitive methods give a higher yield of positive results (Baxby & Blundell 1983). Alternatively, the parasites can be demonstrated histologically in fresh necropsy or jejunal biopsy material, although the small ovoid organisms are easily missed; transmission to suckling mice is possible.

Cryptosporidiosis is clearly important in immunosuppressed individuals (Clinicopathological Conference, 1980, Sloper et al. 1982, Current et al. 1983, Schultz 1983) and in sufferers from the acquired immunodeficiency syndrome (AIDS) (Andreani et al. 1983, Jonas et al. 1983, Malebranche et al. 1983, Pape et al. 1983). It may also be an important cause of diarrhoea in children with measles in the developing world where there is depression of cellular immunity (DeMol et al. 1984). Recently it has been shown to occur frequently in normal children and adults (Casemore & Jackson 1983, Current et al. 1983, Ericsson & DuPont 1983, Jokipii et al. 1983), in whom a syndrome of mild fever, diarrhoea, abdominal pain, sweating and severe headache lasting up to several weeks has been reported. The illness, however, is self-limiting and contrasts with the severe prolonged diarrhoea in immunocompromised patients. Clinically, the disease cannot be distinguished from giardiasis, although its duration is usually shorter, and while abdominal pain and cramps are more common, bloating, anorexia and weakness are less so. A history of contact with calves is usual, although person-to-person transmission is possible. The overall role of the parasite in human diarrhoeal disease has not been adequately assessed. No specific therapy or chemoprophylaxis has yet been found effective.

Sarcocystosis and isosporiasis

The protozoan parasites *Sarcocystis hominis* (previously known as *Isospora hominis*) and *Isospora belli* occur in pockets throughout tropical countries. Infection is from undercooked pork and beef. Clear association with malabsorption has been demonstrated (Bunyaratvej et al. 1982). The organisms replicate within the enterocytes in a way comparable to that of plasmodia (the agents responsible for malaria) in red blood cells. Treatment is unsatisfactory but pyrimethamin+sulphadiazine and cotrimoxazole+nitrofurantoin have been used successfully.

Acknowledgement

I am most grateful to Mr C. James Webb FIST, London School of Hygiene and Tropical Medicine, for the photographs.

References

Ackers J.P. (1980) Giardiasis: basic pathology. *Trans. Roy. Soc. Trop. Med. Hyg.* **74**, 427–429.

Anderson R.M. & May R.M. (1982) Population dynamics of human helminth infections: control by chemotherapy. *Nature, (Lond.)* **297**, 557–563.

Andreani T., Midigliani R., Le Charpentier Y., Galian A., Brouet J.-C., Liance M., Lachance J.-R., Messing B. & Vernisse B. (1983) Acquired immunodeficiency with intestinal cryptosporidiosis: possible transmission by Haitian whole blood. *Lancet,* **i**, 1187–1191.

Angus K.W. (1983) Cryptosporidiosis in man, domestic animals and birds: a review. *J. Roy. Soc. Med.* **76**, 62–70.

Ashford R.W., Hall A.J. & Babona D (1981) Distribution and abundance of intestinal helminths in man in western Papua New Guinea with special reference to *Strongyloides. Ann. Trop. Med. Parasit.* **75**, 269–279.

Baxby D. & Blundell N. (1983) Sensitive, rapid, simple methods for detecting cryptosporidium in faeces. *Lancet,* **ii**, 1149.

Bellander B.T.D., Hagmar L.E. & Österdahl B.-G. (1981) Nitrosation of piperazine in the stomach. *Lancet,* **ii**, 372.

Blumenthal D.S. (1977) Intestinal nematodes in the U.S. *New Engl. J. Med.* **297**, 1437–1439.

Booth C.C. (1964) The first description of tropical sprue. *Gut,* **5**, 45–50.

Botero D. & Castaño S. (1982) Treatment of cysticercosis with praziquantel in Columbia. *Amer. J. Trop. Med. Hyg.* **31**, 811–821.

Brady P.G. & Wolfe J.C. (1974) Waterborne giardiasis. *Ann. Intern. Med.* **81**, 498–499.

Briaud M., Morichau-Beauchant M., Matuchanski C., Touchard G. & Babin P. (1981) Intestinal immune response in giardiasis. *Lancet,* **ii**, 358.

Brodsky R.E., Spencer H.C. & Schultz M.G. (1974) Giardiasis in American travelers to the Soviet Union. *J. Infect. Dis.* **130**, 319–323.

Brown H.W. & Perna V.P. (1958) An overwhelming Strongyloides infection. *J. Amer. Med. Ass.* **168**, 1648–1651.

Bunyaratvej S., Bunyawongwiroj P. & Nitiyanant P. (1982) Human intestinal sarcosporidiosis: report of six cases. *Amer. J. Trop. Med. Hyg.* **31**, 36–41.

Cabrera B.D. & Arambulo P.V. (1977) Studies on the epidemiology and transmission of human taeniasis in the Philippines — a paradoxical public health problem. *J. Philipp. Med. Ass.* **53**, 105–130.

Carroll S.M., Karthigasu K.T., & Grove D.I. (1981) Serodiagnosis of human strongyloidiasis by an enzyme-linked immunosorbent assay. *Trans. Roy. Soc. Trop. Med. Hyg.* **75**, 706–709.

Carter E.A., Bloch K.J., Cohen S., Isselbacher K.J. & Walker W.A. (1981) Use of hydrogen gas (H_2) analysis to assess intestinal absorption. Studies in normal rats and in rats infected with the nematode, *Nippostrongylus brasiliensis. Gastroenterol.* **81**, 1091–1097.

Casemore D.P. & Jackson B (1983) Sporadic cryptosporidiosis in children. *Lancet,* **ii**, 679.

Cello J.P. (1979) Eosinophilic gastroenteritis — a complex disease entity. *Amer. J. Med.* **67**, 1097–1104.

Cerf B.J., Rohde J.E. & Soesanto T. (1981) Ascaris and malnutrition in a Balinese village: a conditional relationship. *Trop. Geogr. Med.* **33**, 367–373.

Clinico-pathological Conference (1980) Immunodeficiency and cryptosporidiosis. *Brit. Med. J.* **281**, 1123–1127.

Cockburn A. (1981) Ancient parasites on the west-bank of the Nile. *Lancet,* **ii**, 938.

Cohen S. & Warren K.S. (1982) *Immunology of Parasitic Infections*, 2nd ed., pp. 848. Blackwell Scientific Publications, Oxford.

Cole T.J., Salem S.I., Hafez A.S., Galal O.M. & Massoud A. (1982) Plasma albumin, parasitic infection and pubertal development in Egyptian boys. *Trans. Roy. Soc. Trop. Med. Hyg.* **76**, 17–20.

Cook G.C. (1974) Malabsorption in Africa. *Trans. Roy. Soc. Trop. Med. Hyg.* **68**, 419–436.

Cook G.C. (1980) *Tropical Gastroenterology*, pp. 254–270, 271–278, 304–324. Oxford University Press, Oxford.

Corachan M., Oomen H.A.P.C. & Sutorius F.J.M. (1981) Parasitic duodenitis. *Trans. Roy. Soc. Trop. Med. Hyg.* **75**, 385–388.

Croll N.A., Anderson R.M., Gyorkos T.W. & Ghadirian E. (1982) The population biology and control of *Ascaris lumbricoides* in a rural community in Iran. *Trans. Roy. Soc. Trop. Med. Hyg.* **76**, 187–197.

Cross J.H. & Basaca-Sevilla V. (1983) Experimental transmission of *Capillaria philippinensis* to birds. *Trans. Roy. Soc. Trop. Med. Hyg.* **77**, 511–514.

Cruickshank J.K. & Mackenzie C. (1981) Immunodiagnosis in parasitic disease. *Brit. Med. J.* **283**, 1349–1350.

Current W.L., Reese N.C., Ernst J.V., Bailey W.S., Heyman M.B. & Weinstein W.M. (1983) Human cryptosporidiosis in immunocompetent and immunodeficient persons. Studies of an outbreak and experimental transmission. *New Engl. J. Med.* **308**, 1252–1257.

DeMol P., Mukashema S., Bogaerts J., Hemelhof W. & Butzler J.P. (1984). Cryptosporidium related to measles diarrhoea in Rwanda. *Lancet,* **ii**, 42–43.

Diwan A.R., Coker-Vann M., Brown P., Subianto D.B., Yolken R., Desowitz R., Escobar A., Gibbs C.J. & Gajdusek D.C. (1982) Enzyme-linked immunosorbent assay (ELISA) for the detection of antibody to cysticerci of *Taenia solium. Amer. J. Trop. Med. Hyg.* **31**, 364–369.

Ericsson C.D. & DuPont H.L. (1983) Cryptosporidium and diarrhoea. *Lancet*, **ii**, 914.

Fantham H.B. (1916) Remarks on the nature and distribution of the parasites observed in the stools of 1305 dysenteric patients. *Lancet*, **i**, 1165–1166.

Feldmeier H., Bienzle U., Döhring E. & Dietrich M. (1982) Flubendazole versus mebendazole in intestinal helminthic infections. *Acta trop.* **39**, 185–189.

Ferguson A., Gillon J. & al Thamery D. (1980) Intestinal abnormalities in murine giardiasis. *Trans. Roy. Soc. Trop. Med. Hyg.* **74**, 445–448.

Gill G.V. (1980) *Strongyloides* and asthma. *Trans. Roy. Soc. Trop. Med. Hyg.* **74**, 426.

Gill G.V. & Bell D.R. (1982) Long-standing tropical infections amongst former war prisoners of the Japanese. *Lancet*, **i**, 958–959.

Gilles H.M., Watson Williams E.J. & Ball P.A.J. (1964) Hookworm infection and anaemia. An epidemiological, clinical and laboratory study. *Quart. J. Med.* **33**, 1–24.

Gilman R.H., Mondal G., Maksud M., Alam K., Rutherford E., Gilman J.B. & Khan M.U. (1982) Endemic focus of *Fasciolopsis buski* infection in Bangladesh. *Amer. J. Trop. Med. Hyg.* **31**, 796–802.

Grant A. (1854) Remarks on hill diarrhoea and dysentery with brief notices of some of the Himalayan sanataria. *Indian Annals of Medical Science*, vol. 1, 2nd Ed. p. 311–348. R.C. Lepage & Co. Calcutta and London.

Greenberg B.L., Gilman R.H., Shapiro H., Gilman J.B., Mondal G., Maksud M., Khatoon H. & Chowdhury J. (1981) Single dose piperazine therapy for *Ascaris lumbricoides*: an unsuccessful method of promoting growth. *Amer. J. Clin. Nutr.* **34**, 2508–2516.

Griffin L., Okello G.B.A. & Pamba H.O. (1982) Mebendazole: a preliminary study comparing its efficacy against hookworm with pyrantel pamoate (Combantrin) and bephenium hydroxynaphthoate (Alcopar) in patients at Kenyatta National Hospital. *E. Afr. Med. J.* **59**, 214–219.

Groupe de travail scientifique de l 'OMS (1981) Diarrhées d'origine parasitaire. *Bull WHO*, **59**, 175–187.

Grove D.I. (1982a) Treatment of strongyloidiasis with thiabendazole: an analysis of toxicity and effectiveness. *Trans. Roy. Soc. Trop. Med. Hyg.* **76**, 114–118.

Grove D.I. (1982b) *Strongyloides ratti* and *S. stercoralis*: the effects of thiabendazole, mebendazole and cambendazole in infected mice. *Amer. J. Trop. Med. Hyg.* **31**, 469–476.

Grove D.I. & Blair A.J. (1981) Diagnosis of human strongyloidiasis by immunofluorescence, using *Strongyloides ratti* and *S. stercoralis* larvae. *Amer. J. Trop. Med. Hyg.* **30**, 344–349.

Gupta M.C. & Urrutia J.J. (1982) Effect of periodic antiascaris and antigiardia treatment on nutritional status of preschool children. *Amer. J. Clin. Nutr.* **36**, 79–86.

Hadidjaja P., Dahri H.M., Roesin R., Margono S.S., Djalins J. & Hanafiah M. (1982) First autochthonous case of *Fasciolopsis buski* infection in Indonesia. *Amer. J. Trop. Med. Hyg.* **31**, 1065.

Hall A. (1983) Dietary protein and the growth of rats infected with the tapeworm *Hymenolepis diminuta*. *Brit. J. Nutr.* **49**, 59–65.

Hoy W.E., Roberts N.J., Bryson M.F., Bowles C., Lee J.C.K., Rivero A.J. & Ritterson A.L. (1981) Transmission of strongyloidiasis by kidney transplant? Disseminated strongyloidiasis in both recipients of kidney allografts from a single cadaver donor. *J. Amer. Med. Ass.* **246**, 1937–1939.

Jeliffe E.F.P. & Jeliffe D.B. (1981) Ascariasis and malnutrition: a worm's eye view. *Amer. J. Clin. Nutr.* **34**, 1976–1977.

Jokipii A.M.M. & Jokipii L. (1982a) Serum IgG, IgA, IgM and IgD in giardiasis: the most severely ill patients have little IgD. *J. Infect.* **5**, 189–193.

Jokipii L. & Jokipii A.M.M. (1982b) Treatment of giardiasis: comparative evaluation of ornidazole and tinidazole as a single oral dose. *Gastroenterol.* **83**, 399–404.

Jokipii L., Pohjola S. & Jokipii A.M.M. (1983) Cryptosporidium: a frequent finding in patients with gastrointestinal symptoms. *Lancet*, **ii**, 358–361.

Jonas C., Deprez C., De Maubeuge J., Taelman H., Panzer J.M. & Deltenre M. (1983) Cryptosporidium in patients with aquired immunodeficiency syndrome. *Lancet*, **ii**, 964.

Joss V. & Brueton M.J. (1981) Unsuspected giardiasis. *Lancet*, **ii**, 996.

Kan S.P. (1983) The antihelmintic effects of flubendazole on *Trichuris trichiura* and *Ascaris lumbricoides*. *Trans. Roy. Soc. Trop. Med. Hyg.* **77**, 668–670.

Kan S.K.P., Kok R.T.C., Marto S., Thomas I. & Teo W.W. (1981) The first report of *Hymenolepis diminuta* infection in Sabah, Malaysia. *Trans. Roy. Soc. Trop. Med. Hyg.* **75**, 609.

Kennedy A.M. & Rosewarne D.D. (1916) *Lamblia intestinalis* infections from Gallipoli. *Lancet*, **i**, 1163–1165.

Lancet (1982) Battles against giardia in gut mucosa. *Lancet*, **ii**, 527–528.

Lloyd D.A. (1981) Massive hepatobiliary ascariasis in childhood. *Brit. J. Surg.* **68**, 468–473.

Lopez-Brea M. (1982) *Giardia lamblia*: incidence in man and dogs. *Trans. Roy. Soc. Trop. Med. Hyg.* **76**, 565.

Malebranche R., Arnoux E., Guérin J.M., Pierre G.D., Laroche A.C., Péan-Guichard C., Elie R., Morisset P.H., Spira T., Mandeville R., Drotman P., Seemayer T. & Dupuy J.-M. (1983) Aquired immunodeficiency syndrome with severe gastrointestinal manifestations in Haiti. *Lancet*, **ii**, 873–878.

Mendelson R.M. (1980) The treatment of giardiasis. *Trans. Roy. Soc. Trop. Med. Hyg.* **74**, 438–439.

Merson M.H., Morris G.K., Sack D.A., Wells J.G.,

Freeley J.C., Bradley Sack R., Creech W.B., Kapikian A.Z. & Gangarosa E.J. (1976) Travelers' diarrhoea in Mexico. A prospective study of physicians and family members attending a congress. *New Engl. J. Med.* **294**, 1299–1305.

Milder J.E., Walzer P.D., Kilgore G., Rutherford I. & Klein M. (1981) Clinical features of *Strongyloides stercoralis* infection in an endemic area of the United States. *Gastroenterol.* **80**, 1481–1488.

Moody A.H., Ridley D.S., Tomkins A.M. & Wright S.G. (1982) The specificity of serum antibodies to *Giardia lamblia* and to enterobacteria in gastrointestinal disease. *Trans. Roy. Soc. Trop. Med. Hyg.* **76**, 630–632.

Moore G.T., Cross W.M., McGuire D. Mollohan C.S., Gleason N.N., Healy G.R. & Newton L.H. (1969) Epidemic giardiasis at a ski resort. *New Engl. J. Med.* **281**, 402–407.

Mowat A.McI. & Ferguson A. (1981) Hypersensitivity reactions in the small intestine. 6. Pathogenesis of the graft-versus-host reaction in the small intestinal mucosa of the mouse. *Transplant.* **32**, 238–243.

Muigai R., Gatei D.G., Shaunak, S. Wozniak A. & Bryceson A.D.M. (1983) Jejunal function and pathology in visceral leishmaniasis. *Lancet*, **ii**, 476–479.

Murray M.J., Murray A.B., Murray M.B. & Murray C.J. (1978a) The adverse effect of iron repletion on the course of certain infections. *Brit. Med. J.* **ii**, 1113–1115.

Murray J., Murray A., Murray M. & Murray C. (1978b) The biological suppression of malaria: an ecological and nutritional interrelationship of a host and two parasites. *Amer. J. Clin. Nutr.* **31**, 1363–1366.

Nair K.V., Gillon J. & Ferguson A. (1981) Corticosteroid treatment increases parasite numbers in murine giardiasis. *Gut*, **22**, 475–480.

Ochola-Abila P. & Barrack S.M. (1982) Roundworm intestinal obstruction in children at Kenyatta National Hospital Nairobi. *E. Afr. Med. J.* **59**, 113–117.

Olveda R.K., Andrews J.S. & Hewlett E.L. (1982) Murine giardiasis: localization of trophozoites and small bowel histopathology during the course of infection. *Amer. J. Trop. Med. Hyg.* **31**, 60–66.

Owen R.L. (1980a) The ultrastructural basis of *Giardia*. *Trans. Roy. Soc. Trop. Med. Hyg.* **74**, 429–433.

Owen R.L. (1980b) The immune response in clinical and experimental giardiasis. *Trans. Roy. Soc. Trop. Med. Hyg.* **74**, 443–445.

Pape J.W., Liauthaud B., Thomas F., Mathurin J.-R., St Amand M.-M. A., Boncy M., Pean V., Pamphile M., Laroche A.C. & Johnson W.D. (1983) Characteristics of the aquired immunodeficiency syndrome (AIDS) in Haiti. *New Engl. J. Med.* **309**, 945–950.

Pearce R.B. (1983). Intestinal protozoal infections and AIDS. *Lancet*, **ii**, 51.

Pene P., Mojon M., Garin J.P., Coulaud J.P. & Rossignol J.F. (1982) Albendazole: a new broad spectrum anthelminthic. Double-blind multicenter clinical trial. *Amer. J. Trop. Med. Hyg.* **31**, 263–266.

Phillips S.C., Mildvan D., William D.C., Gelb A.M. & White M.C. (1981) Sexual transmission of enteric protozoa and helminths in a venereal-disease-clinic population. *New Engl. J. Med.* **305**, 603–606.

Porter A. (1916) An enumerative study of the cysts of giardia (lamblia) intestinalis in human dysenteric faeces. *Lancet*, **i**, 1166–1169.

Ray D.K. & Shrivastava V.B. (1981) The infectivity of ingested adult hookworms. *Trans. Roy. Soc. Trop. Med. Hyg.* **75**, 566–567.

Ridley M.J. & Ridley D.S. (1976) Serum antibodies and jejunal histology in giardiasis associated with malabsorption. *J. Clin. Path.* **29**, 30–34.

Roberts-Thomson I.C., Mitchell G.F., Anders R.F., Tait B.D., Kerlin P., Kerr-Grant A. & Cavanagh P. (1980) Genetic studies in human and murine giardiasis. *Gut*, **21**, 397–401.

Rossignol J.F. & Maisonneuve H. (1983) Albendazole: placebo-controlled study in 870 patients with intestinal helminthiasis. *Trans. Roy. Soc. Trop. Med. Hyg.* **77**, 707–711.

Schultz M.G. (1975) Giardiasis. *J. Amer. Med. Ass.* **233**, 1383–1384.

Schultz M.G. (1983) Emerging zoonoses. *New Engl. J. Med.* **308**, 1285–1286.

Schuman S.H., Arnold A.T. & Rowe J.R. (1982) Giardiasis by inhalation? *Lancet*, **i**, 53.

Shelhamer J.H., Neva F.A. & Finn D.R. (1982) Persistent strongyloidiasis in an immunodeficient patient. *Amer. J. Trop. Med. Hyg.* **31**, 746–751.

Singson C.N., Banzon T.C. & Cross J.H. (1975) Mebendazole in the treatment of intestinal capillariasis. *Amer. J. Trop. Med. Hyg.* **24**, 932–934.

Singson C.N., Banzon T.C. & Cross J.H. (1977) Short-term mebendazole treatment for Capillariasis Philippinensis. *J. Philippin. Med. Ass.* **53**, 31–33.

Sloper K.S., Dourmashkin R.R., Bird R.B., Slavin G. & Webster A.D.B. (1982) Chronic malabsorption due to cryptosporidiosis in a child with immunoglobulin deficiency. *Gut*, **23**, 80–82.

Smith P.D., Gillin F.D., Brown W.R. & Nash T.E. (1981a) IgG antibody to *Giardia lamblia* detected by enzyme-linked immunosorbent assay. *Gastroenterol.* **80**, 1476–1480.

Smith P.D., Horsburgh C.R. & Brown W.R. (1981b) In vitro studies on bile acid deconjugation and lipolysis inhibition by *Giardia lamblia*. *Dig. Dis. Sci.* **26**, 700–704.

Smith P.D., Gillin F.D., Spira W.M. & Nash T.E. (1982) Chronic giardiasis: studies on drug sensitivity, toxin production, and host immune response. *Gastroenterol.* **83**, 797–803.

Sorvillo F. & Ash L.R. (1982) Parasitic diseases in Karamoja, Uganda. *Lancet*, **i**, 912–913.

Sotelo J., Escobedo F., Rodriguez-Carbajal J., Torres B. & Rubio-Donnadiev F. (1984). Therapy of parenchymal brain cysticercosis with praziquantel. *New Engl. J. Med.* **310**, 1001–1007.

Spina-França A., Nobrega J.P.S., Livramento J.A. & Machado L.R. (1982) Administration of praziquantel in neurocysticercosis. *Tropenmed. Parasit.* **33**, 1–4.

Subianto D.B., Tumada L.R. & Margono S.S. (1978) Burns and epileptic fits associated with cysticercosis in mountain people of Irian Jaya. *Trop. Geogr. Med.* **30**, 275–278.

Thomas H., Andrews P. & Mehlhorn H. (1982) New results on the effect of praziquantel in experimental cysticercosis. *Amer. J. Trop. Med. Hyg.* **31**, 803–810.

Tjahjadi G., Subianto D.B., Endardjo S. & Margono S.S. (1978) Cysticercosis cerebri in Irian Jaya. A case report. *Trop. Geogr. Med.* **30**, 279–283.

Toh, C.C.S. & Chow, K.W. (1969) Malabsorption syndrome in a patient infected with *Strongyloides stercoralis*. *Ann. Trop. Med. Parasit.* **63**, 493–497.

Tomkins A.M., Smith T. & Wright S.G. (1978a) Assessment of early and delayed responses in vitamin B_{12} absorption during antibiotic therapy in tropical malabsorption. *Clin. Sci. Molec. Med.* **55**, 533–539.

Tomkins A.M., Wright S.G., Drasar B.S. & James W.P.T. (1978b) Bacterial colonisation of jejunal mucosa in giardiasis. *Trans. Roy. Soc. Trop. Med. Hyg.* **72**, 33–36.

Tomkins A.M., Madi K. & Ogilvie B.M. (1978b) Effect of marginal protein malnutrition on repeated nematode infection of the small intestine. *Proc. Nutr. Soc.* **37**, 10A.

Tzipori S., Angus K.W., Campbell I. & Gray E.W. (1982) Experimental infection of lambs with cryptosporidium isolated from a human patient with diarrhoea. *Gut*, **23**, 71–74.

Valdiserri R.O. (1981) Intestinal anisakiasis. Report of a case and recovery of larvae from market fish. *Amer. J. Clin. Path.* **76**, 329–333.

Vasudev V., Ganguly N.K., Anand B.S., Krishna V.R., Dilawari J.B. & Mahajan R.C. (1982) A study of *Giardia* infection in irradiated and thymectomized mice. *J. Trop. Med. Hyg.* **85**, 119–122.

Walker-Smith J.A., McMillan B., Middleton A.W., Robertson S. & Hopcroft A. (1969) Strongyloidiasis causing small bowel obstruction in an Aboriginal infant. *Med. J. Aust.* **2**, 1263–1265.

Walzer P.D., Milder J.E., Banwell J.G., Kilgore G., Klein M. & Parker R. (1982) Epidemiologic features of *Strongyloides stercoralis* infection in an epidemic area of the United States. *Amer. J. Trop. Med. Hyg.* **31**, 313–319.

Webster A.D.B. (1980) Giardiasis and immunodeficiency diseases. *Trans. Roy. Soc. Trop. Med. Hyg.* **74**, 440–443.

WHO (1981) Intestinal protozoan and helminthic infections. Report of a WHO Scientific group. *Techn. Rep. Ser.*, no. 666, pp. 150. WHO, Geneva.

Wolfe M.S. (1978) Giardiasis. *New Engl. J. Med.* **298**, 319–321.

Chapter 18
Effects of Nutritional Deficiency

DEVHUTI VYAS AND R.K. CHANDRA

Introduction 299
Protein–calorie malnutrition 299
Effects of deficiencies of other nutrients on
  the small intestine 307
Effects of intra-uterine growth retardation on
  the small intestine 308

Introduction

Malnutrition is common. It is estimated that more than 500 million people suffer from the ill-effects of protein-caloric malnutrition (PCM), a disease complex primarily of children in underdeveloped tropical and sub-tropical countries. Both kwashiorkor (syndrome of predominant protein deficiency) and marasmus (syndrome of predominant energy deficiency) are associated with high morbidity and mortality. In these conditions most organs are affected adversely either as a result of malnutrition itself or because of associated infection. Malabsorption of nutrients from the malnourished gastrointestinal tract may exacerbate PCM. Moreover the combination of structural damage to the gut and the impairment of immune competence caused by malnutrition may increase the risk of infection. As a result diarrhoeal illnesses are common.

Marginal undernutrition affects a large percentage of the world population even in affluent countries. Surveys suggest as many as 10–20% of the general population in North America have overt or latent deficiencies of various nutrients (Ten-State Survey, 1972; Nutrition Canada 1973), but little is known of the functional significance of such deficiencies. In this chapter we shall concentrate primarily on the effect of PCM on small intestinal structure and function. Even with this limited brief the available evidence regarding the effects of malnutrition on the small intestine is fragmentary and difficult to interpret.

Protein–calorie malnutrition

Morphology of the small intestine

The intestinal mucosa with its rapid turnover of epithelial cells may be profoundly affected by protein–calorie malnutrition (PCM). Pathological changes in intestinal structure are described both in experimental animals and in humans.

Animal studies

In animals the gross effects of malnutrition are best seen in protein-deficient weanling rats, themselves the offspring of mothers also fed a low protein diet. In such animals small intestinal length, wet weight, mucosal wet weight and wet weight/cm, and length ratio are all significantly reduced (Table 18.1). The small intestine is uniformly affected throughout its length and the mucosa is atrophic.

Changes in the small intestine of animals deprived of protein under alternative experimental conditions may be much less marked. Mucosal appearances vary from near normal (Prosper *et al.* 1968, Sriratanaban & Thayer 1971) to partial villous atrophy (Jambunathan *et al.* 1981). In adult rats, villi are usually shorter and patches of mucosa may be almost flat. Epithelial cells become cuboidal with centrally placed nuclei and thinner brush borders. Goblet cells decrease in number and Paneth cells show degranulation. The villus/crypt length ratio is reversed (it approximates 1:3 in the protein-deficient animal whereas it is 3:1 in well nourished and pair-fed controls). Mitotic indices are low. The muscular layer also shows atrophic changes (Takano, 1964).

Electron microscopy reveals defects in microvilli. They are less numerous, irregular

Table 18.1. Effect of protein deprivation on small intestinal size and villus height.

Group	Intestinal weight (g)	Intestinal length (cm)	Jejunal villus height (mm)
4% Protein diet	2.7±0.4	69.1±7.3	0.6±0.12
Pair-fed controls	5.5±0.6	85.0±6.1	0.9±0.11
21% Protein diet	7.1±0.5	98.0±4.2	1.1±0.06

Groups of 3-week-old weanling rats were given low protein or normal diet and killed after 28 days. Values are given as mean ± SE. Unpublished data of S. Prasad, S. Sharma and R.K. Chandra.

in length and diameter, damaged, blunt and disoriented. The terminal web is absent. Mitochondria of enterocytes show swelling, ribosomes are sparse and the protein matrix reveals lipoidal degeneration. Crypt cells show a decrease in RNA granules whereas the Golgi complex appears normal (Ramalingaswami 1964, Takano 1964).

In weanling rats protein deprivation causes less severe abnormalities. No change in crypt size has been reported, although mitoses are reduced in number. The villous height is reduced, epithelial cells reveal a slight excess of autophagic vacuoles but other ultra-structural lesions, such as fusion of villi, are generally not observed (Hill et al. 1968).

Deo & Ramalingaswami (1965) have shown reduced cell proliferation in the intestine of the protein malnourished Rhesus monkey. They observed that the S-phase of the cell cycle of crypt cells is elongated and that this leads to an increase in labelling index (with ^{3}H-thymidine) in the crypts. Moreover, the time required by cells to reach the tip of the villus increases, so that epithelial cells survive longer. Similarly, Hopper et al. (1972) have shown that in protein-depleted animals the migration time required by crypt cells to appear on the villus is longer than in control animals. Increased migration time and decreased cellular proliferation may be an adaptation to protein deficiency but at the same time it may allow mucosal damage by delaying repair after injury.

Changes in the small intestine of protein-malnourished humans

In both children and adults with protein malnutrition radiological studies of the small intestine show variable abnormalities such as thickened folds with a coarse mucosal pattern, segmentation of contrast medium and decreased transit time. These changes revert to normal after nutritional rehabilitation (Mayoral et al. 1972).

The histological appearances of the small intestinal mucosa of the protein-malnourished vary considerably. New cells formed in the mucosal crypts move up from the base of the villus to the tip and are continuously shed off into the lumen of the bowel. This continuous wear and tear requires nucleic acid synthesis. In malnutrition when the supply of nutrients is limited, it is logical to expect that an energy-requiring process like cellular proliferation would be hampered. The mitotic index in the intestine of marasmic children is reduced (Brunser et al. 1968) rather surprisingly to a greater degree than that described in kwashiorkor. It is difficult to be dogmatic regarding the significance of some of the findings because in most cases subjects are suffering from more than one condition. Often the intestine itself has an associated pathology such as parasitic infestation, bacterial overgrowth or enteric viral infection. Thus the changes are rarely due to uncomplicated protein–calorie malnutrition.

Mucosal appearances in adults

In protein malnutrition epithelial cell height is decreased, the cytoplasm is increased and the nuclei are arranged irregularly. The lamina propria is infiltrated with mononuclear cells and the basement membrane is thickened. In contrast to rather characteristic changes in villous morphology, the crypts do not show a uniform appearance. In some cases they appear atrophic, in others they are clearly normal or hyperplastic (Duque et al. 1975). Of nine patients studied, histological abnormalities of the mucosa of the small intestine were moderate in one and slight in eight. The mean villus height was 248 μ (range 182–326 μ), mean crypt depth 141 μ (range 86–199 μ), and total mucosal thickness 418 μ (range 309–587 μ).

Under the electron microscope the enterocyte from the protein-malnourished adult shows only minor abnormalities. Microvilli are fewer, shorter and deformed with branching or fusion. Lysosomal bodies are often increased but other ultracellular structures (such as tight junctions, mitochondria, endoplasmic reticulum, Golgi apparatus and nuclei) look normal. The subepithelial region shows a finely granular material with increased density of collagen (Mayoral *et al.* 1972, Duque *et al.* 1975).

Mucosal appearances in infants and children

In *marasmus* the histological appearances of the small intestine are very similar to those in the protein-malnourished adult. The epithelial cell height is decreased, the cytoplasm is basophilic, the nuclei irregularly arranged, the brush border is thinned, the basement membrane thickened and there are more lymphocytes and plasma cells in the lamina propria (Fig. 18.1a) (Chandra 1979a), but the changes are patchy and biopsy appearances may be normal or show only minor changes (Fig. 18.1b). In two separate studies, Brunser and his colleagues (1968, 1976) reported that out of eighteen marasmic infants, one had a flat mucosa with few and short villi, four had short and broad villi in some areas only, whereas the remaining thirteen had mucosal biopsies which appeared normal. In their second investigation of seven marasmic children four had a relatively normal mucosal structure, whereas in three there were minor changes as described above. In another study of seven marasmic patients, three had normal-sized villi and four had partial villous atrophy (Campos *et al.* 1979). A thickened basement membrane was the only consistent abnormality in all patients.

Under the electron microscope the microvilli show irregularities including a decreased length, an increased width, branched microvilli, and occasionally loss of the glycocalyx. Epithelial cells show nuclear irregularity and increased cell extrusion. Sometimes, they detach themselves from adjacent cells and protrude into the lumen of the bowel. Supranuclear regions show large autophagosomes containing various cellular organelles (Fig. 18.2). Mitochondria degenerate with a swollen appearance and ruptured membranes. Residual bodies appear in the cytoplasm. The terminal web is reduced and invaded by organelles. On the other hand undifferentiated epithelial cells, Paneth cells and goblet cells appear morphologically normal. The density of connective tissue fibrils increases with deposition of collagen (Fig. 18.3) associated with fine fat droplets. The epithelial cells of the crypt show degenerative changes with few autophagosomes

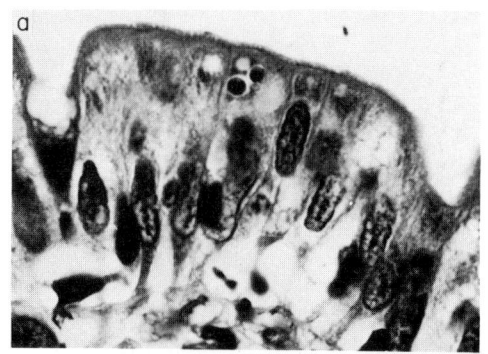

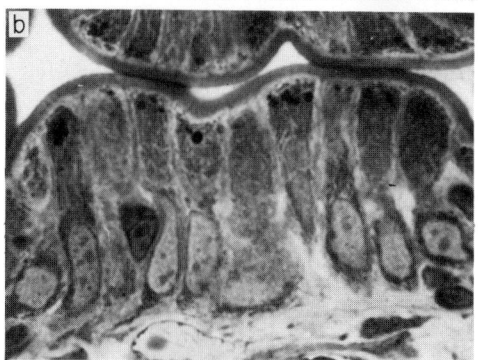

Fig. 18.1. Marasmus. (a) Moderately damaged absorptive epithelium from the middle third of a villus. The brush border is somewhat sparse; nuclei are distributed in a disorderly fashion. The supranuclear cytoplasm of some cells contains dense bodies and vacuoles (paraffin, H & E, × 1200). (b) In this specimen, the structure of the absorptive epithelium is well preserved. Almost every cell has one or more dark staining bodies in the apical cytoplasm, some being more than 1 μm in diameter (Epon, methylene azure II, × 1200). (Courtesy of Professor O. Brunser.)

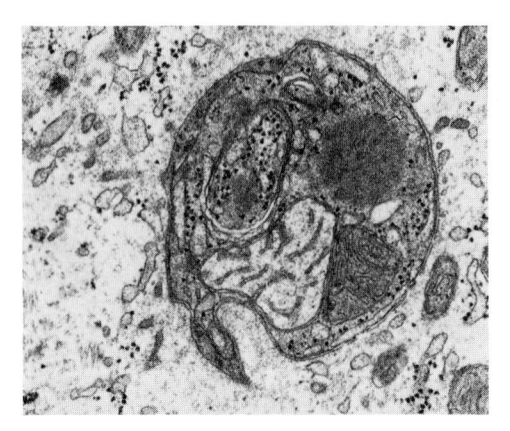

Fig. 18.2. Large autophagosome in the supranuclear cytoplasm of an absorptive cell. It is surrounded by a double membrane and contains mitochondria in various stages of degradation, cisternae of the endoplasmic reticulum, ribosomes, and vacuoles (× 36,000). (From Brunser et al. 1976.)

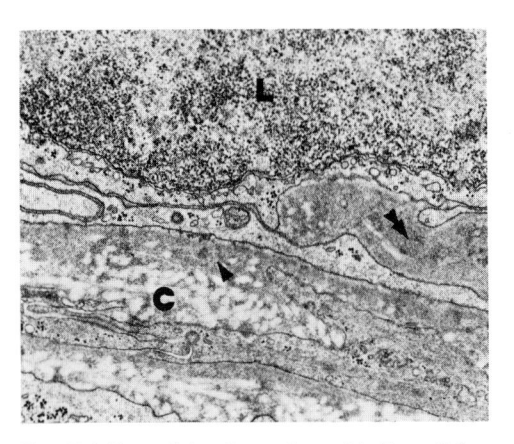

Fig. 18.3. Base of the absorptive epithelium. Below the basement lamella, there are deposits of collagen (C) and dense, finely granular material (▶). Some material with the same characteristics is present in the intercellular space of the epithelium (▶▶) between the lymphocyte (L) and the foot processes of the absorptive cells (×26,000). (Courtesy of Professor O. Brunser.)

and residual bodies. The B lymphocytes of the mucosa are abnormal with collapsed cisternae of the endoplasmic reticulum, indicating reduced or absent synthesis of proteins (presumably immunoglobulins) (Brunser et al. 1976, Campos et al. 1979; Chandra, 1979a).

In *kwashiorkor* the pathological lesions in the small intestine are much more severe than in marasmus. The extent of abnormality is variable but appearances are rarely normal. In the occasional severely affected intestine the mucosa is flat; in the moderate lesion there are some areas with broad and short villi and some flat areas without villi (Figs. 18.4). Crypts appear coiled with a relative increase in length. Crypt cells appear normal but have a lower than normal mitotic index which, however, is higher than that seen in marasmic infants. The lamina propria shows large numbers of lymphocytes, plasma cells and polymorphs, indicating the frequent prevalence of concomitant infection.

Under the electron microscope the surface epithelium of the small intestine from the child with kwashiorkor shows extensive damage although there is relative sparing of crypt cells (Chandra 1979). There is a marked reduction in free ribosomes and in smooth and rough endoplasmic reticulum. Membrane-bound lipid bodies are increased and dispersed throughout the cytoplasm, including the endoplasmic reticulum, the Golgi apparatus, the intercellular spaces, and the lamina propria. Fat accumulates in the intestinal mucosa in a manner analogous to that in the liver (Chandra, 1979c). The hepatic synthesis of β-lipoproteins is decreased. This results in an excessive deposit of neutral fat, which is rapidly remobilized when nutritional supplementation accelerates the production of β-lipoproteins. The similarity of the histochemical lesions in kwashiorkor and in inherited abetalipoproteinaemia lends further support to this concept.

Intestinal physiology in protein calorie malnutrition

The extent of the functional defects of the small intestine associated with the structural changes of PCM is variable although abnormal small bowel function is usual in severely undernourished patients, especially children. Diarrhoea, lactose intolerance and steatorrhea are common.

Absorption of carbohydrate

Human studies: In adults, severe protein

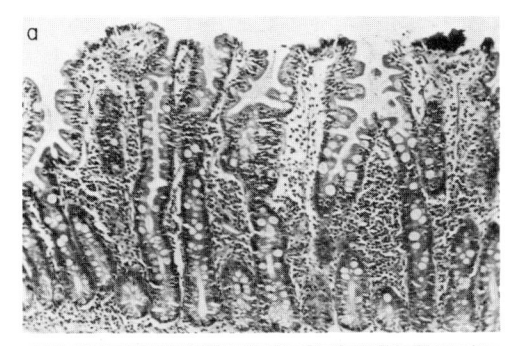

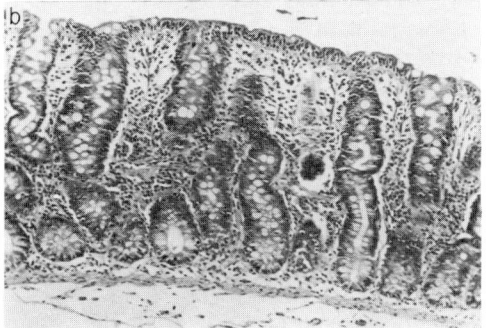

Fig. 18.4. Jejunal mucosa in healthy (a), and undernourished children (b). The variability in structural changes is illustrated. Villi are shorter and blunt. There is mononuclear cell infiltration (H & E × 60).

Table 18.2. Disaccharidase activities of jejunal mucosa (μmoles disaccharide hydrolysed/min at 37°C/g wet weight of mucosa) from malnourished (M) and recovered children (R) grouped according to clinical diagnosis on admission.

	Marasmic		Marasmic-kwashiorkor and Kwashiorkor	
	M (8)	R (6)	M (9)	R (9)
Lactase	4.1±1.4*	5.1±1.1	1.5±0.4	2.6±0.6
Sucrase	5.2±1.1	9.4±2.4	3.6±0.9	8.9±1.8
Maltase	22.0±4.4	29.6±11.0	12.2±3.5	29.3±7.0

*Means ± SEM. Figures in brackets indicate number in each group. (From James (1971b).)

malnutrition is associated with defective D-xylose absorption (Mayoral et al. 1972). In children with severe PCM the absorption of glucose and other monosaccharides is decreased along with that of D-xylose (Bowie et al. 1967, Chandra et al. 1968).

Disaccharide malabsorption almost always accompanies malnutrition in children. Disaccharidase activities are reduced especially in kwashiorkor (Table 18.2) (Chandra et al. 1968, James 1971a). Lactose intolerance during infancy, when milk is the major food consumed, may result in diarrhoea (Chandra et al. 1968, Bilir 1972), although small quantities of lactose and other disaccharides are often well tolerated. In breast-fed infants, the presence of mild–moderate lactose malabsorption is not a contra-indication to continuing breast-feeding.

Animal studies: The results of animal studies are variable possibly because of the differences in experimental protocols and other confounding factors. In most studies of malnourished adult, weanling or suckling rats, the specific activities of mucosal disaccharidases are either unchanged or increased (Prosper et al. 1968, Solimano et al. 1967, Adams & Leichter 1973, Kumar et al. 1971, Jambunathan et al. 1981). In these studies rats were usually given a low or protein-free diet *ad libitum* with added sucrose. Thus, the food was deficient in protein but rich in carbohydrates. Unlike underprivileged malnourished children the animals were not deprived of food. Moreover the experiments were of short duration in contrast to the prolonged deprivation of food in subjects with PCM. Jambunathan et al. (1981) studied rats given a diet containing 6% protein and 61% sucrose. Similarly Prosper et al. (1968) used protein-deprived rats fed a diet containing 70% corn starch. In another study (Lifshitz et al. 1972), animals were given a low protein or a low protein-low carbohydrate diet with non-nutritive cellulose making up the difference. The specific activities of intestinal disaccharidases were not altered and the transport rates of sucrose, maltose and glucose did not change after an experiment lasting 28 days. In contrast to this, when the rats were deprived nutritionally by allowing large litters and limiting the total amount of food available (Hatch et al. 1979), specific activities for sucrase and maltase were lower but that of lactase was increased.

Nevertheless in all studies the wet weight of the intestine as a whole decreased and if disaccharidase activity is calculated as total activity per organ instead of activity per g protein or per unit wet weight of intestine there is a striking reduction. It is possible that the amount of available enzyme becomes rate-limiting with respect to the digestion and absorption of disaccharides although the healthy animal appears to have a considerable reserve.

Absorption of nitrogen

Pancreatic enzymes are reduced in PCM (Barbezat & Hansen 1977, Thompson & Trowell 1952), and various mucosal dipeptidases are also decreased in adults, in children and in laboratory animals (Solimano et al. 1967, Kumar & Chase 1971, Kumar et al. 1971, Hazuria et al. 1974, Gjessing et al. 1977). In addition the absorption of amino acids such as threonine and leucine is reduced in starvation. Even an isocaloric protein-free diet alters the absorption of essential amino acids. At low concentration (5 mM) there is no significant difference from controls but as the concentration increases to 10, 15 and 20 mM absorption is impaired (Adibi & Allen 1970). In rats the transport of lysine decreases, that of phenylalanine and glycine remains unaltered, whereas that of tyrosine increases (Wapnir & Lifshitz 1974). A low protein diet for a relatively short period of time, 7–9 days, has been shown to increase the rate of transport of L-histidine in the intestine of the rat and the guinea-pig whereas no change was observed in the transport by the intestine of the golden hamster (Kreshaw et al. 1960, Hindmarsh et al. 1967, Nakamura et al. 1972).

The increased rate of absorption of amino acids after dietary protein deprivation may be an adaptive mechanism which can be maintained for short periods. In contrast to the activities of the disaccharidases protein deprivation always leads to reduced activities of the mucosal dipeptidases. This may be an adaptive phenomenon with disaccharidase activities maintained by enzyme induction.

Fat absorption

Children with marasmus may have steatorrhoea (Chandra et al. 1968). In one study average fat absorption was only 80% in malnourished children (Holemans & Lambrechts 1977). Absorption of dietary lipids requires normal pancreatic, hepatic and small intestinal functions. Pancreatic insufficiency and decreased levels of conjugated bile acids may impair the micellar solubilization of fat and reduce lipid absorption in the malnourished (Underwood et al. 1967, Schneider & Viteri 1974). The total activity of mucosal fatty acid CoA lipase and acyl CoA monoglyceride acyltransferase were reduced in the intestine of rats fed a protein-deficient diet for 4 days, whereas the specific activities of both enzymes were unchanged from those of the intestine of control rats. Although triglyceride appeared to be absorbed normally up to 8 hours, total ^{14}C-oleic acid absorption was found to be low in the protein-deficient rat (Rodgers 1970).

B_{12} absorption

Vitamin B_{12} absorption is impaired in protein-deficient monkeys (Ramalingaswami 1964).

Water and electrolyte fluxes

The transport of Na, K, Ca, Mg, P, Cu, Zn, Mn and Cr has been shown to be normal in kwashiorkor (McCance et al. 1970). On the other hand, osmotic stress from unabsorbed nutrients (especially sugars) increases adenyl cyclase and C-AMP levels without changes in mucosal phosphodiesterase, Na^+, K^+-ATPase and GPT. Water and sodium cross the intestinal mucosa (Lifshitz et al. 1981) in sufficient quantities to cause diarrhoea (James 1970).

Effect of PCM on intestinal development in the peri-natal period

There are comparatively few data on the intestinal response to immediate post-natal malnutrition. There are distinct and characteristic developmental changes in small intestinal structure, enzyme activity and function in the perinatal period. There is an increase in intestinal weight which parallels the increase in body weight. In developing rodents, new enzymes appear in clusters dur-

Table 18.3. Size of tonsils.

Group	No. of children	Barely visible	Visible but not enlarged	Enlarged beyond faucial arch	Massive Enlargement
Healthy	100	11	55	25	9
Malnourished	90	47	37	4	2

From Chandra (1972).

Table 18.4. Number,* by immunologic class, of plasma cells (mean ± SD) in the jejunal mucosa.

	IgA	IgM	IgG
Malnourished persons	52±15 (57±16)	31±10 (33±11)	9±3 (10±3)
Well-nourished persons	91±17 (80±15)	19±5 (18±4)	4±2 (4±2)

*Number of cells per tissue segment of 6 × 500 µm. Figures in parentheses are percentages of all plasma cells. From Chandra (1979b).

ing the late fetal, neonatal and late suckling periods in a pattern suggestive of a pre-programmed developmental clock mechanism (Hatch et al. 1979). Changes in litter size have been used to study the effect of undernutrition on the neo-natal rat small intestine. The DNA and protein content expressed per gram wet tissue were unchanged although intestinal weight and total DNA were reduced. The mean specific activities of sucrase and maltase were reduced to 20 and 50% of control values respectively and although the specific activity of lactase was increased the total lactase activity per organ was unchanged. The specific activity and total organ activity of enterokinase were significantly higher in the undernourished group. These findings may be important in relation to perinatal nutritional problems in man.

The immunology of protein−calorie malnutrition

Protein−calorie malnutrition makes the host susceptible to GI tract and systemic infections by compromising various host defence mechanisms. The important effects of PCM on mucosal immunity have been reviewed elsewhere (Chandra 1980, 1983a, b). In PCM the gut-associated lymphoid tissues atrophy (Chandra 1980). The small size of tonsils may be a useful clinical sign of these changes (Table 18.3). Rosette-forming lymphocytes, intraepithelial lymphocytes, SIgA-bearing B cells and IgA plasma cells are reduced in the intestinal mucosa (Table 18.4). In PCM, secretory IgA levels are low (Table 18.5) (Chandra 1975a, Sirinsiha et al. 1975, Reddy et al. 1976). Both IgA production and the amount of available secretory component may be affected. After antigenic challenge, the secretion of IgA antibody to poliovirus and measles vaccines is lower in malnourished children (Fig. 18.5) (Chandra 1975). SIgA is a dimeric molecule and may adhere to the epithelial surface in the glycocalyx, thereby blocking the capacity of pathogens to attach and stimulate the metabolic processes which cause diarrhoea. Micro-organisms more easily colonize the gut if there is IgA deficiency. A reduced number of IgA-bearing cells, inactive plasma cells, a reduced glycocalyx, and injured epithelium with a lower capacity for repair, may favour not only bacterial colonization of the small intestine but also penetration of pathogens and antigen through the wall of the gut. Macromolecular absorption is increased (Fig. 18.6), and may result in production of food antibodies (Chandra 1975b). Immunologic effector mechanisms may be activated according to the immunoglobin antibody isotype thereby producing clinical manifestations. A high concentration of deconjugated bile acids in PCM can also injure the gut wall and increase the permeability of the intestine to macromolecules as shown by the augmented uptake of horse-radish peroxidase by the epithelial cells of PCM rats (Teichberg et al. 1981). The injurious effects of bile acids are further aggravated by a decreased mitotic

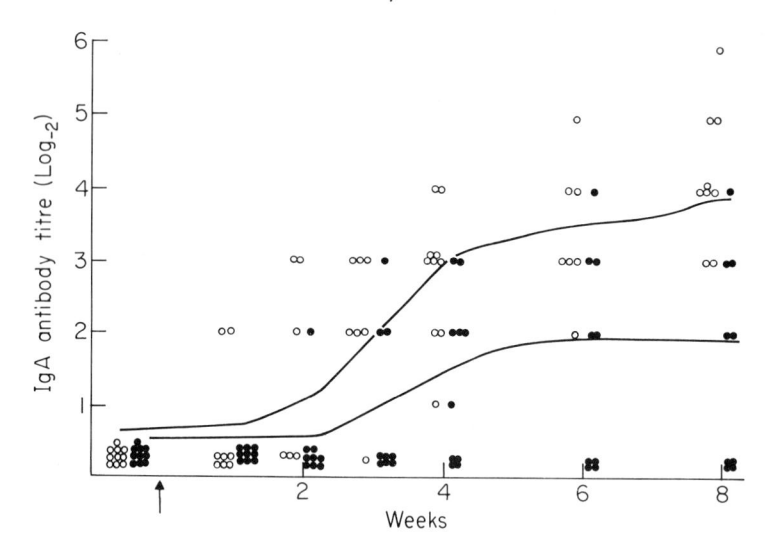

Fig. 18.5. Secretory IgA antibody response to live attenuated poliovirus vaccine in healthy (O) and in malnourished (●) children. The two lines represent mean values. (From Chandra 1975a.)

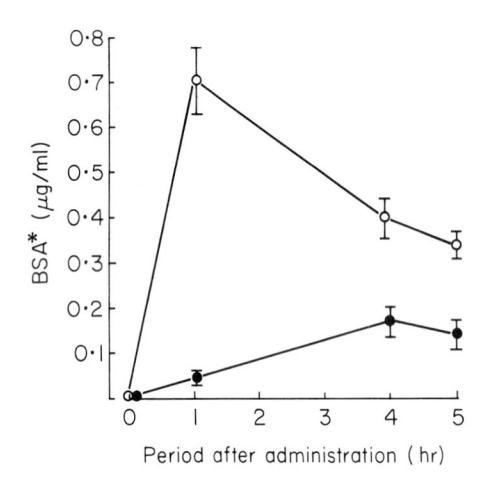

Fig. 18.6. Absorption of radiolabelled bovine serum albumin (BSA) in the gut of protein-deficient (O) and control (●) rats. One milligram of BSA was given by gavage and the blood levels measured periodically for 5 h.

index and an increased transit time of epithelial cells. Infectious agents may be helped not only by an increased gut permeability but also by a reduced rate of epithelial exfoliation, which will favour local colonization.

Gut microflora in protein–calorie malnutrition

The number and type of micro-organisms colonizing the small intestine and their sites of residence are altered in protein–calorie malnutrition (Mata et al. 1972, Gracey et al. 1973). Aspirates from the duodenum and jejunum of many malnourished children often show bacterial contamination. It has been suggested that bacterial colonization of the upper gastrointestinal tract may contribute to the high prevalence of gastroenteritis and malabsorption. 'Weanling diarrhoea' may be the result of synergism between malnutrition and infection. Bacteria in the jejunum may aggravate nutritional deficiency by deaminating and degrading bile salts thereby causing steatorrhoea. The interpretation of observations on luminal bacteria is difficult, however, since there are few control data on well-nourished children living in the same ecologic environment. Critical evaluation of the reported literature suggests that bacterial colonization of the upper gut correlates more with the microbiologic environment than with the nutritional status of the individual. There is a need for defining the precise relationship between the intestinal microflora and the immuno-

Table 18.5. Levels of total proteins, albumin and secretory IgA in nasopharyngeal secretions*.

	Total proteins (g/l)	Albumin (g/l)	SIgA (g/l)
Malnourished	0.887±0.098	0.121±0.016	0.156±0.019
Healthy	1.078±0.163	0.152±0.027	0.281±0.027

*Values are expressed as mean ±SD. From Chandra (1975a).

logic integrity of the gut.

Intestinal parasites are often found in association with PCM. This may be both the cause and effect of nutritional deficiencies. Small intestinal mucosal biopsies obtained from children with PCM often reveal unsuspected Giardia infection. The interrelationships between nutrition, immunity and parasites has been reviewed recently (Chandra 1982).

Recovery from protein–calorie malnutrition

Structural and functional anomalies observed during PCM are not specific. Similar structural alterations are also encountered in coeliac disease and in tropical sprue. After nutritional rehabilitation, clinical recovery is usually fast but changes in the small intestine may persist. Cook & Lee (1966) reported a complete recovery of intestinal structure in children 5.5 years after treatment for kwashiorkor. The level of lactase activity, however, remained depressed. Similarly Bowie et al. (1967) showed that of five children treated for PCM only one regained a normal tolerance for lactose, three showed slight improvement and in the other the defect persisted. In other studies, sucrase, maltase and lactase activity rose significantly after 3 months of treatment (James, 1971) and normal absorption of disaccharides has been found after a few weeks of therapy (Chandra et al. 1968). The mucosal thickness, villus height and dipeptide hydrolase activity did not return to normal after 6–150 days of dietary treatment of protein-malnourished adults (Gjessing et al. 1977). During nutritional treatment, absorption of nitrogen, D-xylose and vitamin A palmitate recovers first whereas absorption of vitamin B_{12} and fat improves more slowly (Viteri et al. 1973).

In experiments using protein-deficient rats which were then fed the normal diet for 22 days, Solimano et al. (1967) found either normal or higher than normal activities of lactase, maltase, sucrase and dipeptidases.

Effects of deficiencies of other nutrients on the small intestine

Deficiencies of nutrients other than protein and calories have been reported to impair the structure and function of the small intestine.

Vitamin B_{12}

Deficiency of vitamin B_{12} causes megaloblastic and megalocytic changes in the epithelial cells. Nuclei become hyperchromatic. The intestine of patients with untreated pernicious anaemia shows shorter villi and reduced mucosal thickness. The number of mitoses is reduced and the lamina propria is infiltrated with plasma cells and lymphocytes (Foroozan & Trier 1967).

Iron

In man, iron deficiency is associated with a variety of clinical manifestations pertaining to the GI tract (Vyas & Chandra 1983). These may be both the cause and the effect of iron deficiency. Buccal and oesophageal mucosae show epithelial metaplasia and a reduced content of cytochrome and other enzymes. Hypochlorhydria is common. The extent of villous change in the jejunum varies from mild to moderate. Faecal occult blood is detected more often in iron-deficient subjects than in controls. There is a higher incidence of beeturia but the functional significance of this observation is not clear. The small intestinal mucosa of iron-deficient rats or puppies does not show changes under the light microscope but disaccharidase activities are reduced (Hoffbrand & Broitman 1969, Sriratanaban & Thayer 1971).

Vitamin A

Vitamin A deficiency is reported to reduce the number and differentiation of goblet cells and to affect protein synthesis and proliferation of mucosal cells (DeLuca et al. 1969, Zile et al. 1977, Rojanapo et al. 1980, Olson et al. 1981). The functional significance of these findings requires further study.

Effects of intra-uterine growth retardation (IUGR) on the small intestine

Maternal deficiency of protein, zinc, pyridoxine and other nutrients during gestation results in low birth weight with a high mortality rate. Intra-uterine protein deprivation causes a reduction in the height and number of villi and also decreases the length and diameter of the intestine. Villi in IUGR pups are less numerous, inter-villus space is much wider and short bud-like villiform projections without connective tissue core are more frequent (Younoszai & Ranshaw 1973). Epithelial cells are columnar with vesicular cytoplasm and oval nuclei. Crypt cells are indistinguishable from the cells lining the villi. Moreover, levels of thymidine kinase and rate of epithelial cell migration and incorporation of ^{3}H-thymidine diminish in protein deprivation (Guiraldes & Hamilton 1981). Microvilli are present only in the apical cells of the villi. Goblet cells are fewer in number (Shrader & Zeman 1969, Loh et al. 1971, Shrader et al. 1977). The amount of DNA per cm length of intestine is less in IUGR pups (Guiraldes & Hamilton 1981) which is indicative of reduced cellularity. The number of epithelial cells is less which directly affects the absorptive process for protein and fat. In some studies the cellular uptake and transport of fatty acids appears to be different between IUGR and control pups but overall absorption is reduced because there are fewer cells (Zeman & Fratzke, 1976). Disaccharidase specific activities are similar to controls but the total activity is reduced 50% because of intestinal atrophy (Jambunathan et al. 1981, Guiraldes & Hamilton 1981). Protein deprivation during gestation and immediately after birth also impairs maturation patterns. At weaning, the array of enzymes may still show an immature pattern. Changes in the young of protein-deprived mothers disappear if they are fed by a foster mother or are given a normal protein diet (Shrader et al. 1977).

References

Adams J.L. & Leichter J. (1973) Effect of protein-deficient diets with various amounts of carbohydrate on intestinal disaccharidase activities in the rat. *J. Nutr.* **103**, 1716–1722.

Adibi S.A. & Allen E.R. (1970) Impaired jejunal absorption rates of essential amino acids induced by either caloric or protein deprivation in man. *Gastroenterol.* **59**, 404–413.

Barbezat G.O. & Hansen J.D.L. (1977) The exocrine pancreas and calorie–protein malnutrition. *Pediat.* **42**, 77.

Bilir S. (1972) Acquired disaccharide intolerance in children with malnutrition. *Amer. J. Clin. Nutr.* **25**, 664–671.

Bowie M.D., Barbezat G.O. Hansen J.D.L. (1967) Garbohydrate absorption in malnourished children. *Amer. J. Clin. Nutri.* **20**, 89–97.

Brunser O., Reid A. & Monckeberg F. (1968) Jejunal mucosa in infant malnutrition. *Amer. J. Clin. Nutr.* **21**, 976–983.

Brunser O., Castillo C. & Araza M. (1976) Fine structure of the small intestinal mucosa in infantile marasmic malnutrition. *Gastroenterol.* **70**, 495–507.

Campos J.V.M., Neto V.F., Wehba P.J., Carvalho A.A. & Shiner M. (1979) Jejunal mucosa in marasmic children, clinical, pathological and fine structural evaluation of the effect of protein-energy malnutrition and environmental contamination. *Amer. J. Clin. Nutr.* **32**, 1575–1591.

Chandra R.K. (1975a) Food antibodies in malnutrition. *Arch. Dis. Child.* **50**, 532.

Chandra R.K. (1975b) Reduced secretory antibody response to live attenuated measles and poliovirus vaccines in malnourished children. *Brit. Med. J.* **57**, 583–585.

Chandra R.K. (1979a) Nutrition and gastrointestinal tract. In *Practice of Pediatrics*, Chapter 31, pp. 1–17. (Ed. by V.C. Kelley). Harper & Row, Hagerstown.

Chandra R.K. (1979b) Nutritional deficiency and susceptibility to infection. *Bull. WHO* **57**, 167–178.

Chandra R.K. (1979c) Nutritional liver disease. In *The Liver and Biliary System in Infants and Children*. Churchill Livingstone, Edinburgh.

Chandra R.K. (1980) *Immunology of Nutritional Disorders*. Edward Arnold, London.

Chandra R.K. (1982) Immune responses in parasitic diseases. Part B: mechanisms. *Rev. Infect. Dis.* **4**, 756–762.

Chandra, R.K. (1983a) Malnutrition. In *Primary and Secondary Disorders*. Churchill Livingstone, Edinburgh.

Chandra R.K. (1983b) Mucosal immunity in nutrition deficiency. In The Secretory Immune System in Health and Disease. *Annals N.Y. Acad. Sci.* **409**, 345–352.

Chandra R.K., Pawa R.R. & Ghai O.P. (1968) Sugar intolerance in malnourished infants and children. *Brit. Med. J.* **4**, 611.

Cook G.C. & Lee F.D. (1966). The jejunum after kwashiorkor. *Lancet*, **2**, 1263–1267.

DeLuca L., Little E.P. & Wolf G. (1969) Vitamin A and protein synthesis by rat intestinal mucosa. *J. Biol. Chem.* **244**, 701–708.

Deo M.G. & Ramalingaswami V. (1965) Reaction of the small intestine to induced protein malnutrition in rhesus monkeys: a study of cell population kinetics in the jejunum. *Gastroenterol.* **49**, 150–157.

Duque E., Bolanos O., Lotero H. & Mayoral L.G. (1975) Enteropathy in adult protein malnutrition: light microscopic findings. *Amer. J. Clin. Nutr.* **28**, 901–913.

Foroozan P. & Trier J.S. (1967) Mucosa of the small intestine in pernicious anemia. *N. Engl. J. Med.* **277**, 553.

Gjessing E.C., Villanueva D., Duque E., Bolanos O. & Mayoral L.G. (1977) Dipeptide hydrolase activity of the intestinal mucosa from protein-malnourished adult patients and controls. *Amer. J. Clin. Nutr.* **30**, 1044–1052.

Gracey M., Suharjono Sunoto & Stone, D.E. (1973) Bacterial contamination of the gut: another feature of malnutrition. *Amer. J. Clin. Nutr.* **26**, 1170.

Guiraldes E. & Hamilton R.J. (1981) Effect of chronic malnutrition on intestinal structure, epithelial renewal and enzymes in suckling rats. *Pediat. Res.* **15**, 930–934.

Hatch T., Lebenthal E., Branski D. & Kranser J. (1979) The effect of early postnatal acquired malnutrition on intestinal growth, disaccharidases and enterokinase. *J. Nutr.* **109**, 1874–1879.

Hazuria R.S., Sarin G.S., Srivastava P.N., Misra R.C., Bhatt I.N. & Chuttani H.K. (1974) Intestinal dipeptidases in primary malnutrition. *Amer. J. Clin. Nutr.* **27**, 760.

Hill Jr R.B., Prosper J., Hirschfield J.S. & Kern Jr F. (1968) Protein starvation and the small intestine. I. The growth and morphology of the small intestine in weanling rats. *Exp. Mol. Path.* **8**, 66–74.

Hindmarsh J.T., Kilby D., Ross B. & Wiseman G. (1967) Further studies on intestinal active transport during semistarvation. *J. Physiol.* **188**, 207–218.

Hoffbrand A.V. & Broitman S.A. (1969) Effect of chronic nutritional iron deficiency on the small intestinal disaccharidase activities of growing dogs. *Proc. Soc. Expt. Biol. Med.* **130**, 595–602.

Holemans K. & Lambrechts A. (1977) Nitrogen metabolism and fat absorption in malnutrition and kwashiorkor. *J. Nutr.* **56**, 477–494.

Hopper A.F., Rose R.M. & Wannemacher Jr R.W. (1972) Cell population changes in the intestinal mucosa of protein-depleted or starved rats. II. Changes in cellular migration rates. *J. Cell. Biol.* **53**, 225–230.

Jambunathan L.R. Neuhoff D. & Younoszai M.K. (1981) Intestinal disaccharidases in malnourished infant rats. *Amer. J. Clin. Nutr.* **34**, 1879–1884.

James W.P.T. (1970) Sugar absorption and intestinal motility in children when malnourished and after treatment. *Clin. Sci.* **39**, 305–318.

James W.P.T. (1971) Effects of protein-calorie malnutrition on intestinal absorption. *Ann. N.Y. Acad. Sci.* **176**, 244.

James W.P.T. (1971a) Jejunal disaccharidase activities in children with marasmus and with kwashiorkor. *Arch. Dis. Child.* **46**, 218–220.

Kimura T., Seto A. & Yoshida A. (1978) Effect of diets on intestinal disaccharidase and leucineaminopeptidase activities in refed rats. *J. Nutr.* **108**, 1087–1097.

Kreshaw T.G., Neame K.D. & Wiseman G. (1960) The effect of semistarvation on absorption of the rat small intestine *in vitro* and *in vivo*. *J. Physiol.* **152**, 182–196.

Kumar V. & Chase H.P. (1971) Undernutrition and intestinal dipeptide hydrolase activity in the rat. *J. Nutr.* **101**, 1509–1514.

Kumar V., Ghai O.P. & Chase H.P. (1971) Intestinal dipeptide hydrolase activities in undernourished children. *Arch. Dis. Child.* **46**, 801.

Lifshitz F., Hawkins R.L., Diaz-Bensussen S. & Wapnir R.A. (1972) Absorption of carbohydrate in malnourished rats. *J. Nutr.* **102**, 1303–1310.

Lifshitz F. & Holman G.H. (1964) Disaccharidase deficiencies with steatorrhea. *J. Pediat.* **64**, 34.

Lifshitz F., Teichberg S. & Wapnir R.A. (1981) Malnutrition and the intestine. *Nutrition and Child Health: Symposia from the XII International Congress of Nutrition. Perspectives for the 1980s*, pp. 1–24. Alan R. Liss, New York.

Loh K.R., Shrader R.E. & Zeman F.J. (1971) Effect of maternal protein deprivation on neonatal intestinal absorption in rats. *J. Nutr.* **101**, 1663–1672.

Mata L.J., Jimenez F., Cordon M., Rosales R., Prera E., Schneider R.E. & Viteri F.E. (1972) Gastrointestinal flora of children with protein–calorie malnutrition. *Amer. J. Clin. Nutr.* **25**, 1118.

Mayoral L.G., Tripathy K., Bolanos O., Lotero H., Duque E., Garcia F.T. & Ghitis J. (1972) Intestinal functional and morphologic abnormalities in severely protein-malnourished adults. *Amer. J. Clin. Nutr.* **25**, 1084.

Mayoral, L.G., Bolanos, O., Lotero, H. and Duque,

E. (1975) Enteropathy in adult protein malnutrition: a review of cali experience. *Amer. J. Clin. Nutri.* **28**, 894–900.

McCance R.A., Rutishauser I.H.E. & Boozer C.N. (1970) Effect of kwashiorkor on absorption and excretion of nitrogen, fat and minerals. *Arch. Dis. Child.* **45**, 410–416.

Nakamura Y., Yasumoto K. & Mitsuda H. (1972) Effect of excess L-histidine diet on active transport of L-histidine by isolated rat small intestine. *J. Nutr.* **102**, 359–364.

Nutrition Canada (1973) *Nutrition: A National Priority.* Information Canada. Ottawa.

Olson J.A., Rojanapo W. & Lamb A.J. (1981) The effect of vitamin A status on the differentiation and function of goblet cells in the rat intestine. *Ann. N.Y. Acad. Sci.* **359**, 181–191.

Prosper J., Murry R.L. & Kern F. (1968) Protein starvation and the small intestine. II. Disaccharidase activities. *Gastroenterol.* **55**, 223–228.

Ramalingaswami V. (1964) Perspectives in malnutrition. *Nature*, **201**, 546–551.

Reddy V., Raghuramulu N. & Bhaskaram C. (1976) Secretory IgA in protein-calorie malnutrition. *Arch. Dis. Child.* **51**, 871–874.

Rodgers J.B. (1970) Lipid absorption and lipid-reesterifying enzyme activity in small bowel of the protein-deficient rat. *Amer. J. Clin. Nutr.* **23**, 1331–1338.

Rojanapo W., Lamb A.J. & Olson J.A. (1980) Prevalence, metabolism and migration of goblet cells in rat intestine following the induction of rapid synchronous Vitamin A deficiency. *J. Nutr.* **110**, 178–188.

Schneider R.E. & Viteri F.E. (1974) Luminal events of lipid absorption in protein-calorie malnourished children; relationship with nutritional recovery and diarrhea. I. Capacity of the duodenal content to achieve micellar solubilization of lipids. *Amer. J. Clin. Nutr.* **27**, 777–787.

Schneider R.E. & Viteri F.E. (1974) Luminal events of lipid absorption in protein-calorie malnourished children; relationship with nutritional recovery and diarrhea. II. Alteration in bile acid content of duodenal aspirates. *Amer. J. Clin. Nutr.* **27**, 788–796.

Shrader R.E., Ferlatte M.I. & Zeman F.J. (1977) Early postnatal development of the intestine in progeny of protein-deprived rats. *Biol. Neonate* **31**, 181–198.

Shrader R.E. & Zeman F.J. (1969) Effect of maternal protein deprivation on morphological and enzymatic development of neonatal rat tissue. *J. Nutr.* **99**, 401–412.

Sirisiha S., Suskind R., Edelman R. Asvapaka C. & Olson R.E. (1974) Secretory and serum IgA in children with protein-calorie malnutrition. *Adv. Exp. Med. Biol.* **45**, 389–398.

Solimano G., Burgess E.A. & Levin B. (1967) Protein-calorie malnutrition: Effect of deficient diets on enzyme levels of jejunal mucosa of rats. *Brit. J. Nutr.* **21**, 55–68.

Sriratanaban S. & Thayer W.R. (1971) Small intestinal disaccharidase activities in experimental iron and protein deficiency. *Amer. J. Clin. Nutr.* **24**, 411–415.

Takano J. (1964) Intestinal changes in protein deficient rats. *Exp. Mol. Pathol.* **3**, 224–231.

Teichberg S., Fagundes-Neto U., Bayne M.A. & Lifshitz F. (1981) Jejunal macromolecular absorption and bile salt deconjugation in protein-energy malnourished rats. *Amer. J. Clin. Nutr.* **34**, 1281–1291.

Ten-State Nutrition Survey 1968–1970 (1972) *DWEH Publication No. HSM 72-8130.* Center for Disease Control, Atlanta.

Thompson M.D. & Trowell H.C. (1952) Pancreatic enzyme activity in duodenal contents of children with a type of kwashiorkor. *Lancet*, i, 1031.

Underwood B.A., Hashim S.A. & Sebrell W.R. (1967) Fatty acid absorption and metabolism in protein calorie malnutrition. *Amer. J. Clin. Nutr.* **20**, 226.

Viteri F.E., Flores J.M., Alvarado J. & Behar M. (1973) Intestinal malabsorption in malnourished children before and during recovery. *Dig. Dis.* **18**, 201–211.

Vyas D. & Chandra R.K. (1983) Functional significance of iron deficiency. In *Iron Deficiency in Infancy and Childhood.* (Ed. by A. Stekel & P. Guesry). Raven Press, New York.

Wapnir R.A. & Lifshitz F. (1974) Absorption of amino acids in malnourished rats. *J. Nutr.* **104**, 843–849.

Younoszai M.K. & Ranshaw J. (1973) Gastrointestinal growth in the fetus and suckling rat pups: effect of maternal dietary protein. *J. Nutr.* **103**, 454–461.

Zeman F.J. & Fratzke M.K. (1976) Lipid absorption in the young of protein-deficient rats. *Lipids*, **11**, 652–661.

Zile M., Bunge E.C. & DeLuca H.F. (1977) Effect of vitamin A deficiency on intestinal cell proliferation in the rat. *J. Nutr.* **107**, 522–560.

Chapter 19
Tropical Sprue

ANDREW TOMKINS AND CHRISTOPHER C. BOOTH

History 311
Epidemiology 315
Pathology 315
Motility 318
Microbiology 319
Absorption tests 320
Clinical features and treatment 322
Aetiology 328
Tropical enteropathy 329

History

Tropical sprue has been recognized by medical practitioners in India since at least 600 BC. In Charaka Samhita, a textbook dating from between 1300 and 600 BC, the condition is described as 'grahini ryadhi'. The disease was thought to be due to 'a weakness in the digestive fire' leading to 'impaired assimilation of ingested food', a perceptive analysis (Mathan 1978). It is also described in ancient Tamil texts as 'ubbumariyayae' which means a visitation by the goddess of distension, one of the cardinal symptoms of the disorder. The earliest European description of tropical sprue was by William Hillary who reported the features of the disease among planters and settlers in the Caribbean island of Barbados in 1759 (Hillary 1759, Booth 1963).

During the nineteenth century, physicians who accompanied the colonizing maritime powers from Europe to India, South-east Asia and the Far East became familiar with a form of chronic diarrhoea, similar to that described by Hillary, which was accompanied by severe weight loss, glossitis, anaemia and sometimes death. In 1818, Ballingal, surgeon to H.M. 33rd Regiment of Foot, described persistent diarrhoea with white, frothy stools in British soldiers in Bengal and similar symptoms were reported among European merchants in Calcutta (Twining 1832). Most individuals appeared to have an intestinal disorder, the 'diarrhoea alba' or 'white flux', but Ballingal also used the term 'hepatic flux' to suggest an alternative aetiology. Some of Ballingal's patients had dysentery and others had severe abdominal pain. Parasitological examination was not performed so it is impossible now to know how many of these patients had infection with *Strongyloides stercoralis*, giardia or *Entamoeba histolytica*. A further variety of the condition was 'hill diarrhoea' (Grant 1853). Expatriate personnel escaping from the heat of the plains of India to the cool of the mountainous areas developed acute watery diarrhoea with flatulence, soon progressing to steatorrhoea. Retrospective diagnosis suggests the possibility that some patients with 'hill station diarrhoea' may have had giardiasis. Tropical sprue was often self-limiting after a few months but relapses occurred. There was a significant mortality unless the sufferer was repatriated to a temperate climate.

A characteristic feature of the condition was the occurrence of nutritional deficiency. Weight loss and weakness were common and associated with anaemia. Severe pallor and glossitis were sometimes complicated by monilial infections of the mouth. The Dutch word 'sprouw', which Manson (1880) Anglicized to 'sprue', was used to describe oral lesions in association with diarrhoea. Severe anorexia has been consistently described in tropical sprue and may have frequently contributed to the development of nutritional deficiency.

Macrocytic and megaloblastic anaemia were found to be an almost constant feature of long-standing tropical sprue (Thin 1897). In early sprue, there was often no gross haematological abnormality but in later stages of the disorder, megaloblastic anaemia might be severe and was indistinguishable from that seen in Addisonian pernicious anaemia. Rarely there might be terminal transformation to an aplastic marrow. At first, many authors considered the anaemia to be due to intestinal toxaemia, as had also been proposed as an explanation for the megaloblastic anaemia associated with the stagnant loop syndrome (cf. Chapter 15). Liver soup was used in the treatment of sprue in the early days and may have induced remission in some cases, but it was the successful use of liver extract in the treatment of the megaloblastic anaemia of sprue which followed the discovery by Minot & Murphy (1926) of the efficacy of liver in the treatment of Addisonian pernicious anaemia, that established that nutritional deficiency was the cause of the megaloblastic anaemia. Castle's demonstration in 1929 of the need for an intrinsic factor to ensure the absorption of the haemopoietic principle necessary for normal blood formation (Castle 1929, Castle & Townsend 1929) led to the realization that malabsorption was the cause of megaloblastic anaemia in sprue. Subsequent work following the isolation of folic acid in 1945 and of vitamin B_{12} in 1948 established that the anaemia was due to deficiency of vitamin B_{12} and folic acid and that this was due to malabsorption of these substances (Spies *et al.* 1946, Spies & Suarez 1948).

During the Second World War there were repeated outbreaks of tropical sprue among British and Commonweath military personnel involved in campaigns in India, Burma and South-east Asia. An interesting feature was the apparent absence of tropical sprue among African soldiers serving in India and Burma. During this period, the largest study was performed by Stefanini (1948) who described a thousand cases of tropical sprue among Italian prisoners of war in camps in North India. He documented three stages of the disorder. Firstly, there was diarrhoea, flatulence and weight loss, together with steatorrhoea which was accompanied within a few weeks of onset by anorexia, severe weakness and loss of weight. Secondly, when the symptoms were more prolonged, glossitis and pigmentation accompanied the steatorrhoea. Thirdly, macrocytic anaemia

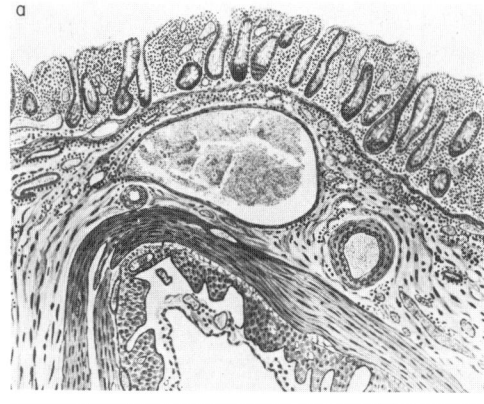

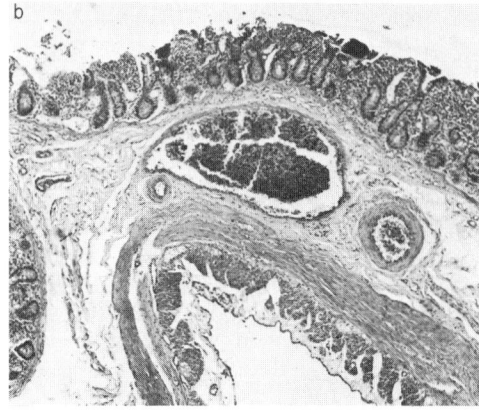

Fig. 19.1. Histopathological section of the ileum obtained at autopsy from a 36-year-old Caucasian woman who died in Colombo in 1913. (a) Drawing made by Sir Philip Manson-Bahr (Bahr 1915, Plate VI). (b) Photomicrograph from the original slide; Sir Philip had written 'Draw!!' upon the labels (H & E, × 50).

developed. Nearly all patients responded well to treatment with sulphonamides, together with liver extract and yeast.

Before the introduction of jejunal biopsy techniques in the 1950s there was considerable controversy as to whether there were any pathological lesions of the small intestine in sprue. Begg, working in China, described autopsy findings in sprue in 1912. The intestine was found to be lined with a thick layer of mucous material within which there were enormous numbers of rod-shaped bacteria. The mucous membrane showed an inflammatory cell infiltration, most marked in the ileum. Soon afterwards Bahr (later Sir Philip Manson-Bahr), working under the auspices of the Ceylon Tea Planation Association, confirmed that at autopsy undertaken as soon as 2 h after death the whole of the intestinal canal was covered by a thick layer of mucus (Bahr 1915). Microscopically the intestinal mucous membrane was infiltrated with round cells, leucocytes and plasma cells. In the ileum there were striking changes in the mucous membrane of the small intestine, the villi being shrunken and atrophic (Fig. 19.1). These observations were clearly of great importance but Bahr himself was not at that time convinced by the pathological appearance of the bowel. He concluded that 'there is no more evidence for regarding the loss of surface epithelium and the attenuation of the gut as being any more characteristic of sprue than it is of any other diarrhoea' (Bahr 1915). The specimen of the ileum illustrated in Fig. 19.1 emphasizes the difficulty encountered by investigators of that era in excluding agonal changes or post-mortem artefacts in the study of the intestine in sprue at autopsy. By 1924, however, Manson-Bahr stated that 'evidence is now accumulating that the essential primary lesion of sprue is an ulceration of the small intestine, chiefly affecting the lower end of the ileum' (Manson-Bahr 1924). Others challenged this view. Thaysen (1931) found no abnormality in the small intestine in sprue and dismissed any abnormal findings at autopsy as post-mortem artefact. Although Fairley and his colleagues had described a condition of withering of the intestinal villi at autopsy in Bombay (Mackie & Fairley 1928−29), later studies of two patients dying of sprue in London failed to reveal any abnormality of the small intestine and they therefore supported Thaysen's conclusion (Mackie & Fairley 1933−34). The characteristic mucosal abnormality in tropical sprue was not clearly defined until further studies were carried out in autopsy material in Puerto Rico (Suarez et al. 1947), on biopsies taken at laparotomy in Cuba (Milanes et al. 1951) and particularly on mucosal biopsies obtained by peroral intubation techniques (Fig. 19.2) (Shiner 1956, Shiner & Doniach 1960, Crosby & Kugler 1957, Swanson & Thomassen 1963).

A review of the epidemiological features of tropical sprue in the last 100 years strongly suggests an infective aetiology, but no bac-

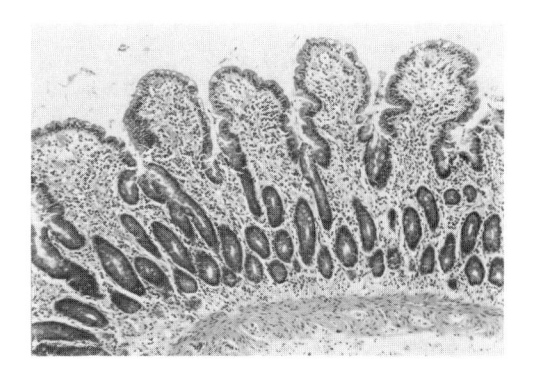

Fig. 19.2. The first peroral jejunal biopsy in untreated tropical sprue, showing partial villous atrophy in a 55-year-old Anglo-Indian lady who developed symptoms in England in 1956, 11 months after emigrating from India where she had lived near Madras (H & E, × 80). (Courtesy of Dr Margot Shiner.)

terial, viral or parasitic organism has been found and the aetiology therefore remains uncertain. Nevertheless, the early clinical and autopsy studies were interesting. Begg's observation of excessive mucus in the ileum in which he found large numbers of bacteria led to his inclusion of the antiseptic substance, santonin, in the treatment of sprue, the mainstays of which at that time comprised liver soup, yeast and spinach. In the early years of this century, he did not have to repatriate a patient from China during 13 years of clinical practice using this regime (Begg 1912). Bahr had also shown bacteria embedded in the mucus overlying the intestinal mucosa. Mackie et al. (1928) cultured large numbers of intestinal bacteria from duodenal fluid and later Rogers (1938) reported the improvement of diarrhoea after treatment with Prontosil, an antiseptic which had in fact been originally prescribed for a respiratory infection. Subsequently, treatment with combinations of oral broad spectrum antibiotics were shown to be beneficial in sprue (French et al. 1956), suggesting that micro-organisms might be involved in the pathogenesis of sprue in some unknown way.

Many of the early reports of tropical sprue described the condition among expatriate Caucasians living in India and the Far East, but there were also reports from India emphasizing that the condition was common among the indigenous population (Morehead 1860). Since the end of the Second World War detailed studies of endemic and epidemic sprue have been reported from India and the Caribbean. Baker & Mathan (1970) described the clinical features of large numbers of Indian patients seen in Vellore, South India. There were considerable variations in clinical presentation. In some there was an epidemic form with a severe, acute watery diarrhoea which progressed to malabsorption. Others had milder symptoms yet objective tests of intestinal absorption were as severe as those with marked diarrhoea. Severe nutritional disturbances also occurred but there might be minimal intestinal symptoms even in the presence of severe malabsorption. A feature of the Indian patients was the intermittent nature of the diarrhoea with occasional spontaneous remissions and relapses. The response to antibiotics at Vellore was often disappointing.

Most of these Indian patients with tropical sprue had an abnormal jejunal mucosa on biopsy. Interpretation was difficult. Many asymptomatic individuals living in South India also had abnormal jejunal mucosa when compared with normal biopsies from temperate zones. In many developing countries it was also found that the jejunal mucosa might show similar abnormalities. Furthermore, changes in the intestinal mucosa were noted among American Peace Corps volunteers living in Asia for some months and these abnormalities reverted to normal when individuals returned to the USA (Lindenbaum 1968). This condition has been defined as 'tropical enteropathy' (p. 328).

Sprue had been described among residents of certain Caribbean islands and Central America since the early years of this century (Ashford 1913, 1917, Gardner 1956, Sheehy et al. 1965) and detailed studies were published by Klipstein among patients investigated in New York City who had arrived from Puerto Rico, Cuba, Guatemala and the Dominican Republic (Klipstein 1964, Klipstein & Falaiye 1969). In addition, there were patients with tropical sprue seen in Haiti (Klipstein et al. 1968), many of whom had a severe megaloblastic anaemia resembling that seen in New York in patients with particularly protracted symptoms. In these patients, antibiotic therapy seemed to be more effective than folic acid, in contrast to observations made in South India.

Table 19.1. Countries in which tropical sprue has been described.

Region	Country
Asia	China
	Indonesia
	Philippines
	Hong Kong
	Malaya
	Singapore
	Borneo
	Vietnam
	Burma
	Thailand
	India
	Afghanistan
	Nepal
Middle East	Yemen
	Egypt
	Lebanon
Caribbean	Haiti
	Puerto Rico
	Cuba
	Dominican Republic
Central and South America	Guatemala
	Colombia
	Venezuela
	Mexico
Africa	South Africa
	Zimbabwe
	Nigeria

The Wellcome Trust collaborative study 'Tropical Sprue and Megaloblastic Anaemia' published in 1971 described the history of tropical sprue, its acute occurrence among British expatriates in Singapore and Malaysia and the features of chronic sprue in patients seen in London. Observations in these groups of patients were compared with studies of tropical sprue in South India and the Caribbean. These detailed studies led to a tentative definition of the disorder as *a syndrome of intestinal malabsorption which occurs among residents in or visitors to certain regions of the tropics*. Baker & Mathan (1971) emphasized that there should be malabsorption of two substances and that all other causes of malabsorption should be excluded. The aetiology of the disease, however,

Epidemiology

The most striking feature of tropical sprue is its geographical distribution. The countries from which it has been described are shown in Table 19.1. It occurs particularly in the Indian subcontinent and the Far East and many individuals from Europe and the USA have developed their disorder when visiting India, Sri Lanka, Bangladesh or Nepal. The condition was also common among US personnel in the Philippines and Vietnam. Tropical sprue occurs selectively in the Caribbean. It is prevalent in Puerto Rico, where extensive studies have been carried out, and in Haiti. It has never been described in Jamaica and no case has been reported from Barbados since Hillary's original description. It occurs in Guatemala, Colombia, Venezuela and Mexico but reports suggest that it is becoming less frequent in these areas, possibly as a result of the increasing use of antibiotics for attacks of diarrhoea. Sprue has also been recognized in certain countries in the Middle East. For many years, it was considered not to occur in Africa south of the Sahara. In striking contrast to clinical experience with their countrymen resident in India and the Far East, British physicians have not encountered tropical sprue among the large number of expatriates who spent large parts of their lives in African countries during the colonial era. With the exception of the occasional report (Manson-Bahr 1928), experienced physicians have in the past repeatedly stated their belief that sprue does not occur in Africa. Moshal et al. (1975), however, have described a syndrome of malabsorption, often involving fat and vitamin B_{12}, together with megaloblastic anaemia among Africans living in or around Durban, a city with a high Asian population. Similar observations have been made in Zimbabwe (Thomas & Clain 1976). Falaiye (1970) has also claimed that sprue may occur in Nigeria but his report from Lagos has not been confirmed in other centres in West Africa.

The epidemic nature of tropical sprue has been recognized since the earliest descriptions. Epidemics were a major clinical problem in north-east India and the Burma theatre during the Second World War. In South India, several large epidemics have been reported. Between 1960 and 1962, Baker & Mathan (1970) estimated that 100,000 people were affected and that at least 30,000 may have died. There was no relationship of the epidemic to any season of the year. Diet, sanitation, type of housing and drinking water had no influence on the development of the disease. Certain compounds, however, might be associated with the disorder, recalling the 'sprue houses' which were thought to encourage the development of tropical sprue in an earlier era. A particular feature of epidemics is that adults are affected earlier than children, and among expatriates living in an endemic area the condition is exceptionally rare in children. In Puerto Rico, there is an impressive but unexplained seasonality in the occurrence of tropical sprue, a high proportion of cases presenting in the months following the Christmas festivities.

The prevalence of endemic tropical sprue in any community is uncertain. Bahr (1915) carried out a field study and found thirty-six cases of tropical sprue among 7592 Europeans living in Ceylon, a prevalence of 4.7/1000. In Puerto Rico, Sheehy et al. (1965) noted a 6% incidence of tropical sprue among North Americans living on that island who developed diarrhoea. In India, it seems likely that the prevalence in the indigenous populations is higher than this.

Pathology

Whatever the cause of tropical sprue, the primary abnormality is in the mucosa of the small intestine and malabsorption and malnutrition are secondary to this. The lesion appears first to affect the jejunum but in chronic cases spreads distally to involve the ileum.

Jejunum

In the earliest stages of the disease, when symptoms have been present for no longer than a month or two, the jejunal mucosa may be normal, or there may be only slight ab-

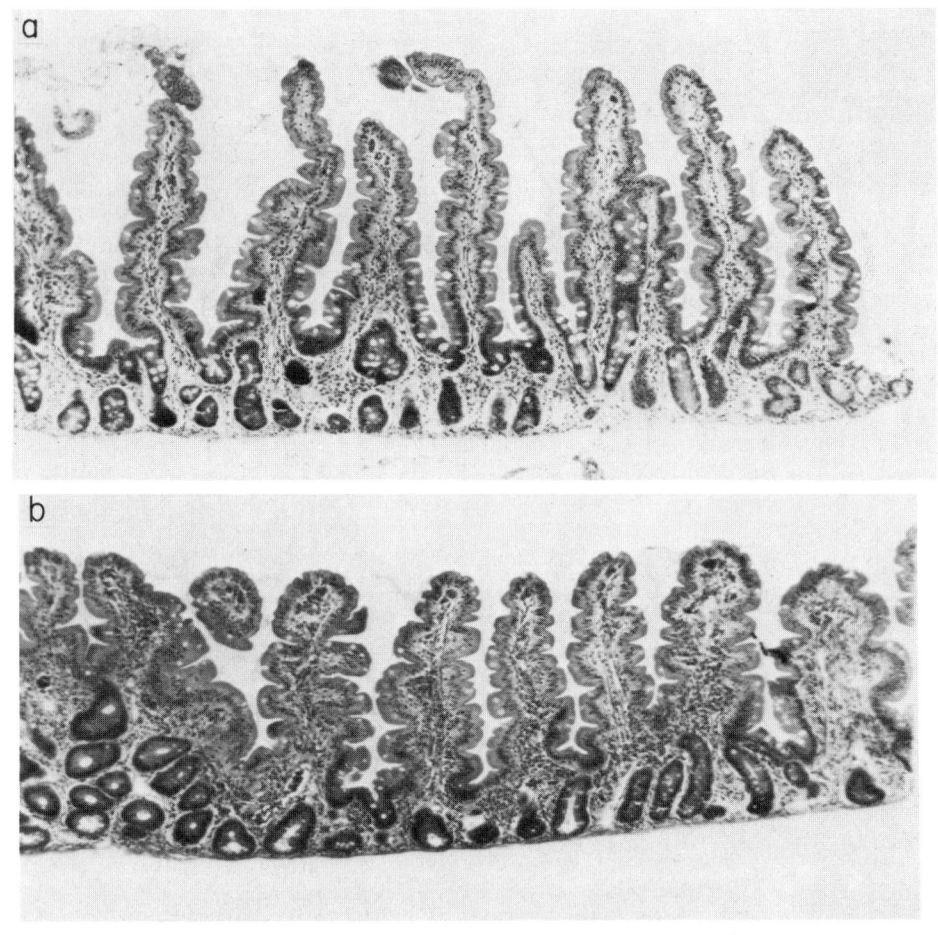

Fig. 19.3. Jejunal biopsy in overland travellers to India. (a) Normal intestinal morphology with minimal symptoms without malabsorption (H & E, × 100). (b) Mild shortening of villi in a patient with tropical sprue of 3 months' duration (H & E, × 100).

normalities, with cellular infiltration, increased numbers of intraepithelial lymphocytes but no recognizable damage to villi or enterocytes either on dissecting microscopy or histologically (Fig. 19.3 a and b).

If symptoms have been present for 3 months or more, however, the jejunal mucosa is usually abnormal. Dissecting microscopy is particularly helpful in recognizing the characteristic appearance of tropical sprue. The mucosa typically shows a convoluted appearance (Fig. 19.4a) and on histological examination there is partial villous atrophy (Fig. 19.4b). The overall thickness of the mucosa is usually normal but the villi are shortened and the crypts increased in depth. The enterocytes may show abnormalities, the cells being cuboidal, but the lesion of the enterocyte is less severe than that seen in coeliac disease. There are also abnormalities that suggest a defect in fat transport by the enterocytes. Biopsies from patients with tropical sprue in Puerto Rico, Haiti and India show an accumulation of lipid droplets adjacent to the basement membrane, even after 12 to 18 h of fasting (Schenk et al. 1965).

Using electron microscopy, ultra-structural changes have also been described (Mathan et al. 1975). The enterocyte abnormalities include disruption of microvilli, with an increase in lysosomes and degeneration of the rough endoplasmic reticulum and mitochondria. There are also pale staining degenerating cells in the crypt zone with vacuolization

Tropical Sprue

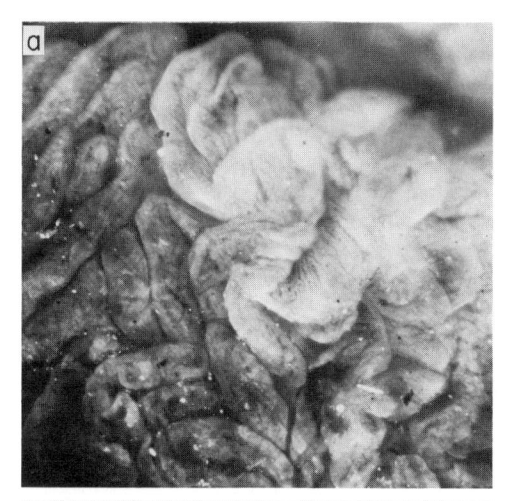

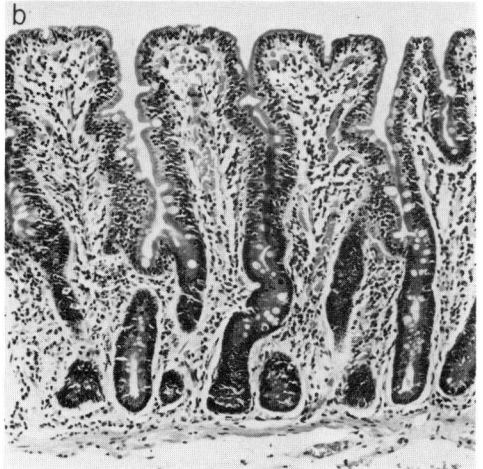

Fig. 19.4. Jejunal mucosa from a 40-year-old nursing sister who developed tropical sprue in Hong Kong. (a) Dissecting microscopy showing convoluted mucosa (× 50) (after treatment with folic acid 30 mg daily for 2 months). (b) Histological section of biopsy shown in Fig. 19.4a (H & E × 150).

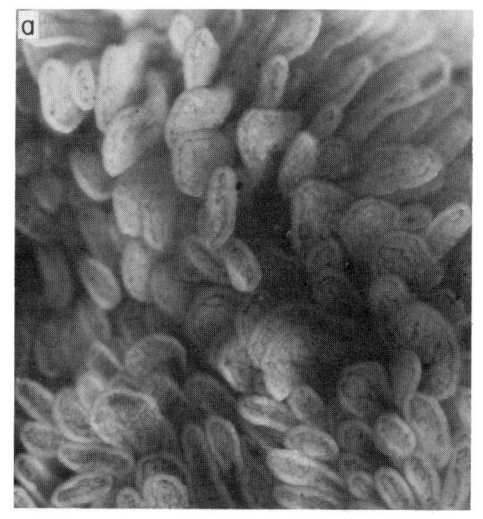

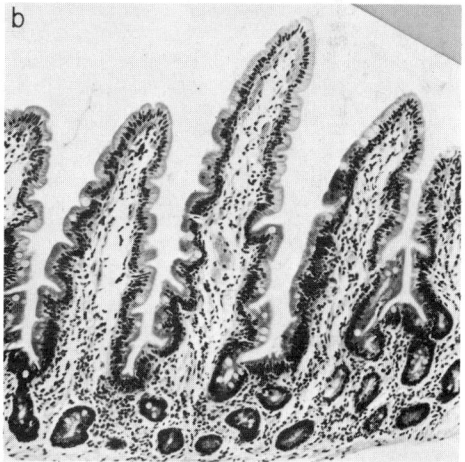

Fig. 19.5. Jejunal mucosa 4 months after treatment with oral broad spectrum antibiotics from the patient whose pre-treatment biopsy is shown in Fig. 19.4. (a) Normal finger and leaf-shaped villi (× 50). (b) Histology (H & E × 150).

and changes in mitochondria and nuclei.

Individuals with tropical sprue may not respond satisfactorily to treatment in the early stages, particularly if treated with folic acid alone, and the condition may then become chronic. The mucosal lesion in the jejunum, however, does not appear to progress and even when sprue has been present for as long as 10 years or more the mucosa usually continues to show a convoluted appearance on dissecting microscopy with partial villous atrophy on light microscopy.

The lesion of chronic sprue is reversible following treatment with antibiotics, as illustrated in Fig. 19.5.

The severe flat mucosa of coeliac disease, with its characteristic mosaic pattern (Chapter 9, Fig 9.1) is rarely seen in tropical sprue. If subtotal villous atrophy and a flat mucosa is found during the investigation of a patient for possible sprue, the diagnosis of coeliac disease should be suspected. This condition may present in an endemic area in the tropics or may be activated in a pre-

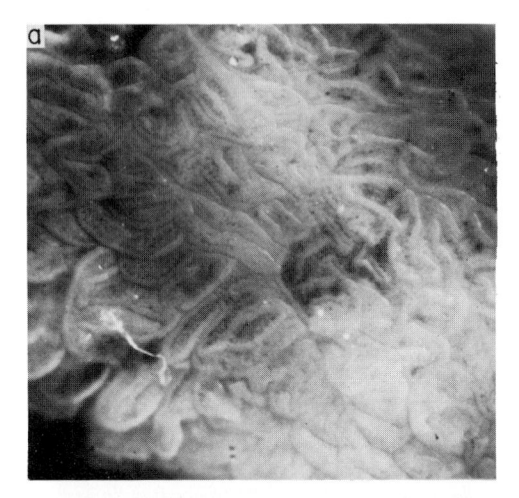

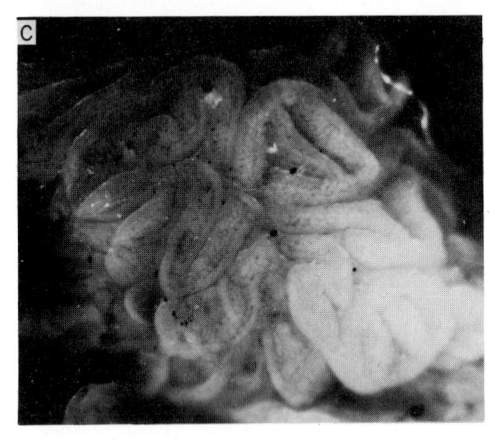

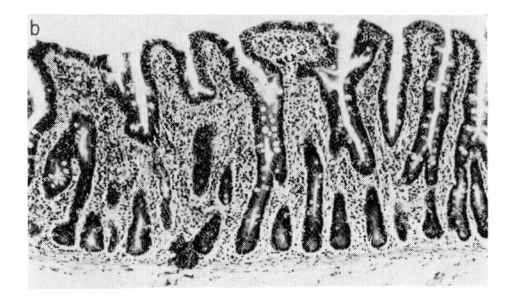

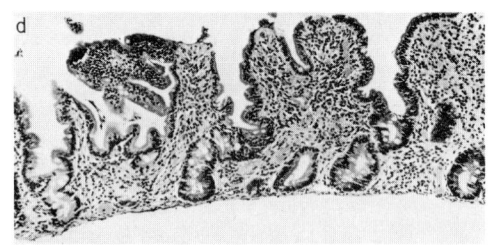

Fig. 19.6. Intestinal biopsies in chronic tropical sprue of 15 years duration. (a) Convoluted jejunal mucosa (× 40). (b) Histology of jejunal mucosa (H & E × 150). (c) Ileal mucosa in the same patient (× 50). (d) Histology of the ileum (H & E × 150) (Mollin & Booth 1971).

viously asymptomatic individual by an intercurrent gastrointestinal infection.

In endemic sprue in south India, the mucosal lesion may show a wide range of abnormalities ranging from minimal changes to a severely flattened mucosa. This variability in pathology of the intestinal mucosa may reflect differences in duration of a disease which in an indigenous population characteristically undergoes spontaneous remission and relapse. It may also be due to differences in immune response in indigenous populations.

Ileum

In the early stages of tropical sprue, within the first 2–3 months of the development of the disorder, the ileum may be normal or less severely involved than the jejunum (O'Brien & England 1971). As the disorder progresses, however, the ileum appears to develop the same convoluted mucosa and partial villous atrophy as the jejunum (Bayless et al. 1968, Wheby et al. 1971). In patients studied in London with tropical sprue which had become chronic despite treatment with folic acid for many years, the ileum was found to be as severely involved as the jejunum (Fig. 19.6) (Mollin & Booth 1971). The abnormality of the ileum may become more marked as time goes on and in fatal sprue the severity of the ileal lesion is illustrated by the autopsy studies carried out by Begg (1912) and Bahr (1915) in the early years of this century (Fig. 19.1).

Motility

Radiological studies show marked dilatation of the small intestine in the acute phase of tropical sprue and the changes are in general related to the severity of the illness. There is also a prolongation of the transit time of the barium through the small intestine. This abnormality has been assessed further by studying the time of appearance of hydrogen in the breath after oral lactulose. In acute tropical sprue studied in London most patients had delayed small intestinal transit which returned to normal after recovery. (Cook 1978).

Relationship to gut hormone profile

Plasma levels of gut hormones have been measured after a standard meal in British patients with acute tropical sprue (Chapter 23, Besterman et al. 1979). The fasting levels of motilin and enteroglucagon were markedly increased and they rose to high levels after the oral test meal. By contrast, levels of gastric inhibitory polypeptide and insulin were reduced. These findings are different from those in coeliac disease in whom there are normal levels of motilin in the fasting state and only slightly increased basal enteroglucagon levels.

There is a correlation between the plasma enteroglucagon level and the time of appearance of hydrogen in the breath after oral lactulose, suggesting that the prolongation of intestinal transit time in tropical sprue is due to an inhibitory effect of enteroglucagon on gut motility. The possible effect of this regulatory peptide on intestinal mucosal growth in sprue remains speculative.

Microbiology

Among Caucasian subjects living in Europe or North America there is an autochthonous flora introduced soon after birth consisting of lactobacilli and streptococci (Chapter 14). Enterobacteriaceae are rarely present in the upper intestine and even in the lower small intestine are found in low numbers. A similar microflora occurs in healthy indigenous adults studied in Costa Rica (Jarumilinta et al. 1976), North India (Gorbach et al. 1970), Haiti (Klipstein et al. 1976), and in expatriates without malabsorption returned from visits to India (Tomkins et al. 1976). On the other hand, enterobacteria have been identified in the upper intestine of a few control subjects in South America (Cain et al. 1976) and were present in nearly all control subjects in South India where anaerobic organisms were also isolated from the upper small intestine (Bhat et al. 1972).

During an acute diarrhoeal episode one or more of a variety of enteropathogens may be found in the upper intestine both in samples of luminal fluid obtained by intubation and attached to the intestinal mucosa. In most individuals there is effective microbial clearance of the intestine by the time that intubation is repeated after recovery. By contrast, in tropical sprue the upper intestine appears to be persistently colonized by enterobacteria (Gorbach et al. 1970, Tomkins et al. 1975). There is no single bacterium which is common to all patients but it is remarkable how a limited number of species of enterobacteriaceae (*E. coli, Klebsiella pneumonia, Enterobacter cloacae*) are present in most cases. These species have not been regarded as classical enteropathogens in the past but several studies have indicated that they produce enterotoxins (Klipstein et al. 1973) which have morphological and physiological effects on the small intestine (Klipstein et al. 1975). Both heat-stable and heat-labile enterotoxins have been identified which stimulate fluid secretion in ligated loops of rabbit ileum and in the perfused rat jejunum. Transport of amino acids may also be impaired. The role of these bacteria in the mucosal damage is not so clearly defined but crude broth filtrates of enterobacteria isolated from patients with tropical sprue in Haiti have caused villous changes when instilled into ileal loops of rabbits (Klipstein & Schenk 1975). Further, a series of enterotoxins having a cytopathic effect on tissue culture cells have been prepared from enterobacteria isolated from British subjects who developed acute tropical sprue in India. (Drasar et al. 1980). The absence of enterotoxins in filtrates of enterobacteria obtained from the upper intestine of patients with the blind loop syndrome suggests that the bacteria which colonize in sprue may have plasmids which encode for toxin production, rather like the toxins of *E. coli*.

Bacterial colonization of the small intestine in tropical sprue does not appear to be a mere epiphenomenon, at least in the acute phase of the disorder (Simon & Gorbach

1984). Administration of oral broad spectrum antibiotics results in increased appetite and there is immediate improvement in the absorption of fat and vitamin B_{12}. At the same time, water and electrolyte absorption in the upper small bowel improves. In the later stages of chronic sprue, antibiotics are not so immediately effective, whether in endemic sprue in India or in chronic long-standing cases in temperate climates.

A key question is why organisms colonize the upper intestine. The close association of the enterobacteria with the mucosal surface suggests that adhesion appears to be important, perhaps by pili or a colonization factor antigen. Of the various host factors which favour colonization hypochlorrhydria is important. The presence of atrophy of the gastric mucosa and reduced gastric acidity is well described in malnourished children and adults, which may explain why so many control subjects in South India have bacterial colonization of the small intestine.

The studies of breath hydrogen levels after orally ingested carbohydrate which suggest that there is a prolongation of the small intestinal transit time in tropical sprue, indicate that stasis could contribute to bacterial colonization. In patients with the stagnant loop syndrome due to stasis, however, the intestinal microflora is quite different from that of tropical sprue. Whereas it is an anaerobic flora that colonizes the gut in patients with the stagnant loop syndrome, the microflora in tropical sprue is predominantly aerobic. Furthermore, the mucosal abnormalities in the two conditions are different. In tropical sprue there is a generalized abnormality of the intestinal mucosa, of varying degree; in the stagnant loop syndrome in man, on the other hand, mucosal changes are either not present or restricted to local areas of ulceration within obstructed loops (Booth et al. 1968, Chapter 15, Fig. 15.6).

The faecal microflora of patients with tropical sprue is also markedly different from that in normal individuals. In sprue, aerobic organisms are apparently present in higher concentration than anaerobes, a striking reversal of the normal situation (Bhat et al. 1972).

The search for a possible virus in tropical sprue has so far been unrewarding. No known virus such as the rotavirus or Norwalk agent has been found in adults or children with tropical sprue. Faecal samples and jejunal biopsy specimens have been examined for the presence of other viruses and coronavirus-like particles (CVLP) have been found in the stool of a proportion of patients with tropical sprue in South India (Mathan et al. 1975). A similar proportion of control subjects also have CVLP in their stools. There is, however, doubt whether these particles are coronaviruses (MacNaughton & Davies 1981). A few reports have described the presence of algae in stool samples from patients with tropical sprue but these have not been identified in subsequent studies. No known parasite has been uniformly present in cases of tropical sprue.

Absorption tests

From the onset of tropical sprue there are defects of absorption often involving the entire small intestine. In general, these defects reflect the mucosal abnormality. Even at the earliest stage of tropical sprue, however, when the intestinal mucosa is normal or only mildly abnormal, there may be steatorrhoea or vitamin B_{12} malabsorption. The progressive development of mucosal abnormalities in the ileum provides an explanation for the persistent defect in B_{12} absorption which is so common in patients with long-continued and chronic disease.

Fluid and electrolytes

Studies of fluid and electrolyte transfer in the upper small intestine have been carried out using intraluminal perfusion techniques (Tomkins 1981). Many patients with tropical sprue studied in Puerto Rico and Bengal were found to be in a net secretory state. When the patients in Bengal were restudied following antibiotic therapy, which reduced the numbers of intestinal enterobacteria, net fluid secretion was markedly reduced (Gorbach et al. 1970, Banwell et al. 1970). This suggests that fluid secretion into the gut lumen may be induced by bacterial enterotoxins.

Patients with tropical sprue in South India appear to be different (Hellier et al. 1977) in that they are not in a net secretory phase and their fluid and electrolyte absorption is similar to that of control subjects from local villages, many of whom may have similar bacterial colonization of the small intestine to that of the sprue patients. It may be that these individuals represent a more chronic form of the disorder than that studied elsewhere in India or the Caribbean. Despite the similarity in water and electrolyte absorption in the perfused segment of the jejunum in those with tropical sprue and the control subjects in South India, the sprue patients had larger stool volumes than the controls, indicating a possible defect in colonic function. Further studies have in fact shown a defect of colonic sodium and water absorption in tropical sprue. There was also increased faecal excretion of unsaturated fatty acids, especially oleic acid, and faecal weight correlated closely with the quality of the faecal fatty acids (Tirrupathi et al. 1983). It has been proposed that these fatty acids inhibited the ATP-ases located in the basolateral membrane of isolated rat colonocytes and thereby increased the intestinal losses of fluid and electrolytes. The larger chain fatty acids (linoleic C-18, linolenic C-18 and arachidonic acid C-20) reduce Na K-ATP-ase activity by about a half, whereas the shorter chain fatty acids (lauric C-12, myristic C-14) are less inhibitory. These deficiencies in Na K-ATP-ase activity may be enhanced in the presence of folate deficiency, which is so constant a feature of established tropical sprue.

Aminoacids and peptides

Malabsorption of glycine has been reported in India and Puerto Rico and in addition impaired absorption of methionine, leucine and valine has been observed in Puerto Rico (Klipstein & Corcino 1975). The absorption of the dipeptide glycyl-glycine may also be impaired at high concentrations (Hellier et al. 1980).

Carbohydrate

Xylose

Xylose absorption is frequently reduced. This reflects upper small intestinal damage as there is a close correlation between the severity of jejunal villous atrophy and xylose absorption. Impaired absorption of glucose has also been reported in perfused segments of the upper intestine of adult British subjects with tropical sprue (Cook 1981).

Lactose

Secondary hypolactasia may occur in tropical sprue, a high proportion of patients with acute sprue studied in the UK showing abnormal lactose tolerance (Tomkins et al. 1974). Disaccharidase levels in jejunal biopsy samples are also low (Swaminathan et al. 1970).

Fat

Faecal fat excretion is almost always increased in patients with tropical sprue. In more than 90% of subjects studied in South India and in the majority of sprue patients in Puerto Rico and New York City, there was steatorrhoea. At the earliest phase of the disorder, steatorrhoea may be mild, but even in patients with a normal or almost normal intestinal jejunal biopsy, steatorrhoea is usually present (O'Brien & England 1971). As the disease progresses, steatorrhoea becomes more marked (Table 19.2). In endemic sprue in indigenous populations, there may be considerable variation in the severity of the disease and in the amount of steatorrhoea. In general, however, the degree of steatorrhoea reflects the severity and extent of the intestinal mucosal lesion.

Bile acids

Although concentrations of bile salts have been found to be low in the jejunal lumen in tropical sprue, there has been no evidence of bile salt deconjugation, in contrast to the stagnant loop syndrome. Furthermore, there appears to be no malabsorption of bile salts (Bevan et al. 1974).

Table 19.2. Mean faecal fat and xylose excretion related to duration of symptoms in patients with tropical sprue.

	Duration of disease (months)		
	1–2	3–4	5 or more
Mean faecal fat (g/day) (50 patients)	14.8	19.6	21.8
Range	9.0–22.7	8.6–34.9	9.2–43.7
Mean xylose excretion (g/5 h) (38 patients)	15.8	10.1	7.5
Range	8.4–24.0	7.0–18.0	2.7–12.0

(O'Brien & England 1971)

Folic acid

There is little doubt that there is malabsorption of folic acid in tropical sprue. Studies with ^{3}H-labelled folic acid (PG-1) using plasma levels after an oral dose, have shown impaired absorption (Halsted 1980). The development of radioactively labelled polyglutamate (C^{14} PG-7), however, has made possible the study of absorption of dietary forms of folate conjugates. Puerto Ricans with tropical sprue had impaired absorption of both ^{3}H PG-1 and ^{14}C PG-7 when tested individually in a perfusion system (Corcino et al. 1976). When ^{14}C PG-7 was infused, however, considerable quantities of ^{14}C PG-1 were obtained in the aspirated perfusate. This suggests that the polyglutamate is adequately hydrolysed by folate conjugate in the mucosa and PG-1 then diffuses back into the intestinal lumen to be absorbed, albeit at a low rate.

Vitamin B$_{12}$

Even in the earliest phase of tropical sprue, the majority of patients may fail to absorb the B$_{12}$-intrinsic factor complex. O'Brien & England (1971) found that thirty-two of thirty-eight patients with acute tropical sprue failed to absorb vitamin B$_{12}$. At this stage of the disease, when the histological appearance of the ileum may still be normal, there may be a rapid improvement in vitamin B$_{12}$ absorption following treatment with oral broad spectrum antibiotics, suggesting that bacterial overgrowth within the gut lumen may be responsible for malabsorption at this stage. (O'Brien & England 1971, Tomkins et al. 1978). The response at this early phase is similar to that seen in the stagnant loop syndrome (Chapter 15, p. 259) in which bacterial uptake of the B$_{12}$-IF complex inhibits absorption (Schjønsby et al. 1973).

As the disease progresses, however, and mucosal lesions of the ileum develop, malabsorption of vitamin B$_{12}$ may become a persistent and constant feature of the disorder. This is in striking contrast to the situation in coeliac disease, a proximal intestinal disorder, in which there is rarely significant B$_{12}$ malabsorption even in long-continued disease. When sprue has been present for months or years, there is evidence that the defect in vitamin B$_{12}$ absorption is due to the defect in the intestinal mucosa (Kapadia et al. 1976). At this stage, improvement in absorption following antibiotics takes place only after a considerable time (Table 19.3), presumably a reflection of the time required for the ileal mucosal lesion to recover.

In patients with chronic tropical sprue rendered asymptomatic by treatment, there may be a persistent latent defect in vitamin B$_{12}$ absorption. Rarely this may lead to the development of severe vitamin B$_{12}$ deficiency and megaloblastic anaemia, resembling Addisonian pernicious anaemia, many years after an individual has returned from the tropics to a temperate climate (Mollin & Booth 1971).

Clinical features and treatment

Tropical sprue occurs in three main groups of subjects. The major group includes large numbers of patients among indigenous populations of the world where the disorder occurs in both endemic and epidemic forms. Expatriates living in such areas, such as military or diplomatic personnel, are also subject to the disease. In temperate climates, the disorder is seen most frequently amongst travellers and tourists who have returned

Table 19.3. Serial Schilling tests (oral dose 1 μg ^{57}Co-B$_{12}$) in a patient with chronic tropical sprue treated with oral broad spectrum antibiotics.

	% of dose excreted in urine in 24h*
After folic acid (30 mg daily for 4 months)	1.3
After antibiotics (3 successive 5-day courses of chlortetracycline, chloramphenicol and sulphasuccidine)	
10 days	2.6
4 months	6.2
16 months	4.6
2 years	7.8
3 years	10.2

*Normal should be greater than 10% (Mollin & Booth 1971).

from visits to endemic areas of the world, such as the Indian subcontinent or the Caribbean. A chronic form of the disease may also be encountered among Caucasian ex-residents of endemic areas who have returned to live in the temperate zone. Thirdly, inhabitants of endemic areas who emigrate to temperate climates, for example Indians living in Britain or citizens of Central America or the Caribbean living in the major cities of the USA, may develop symptoms and signs of tropical sprue often some years after leaving the tropics.

Acute tropical sprue

This form of the disease has been repeatedly described in endemic areas among military personnel or volunteer workers who live temporarily in the tropics. It was a major cause of morbidity among British and Indian troops in India and Burma during World War II, in American military personnel in the Philippines, Puerto Rico and Vietnam, and in soldiers and their families in Malaya and Singapore during the 1960s. It also occurs during epidemics of tropical sprue in endemic areas. Individuals travelling overland from Europe to India (Fig 19.7) (Tomkins *et al.* 1974) and tourists after a holiday abroad may also develop tropical sprue. In general, the condition is declining in incidence in Britain, partly as a result of restrictions in overland travel to the Indian subcontinent, but probably also because antibiotics are so frequently prescribed for acute diarrhoeal illnesses.

Symptoms and signs

The main presenting symptom is chronic diarrhoea which is accompanied by gaseous abdominal distension. Some patients identify the start of the illness clearly with an

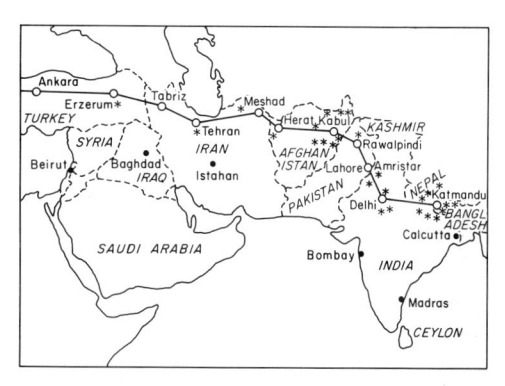

Fig. 19.7. Route taken by overland travellers to India who developed malabsorption. Asterisks indicate the place of onset of symptoms (Tomkins *et al.* 1974).

acute diarrhoeal illness with vomiting, pyrexia and abdominal pain. Others, especially indigenous subjects, experience a more gradual onset of diarrhoea. As the symptoms continue the distension becomes more severe and marked intolerance to milk may occur as lactose intolerance develops. Many expatriates with tropical sprue complain of a worsening of the diarrhoea and unpleasant after-effects following small quantities of alcohol. With progression of symptoms there may be anorexia, sometimes severe, which together with malabsorption is responsible for weight loss and vitamin and mineral deficiencies. In those with severe watery diarrhoea hypokalaemia may occur. Occasionally tetany due to hypocalcaemia or hypomagnesaemia develops.

Depending on the initial nutritional status of the individual, the degree of anorexia, the severity of the malabsorption and the duration of the illness, a variety of nutritional deficiencies ensue. Folate deficiency is usually the first; the serum and red blood cell folate levels fall and blood examination shows macrocytosis. After 3 months or more of symptoms, the tongue may become smooth and painful and megaloblastic anaemia develops. In pregnancy or soon after childbirth, however, megaloblastic anaemia occurs much earlier in the course of the disease.

Diagnosis

This is established by demonstrating the presence of malabsorption using tests of absorption of xylose, fat and vitamin B_{12} and by recognizing the features of tropical sprue on jejunal biopsy. It is also essential to exclude other more common causes of malabsorption and diarrhoea such as bacterial infection (Chapter 14) and parasitological disorders, of which the most important is giardiasis (Chapter 17). Amoebiasis is usually associated with blood and mucus in the stools. Strongyloidiasis usually presents with severe diarrhoea and steatorrhoea, together with a marked eosinophilia in individuals visiting the tropics from the temperate zone. Other conditions of the small intestine causing diarrhoea, such as Crohn's disease or coeliac disease, may present following a visit to the tropics or when living in an area endemic for tropical sprue. Such conditions should be excluded by careful radiological examination and jejunal biopsy.

Treatment

If symptoms are mild and diarrhoea is improving, the patient may be reassured that the natural history is of spontaneous improvement. Symptoms may also be improved by the avoidance of lactose and alcohol. Folic acid (5 mg twice daily for 10 days) ensures full recovery in most patients.

If symptoms are more marked and there is weight loss, poor appetite, a low serum or red cell folate level or macrocytic anaemia, folic acid should be given (5 mg twice daily) together with tetracycline (250 mg four times daily) for 4 weeks. In British servicemen treated with this regime in the Far East (O'Brien & England 1971), recovery was faster than when folic acid was given alone. There have been, however, no carefully controlled clinical trials of antibiotics and folic acid treatment in acute tropical sprue.

In former years, before the availability of antibiotics, there was a risk of relapse of tropical sprue if the patient returned to the endemic area and individuals were often advised against further overseas service. Nowadays, provided that the symptoms, tests of absorption and mucosal histology recover fully following one or possibly two courses of tetracycline and folic acid, there appears to be little evidence of increased risk of further attacks of tropical sprue if the patient returns to his overseas post.

Chronic tropical sprue

If the acute phase of tropical sprue does not remit completely, the condition may become chronic (Mollin & Booth 1971). Patients may have been treated with folic acid (or liver extract in an earlier era) but the symptoms of diarrhoea and steatorrhoea may continue. During the early phase of chronic sprue, within the first 2–5 years after symptoms develop, folic acid deficiency is the major nutritional problem. Untreated patients may therefore develop megaloblastic anaemia, sometimes of severe degree, due to folic acid deficiency. If the condition has been treated with folic acid, however, there is usually no megaloblastic anaemia until much later in the disease. The mucosal lesion in the small intestine and particularly in the ileum may persist, however, and both steatorrhoea and defective absorption of vitamin B_{12} may continue. As time goes on, deficiency of vitamin B_{12} may therefore become a major feature of the disease. This does not occur until 4 or 5 years after the condition has been established and often much larger. Thereafter, if treatment with vitamin B_{12} is not given, B_{12} deficiency may be sufficiently severe to cause neurological signs of subacute combined degeneration of the spinal cord.

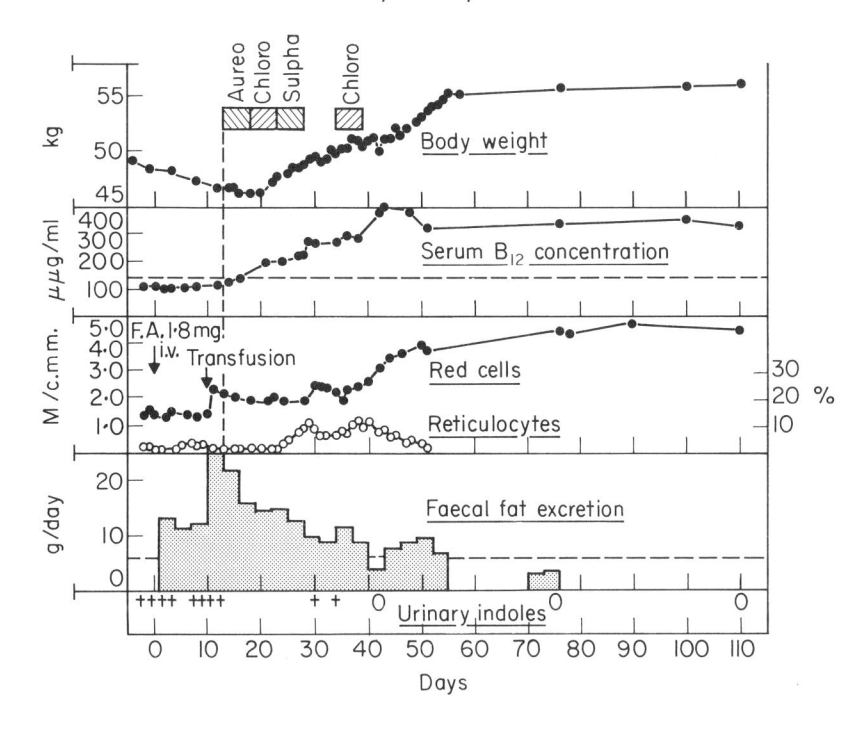

Fig. 19.8. Response to treatment with oral broad spectrum antibiotics (chlortetracycline 250 mg 6-hourly, chloramphenicol 250 mg 6-hourly and succinyl sulphathiazole 10 g daily for each of 5 days) in an Anglo-Indian patient who developed tropical sprue and severe megaloblastic anaemia 3 months after emigrating to England (Booth et al. 1968).

Treatment

Chronic sprue should be treated first by correction of nutritional deficiencies. Folic acid (5 mg twice daily) for 1 month is usually sufficient to correct deficiency; if vitamin B_{12} deficiency has developed, as evidenced by a low serum B_{12} level, parenteral injections of vitamin B_{12} should be given. Oral broad spectrum antibiotics (chlortetracycline, chloramphenicol and suplhasuccidine given in divided dosage for each of 5 days) may be followed by a slow but progressive improvement in intestinal function (Fig. 19.8), the response sometimes taking months before steatorrhoea or xylose absorption returns to normal. Vitamin B_{12} absorption returns to normal even more slowly and may never be completely normal, as illustrated by the following case history:

> E.H., a 62-year-old retired teacher and missionary, born in 1899, was referred to Hammersmith Hospital in 1961 because she had developed severe vitamin B_{12} deficiency. She had lived in India from 1929 until 1949 and had been well until 1947 when she first had an attack of diarrhoea and vomiting. She developed bulky, loose, offensive stools and lost some 13 kg in weight during the next 2 years. She returned to England in 1949 and remained reasonably well on treatment with a low fat diet and folic acid (20 mg daily). Diarrhoea continued, however, and she never felt well. In 1961 she became aware of an unpleasant numb feeling in the fingers and toes and fine movements had become increasingly clumsy. Her serum B_{12} concentration was almost unmeasurable (10 pg/ml). Intestinal biopsies showed a convoluted appearance in the jejunum and the same appearances were found in the ileum. Both jejunum and ileum showed the same degree of partial villous atrophy. Intestinal function tests showed that

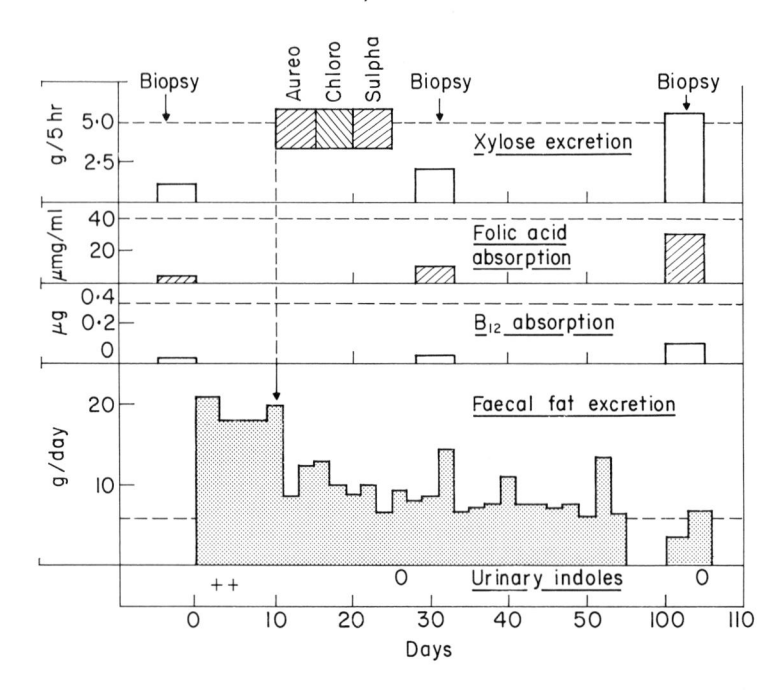

Fig. 19.9. Response of intestinal function tests to treatment with oral broad spectrum antibiotics (as described in Fig. 19.8) in a 62-year-old Englishwoman who had suffered from chronic sprue for 14 years despite continuous treatment with folic acid (Booth et al. 1968).

xylose absorption was markedly reduced, as was folic acid absorption. Faecal fat excretion ranged from 18–21 g per day during successive balance periods. Absorption or radioactive vitamin B_{12} was markedly reduced, being 0.01 µg from an oral dose of 1 µg given with intrinsic factor.

Treatment and progress. After preliminary observation, she was treated with a course of oral broad spectrum antimicrobial drugs (chlortetracycline, chloramphenicol and sulphasuccidine, each for 5 days). The initial response of her intestinal function tests and her jejunal mucosa are shown in Fig. 19.9. Soon after the antibiotics were started, there was a dramatic fall in faecal fat excretion and considerable symptomatic improvement, the stools being reduced to one to two daily. However, the jejunal biopsy and vitamin B_{12} absorption were unchanged some 25 days after initiation of treatment, although the absorption of xylose and folic acid were significantly improved. Reassessment 3 months after treatment was given showed a normal xylose absorption and almost normal folic acid absorption. There was no steatorrhoea but vitamin B_{12} absorption was still grossly abnormal. The jejunal biopsy also remained abnormal, the mucosa still showing a convoluted appearance and partial villous atrophy. Eight months later, the jejunal biopsy showed interlacing leaf-shaped villi under the dissecting microscope but histology still showed a mild, partial villous atrophy. Vitamin B_{12} absorption remained subnormal. Two years later, her jejunal biopsy was entirely normal and the only abnormality was a persistent defect in vitamin B_{12} absorption, only 3.5% of the dose given with intrinsic factor being excreted in a Schilling test. Three and a half years after treatment the Schilling test showed that she still excreted only 4.5% of the dose given with intrinsic factor, but she was now extremely well and had no intestinal symptoms.

As is illustrated by this patient, the response of the jejunal mucosa is often slow and B_{12} absorption recovers even more slowly. In chronic sprue, treatment with oral broad spectrum antibiotics for only 3 weeks (Sheehy & Perez-Santiago 1962) may be very effective but continued treatment with tetracycline (1 g daily in divided dosage) for six months or more results in a return of the intestinal lesion to normal in a high proportion of cases (Guerra et al. 1965, Maldonado et al. 1969).

Latent sprue

Sprue may be virtually symptomless when first acquired, or it may become latent after an initially mild illness. Symptoms and signs of diarrhoea, steatorrhoea and megaloblastic anaemia may therefore only develop at a later stage. An individual who has lived in the tropics and emigrated to a temperate climate may develop sprue months or years after leaving the tropical area where sprue is endemic. Such a presentation of tropical sprue has been described by Klipstein (1964) among Puerto Ricans living in New York City and by Mollin & Booth (1971) among Anglo-Indians in London. Such patients usually present with steatorrhoea and megaloblastic anaemia due to folic acid deficiency in the early years after leaving the tropics. There are other patients, however, in whom the major intestinal lesion involves the ileum. This may cause malabsorption of vitamin B_{12}, with only minimal steatorrhoea and therefore no signficant diarrhoea. Such patients may present many years after leaving the tropics with deficiency of vitamin B_{12} causing megaloblastic anaemia which is virtually indistinguishable from Addisonian pernicious anaemia. Only when the history of previous residence in an area endemic for tropical sprue is revealed, and when vitamin B_{12} absorption tests show an intestinal rather than a gastric lesion, is the true diagnosis suspected.

Indigenous sprue

In indigenous populations afflicted by tropical sprue, there is the same wide variety of symptoms as may occur in expatriates who contract the disorder in an endemic area. The most extensive studies have been carried out in South India (Baker & Mathan 1971) where patients with the disease have been investigated over long periods of time and where control subjects living in their normal environment have also been assessed.

The majority of patients complain of diarrhoea, anorexia and abdominal distension. Depending on the state of nutrition of the affected individuals when the disease is contracted, there may be symptoms of nutritional deficiency, especially pallor, weakness, sore tongue and mouth, oedema and sometimes night blindness. Studies of asymptomatic control subjects have revealed evidence of jejunal mucosal abnormalities, sometimes as severe as are seen in fully developed sprue, as well as bacterial overgrowth in the small intestine and malabsorption. These findings show that there may be a considerable number of individuals suffering from latent sprue in any endemic area and that within this population the fully developed syndrome of malabsorption and malnutrition may occur either sporadically or in epidemic form. A few patients may present with only isolated sequelae of malabsorption, such as megaloblastic anaemia, which was thought in the past to be due to nutritional deficiency; absorption studies have established that such patients may have malabsorption due to latent sprue.

Patients affected in an epidemic and some with endemic sprue may be able to remember the day and hour of onset of their symptoms. There is sometimes fever, malaise and anorexia. Thereafter, the course of the illness is determined by the severity of malabsorption and resultant malnutrition. Stools are usually watery at the onset and there may also be flecks of blood and mucus. Anorexia is often striking at the onset and the abdomen is distended. Loss of weight, anaemia, mucosal pigmentation, glossitis and angular stomatitis are the major symptoms of nutritional deficiency. Occasionally, severe hypoproteinaemia and a clinical syndrome resembling kwashiorkor may develop, particularly in severely malnourished populations as in Haiti (Klipstein et al. 1968).

Hypocalcaemia and tetany are rarely seen in sprue in South India.

Differential diagnosis

In the tropical environment, parasitic and other infections of the gastrointestinal tract must be carefully excluded. In endemic areas intestinal tuberculosis remains the most important differential diagnosis. Careful radiological examination is essential in detecting tuberculous strictures or ulceration, as well as other lesions such as lymphoma. Coeliac disease may also occur in traditional rice-eating populations whose diet increasingly includes wheat or wheat-based products.

Treatment (Mathan 1978)

Diarrhoea can usually be controlled by Loperamide (2.5—5.0 mg three or four times daily). Dehydration, electrolyte depletion and other deficiencies should be corrected. Using these simple techniques, the mortality in epidemic tropical sprue has been reduced to less than 1%. Iron and folic acid may be given orally, but vitamin B_{12} should be given parenterally since there is B_{12} malabsorption in as many as 60% of patients. In indigenous populations with sprue, the improvement in intestinal absorption following treatment with folic acid or vitamin B_{12} is no better than in control groups not so treated. Short-term antibiotic therapy (for 2 weeks) is rarely found to be effective in South India. Forty eight per cent of forty-eight patients treated with antibiotics achieved normal fat absorption but in fifty-seven control patients not treated with B_{12}, folic acid or antibiotics, the faecal fat excretion became normal in 50%. Longer-term antibiotic therapy, as recommended by Guerra *et al.* (1965), may possibly be more helpful in indigenous populations. Guerra's results in Puerto Rico showed that forteen of fifteen patients with chronic indigenous sprue improved after treatment with tetracycline (1 g daily in divided dosage) for 6 months. Spontaneous remission and relapse, however, is a frequent feature of indigenous sprue, emphasizing the need for control studies. Nevertheless, the South Indian experience shows clearly that if diarrhoea is controlled and nutritional deficiencies corrected, the patient may lead a normal life whatever the state of the jejunal mucosa.

Aetiology

The frequent accounts of nutritional deficiency in tropical sprue, particularly of folic acid and vitamin B_{12}, and the improvement in intestinal function that may follow correction of nutritional deficiency, have suggested that the condition may be basically a nutritional disease. There is no evidence to support this view. Tropical sprue afflicts individuals who are well nourished. The intestinal defect clearly leads to nutritional deficiency rather than the other way round, since deficiency states increase in severity with increasing duration of the illness. Furthermore, correction of nutritional deficiency does not invariably cure the disease. Experimental folic acid deficiency may cause abnormalities in morphology and function of the small intestine and deficiency of folate, once established, may therefore play a role in perpetuating the condition. A primary role for nutritional deficiency as a cause for tropical sprue is highly unlikely, particularly in view of the epidemiological data.

The overwhelming evidence suggests that the disorder is due to an infection with a hitherto undiscovered agent. There is clearly a large reservoir of tropical sprue among indigenous populations, particularly in the Indian subcontinent where it is likely that the condition may be latent and involve asymptomatic subjects. The pattern of the disorder with relapses and remissions, the epidemic nature of the disease, the association with particular households, the carriage to temperate zones by individuals from endemic areas, and the transmission of the disorder to visitors and travellers in the endemic area are also in keeping with an intestinal infection. If the condition is infective in origin, the aetiological agent must be capable of lying dormant for long periods, as in herpetic infections, and tropical sprue can occur many years after initial exposure.

No clear evidence exists to implicate a

particular micro-organism in tropical sprue. The role of toxigenic bacteria in the pathogenesis of the disorder is ill-defined. The dramatic improvement in intestinal function that may follow treatment with antibiotics strongly suggests that these bacteria are not 'idle by-standers' (Simon & Gorbach 1984). The basic cause of tropical sprue, however, remains as enigmatic as it was to investigators a century ago.

Tropical enteropathy

Following the development of jejunal biopsy techniques and tests of intestinal absorption, it became possible to assess the structure and function of the small intestine in asymptomatic subjects in populations of many countries. It was soon apparent that there were jejunal abnormalities among many apparently healthy, well-nourished individuals in developing countries, when compared with Caucasians living in Western Europe or North America.

Intestinal structure

The typical finger-like villi found in Caucasian subjects are present in new-born infants in the developing world. By 4–6 months of age, however, the villi in infants in developing countries are distinctly flattened, becoming 'leaf'- or ridge-shaped, with an increase in inflammatory cell infiltrate in the lamina propria and in the number of intraepithelial cell lymphocytes. These changes also occur in American Peace Corps volunteers after living in Asia for some months. Conversely the 'tropical' appearance of the villi changes to a 'Western' pattern in Asians who leave their country to work in the USA. In Zimbabwe the mucosal lesions are more prominent among those who live in villages with unprotected water supply than in those who live in towns. Similarly, mucosal lesions are more marked in American volunteers living in villages compared with diplomats in a more protected environment.

Intestinal absorption

Using the xylose absorption test it is possible to demonstrate abnormalities, by Western standards, in a similar way to those demonstrated by histological studies. In addition there may be increased excretion of faecal fat and decreased absorption of vitamin B_{12} in asymptomatic subjects in the developing world. A study of dipeptide absorption using intestinal perfusion in asymptomatic subjects in South India showed impaired absorption of glycine and glycyl-glycine compared with healthy subjects in Britain. Studies in India, Guatemala and Zimbabwe have shown that urban subjects of higher social class have better absorption of xylose than their rural countrymen. When a protected water supply was introduced into a rural Guatemalan area, the xylose absorption apparently improved.

Aetiology

Two main hypotheses have been advanced to explain these structural and functional abnormalities, usually called tropical enteropathy. These are malnutrition and infection. Malnutrition is an unlikely cause of mild small intestinal abnormalities, for many asymptomatic adults are relatively well nourished. It seems more likely that repeated intestinal infections are the important factor and studies in Bangladesh, South India and Zimbabwe show a more marked mucosal lesion in those with the greatest number of attacks of diarrhoea. No study, however, has shown the consistent presence of a single enteropathogen. This is hardly surprising as longitudinal studies have shown that enteropathogens such as rotavirus may be present for less than 1 week after an initial infection, whereas mucosal regeneration and recovery of absorption may not occur for several months. Tropical enteropathy may therefore represent a non-specific response to repeated infections by enteropathogens which damage the intestinal mucosa.

A key question is the relationship between tropical enteropathy and tropical sprue. Table 19.4 shows the large number of countries where tropical enteropathy has been

Table 19.4. Countries in which tropical enteropathy has been described.

Region	Country
Asia	Bangladesh
	India
	Thailand
	Singapore
	Pakistan
	Vietnam
Caribbean	Haiti
	Dominican Republic
	Puerto Rico
Central and South America	Mexico
	Venezuela
	Guatemala
	Peru
Africa	Nigeria
	Liberia
	Zimbabwe
	Zambia
	Egypt
Middle East	Iran

described. The geographical distribution of this seemingly ubiquitous disorder appears only to be limited by the enterprise of investigators in different countries and abnormalities of jejunal structure and function have been described in virtually every Third World country in which they have been sought.

References

Ashford B.K. (1913) Notes on sprue in Porto Rico and the result of treatment with yellow Santonin. *Amer. J. Trop. Med.* **1**, 146–158.

Ashford B.K. (1917) The etiology of tropical sprue. *Amer. J. Med. Sci.* **154**, 157–176.

Bahr P.H. (1915) *A Report on Researches in Sprue in Ceylon, 1912–1914*. Cambridge University Press, Cambridge.

Baker S.J. & Mathan V.I. (1970) Epidemic tropical sprue. Pt. II. Epidemiology. *Ann. Trop. Med. Parasit.* **64**, 453–467.

Baker S.J. & Mathan V.I. (1971) Tropical sprue in Southern India. In *Wellcome Trust Collaboration Study 1961–1969*, pp. 189–260. Wellcome Trust, Churchill Livingstone, London.

Banwell J.G., Gorbach S.L., Mitra R., Casselles J.S., Guha-Mazumder D.N., Thomas J. & Yardley J.H. (1970) Tropical sprue and malnutrition in West Bengal. II. Fluid and electrolyte transport in the small intestine. *Amer. J. Clin. Nutrit.*, **23**, 1559–1568.

Bayless T.M., Wheby M.S. & Swanson V.L. (1968) Tropical sprue in Puerto Rico. *Amer. J. Clin. Nutrit.* **21**, 1030–1041.

Begg C. (1912) *Sprue, its Diagnosis and Treatment*. John Wright & Sons, Bristol.

Bellingal G. (1818) *Practical observations on Fever, Dysentery and Liver Complaints as they occurred amongst European troops in India*. T. and C. Underwood, London.

Besterman H.S., Cook G.C., Sarson D.L., Christofides N.D., Bryant M.G., Gregor M. & Bloom S.R. (1979) Gut hormones in tropical malabsorption. *Brit. Med. J.* **2**, 1252–1255.

Bevan G., Engert R., Klipstein F.A., Maldonado B., Rubulis A. & Turner M.D. (1974) Bile salt metabolism in tropical sprue. *Gut*, **15**, 254–259.

Bhat P., Shantakamusi S., Rajan D., Mathan V.I., Kapadia C.R., Swarnabai C. & Baker S.J. (1972) Bacterial flora of the gastrointestinal tract in Southern Indian control subjects and patients with tropical sprue. *Gastroenterol.* **62**, 11–21.

Booth C.C. (1963) William Hillary: a pupil of Boerhaave. *Med. Hist.* **7**, 297–316.

Booth C.C., Tabaqchali S. & Mollin D.L. (1968) Comparison of stagnant loop syndrome with chronic tropical sprue. *Amer. J. Clin. Nutrit.* **21**, 1097–1109.

Cain J.R., Mayoral L.G., Lotero H., Bolanos O. & Buque E. (1976) Enterobacteriaceae in the jejunal microflora: prevalence and relationship to biochemical and histological evaluations in healthy Columbian men. *Amer. J. Clin. Nutrit.*, **29**, 1397–1403.

Castle W.B. (1929) Observations on the etiologic relationship of achylia gastrica in pernicious anaemia. I. The effect of the administration to patients with pernicious anaemia of the contents of the normal stomach recovered after the ingestion of beef muscle. *Amer. J. Med. Sci.* **178**, 748–764.

Castle W.B. & Townsend W.C. (1929) Observations on the etiologic relationship of achylia gastrica in pernicious anaemia. II. The effect of administration to patients with pernicious anaemia of beef muscle after incubation with normal human gastric juice. *Amer. J. Med. Sci.* **178**, 764–777.

Cook G.C. (1981) Jejunal absorption rates of glucose and glycine in post-infective tropical malabsorption. *Trans. Roy. Soc. Trop. Med. Hyg.* **75**, 378–384.

Cook G.C. (1978) Delayed small intestinal transit in tropical malabsorption. *Brit. Med. J.* **ii**, 238–240.

Corcino J.J., Maldonado M. & Klipstein F.A. (1973) Intestinal perfusion studies in tropical sprue. I. Transport of water, electrolytes and d-xylose. *Gastroenterol.* **65**, 192–198.

Corcino J.J., Reisenaver A.M. & Halsted C.H. (1976) Jejunal perfusion of simple and conjugated folates in tropical sprue. *J. Clin. Invest.* **58**, 298–305.

Crosby W.H. & Kugler H.W. (1957) Intraluminal biopsy of the small intestine, the intestine biopsy capsule. *Amer. J. Digest. Dis. N.S.* **2**, 236–241.

Drasar B.S., Gyselynck S. & Tomkins A.M. (1980) Toxin production by enterobacteria in tropical malabsorption but not in blind loop syndrome. *Gut*, **21** A926–927.

Falaiye J.M. (1970) Tropical sprue in Nigeria. *J. Trop. Med. Hyg.* **73**, 119–125.

French J.M., Gaddie R. & Smith N.M. (1956) Tropical sprue, a study of seven cases and their response to combined chemotherapy. *Quart. J. Med.* **25**, 333–351.

Gardner F. (1956) A malabsorption syndrome in military personnel in Puerto Rico. *Arch. Intern. Med.* **98**, 44–60.

Gorbach S.L., Banwell J.G., Jacobs B., Chatterjee B.D., Mitra R., Sen N.N. & Guha Mazumder D.N. (1970) Tropical sprue and malnutrition in West Bengal. I. Intestinal microflora and absorptions. *Amer. J. Clin. Nutrit.* **23**, 1545–1558.

Gorbach S.L., Mitra R., Jacobs B., Banwell J.G., Chatterjee B.D. & Guha Mazumder D.N. (1969) Bacterial contamination of the upper small bowel in tropical sprue. *Lancet*, **i**, 74–77.

Grant A. (1853) Remarks on hill diarrhoea and dysentery. *Ind. Ann. Med. Sci.*, **1**, 311–348.

Guerra R., Wheby M.S. & Bayless T.M. (1965) Long-term antibiotic therapy in tropical sprue. *Ann. Intern. Med.* **63**, 619–634.

Halsted C.H. (1980) Intestinal absorption and malabsorption of folates. *Ann. Rev. Med.* **31**, 79–87.

Hellier M.D., Radhakrishnan A.N., Ganapathy V., Mathan V.I. & Baker S.J. (1976) Intestinal perfusion studies in tropical sprue. 1. Aminoacid and dipeptide absorption. *Gut*, **17**, 511–516.

Hellier M.D., Bhat P., Albert J. & Baker S.J. (1977) Intestinal perfusion studies in tropical sprue. 2. Movement of water and electrolytes. *Gut*, **18**, 480–483.

Hellier M.D., Ganapathy C., Gammon A., Mathan V.I. & Radhakrishnan A.M. (1980) Impaired intestinal absorption of dipeptide in tropical sprue patients in India. *Clin. Sci.* **58**, 431–433.

Hillary W. (1759) *Observations on the Change in the Air and the Concomitant Epidemical Disease in the Island of Barbados*. Hitch and Hawes, London.

Jarumilinta R., Miranda M. & Villarejos V.M. (1976) A bacteriological study of the intestinal mucosa and luminal fluid of adults with acute diarrhoea. *Ann. Trop. Med. Parasitol.* **70**, 165–179.

Kapadia C.R., Bhat P., Jacob E. & Baker S.J. (1976) Vitamin B_{12} malabsorption. A study of intraluminal events in control subjects and patients with tropical sprue. *Gut*, **16**, 988–993.

Klipstein F.A. (1964) Tropical sprue in New York City. *Gastroenterol.* **47**, 457–470.

Klipstein F.A., Samloff I.M., Smarth G. & Schenk E.A. (1968) Malabsorption and malnutrition in rural Haiti. *Amer. J. Clin. Nutrit.* **21**, 1042–1052.

Klipstein F.A. & Falaiye J. (1969) Tropical sprue in expatriates from the tropics living in the continental United States. *Med. (Balt.)* **48**, 475–491.

Klipstein F.A., Haldeman L.V., Corcino J.J. & Moore W.E.C. (1973) Enterotoxigenic intestinal bacteria in tropical sprue. *Ann. Intern. Med.* **79**, 632–641.

Klipstein F.A. & Corcino J.J. (1975) Malabsorption of essential amino acids in tropical sprue. *Gastroenterol.* **68**, 239–244.

Klipstein F.A., Horowitz I.R., Engert R.F. & Schenk E.A. (1975) Effect of *Klebsiella pneumoniae* enterotoxin on intestinal transport in the rat. *J. Clin. Invest.* **56**, 799–807.

Klipstein F.A. & Schenk E.A. (1975) Enterotoxigenic intestinal bacteria in tropical sprue. II. Effect of the bacteria and their enterotoxins on intestinal structure. *Gastroenterol.* **68**, 642–655.

Klipstein F.A., Short H.B., Engert R.F., Jean L. & Weaver G.A. (1976) Contamination of the small intestine by enterotoxigenic coliform bacteria among the rural population of Haiti. *Gastroenterol.* **70**, 1035–1041.

Klipstein F.A., Goetsch C.A., Engert R.F., Short H.B. & Schenk E.A. (1979) Effect of monocontamination of germ-free rats by enterotoxigenic coliform bacilii. *Gastroenterol.* **76**, 341–348.

Lindenbaum J. (1968) Small intestinal dysfunction in Pakistanis and Americans resident in Pakistan. *Amer. J. Clin. Nutrit.* **21**, 1023–1029.

Mackie F.P. & Fairley N.H. (1928-29) The morbid anatomy of sprue. *Ind. J. Med. Res.* **16**, 799–811.

Mackie F.P. & Fairley N.H. (1933-34) Gross and microscopic anatomy of the intestinal canal from two cases of sprue. *Trans. Roy. Soc. Trop. Med. Hyg.* **23**, 340.

Mackie F.P., Gore S.N. & Wadia J.H. (1928) The bacteriology of sprue. *Ind. J. Med. Res.* **16**, 95–108.

Macnaughton M.R. & Davies H.A. (1981) Human enteric Coronaviruses. *Arch. Virol.* **70**, 301–313.

Maldonado N., Horta E., Guerra R. & Perez-Santiago E. (1969) Poorly absorbed sulfonamides in the treatment of tropical sprue. *Gastroenterol.* **57**, 559–568.

Manson P. (1880) Notes on sprue. *Med. Rep. China Imp. Marit. Customs*, **19**, 33–37.

Manson-Bahr P.H. (1924) The morbid anatomy and pathology of sprue and their bearing upon aetiology. *Lancet*, **i**, 1148–1151.

Manson-Bahr P.H. (1928) Sprue indigenous to Nyasaland. *Trans. Roy. Soc. Trop. Med. Hyg.* **22**, 81–82.

Mathan V.I. & Baker S.J. (1971) The epidemiology of tropical sprue. In *Wellcome Trust Collaborative study 1961–69*, pp. 159–188. Wellcome Trust, Churchill Livingstone, London.

Mathan V.I. (1978) Tropical sprue. In *Gastrointestinal Diseases*. 2nd ed., pp. 1143–1154. (Ed. by M.H. Sleisenger & J.S. Fordtran). W.B. Saunders Co., Philadelphia.

Mathan M., Mathan V.I. & Baker S.J. (1975) An electron microscope study of jejunal mucosal morphology in control subjects and in patients with tropical sprue in Southern India. *Gas-*

troenterol. **68**, 17−32.

Milanes F., Leon P. & Cause A. (1951) Jejunal histopathological studies through surgical biopsy in a case of tropical sprue in relapse. *Rexista Gastroent. Mex.* **18**, 182.

Minot G.R. & Murphy W.P. (1926) Treatment of pernicious anaemia by a special diet. *J. Amer. Med. Assoc.* **87**, 470−476.

Mollin D.L. & Booth C.C. (1971) Chronic tropical sprue in London. In *Wellcome Trust Collaborative Study 1961−69*, pp. 61−127. Wellcome Trust, Churchill Livingstone London.

Morehead C. (1860) *Clinical Researches in Diseases in India*, 2nd ed. Longman and Roberts, London.

Moshal M.G., Hirst W., Kallicburum S. & Pillay K. (1975) Enteric tropical sprue in Africa. *J. Trop. Med. Hyg.* **78**, 2−5.

O'Brien W. & England N.W.J. (1971) Tropical sprue amongst British Servicemen and their families in South-east Asia. In *Wellcome Trust Collaborative Study 1961−69*, pp. 25−60. Wellcome Trust, Churchill Livingstone London.

Ramakrishna B.S. & Mathan V.I. (1982) Water and electrolyte absorption by the colon in tropical sprue. *Gut*, **23**, 843−846.

Rogers L. (1938) The use of prontosil in sprue. *Brit. Med. J.* **ii**, 943−944.

Schenk E.A., Samloff I.M. & Klipstein F.A. (1965) Morphological characteristics of jejunal biopsies in celiac disease and tropical sprue. *Amer. J. Path.* **47**, 765−782.

Schjønsby H., Drasar B.S., Tabaqchali S. & Booth C.C. (1973) Uptake of vitamin B_{12} by intestinal bacteria in the stagnant loop syndrome. *Scand. J. Gastroent.* **8**, 41−47.

Sheehy T.W. & Perez-Santiago E. (1961) Antibiotic therapy in tropical sprue. *Gastroenterol.* **41**, 208−214.

Sheehy T.W., Cohen W.H., Wallace D.K. & Legtens L.J. (1965) Tropical sprue in North Americans. *J. Amer. Med. Assoc.* **194**, 1069−1076.

Shiner M. (1956) Jejunal-biopsy tube. *Lancet*, **i**, 85.

Shiner M. & Doniach J. (1960) Histopathological studies in steatorrhoea. *Gastroenterol.* **38**, 419−440.

Simon G.L. & Gorbach S.L. (1984) Intestinal flora in health and disease. *Gastroenterol.* **86**, 174−93.

Spies T.D., Milanes F., Menandez A., Koch M.B. & Minnich V. (1946) Observations on treatment of tropical sprue with folic acid. *J. Lab. Clin. Med.* **31**, 223−241.

Spies T.D. & Suarez R.M. (1948) Responses of tropical sprue to vitamin B_{12}. *Blood*, **3**, 1213−1220.

Stefanini M. (1948) Clinical features and pathogenesis of tropical sprue: observations on a series of cases among Italian prisoners of war in India. *Med. (Balt).* **27**, 379−427.

Suarez R.M., Spies T.D. & Suarez Jr R.M. (1947) Use of folic acid in sprue. *Ann. Intern. Med.* **26**, 643−677.

Swaminathan N., Mathan V.I., Baker S.J. & Radakrishnan A.N. (1970) Disaccharidase levels in jejunal biopsy specimens from American and South Indian control subjects and patients with tropical sprue. *Clinica Clinica Acta.* **30**, 707−712.

Swanson V.L. & Thomassen R.W. (1963) Pathology of the jejunal mucosa in tropical sprue. *Amer. J. Path.* **46**, 511−551.

Thaysen T.E.H. (1931) Pathological anatomy of the intestinal tract in tropical sprue. *Trans. Roy. Soc. Trop. Med. Hyg.* **24**, 539−548.

Thin G. (1897) *Psilosis or Sprue*. Churchill, London.

Tirruppathi C., Balasubramanian K.A., Hill P.G. & Mathan V.I. (1983) Faecal-free fatty acids in tropical sprue and their possible role in the production of diarrhoea by an inhibition of ATPases. *Gut*, **24**, 300−305.

Thomas G. & Clain D.J. (1976) Endemic tropical sprue in Rhodesia. *Gut*, **12**, 877−887.

Tomkins A.M. (1981) Tropical malabsorption: recent concepts in pathogenesis and nutritional significance. *Clin. Sci.* **60**, 131−137.

Tomkins A.M., James W.P.T., Cole A.C.E. & Walters J.H. (1974) Malabsorption in overland travellers to India. *Brit. Med. J.* **3**, 380−384.

Tomkins A.M., Drasar B.S. & James W.P.T. (1975) Bacterial colonisation of jejunal mucosa in acute tropical sprue. *Lancet*, **i**, 59−62.

Tomkins A.M., Smith R. & Wright S.G. (1978) Assessment of early and delayed responses in vitamin B_{12} absorption during antibiotic therapy in tropical malabsorption. *Clin. Sci. Mol. Med.* **55**, 533−539.

Tomkins A.M., Wright S.G. & Drasar B.S. (1980) Bacterial colonisation of the upper intestine in mild tropical malabsorption. *Trans. Roy. Soc. Trop. Med. Hyg.* **74**, 752−755.

Twining W. (1832) *Clinical Illustrations of the Most Important Disease of Bengal*, p. 106. Parbury, Allen, Calcutta.

Wellcome Trust Collaborative Study 1961−1969 (1971) *Tropical Sprue and Megaloblastic Anaemia*. Churchill Livingstone, Edinburgh.

Wheby M.S., Swanson V.L. & Bayless T.M. (1971) Comparison of ileal and jejunal biopsies in tropical sprue. *Amer. J. Clin. Nutrit.* **24**, 117−123.

Chapter 20
Vascular Abnormalities

GRAHAM NEALE

The mesenteric circulation 333
Experimental intestinal ischaemia 334
Disease of large arteries 335
Clinical features of ischaemia 336
Diseases of small arteries 338
Other ischaemic disorders of the small
  intestine 342
Vascular malformations 343

Disorders of blood vessels supplying the small intestine can cause dramatic disease. The end result may be infarcted bowel or severe intestinal haemorrhage. The spectrum of disease is broad. Short-lived ischaemia causes transient mucosal damage with ulceration, but this may be followed by rapid healing and total recovery of gut structure and function. Prolonged ischaemia causes necrosis of submucosal tissue which, if transmural, results in gangrene and ultimately perforation of the gut. An episode of intermediate severity leads to tissue damage, which may heal by fibrosis, and results in the formation of strictures.

The mesenteric circulation

Anatomy

The splanchnic arterial tree consists of the main vessels (which for the small intestine comprise the coeliac axis and its major branches and the superior mesenteric artery), the intermediate vessels and the microcirculation which is particularly important at the mucosal interface. The jejunal and ileal circulation comes from the superior mesenteric artery via the intestinal arteries which vary in number from five to twenty and which form a series of vascular arcades increasing in number and complexity towards the ileum. From the arcades arise vessels which pierce the muscular wall of the small intestine to feed a submucosal plexus which provides a rectilinear network of arterioles extending along the whole small intestine. From this plexus spring the arterioles which supply the villi.

The mucosal plexus is richer and better developed than in the large intestine which may help explain its greater ability to withstand ischaemic insult. A reduced blood flow through the superior mesenteric artery is usually readily compensated by anastomotic flow from the territories of adjacent arteries. Thus even acute occlusion of the superior mesenteric artery will usually leave a critical 25–30 cm of viable jejunum which is often sufficient to maintain nutritional requirements (cf. Chapter 6).

Physiology

The factors which control the blood supply to the mucosa of the small intestine are still poorly understood despite considerable advances in knowledge over the past decade.

The splanchnic blood volume in a 70-kg man is estimated to be approximately 1500 ml with a flow of perhaps 1 l/min. Following a meal the flow of blood in the superior mesenteric artery increases by 50% or more above resting values ('digestive hyperaemia'). This appears to be mediated by the gastrointestinal hormones gastrin, secretin and cholecystokinin and by local autonomic reflexes.

The physiological factors which determine the flow of blood to the intestine and its distribution inter-react in a complex manner. Some are centrally determined (cardiac output, central arterial pressure, central autonomic control), others appear to operate at the gut level (neurohormonal messengers and biochemical factors) and in addition there are local mechanical factors and reflexes (Marston 1977a).

Of the various layers of the wall of the small intestine the mucosa has by far the greatest need for blood. Oxygen is needed to maintain the metabolic activities of the enterocytes and a constant flow of plasma is necessary to carry nutrients from the lumen of the intestine. Blood can be redistributed from one layer of the intestine to another by the operation of variable vascular resistances within the gut wall (Folkow 1967). Moreover a counter current system has been shown to operate within the intestinal villus (Lundgren 1974), creating a zone of hyperosmolarity at its tip. These mechanisms are of considerable importance in understanding the effects of ischaemia. The cells at the tips of the villi are peculiarly vulnerable to ischaemic damage because of the shunting of oxygen; basal villus and crypt cells are better protected and provide a means of mucosal regeneration after damage.

Experimental intestinal ischaemia

It is not easy to produce an experimental model for the study of ischaemic small intestine. Many studies have been undertaken but it is almost impossible to extrapolate from data obtained in experimental animals to human pathology. Firstly there are important inter-species differences in the anatomy of the circulation to the small intestine; secondly it is difficult to mimic human vascular pathology (especially that of atheromatous disease); and finally the response to low flow states may be very different depending on factors which are impossible to control (e.g. neurohormonal responses, bacterial and enzyme contents of the small intestine).

Acute vascular occlusion

Structural damage to the mucosa of the small intestine occurs within minutes of total circulatory arrest. Under the electron microscope the microvilli of enterocytes at the tips of villi show the first signs of damage (Varkonyi *et al.* 1977) and by light microscopy the epithelial cells are seen to become detached from the basement membrane (Wagner *et al.* 1979). Within 30–60 min the upper two-thirds of the villi are denuded of cells (Robinson & Mirkovitch 1972) whereas crypt cells remain *in situ* and show little change.

Cytochemical changes (Robinson *et al.* 1981) appear to correlate well with morphological appearances. Brush border enzyme activity is reduced and within an hour of ischaemia the mucosa has lost its capacity for the active transport of sugars and amino acids. The mechanism of the early cell damage remains uncertain but is probably due to a loss of energy-dependent processes. This may explain not only the seepage of fluid into subepithelial spaces and the associated detachment of cells (Wagner *et al.* 1979) but also the reduction in concentrations of key enzymes as regenerative processes fail to keep pace with the catabolic effect of the intraluminal digestive enzymes (Bounous *et al.* 1979).

The recovery of the mucosa of the small intestine after an acute ischaemic insult is equally remarkable. The damage caused by total ischaemia for 1 h may be reversed in 2–3 days. If the blood supply is cut off for 2 h the dying mucosa may take a week to recover. In dogs the intestinal mucosa may still regenerate after periods of ischaemia lasting 7 h (Glotzer *et al.* 1962). After short periods of ischaemia (say 30 min) the small intestine will have lost most of its normal function and the epithelium from the upper two-thirds of the villi will have been shed. Recovery appears to take place in two phases. Within 24 h a new epithelial covering has been generated by the cells from the lower third of the villi. The new villi are initially stunted and distorted, returning to their normal form as the cells proliferate and migrate upwards from the crypts (Menge & Robinson 1979).

Experimentally, damage to the ischaemic intestinal mucosa can be slowed by intraluminal factors such as the presence of glucose and oxygen in solution (Robinson & Mirkovitch 1977). On the other hand the accumulation of fluid in obstructed intestine does not impair the recovery of ischaemic intestine (Mirkovitch *et al.* 1976).

Chronic intestinal ischaemia

Experimental studies on the effects of chronic intestinal ischaemia are few. In humans the atherosclerotic process rarely leads to chronic ischaemia because of the efficiency of the collateral arterial links which are rarely occluded. In experimental animals it has not proved possible to mimic the generalized lesions necessary to slow the blood supply to the small intestine to what is probably a fairly exact critical level (Robinson et al. 1981).

Non-occlusive intestinal infarction

The effects of profound hypotension on perfusion of the small intestine have been studied in the experimental animal (Wolf & Sumner 1973). During shock the actively perfused microcirculation of the mucosa and submucosa is decreased by more than 80% and of the muscle layers by more than 50%. The development of shallow ulcers in the small intestine in severe shock is probably not uncommon although less well recognized than similar changes in the stomach (Schellerer 1974).

Little is known about blood flow to the small intestine and its distribution under other circumstances but no significant changes have been reported in experimental infections (Norris & Sumner 1974).

Disease of large arteries

The mesenteric arteries may be occluded by external compression, or by expansion of an intramural atheromatous plaque, thrombosis or emboli. Often more than one process is involved. In most cases symptoms occur only if there is a sudden critical reduction of blood flow, often with extending thrombosis as the final insult.

Compression of mesenteric vessels

Vascular compression is a rare cause of small intestinal ischaemia. It may be caused by retroperitoneal haematomata following trauma or in association with a leaking aneurysm, by neoplastic infiltration, or rarely as a result of proliferating fibrous tissue in retroperitoneal fibrosis or very exceptionally around carcinoid tumours (Anthony 1970).

Atheroma

Atheromatous occlusion of the roots of the major arteries is a common occurrence but the pathological process usually progresses sufficiently slowly to allow for the development of a collateral circulation. Evidence from autopsies and by aortic angiography shows that in the Western world 40% of subjects over the age of 45 and two-thirds over the age of 55 have atheromatous narrowing or occlusion of the coeliac axis or superior mesenteric arteries. The inferior mesenteric artery is less often affected. The lesions are mainly confined to the aortic origins of the vessels and rarely cause overt bowel ischaemia (Derrick et al. 1959, Reiner 1964). Intestinal infarction secondary to atheromatous occlusion of one major vessel is uncommon. Indeed all three major vessels may be occluded without visceral damage (Chiene 1869, Marston 1977b).

Arterial thrombosis

Thrombosis of a large vessel often develops in association with an ulcerated atheromatous plaque but may also occur as a result of such disorders as sickle-cell disease (Matthews 1981), polycythaemia rubra vera, thrombophlebitis migrans (Trousseau's syndrome) (Durham 1955), thrombotic thrombocytopaenic purpura, cryoglobulinaemia, amyloidosis and the use of the contraceptive pill (Martel et al. 1972).

Embolic occlusion

Systemic arterial embolism may account for a third of cases of mesenteric vascular occlusion (Skinner et al. 1974) but this is an artificial statistic because the accuracy of diagnosis is often inadequate. Emboli arise from the heart especially in patients with mitral stenosis and atrial fibrillation but also in those who have endocardial thrombosis following myocardial infarction or bacterial vegetations on damaged valves. Embolism from aortic mural thrombi appears to be a rare occurrence and certainly paradoxical emboli from the systemic venous system through a patent foramen ovale are very uncommon.

Clinical features of ischaemia

Mesenteric vascular insufficiency may cause acute or chronic disease. Acute intestinal ischaemia with actual or threatened gangrene is a surgical emergency; chronic intestinal ischaemia is difficult to recognize but classically causes abdominal angina.

Acute intestinal ischaemia

Ischaemic necrosis of the small intestine occurs especially in the elderly with cardiovascular pathology but may be seen in any age group as a result of the pathological conditions already described. The onset of disease is usually abrupt. Often the patient is under treatment in hospital for a condition associated with vascular insufficiency. Abdominal pain is the key symptom. At the onset it is usually colicky and poorly localized. As the situation progresses the pain becomes constant and unremitting. Initially it is often localized to the right iliac fossa and then spreads over the entire abdomen. Diarrhoea is usual and frequently the stools contain blood. Vomiting may occur but haematemesis is rare.

In the early stages of illness the distress of the patient is out of all proportion to the physical signs. This may mislead the inexperienced clinician who will be inclined to dismiss the symptoms as over-reaction or due to anxiety. There may be slight tenderness in the right iliac fossa and some exaggeration of bowel sounds. As the condition develops over the course of hours, or at the most a day or two, the abdomen becomes distended and silent. There is increasing tenderness and a positive rebound sign. At the same time signs of peripheral circulatory failure appear. The patient becomes pale, anxious, sweating and tachypnoeic. Later as the blood pressure falls, there is cyanosis and anuria. At this stage intestinal necrosis has almost certainly gone beyond the point of recovery.

The diagnosis may be suspected on clinical grounds but is often difficult and delayed. It may depend on the efficiency with which other causes of abdominal catastrophe can be excluded. Needling the peritoneal cavity usually produces blood-stained fluid.

Plain radiographs of the abdomen may show non-specific dilatation of loops of intestine with multiple fluid levels. The presence of gas bubbles in the portal vein is diagnostic of intestinal necrosis but only at a stage when the patient is beyond recovery. The place of pre-operative aortography is not yet clearly defined.

Management

Initially, treatment should deal with losses of water, electrolytes and protein which lead to hypovolaemia and impaired tissue perfusion, bacterial invasion and disseminated intravascular coagulation. Experimental studies indicate that the effects of ischaemia can be ameliorated by the administration of 100% oxygen (Aho et al. 1973). There is little data on the possible benefit of other therapies such as the use of antibiotics and the provision of optimal forms of nutrition for dying mucosal cells.

The value of pharmacological agents such as phenoxybenzamine, glucagon or dopamine to improve the mesenteric circulation remains uncertain. Similarly there is no clear evidence regarding the potential beneficial effect of large doses of corticosteroids.

If full thickness infarction is suspected, the intestine must be inspected surgically. Unfortunately the macroscopic criteria for the viability of an ischaemic segment of intestine (colour, bleeding, peristalsis) are unreliable. Attempts to obtain better indices have provided interesting physiological and pathophysiological data on the effects of ischaemia, such as changes in pH and of electromyographic activity (Katz et al. 1974). Studies describing the clearance of radio-labelled microspheres injected intra-arterially is an interesting approach (Norris 1977) but the technical difficulties of this method have not been solved. Fluorencent techniques offer greater promise (Carter et al. 1984).

If a large vessel is occluded, embolectomy or arterial reconstruction may be possible. In both occlusive and non-occlusive vascular disease it is necessary to decide how much intestine to resect. If there is doubt regarding the viability of the intestine left *in situ* the abdomen should be closed and re-explored 24 h later. Infiltrating the coeliac and mesenteric plexuses with local anaesthetic may help relieve vascular spasm.

The mortality of patients with intestinal necrosis is high (Cooke & Sande 1983). Those who do recover may present major problems in the management of their nutrition status (cf. Chapter 6).

Chronic intestinal ischaemia

All too often warning symptoms of impaired perfusion of the mesenteric vascular bed go unnoticed or undiagnosed. The prodromal period is usually short but the history of a quite characteristic abdominal pain occurring shortly after eating raises the possibility of chronic intestinal ischaemia. Unfortunately in the absence of any test to show functionally significant intestinal ischaemia the diagnosis is often delayed. Classically the patient suffers cramping abdominal pain 20–60 min after eating. This may be relieved by simple analgesics or by vasodilator drugs. As the condition progresses the patient becomes afraid to eat and loses weight.

The finding of a loud systolic bruit on auscultation of abdomen is a doubtfully valid physical sign. Bruits may be detected in normal subjects, young as well as old, and may be absent in patients with severe visceral arterial disease.

In practice, the diagnosis is often made only after excluding other conditions which cause obscure abdominal pain and weight loss. Standard tests of intestinal function are usually normal and are not helpful in assessing intestinal blood flow. For these reasons diagnostic problems are common as shown in the following case report:

> J.A., aged 67, a retired mechanic, who had smoked 10–20 cigarettes a day for 50 years, presented with epigastric pain and weight loss (7 kg in 6 months). He was tender in the epigastrum but physical examination was otherwise unremarkable. The blood pressure was 110/80 and all peripheral pulses were palpable.
> An upper gastrointestinal endoscopic examination revealed pre-pyloric and duodenal ulceration and the patient was given cimetidine. The abdominal pain was partially relieved but routine biochemical tests showed a fall in the concentration of circulating albumin without evidence of liver dysfunction. Within a month the abdominal pain became more severe especially after meals. The patient lost further weight and was thought to have a carcinoma. CT scanning of the abdomen and scintiscanning of the liver revealed no abnormality. The jejunum was abnormal on contrast radiography, showing thickened folds consistent with an infiltrating or an inflammatory process (Fig. 20.1a) but histology of a mucosal biopsy was normal.
> At this stage a diagnosis of ischaemic bowel disease was suggested. Aortography was performed (Fig. 20.1b). This showed extensive atheromatous disease. The coeliac axis could not be identified, although a little contrast leaked through into the hepatic and gastroduodenal arteries. The superior and inferior mesenteric arteries were occluded and on later films a small amount of dilute contrast could be seen in branches of the superior mesenteric artery and the wandering artery of Drummond.
> The patient died with almost total intestinal infarction. As often occurs, the disease caused by vascular insufficiency was obscured by other pathology within the abdomen (Morgan et al. 1982). Collateral channels were identified at angiography and with earlier diagnosis arterial reconstruction should have been possible.

338   *Chapter 20*

splanchnic circulation is usually not long delayed (Marston 1977b). Transluminal angioplasty is being evaluated (Roberts *et al.* 1983).

Coeliac axis compression

Occasionally in young adults with chronic abdominal pain and an abdominal bruit (often stated to be exacerbated by inspiration) aortography shows apparent constriction of the coeliac axis by the median arcuate ligament. It has been claimed that the arteries in the territory of the coeliac axis 'steal' blood from that of the superior mesenteric artery, thereby causing intestinal angina which may be relieved by dividing the median arcuate ligament and possibly by reconstructing the coeliac axis. Unfortunately, this is not supported by good evidence. Indeed coeliac axis 'compression' has been shown to exist in many asymptomatic patients. Moreover, although some patients claim to have been cured by coeliac axis surgery others have not been helped and few gastroenterologists now accept the validity of the syndrome.

Focal ischaemia of the small intestine

Focal ischaemia of the small intestine causes ulceration with subsequent stenosis. It occurs especially following vascular damage by blunt trauma, strangulation of a segment of mesentery and irradiation. It may also occur with minor episodes of occlusive arterial disease, whether these be thrombotic, embolic or inflammatory.

The patient with a stenotic segment of small intestine presents with the classical features of subacute intestinal obstruction. Colicky abdominal pain occurs 2–3 h after meals, associated with nausea, abdominal distension and occasional vomiting. The stricture is located by radiological examination of the small intestine and should be resected surgically.

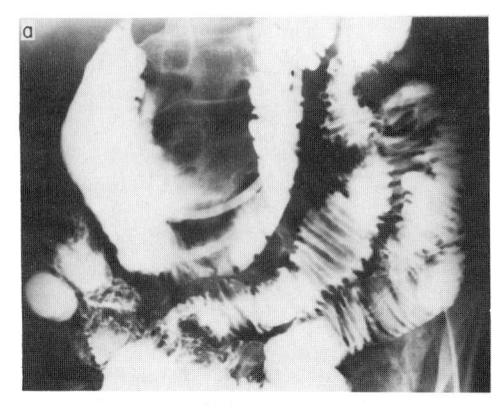

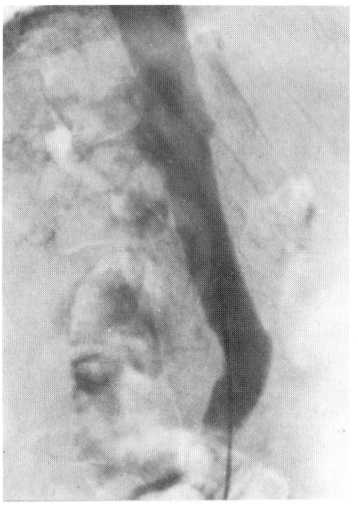

Fig. 20.1. (a) Thickened folds of small intestine on barium follow-through examination in a patient with long-standing mesenteric vascular occlusion causing ischaemia. (b) Aortogram showing occlusion of the origins of the coeliac axis, superior mesenteric and inferior mesenteric arteries. (Courtesy of Dr D. Appleton.)

Management

Chronic intestinal ischaemia secondary to large vessel disease is essentially a surgical problem. The descriptions of methods for the correction of arterial abnormalities are impressive in terms of technical skill and ingenuity. Unfortunately, however, there are very few data on how best to evaluate the results. If surgery is not possible, symptoms may be alleviated by the taking of small frequent meals. But death from vascular occlusion in the cerebral, coronary or

Diseases of small arteries

Vasculitis in the small intestine is seen in many multi-system disorders, especially polyarteritis nodosa and the collagen diseases. The end result may be ulceration, perforation or haemorrhage.

Polyarteritis and associated disorders

Polyarteritis nodosa and more rarely other arteritides such as fibro-elastic hyperplasia and Takayashu's disease affect the small intestine causing perforation and haemorrhage, focal ulceration and subsequently strictures (Rose & Spencer 1957, Carron & Douglas 1965). Köhlmeier−Degos syndrome is a variant of polyarteritis, characterized by a papular skin eruption and occlusive inflammatory lesions of small arteries (Köhlmeier 1941, Degos *et al.* 1942, Strole *et al.* 1967). Malignant granuloma (mid-line granuloma, Wegener's disease) which is associated with lesions similar to those of polyarteritis, may affect the small intestine, as illustrated by the following case report:

> M.H., aged 74, housewife, was admitted to hospital as an emergency with a history of vomiting dark fluid over the previous 24 h. She had a history of chronic bronchitis and had been unwell with cough and shortness of breath for a month following a 'flu-like illness. On examination the patient was frail and ill with a blood pressure of 150/90. She was apyrexial. The abdomen was somewhat distended with tenderness in the left hypochondrium. A straight X-ray showed gaseous distension of the transverse colon. The colonic distension was later confirmed by barium enema. Chest X-ray showed patchy consolidation which was thought to be due to bronchopneumonia or to aspiration. The haemoglobin was 10.4 g/dl, WCC 13 × 10^9/l neutrophils 11.2, lymphocytes 1.0, monocytes 0.65, eosinophils 0.15) and platelets 1170 × 10^9/l; serum proteins 54 g/l (albumin 16), bilirubin 12 µmol/l, alkaline phosphatase 134 u/l, SGOT 12 u/l, amylase 303 u/l. The urine contained albumin (+) and red blood cells but serum creatinine and blood urea remained normal throughout the illness.

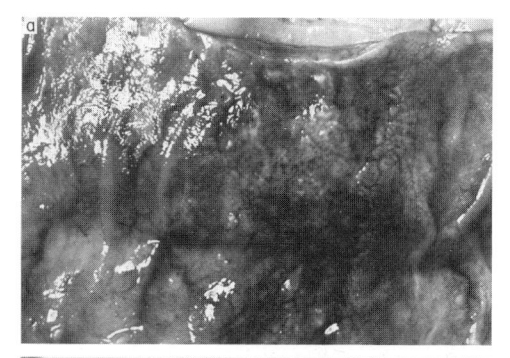

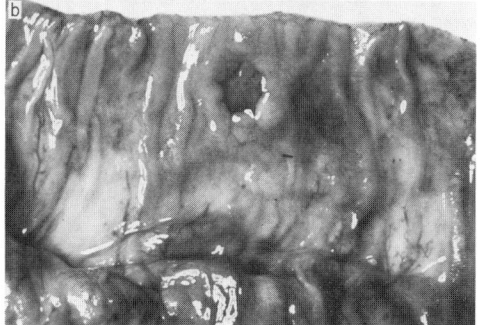

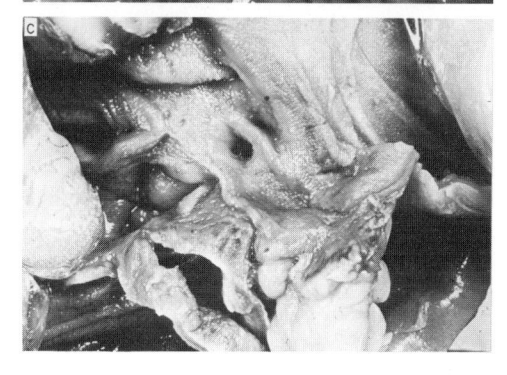

Fig. 20.2. Spectrum of lesions produced by vasculitis affecting the small intestine. (a) Injection of the mucosa and punctate ulceration in jejunum. (b) Deep punched-out ulcer in jejunum. (c) Orifices of a sinus and a fistula in the upper jejunum. The fistula connected to an adjacent loop of small intestine and there was a leak to the peritoneal cavity.

> Intra-abdominal sepsis was suspected but a gallium scan did not show an inflammatory focus.
> The patient was treated with ampicillin, gentamicin and metronidazole and was given supportive care but became progressively weaker. On the tenth hospital day the patient's temperature

rose, she became hypotensive and died within a few hours.

At necropsy, loops of jejunum were adherent in the left hypochondrium. There were three or four deep sinus tracts from the mucosal surface, one of which had perforated into the peritoneum and another had fistulated to adjacent small intestine. The rest of the small intestine appeared normal apart from one small superficial ulcer (Fig. 20.2) and a few patches of inflammation. Histology showed a vasculitis with fibrinoid necrosis affecting arteries and veins (Fig. 20.3). The kidneys were similarly affected, as were the lungs which contained necrotizing granulomata. A similar patient is described by McNabb et al. (1982)

Henoch—Schönlein purpura

Of all the vasculitis disorders, Henoch—Schönlein purpura is the condition in which the small intestine is most commonly involved. Abdominal pain with gastrointestinal bleeding occurs in more than 50% of patients. Intussusception, gross infarction and perforation are rare but well-recognized manifestations of the disease (Cream et al. 1970). The disease process is self-limiting but corticosteroids are sometimes beneficial to patients with serious organ dysfunction (Editorial 1971).

Collagen diseases

Inflammatory vascular pathology also occurs in several multi-system disorders in which there are often striking immunological findings such as systemic lupus erythematosus (SLE), rheumatoid disease, dermatomyositis, anaphylactoid purpura and diffuse systemic sclerosis. In these diseases there may be involvement of visceral muscle as well as focal ischaemic damage to the mucosa of the small intestine. Thus the disorder of the small intestine may include disturbances of motility (Chapter 4), malabsorption and protein-losing enteropathy; and occasionally pneumatosis cystoides intestinalis. In all these conditions involvement of the small intestine is uncommon and gastrointestinal symptoms are more often caused by drugs used to control the inflammatory process than by an associated vasculitis.

Systemic lupus erythematosus

In SLE, gastrointestinal symptoms are common. In most reported series, anorexia and weight loss occur in more than 50% of patients. More specific symptoms such as abdominal pain, vomiting and diarrhoea and gastrointestinal bleeding are described in about one-third of patients (Harvey et al. 1954, Dubois & Tuffanelli 1964, Hoffman & Katz 1980). Abdominal pain is usually mild and non-specific (O'Neill 1961) and dramatic gastrointestinal manifestations are uncommon. Nevertheless mucosal ulceration may cause bleeding or perforation (Dubois & Tuffanelli 1964); lymphadenopathy predisposes to intussusception (Hermann 1967) and venular inflammation is associated with protein-losing enteropathy (Weiser et al. 1981).

Rheumatoid disease

The clinical evidence of vasculitis involving the small intestine of patients with rheumatoid arthritis is similar to that of SLE. The pathology and associated symptoms are usually mild and subacute but diffuse necrosis of intestine may rarely occur (McCurley & Collins 1984). Intestinal manifestations occur especially in long-standing seropositive disease (Wilkinson & Torrance 1967, Bienenstock et al. 1967, Hart 1969). Perforation of the intestine in rheumatoid disease is a rare and usually fatal condition (Tsai 1980).

Dermatomyositis

In dermatomyositis the principal changes in the gut occur in the oesophagus. Nevertheless involvement of smooth muscle may lead to disordered motility in the small intestine and sometimes to pseudo-diverticula (Levesque et al. 1981).

Thrombotic disorders of small vessels

Microthrombosis

Diffuse thrombosis of small intestine may occur as a result of damage to vascular endothelium (as in the Schwartzmann reaction), especially in young children. The cause is not clearly established but circulating endotoxins, localized intravascular coagulation and immunological factors have all been implicated (Goldstein et al. 1979).

Haemolytic–uraemic syndrome (HUS)

The haemolytic–uraemic syndrome is a disease complex of the young in which anaemia, thrombocytopenia and renal failure dominate the clinical picture. Gastrointestinal involvement is common and many cases present with what appears to be an enterocolitis. The large intestine is more frequently involved than the jejunum or ileum but intramural bleeding and focal ulceration in the small intestine are not uncommon. Indeed any of the manifestations of ischaemic bowel disease may occur depending on the site and type of vessels involved (Whitington et al. 1979).

Infection with viruses and enteropathogenic bacteria such as Salmonellae, Shigellae (Koster et al. 1978) and Campylobacter appear to have precipitated the syndrome in several well-documentad cases (Dennenberg et al. 1982). This provides a possible link with the microangiopathy caused experimentally by the Schwartzmann reaction to repeated challenge with endotoxins.

In infants and children the mortality from haemolytic–uraemic syndrome has fallen to less than 5%. Unfavourable prognostic factors include severe gut involvement in the acute phase of the disease (Gianantonia et al. 1964).

Thrombotic thrombocytopenic purpura (TTP)

Diffuse microthrombosis also occurs in thrombotic thrombocytopenic purpura. This is a serious but uncommon disorder of young adults characterized by haemolytic anaemia, thrombocytopenia, neurological

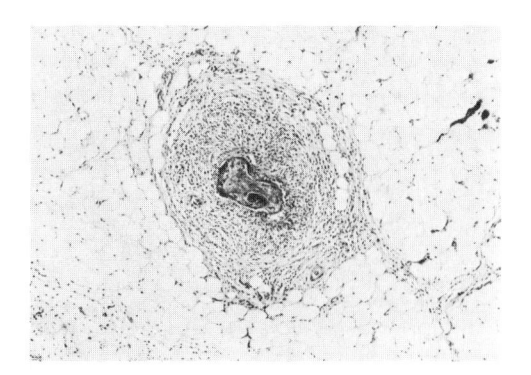

Fig. 20.3. Histology of a small vessel in the mesentery (H & E × 120) showing vasculitis.

involvement, renal disease and fever. The clinical manifestations occur as a result of diffuse disease of small vessels and the condition merges clinically and pathologically with the haemolytic–uraemic syndrome. It differs in that the lesions are more widespread and the mortality rate is higher. Nearly all patients bleed, especially from the intestine, and abdominal pain occurs in about 10% (Amorosi & Ultman 1966).

It has been postulated that patients with TTP, like those with the haemolytic–uraemic syndrome, lack a plasma factor that stimulates endothelial cells to produce prostacyclin, which is an inhibitor of platelet aggregation (Remuzzi et al. 1978, Hensby et al. 1979). The prognosis of TTP has always been considerably worse than that of HUS. Fewer than 10% survived 1 year (Amorosi & Ultman 1966) until the introduction of drugs inhibiting platelets and the use of plasma with or without exchange transfusion. With judicious treatment an increasing number of patients are managing to achieve long-lasting remissions.

Hypertensive vascular disease

Arteriolar damage with intestinal hyperplasia and fibrinoid necrosis occurs in malignant hypertension and sometimes after surgical correction of a coarctation of the aorta (Sealy 1953). The necrotizing arteritis is most marked at vessel bifurcations and appears to be related to the sudden sustained increase in blood pressure. In most cases the damage resolves spontaneously but occasionally intestinal infarction occurs (Reid & Dallachy 1958, Ibarra-Perez & Lillehei 1969).

Other ischaemic disorders of the small intestine

Venous occlusion

Acute mesenteric venous thrombosis occurs less frequently than arterial occlusion. Hypercoagulable states, sepsis, trauma and malignant infiltration predispose to this disorder. It has been reported with the use of the contraceptive pill and also following renal transplantation. In most cases the clinical picture is similar to that of intestinal infarction secondary to arterial occlusion although the onset may be sufficiently slow to allow the development of a serosanguinous ascites. Bleeding into the lumen of the gut is surprisingly rare and in general the outlook is better than that of arterial occlusion (Williams 1971).

Thromboangiitis obliterans (Buerger's disease)

Since Buerger first described the specific clinical and pathological patterns of this disease in 1908 there has been disagreement over its existence as a distinct entity (Wessler et al. 1960). Nevertheless, the pathological process appears to be distinctive. Arterial occlusion is associated with concentric thickening of the intima and transmural inflammation without necrosis or degeneration of the media. There is often associated fibrosis of adjacent veins and nerves (Vink 1973). Patients with this condition are usually heavy smokers and characteristically present with progressive peripheral arterial disease and migratory thrombophlebitis. Involvement of the mesenteric vessels is rare but may occur at any stage of the disease. It causes either low grade intestinal ischaemia with chronic abdominal pain especially after meals and weight loss, or an acute-abdominal emergency secondary to intestinal perforation. The involved segment of bowel may be in the small or large intestine. Visceral involvement in Buerger's disease appears to worsen the prognosis of this unpleasant condition (Deitch & Sikema 1981).

Fabry's disease (angiokeratoma corporis diffusum)

This sex-linked disorder of glycolipid metabolism is due to inadequate ceramide galactaryl hydrolase activity. Glycolipids are deposited in blood vessels, nerves, the cornea and renal epithelium. Most patients die in middle age of renal failure. Deposition of ceramide trihexoside in vessels of the small intestine distorts the vascular architecture and cause inflammation and thrombosis. Localized ischaemic damage causes pain and occasionally bleeding from or perforation of the small intestine (Rowe et al. 1974, Bryan et al. 1977).

Necrotizing enteritis

Sporadic and epidemic cases of necrotizing enteritis have been described in all age groups from premature neonates to the very elderly. Ischaemia is believed to be the underlying and unifying cause of this pathological process but the mechanisms are poorly defined and in most cases vascular occlusion cannot be demonstrated. Disseminated intravascular coagulation often occurs but this may be secondary to the disease process. In premature infants bacterial colonization of the gut may be delayed allowing the proliferation of potentially harmful organisms (Lawrence et al. 1982). Hexosaminadase may be a useful marker in necrotizing enterocolitis of the pre-term infant (Lobe et al. 1984).

Necrotizing enteritis in the elderly

In the Western world infarction of the small intestine without overt vascular occlusion is also recognized especially with severe low output cardiac failure in the elderly and occasionally in badly shocked subjects of any age.

In many elderly patients drugs which reduce the circulating blood volume and cause splanchnic vasoconstriction, such as powerful diuretics, digoxin, and alpha-adrenergic vasoconstrictors, may play a part. Occasionally a precipitating event cannot be identified (Williams 1971).

Angiography is useful in the diagnosis of this syndrome. The branches of the superior mesenteric artery are characteristically narrow and irregular. There may be spasm in arterial arcades, and there is poor filling of intramural vessels (Wittenberg et al. 1973). It is, however, important to exclude a surgically remediable vascular occlusion.

Necrotizing enteritis in the tropics

In tropical and sub-tropical areas the condition occurs in all age groups and may be related to environmental factors including diet, infection and infestation.

Irrespective of the aetiological factor the initial mucosal insult appears to be ischaemic. The necrotizing jejunitis related to pig-feasting (pig bel) in New Guinea is a well-studied example of this group of disorders (Murrell et al. 1966). Nearly a century ago a similar disorder was recognized in Germany. The pathology of this fatal enteritis, known as 'Darmbrand' (fire in the bowels) was not studied in detail until 50 years later (Jeckeln 1947) and was then related to the beta-toxin of *Clostridia welchii* type C. The microvasculature may be affected directly by bacterial cytoxins or indirectly by local hypersensitivity reactions to invading antigens (such as those introduced by migrating parasitic larvae). Subsequently, invading bacteria may cause the necrotic process to extend sometimes to the point of producing rapidly progressive gangrene (Arseculeratne et al. 1980).

Paroxysmal nocturnal haemoglobinuria (PNH)

Abdominal pain is sometimes a distressing symptom in patients with PNH. In a patient described by Lewis & Dacie (1967), the abdominal pain appeared to be associated with spontaneous haemorrhage in the subserosa of the small intestine. This was probably due to thrombocytopenia. In other patients, however, venous thromboses, sometimes causing small areas of necrosis of the small intestine, have been incriminated (Dacie 1967 Doukas et al. 1984).

Vascular malformations

Obscure bleeding from the gut may be due to a vascular malformation (Sheedy et al. 1975). In the small intestine vascular anomalies are difficult to identify but angiographic studies may be helpful (Fig. 20.4). At laparotomy, the lesions are often not visible and in appropriate cases further angiography on the operating table may provide invaluable help. A resected segment of intestine should be examined most carefully after injecting the arteries with colloidal barium sulphate. By this means it is often possible to confirm the presence and nature of the vascular malformation and this is an essential step before cutting the tissue for histological examination (Tarin et al. 1978). Unfortunately, resection is not always successful in controlling haemorrhage since the lesions are often multiple.

In the differential diagnosis it is important to consider vascular tumours such as leiomyomata and bleeding from ectopic gastric mucosa as in a Meckel's diverticulum. Radiolabelled red-cell scanning may give useful information in the patient who is bleeding actively but intermittently. The site of bleeding may be located approximately and this will help direct the attention of the radiologist to the segment of gut for selective and super-selective angiography.

Hereditary haemorrhagic telangiectasia

Vascular lesions of the small intestine are common in fully developed hereditary haemorrhagic telangiectasia (Rendu–Osler–Weber). Identical changes are sometimes seen in association with other conditions, for example Turner's syndrome (Haddad & Wilkins 1959) and von Willebrand's disease (Conlon et al. 1978).

Characteristically the finding of multiple lesions on the skin and buccal mucosa leads to a diagnosis of diffuse telangiectasia. Symptoms are usually delayed until late middle-life when occult bleeding from the gut causing recurrent anaemia may become a

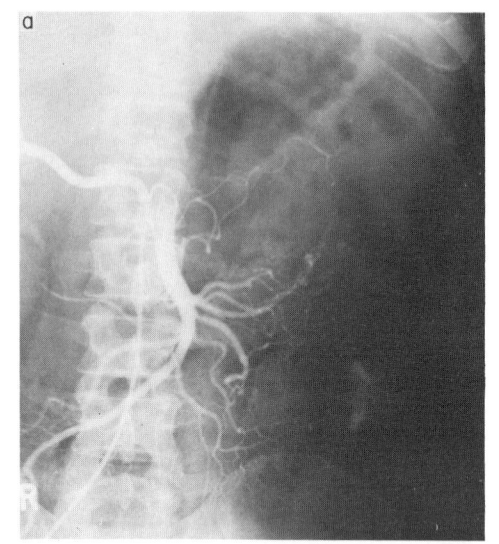

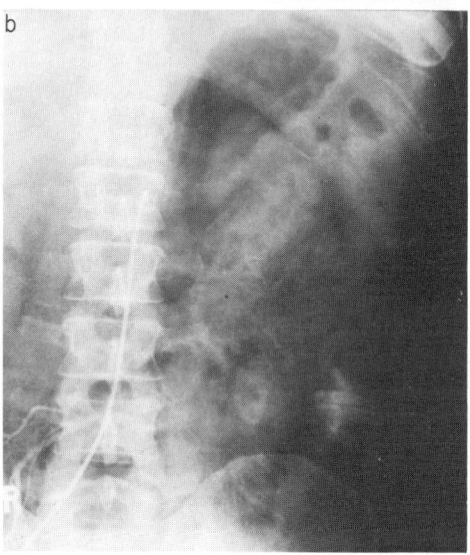

Fig. 20.4. Mesenteric angiography in a 45-year-old man with unexplained gastrointestinal bleeding. (a) Early film showing injection into superior mesenteric artery and contrast collecting in the small intestinal lumen (arrowed). (b) Later film showing residual contrast in the small intestine, outlining the valvulae conniventes. (Courtesy of Dr Anne Hemingway.)

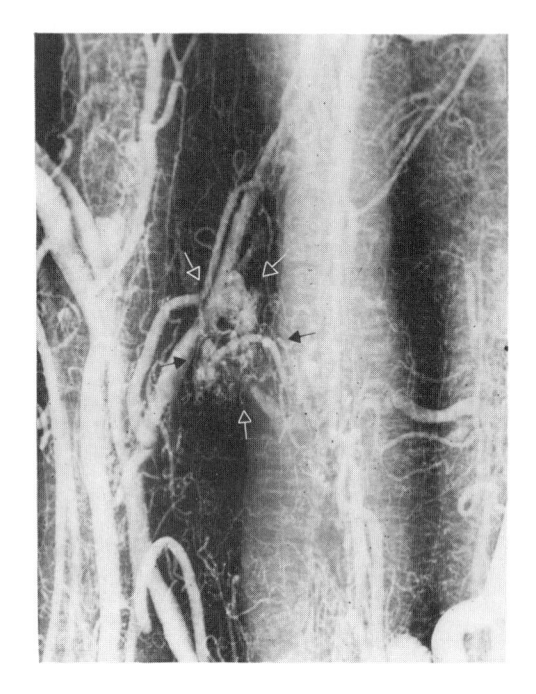

Fig. 20.5. Arteriovenous malformation (angiodysplasia) in the small intestine. Radiograph of resected segment ($\times$ 10) after arterial injection with colloidal barium. Arrows indicate the abnormal vessels. (Courtesy of Dr Anne Hemingway.)

problem. An inherited lack of elastic tissue within capillaries is thought to be the cause of increased vascular fragility, but arterioles and venules also become dilated and histologically it is not possible to distinguish the lesions of hereditary telangiectasis from those of arteriovenous malformations (angiodysplasia).

Other genetic disorders

Benign vascular malformations causing bleeding from the small intestine may occur with pseudoxanthoma elasticum (Sames 1961) and Ehlers−Danlos syndrome (Beighton et al. 1969).

Arterio−venous malformations (angiodysplasia)

Ectatic vascular lesions of the small intestine may be acquired especially in later life. In many cases there are associations with cardiovascular, renal or pulmonary disease (Rogers 1980, Cunningham 1981).

The term 'angiodysplasia' has been used for small lesions which occur especially in the older age group and predominantly in the caecum and ascending colon (Boley et al.

1977). Similar vascular abnormalities may occur in the small intestine (Fig. 20.5). Here the lesions are usually single, may be large enough to be visible at operation and often occur under the age of 50 (Moore et al. 1976).

Mesenteric varices

Patients with cirrhosis of the liver and portal hypertension frequently develop varices in the portal venous system. These rarely affect the small intestine and usually there is a predisposing cause such as intestinal adhesions (Moncure et al. 1976).

References

Aho A.J., Arstila A.U., Ahonen J., Inberg M.V. & Scheinin T.M. (1973) Ultrastructural alterations in ischaemic lesion of small intestinal mucosa in experimental superior mesenteric artery occlusion. Effect of oxygen breathing. *Scand. J. Gastroenterol.* 8, 439–447.

Amorosi E.L. & Ultman J.E. (1966) Thrombotic thrombocytopenic purpura. *Medicine*, 45, 139–159.

Anthony P.P. (1970) Gangrene of the small intestine — a complication of argentaffin carcinoma. *Brit. J. Surg.* 57, 118–122.

Arseculeratne S.N., Panabokke R.G. & Navaratnam C. (1980) Pathogenesis of necrotising enteritis with special reference to intestinal hypersensitivity reactions. *Gut*, 21, 265–278.

Beighton P.H., Murdoch J.L. & Votteler T. (1969). Gastro-intestinal complications of the Ehlers–Danlos syndrome. *Gut*, 10, 1004–1008.

Bienenstock M., Minick R. & Rogoff B. (1967) Mesenteric arteritis and intestinal infarction in rheumatic disease. *Arch. Int. Med.*, 119, 359–364.

Bluestone R., MacMahon M. & Dawson J. (1969) Systemic sclerosis and small intestinal involvement. *Gut*, 10, 185–191.

Boley, S.J. Scott J., Sammartano B.S., Adams A., DiBiase A., Kleinhaus S. & Sprayregen S. (1977) On the nature of vascular ectasias of the colon. *Gastroenterol.* 72, 650–655.

Bounous G., Proulx J., Konok G. & Wollin A. (1979) The role of bile and pancreatic proteases in the pathogenesis of ischemic enteropathy. *Int. J. Clin. Pharmacol. Biopharm.* 17, 317–323.

Bryan A., Knauft R.F. & Burns W.A. (1977) Small bowel perforation in Fabry's disease. *Ann. Int. Med.* 86, 315–316.

Buerger L. (1908) Thrombo-angiitis obliterans. A study of the vascular lesions leading to presenile spontaneous gangrene. *Amer. J. Med. Sci.* 136, 567–580.

Carron D.B. & Douglas A.P. (1965) Steatorrhoea in vascular insufficiency of small intestine. 5 cases of polyarteritis nodosum and allied disorders. *Quart. J. Med.* 34, 331–340.

Carter, M.S., Fantini, G.A., Sammartano, R.J., Mitsudo, S., Silverman, D.G. & Boley, S.J. (1984). Qualitative and quantitative fluorescein fluorescence in determining intestinal viability. *Amer. J. Surg.* 147, 117–123.

Chiene J. (1869) Complete obliteration of the coeliac and mesenteric arteries: the viscera receiving their blood supply through the extrapyramidal system of vessels. *J. Anat. Physiol.* 3, 65–72.

Conlon C.L., Weinger R.S., Cimo P.L., Moake J.L. & Olson J.D. (1978) Telangiectasia and von Willebrand's disease in two families. *Ann. Int. Med.* 89, 921–924.

Cooke, M. & Sande, M.A. (1983) Diagnosis and outcome of bowel infarction on an acute medical service. *Amer. J. Med.* 75, 984–992.

Cream J.J., Gumpel J.M. & Peachey R.D.G. (1970) Schönlein–Henoch purpura in the adult. A study of 77 adults with anaphylactoid or Schönlein–Henoch purpura. *Quart. J. Med.* 39, 461–484.

Cunningham J.T. (1981) Gastric telangiectases in chronic haemodialysis patients: a report of six cases. *Gastroenterol.* 81, 1131–1133.

Dacie J.V. (1967) *The Haemolytic Anaemias. Congenital and Acquired.* Part 4. Drug-induced haemolytic anaemias, 2nd ed. London, J. and A. Churchill. p. 1219.

Degos R., Delort J. & Tricot R. (1942) Dermatite papulo-squameuse atrophiante. *Bull. Soc. Franc. Dermat. Syph.* 49, 148–150; 281. (published in *Ann. Derm. Syph.* 1942, 8th series, vol. 2).

Deitch E.A. & Sikema W.W. (1981) Intestinal manifestations of Buerger's disease. Case report and literature review. *Amer. Surg*, 47, 326–328.

Dennenberg T., Friedberg M., Holmberg L., Mathiasen C., Nilsson K.O., Takolander R. & Walder M. (1982) Combined plasmaphoresis and haemodialysis treatment for severe haemolytic-uraemic syndrome following Campylobacter colitis. *Acta Paediat. Scand.* 71, 243–245.

Derrick J.R., Pollard H.S. & Moore R.M. (1959) The pattern of arterio-sclerotic narrowing of the coeliac and superior mesenteric arteries. *Ann. Surg.* 149, 684–690.

Doukas, M.A., Dihorenzo, P.E. & Mohler, D.N. (1984) Intestinal infarction caused by paroxysmal nocturnal haemoglobinuria. *Amer. J. Hematol.* 16, 75–81.

Dubois E.L. & Tuffanelli D.L. (1964) Clinical manifestations of systemic lupus erythematous. *J. Amer. Med. Ass.* 190, 104–111.

Durham R.H. (1955) Thrombophlebitis migrans and visceral carcinoma. *Arch. Int. Med.* **96**, 380–386.

Editorial (1971) Schönlein–Henoch in adults. *Lancet*, **i**, 437.

Folkow B. (1967) Regional adjustments of intestinal blood flow. *Gastroenterol.* **52**, 423–431.

Gianantonia C., Vitacco M., Mendilaharzu F., Rutty A. & Mendilaharzu J. (1964). The hemolytic-uremic syndrome. *J. Pediat.* **64**, 478–491.

Glotzer D.J., Villegas A.H., Anekamaya S. & Shaw R.S. (1962) Healing of the intestine in experimental bowel infarction. *Ann. Surg.* **155**, 183–190.

Goldstein M.H., Churg J., Strauss L. & Gribetz D. (1979) Hemolytic–uremic syndrome. *Nephron*, **23**, 263–272.

Haddad, H.M., & Wilkins, L. (1959) Congenital abnormalities associated with gonadal aplasia. *Pediat.* **23**, 885–902.

Hart F.D. (1969) Rheumatoid arthritis: Extra-articular manifestations I. *Brit. Med. J.* **iii**, 131–136.

Harvey A.M., Shulman L.E., Tumulty P.A., Conley C.L. & Schoenrich E.H. (1954) Systemic lupus erythematosus. Review of literature and clinical analyses of 138 cases. *Medicine*, **33**, 291–437.

Hensby C.N., Lewis P.J., Hilgard P., Mufti G.J., Hows J. & Webster J. (1979) Prostacyclin deficiency in thrombotic thrombocytopenic purpura. *Lancet*, **ii**, 748.

Hermann G. (1967) Intussusception secondary to mesenteric adenitis. *J. Amer. Med. Assoc.* **200**, 74–75.

Hoffman B.I. & Katz W.A. (1980) The gastro-intestinal manifestations of systemic lupus erythematosus: a review of the literature. *Semin. Arthritis Rheum.* **9**, 237–247.

Ibarra-Perez C. & Lillehei C.W. (1969) Treatment of mesenteric arteritis following resection of co-arctation of aorta. *J. Thor. Cardiovasc. Surg.* **58**, 135–139.

Jeckeln E. (1947) Über 'Darmbrand'; das pathologisch-anatomische Bild des Darmbrandes. *Deutsch med Wohnschr.* **72**, 105–108.

Kahn I.J., Jefferies G.H. & Sleisenger M.H. (1966) Malabsorption in intestinal scleroderma. Correction by antibiotics. *New Eng. J. Med.* **274**, 1339–1343.

Katz S., Wahab A., Murray W. & Williams L.F. (1974) New parameters of viability in ischemic bowel disease. *Amer. J. Surg.* **127**, 136–141.

Köhlmeier W. (1941) Multiple Hautnekrosen bei Thromboangiitis obliterans. *Arch. Dermat. Syph.* **181**, 783–788.

Koster F., Levin J., Walker L., Tung K.S.K., Gilman R.H., Rahaman M.M., Majid M.A., Islam S. & Williams Jr R.C. (1978) Haemolytic–uraemic syndrome after Shigellosis. Relation to endotoxemia and circulating immune complexes. *New Engl. J. Med.* **298**, 927–933.

Lawrence G., Bates J. & Gaul A. (1982) Pathogenesis of neonatal necrotising enterocolitis. *Lancet*, **i**, 137–139.

Levesque M., Fauck C., Mornet P., Barsamian L., Lecronier M. & Vital C. (1981) Manifestations digestives de la dermatomyosite. *J. Radiol.* **62**, 13–18.

Lewis S.M. & Dacie J.V. (1967) The aplastic anaemia-paroxysmal haemoglobulinuria syndrome. *Brit. J. Haemat.* **13**, 236–251.

Lobe, T.E., Richardson, C.J., Rassin, D.K., Mills, R., Schwartz, M. (1984) Hexosaminidase: a biochemical marker for necrotising enterocolitis in the pre-term infant. *Amer. J. Surg.* **147**, 49–52.

Lundgren O. (1974) The circulation of the small bowel mucosa. *Gut*, **15**, 1005–1013.

Marston A. (1977a) Regulation and distribution of intestinal blood flow. In *Intestinal Ischaemia*. Edward Arnold, London pp. 22–42.

Marston A. (1977b) Chronic intestinal ischaemia. In *Intestinal Ischaemia*. Edward Arnold, London pp. 105–131.

Martel A.J., Lillie Jr H.J. & Sawicki J.E. (1972) Haemorrhage and stenosis of the jejunum following course of progestational agent. *Amer. J. Gastroenterol.* **57**, 261–265.

Matthews M.S. (1981) Cholelithiasis: A differential diagnosis in abdominal "crisis" of sickle cell anaemia. *J. Natl. Med. Assoc.* **73**, 271–273.

McCurley, T.L. & Collins, R.D. (1984) Intestinal infarction in rheumatoid arthritis. Three cases due to unusual obliterative vascular lesions. *Arch. Pathol. Lab. Med.* **108**, 125–128.

McNabb W.R., Lenn M.S. & Wedziche J.A. (1982) Small intestinal perforation in Wegener's granulomatosis. *Postgrad. Med. J.* **58**, 123–125.

Menge H. & Robinson J.W.L. (1979) Early phase of jejunal regeneration after short-term ischemia in the rat. *Lab. Invest*, **40**, 25–30.

Mirkovitch V., Robinson J.W.L., Menge H. & Cobo F. (1976) The consequences of ischaemia after mechanical obstruction of the dog ileum. *Res. Exp. Med.* **168**, 45–55.

Moncure A.C., Waltman A.C., Valdersalm T.J., Linton R.R., Levine F.H. & Abbott W.M. (1976) Gastrointestinal hemorrhage from adhesion-related mesenteric varices. *Ann. Surg.* **183**, 24–29.

Moore J.D., Thompson N.W., Appelman H.D. & Foley D. (1976) Arterio-venous malformation of the gastro-intestinal tract. *Arch. Surg.* **111**, 381–389.

Morgan R.J., Russell R.I., Inrie C.W. & Pollack J.G. (1982) Chronic bowel ischaemia presenting as chronic pancreatitis. *Postgrad. Med. J.* **58**, 121–122.

Murrell T.G.C., Roth L., Egerton J., Samuels J. & Walker P.D. (1966) Pig bel: enteritis necroticans. A study in diagnosis and management. *Lancet*, **i**, 217–220.

Norris H.T. (1977) Ischaemic bowel disease: its spectrum. In *The Gastro-intestinal Tract*, pp. 15–30. (Ed. by J.H. Yardley, B.C. Morson &

M.R. Abell). Williams & Wilkins Co., Baltimore.

Norris H.T. & Sumner D.S. (1974) Distribution of blood flow to the layers of the small bowel in experimental cholera. Gastroenterol. 66, 973–981.

O'Neill P.B. (1961) Gastrointestinal abnormalities in collagen disease. Amer. J. Dig. Dis. 6, 1069–1083.

Reid H.C. & Dallachy R. (1958) Infarction of the ileum following resection of co-artation of aorta. Brit. J. Surg. 45, 625–632.

Reiner L. (1964) Mesenteric arterial insufficiency and abdominal angina. Arch. Int. Med. 114, 765–772.

Remuzzi G., Misiani R., Marchesi D., Livio M., Mecca G. de Gaetano G. & Donati M.B. (1978) Haemolytic-uraemic syndrome: deficiency of plasma factors regulating prostacyclin activity? Lancet, ii, 871–872.

Roberts, L.J., Wertman, D.A.J., Mills, S.R., Moore, A.V.J., Heaston, D.K. (1983) Transluminal angioplasty of the superior masenteric artery: an alternative to surgical re-vascularization. Amer. J. Roentgenol. 141, 1039–1042.

Robinson J.W.L. & Mirkovitch V. (1972) The recovery of function and microcirculation in small intestinal loops following ischaemia. Gut, 13, 784–789.

Robinson J.W.L. & Mirkovitch V. (1977) The roles of intraluminal oxygen and glucose in the protection of the rat intestinal mucosa from the effects of ischaemia. Biomed. 27, 60–62.

Robinson J.W.L., Mirkovitch V., Winistörfer B. & Saegesser F. (1981) Response of the intestinal mucosa to ischaemia. Gut, 22, 512–527.

Rogers B.H. (1980) Endoscopic diagnosis and therapy of mucosal vascular abnormalities of the gastro-intestinal tract occurring in elderly patients and associated with cardiac, vascular and pulmonary disease. Gastroint. Endorop. 26, 134–138.

Rose G.A. & Spencer H. (1957) Polyarteritis nodosa. Quart. J. Med. 26, 43–79.

Rowe J.W., Gilliam J.I. & Warthin T.A. (1974) Gastrointestinal manifestations of Fabry's disease. Ann. Int. Med. 81, 628–631.

Sames, C.P. (1961) Pseudo-xanthoma elasticum: severe melaena from the jejunum treated by resection. Proc. Roy. Soc. Med. 54, 519–520.

Schellerer W. (1974) The role of mucosal blood flow in the pathogenesis of stress ulcers. Acta Hepatogastroenterol. (Stutt.) 21, 138–141.

Sealy W.C. (1953) The indications for surgical treatment of co-arctation of aorta. Surg. Gyne. Obs. 97, 301–306.

Sheedy P.F., Fulton R.E. & Atwell D.T. (1975) Angiographic evaluation of patients with chronic gastro-intestinal bleeding. Amer. J. Roentgenol. 123, 338–347.

Skinner D.B., Zarins C. & Moosa A.R. (1974) Mesenteric vascular disease. Amer. J. Surg. 128, 835–839.

Strole W.E., Clark W.H. & Isselbacher K.J. (1967) Progressive arterial occlusive disease Kohlmeier-Degos). New Engl. J. Med. 276, 195–201.

Tarin D., Allison D.A., Modlen P. & Neale G. (1978) Diagnosis and management of obscure gastro-intestinal bleeding. Brit. Med. J. ii, 751–754.

Tsai J.T. (1980) Perforation of the small bowel with rheumatoid arthritis. South. Med. J. 73, 939–940.

Varkonyi T., Wittman T., Varro V. (1977) Effect of local circulatory arrest on the structure of the enterocytes of the isolated intestinal loop. Digest., 15, 295–302.

Vink M. (1973) Symposium on Buerger's disease. J. Cardiovasc. Surg. 14, 1–51.

Wagner R., Gabbert H. & Höhn P. (1979) The mechanism of epithelial shedding after ischemic damage to the small intestinal mucosa. A light and electron microscopic investigation. Virchows. Arch. (Cell Pathol.) 30, 25–31.

Weaver G.A., Alpern H.D., Davis J.J., Ramsey W.H. & Reichelderfer M. (1979) Gastrointestinal angiodysplasia associated with aortic valve disease: Part of a spectrum of angiodysplasia of the gut. Gastroenterol. 77, 1–11.

Weiser M.M., Andres G.A., Brentjens J.R., Evans J.T. & Reichlin M. (1981) Systemic lupus erythematosus and intestinal venulitis. Gastroenterol. 81, 570–579.

Wessler S., Ming S.C., Gurewich V. & Freimand G. (1960) A critical evaluation of thromboangiitis obliterans. The case against Buerger's disease. New. Engl.J. Med., 262, 1149–1160.

Whitington P.F., Friedman A.L. & Chesney R.W. (1979) Gastro-intestinal disease in the haemolytic uraemic syndrome. Gastroenterol., 76, 728–733.

Wilkinson, M. & Torrance, W.N. (1967) Clinical background of rheumatoid vascular disease. Ann. Rheum. Dis. 26, 475–480.

Williams, L.F. Jr (1971) Vascular insufficiency of the intestine. Gastroenterology, 61, 757–777.

Wittenberg, J., Athansoulis, C.A., Shapiro, J.H. & Williams, L.F. Jr. (1973) A radiologic approach to the patient with acute extensive bowel ischaemia. Radiology, 106, 13–24.

Wolf, E.A. Jr & Sumner, D.S. (1973) Redistribution of intestinal blood flow during hypotension. Swg. Forum, 24, 20–22.

Chapter 21
Intestinal Lymphangiectasia

GRAHAM NEALE

History 348
The intestinal lymphatic channels 350
Pathology of lymphangiectasia 350
Natural history and clinical aspects 353

Intestinal lymphangiectasia is of importance because of the light it has shed on the physiology and immunology of the small gut. It has provided a model for determining the nature of protein-losing enteropathy, the pathways of absorption of fat-soluble compounds, and the role of lymphocytes in the immune system.

History

Before 1960, patients severely affected by intestinal lymphangiectasia were probably thought to have hypoalbuminaemia secondary to malabsorption. The less severely affected were simply reassured that intermittent swelling of the ankles was an unimportant benign disorder. In a few patients the concentration of circulating albumin was measured and found to be low (Jungmann 1922, Csèpai 1923, Meyer-Bisch 1925). Such patients might have transient attacks of diarrhoea or a low serum cholesterol (Myers & Taylor 1933). Studies, often extending over many months, included detailed measurements of plasma proteins and biochemical assessment of nitrogen balance under a variety of dietary conditions. They gave disappointing answers. Nitrogen excretion in the faeces was normal and independent of nitrogen intake. Circulating protein concentrations did not respond in a predictable manner to changes in protein intake. Steatorrhoea occurred in some patients and not others. Most workers concluded that the low levels of circulating proteins were due to a failure of hepatic synthesis. Increased catabolism was thought to be highly improbable although there were tantalizing suggestions that other mechanisms might be playing a part. Cope & Goadby (1935) were particularly concerned that 'the condition of the intestinal mucosa could not be investigated'.

Catabolism of albumin

Albright et al. (1949) reported the first convincing evidence of excessive catabolism of albumin in such patients. They used the classical techniques of metabolic balance and demonstrated that albumin administered intravenously to patients with idiopathic hypoproteinaemia was promptly followed by an increase in the excretion of urinary nitrogen. This suggested an increased rate of albumin breakdown. It was not long before this conclusion was confirmed by the demonstration of a reduced half-life of radiolabelled albumin in patients presenting a similar clinical picture (Corbeel et al. 1954) and the term 'idiopathic hypercatabolic hypoproteinaemia' was proposed (Schwartz & Thomsen 1957).

Introduction of ^{131}I-labelled PVP

At the same time Citrin et al. (1957) demonstrated the leakage of radioactive albumin into the stomach of a patient with giant hypertrophy of the gastric mucosa. Subsequently Gordon (1958) conceived the idea of labelling a substance of similar molecular weight to albumin, but one which would not be digested in the gastrointestinal tract. PVP with a molecular weight of 40,000 was already in use as an artificial plasma substitute and seemed to be the ideal compound. It was labelled with ^{131}I and given to nine patients known to have idiopathic hypercatabolic hyperproteinaemia. Excessive losses into the gut were demonstrated but the basis of the disorder remained obscure (Gordon 1959). The *Lancet* proposed that the new designation for the condition should be 'protein-losing gastroenteropathy' (Editorial, 1959).

Pathological findings

Gordon *et al.* (1959) at a clinical staff conference of the National Institute of Health then pointed out that three of the nine patients studied had had spontaneous chylous effusions which led them to suspect a defect in the lymphatic system. This suspicion was supported by their review of reports of up to 100 patients with idiopathic oedema. Not only were chylous effusions common (18%) but in seven patients distended lymphatics had been noted at laparotomy coursing over the serosal surface of the small intestine. They speculated that 'chylous fluid might be lost into the lumen of the intestine' thereby contributing to the steatorrhoea which had been found in some patients and to the reduced values for circulating lipids.

These studies were then extended to cover a total of eighteen patients with hypoproteinaemia shown to be due to protein-losing enteropathy and the anatomical lesion was sought. In twelve, tissue was obtained for pathological examination, in most cases by suction biopsy (twenty-five specimens), but also by removal of tissue at laparotomy or at autopsy. The description of the intestine was exact — 'The affected portions of intestine were oedematous. The serosal surface was dusky and congested with areas of fibrinous exudate. The serosal lymphatic vessels were dilated and in two cases there were yellow nodules less than 5 mm diameter along their course. The mesenteric lymph nodes contained foci of a similar yellow colour'.

The lumen of the intestine was only slightly dilated. The valves of Kerkring were present throughout but in the affected areas they were swollen and broader than normal. The villi had enlarged bulb-like tips imparting a white, pebbly almost papillary appearance to the mucosal surface. There

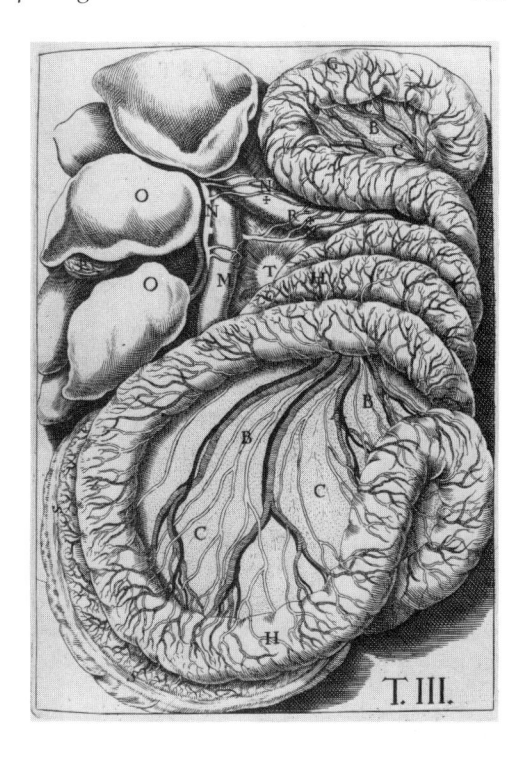

Fig. 21.1. The first illustration of the abdominal lymphatics. From Asellius (1627) (by permission of the Syndics of Cambridge University).

was segmental red-brown pigmentation of the external muscularis. The pigmented areas were not necessarily correlated with the swollen segments. Histologically the pigment was in the cytoplasm of the smooth muscle cells of the external muscularis. Histochemically it reacted as lipofuscin or ceroid.

Microscopically there was a variable degree of dilatation of the lymph vessels of the mucosa and submucosa. The dilated lymph vessels contained foamy lipophages and similar cells were seen in the yellow nodules and lymph nodes. Histochemically the lipid in the macrophages reacted as neutral fat. Unlike the cells in Whipple's disease the lipophages were not periodic acid-Schiff (PAS)-positive in paraffin sections.

The mesenteric lymphatics had a greatly thickened and fragmented elastica interna and there was hypertrophy of the muscular layers of the media. Fibrous tissue, which appeared to be continuous with the adventitia, penetrated the tunica media and narrowed the lumens of the vessels. No inflammatory reaction was seen along the lymphatics. The mesenteric lymph nodes were affected by similar changes. There was hypertrophy of the capsular elastic fibres and the trabeculae were thickened by fibrosis'. The term intestinal lymphangiectasia was proposed in the summary of the paper in which the condition was so clearly described (Waldmann et al. 1961).

The intestinal lymphatic channels

Anatomy

Asellius (1627) first described the intestinal lymphatics (Fig. 21.1). He observed the milkiness of the lacteals in a dog which had been fed a fat meal a short time before and promptly speculated on the role of the lymphatics in the absorption of foodstuffs. Hunter (1784) believed they were the sole channels of absorption. Each villus has a central lymphatic (possibly more than one in broad leaf-shaped structures) which anastomoses with the lymphatic capillary network at the base of the crypts of the small intestine. This plexus rests on the inner surface of the muscularis mucosa and perforating branches with valves provide communication with the submucosal plexus which in turn drains to the intermuscular channels which amalgamate to form mesenteric lymphatics draining to lymph nodes and ultimately into the cisterna chyli.

In the subepithelial framework of the villus are strands of smooth muscle which arise from the muscularis mucosae and are arranged parallel to the axis of the villus around its central lacteal. Rhythmic contractions of the villi occur which may be under the control of villikinin, a substance released by duodenal acidification which has been partially characterized as a small acidic peptide.

In the resting state, villous pressure in lacteals is less than that in arterioles and capillaries (Königes & Otto 1936) but during contraction the flow of blood ceases and tissue pressure exceeds that in the arterioles (Wells & Johnson 1934). Thus the contracting villi have a pumping action which is probably important in the transfer of chylomicra to the circulation.

Physiology

Absorption of all the naturally occurring fat-soluble vitamins occurs predominantly via the lymphatic channels but some absorption of vitamins A and E can occur by way of the portal vein although the importance of this route in man is uncertain (Clark & Harries 1975).

Intestinal lymph flow is markedly influenced by feeding. Experiments in animals indicate that the trans-mucosal transfer of water and fat are the main controlling factors, the absorption of proteins and carbohydrate eliciting little or no increase in lymph flow. Transferred fluid appears to dilute the extravascular fluid in the intestinal mucosa and slightly increases capillary filtration of protein during the process of absorption, which leads to an increased flow of lymph of low protein concentration. On the other hand the absorption of fat greatly increases the turnover of extravascular protein and the enhanced flow of lymph contains protein at concentrations close to those of plasma (Simmonds 1955). It also seems likely that any unchanged molecules of protein crossing the intestinal mucosa subsequently enter both lymphatics and the capillaries (Warshaw & Walker 1974). The lymphatics are also important channels for the circulation of lymphocytes, as described in Chapter 8.

Pathology of lymphangiectasia

Intestinal lymphangiectasia may be primary or secondary; it may be localized to the lamina propria; it may be generalized (involving lamina propria, submucosa, serosa and mesentery; or it may affect only the mesentery (Vardy et al. 1975). The colon is rarely involved (Kingham et al. 1982).

Primary intestinal lymphangiectasia

Primary intestinal lymphangiectasia is

frequently part of a congenital disorder of the lymphatic system as a whole, as suggested by Pomerantz & Waldmann (1963). In one half of their series of sixteen patients there was clinical evidence of extra-intestinal lymphatic abnormalities and in the four patients subjected to peripheral lymphangiography the lymphatics appeared hypoplastic. In addition, in one patient no inguinal, pelvic or retroperitoneal nodes could be demonstrated, and in another the thoracic duct was occluded. There is therefore evidence to support the view that intestinal lymphangiectasia is one facet of a generalized disorder, the manifestations of which are determined by the location and extent of the lymphatic anomalies (Vardy et al. 1975). Nevertheless it is a big conceptual leap to group all cases as variants of 'congenital hereditary lymphoedema' a condition believed to be governed by a simple autosomal dominant gene with incomplete penetrance and variable expressivity, as proposed by Esterly (1965). Milroy's cases of primary lymphoedema (1892) were both congenital and hereditary but in unselected series a family history is found in only 20% (Champion 1972). There are no distinguishing features between familial and apparently non-familial cases. On the other hand, up to 25% of patients with primary lymphoedema of the limbs have been shown to have excess protein loss from the gut (Kinmonth 1982).

Embryologically lymphatic channels develop in confluence with perivenous spaces as an evagination from venous channels. Failure of this process is thought to be responsible for the development of primary lymphoedema and has been described in dogs, cattle and swine as an inherited congenital defect. In such animals, absence or hypoplasia of regional peripheral nodes is one of the manifestations of a more generalized defect in the development of the lymphatic system (Luginbühl et al. 1967).

Primary lymphoedema especially of the lower limbs may be associated with another developmental anomaly in which large tortuous incompetent lymph trunks extend from the cisteria chyli through the retroperitoneal space to the lower limbs and to the serosal surface of the intestine. In many cases the thoracic duct is abnormal and there is also a strong association with congenital vascular anomalies (Kinmonth et al. 1964). Although chylous ascites is common with this disorder, intestinal lymphangiectasia is rarely found.

Table 21.1. Primary intestinal lymphangiectasia and its associations.

Disorder localized to intestinal lymphatics
  Familial (Shani et al. 1974)
  Sporadic (Waldmann 1966)

Widespread lymphatic pathology
  Presenting as congenital hereditary lymphoedema (Milroy's disease) — rare
  Presenting with manifestations of hypoproteinaemia and shown to have widespread lymphatic abnormalities (Pomerantz and Waldmann 1963, Vardy et al. 1975)

In association with other disorders
  Nephrotic syndrome (Salazar De Sousa 1968)
  Noonan's syndrome (Vallet et al. 1972, Herzog et al. 1976)
  Di George syndrome (Vardy et al. 1975)
  Enamel hypoplasia (Dummer 1977)
  ? Metageria (Silver et al. 1972)

Primary intestinal lymphangiectasia has been associated with several conditions, mostly as single case reports of congenital disorders (Table 21.1). Protein-losing enteropathy occurs in severe nephrosis (Royer et al. 1963) and a relationship with lymphangiectasia has been claimed (Salazar De Sousa et al. 1968). Familial intestinal lymphangiectasia has been shown in a family of two sibships. Eight of twenty-eight children had growth retardation, oedema, diarrhoea or abdominal pain in varying combinations. Intestinal protein loss was demonstrated in five and dilated lacteals were found in three intestinal biopsies (Shani et al. 1974). An unusual association of intestinal lymphangiectasia with other congenital abnormalities is described below.

A.J., born 1955, was frail and small in infancy and at age 5 years was noted to have unusual finger-tips. He has a bird-like facies (Fig. 21.2). His height and proportions are on the 15th percentile but his weight is below the 3rd

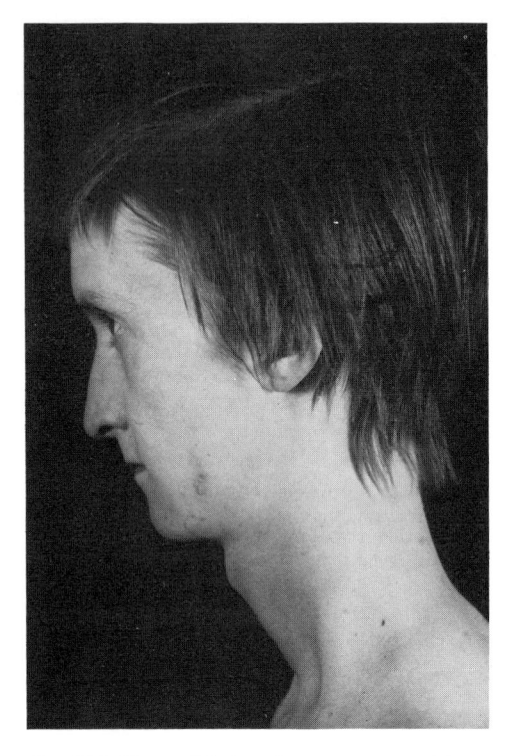

Fig. 21.2. Unusual facies of a young man with multiple congenital abnormalities of skin, connective tissue, skeleton and intestinal lymphatics.

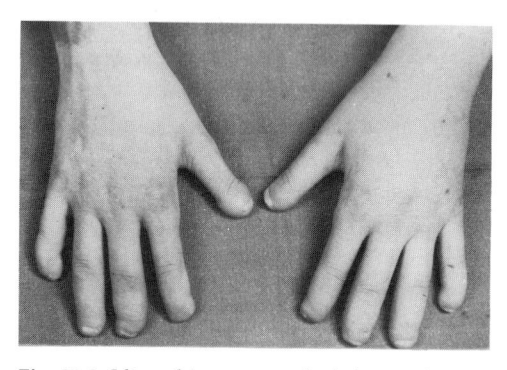

Fig. 21.3. Idiopathic acro-osteolysis in a patient with primary intestinal lymphangiectasia.

percentile (42.5 kg). His skin is thin and he has odd geographic patterns of pigmentation especially on the fore-arms. The digits show recession of the terminal phalanges with pseudo-clubbing (Fig. 21.3).

At about the age of 10 he developed ankle oedema and was subsequently referred to Hammersmith Hospital. Investigation showed: Hb 15 g/dl, WCC 7×10^9/l, albumin 17, globulin 14 g/l (IgG 3.0, IgA 0.8, IgM 0.15). The small bowel was dilated with a coarse mucosal pattern and jejunal biopsy revealed dilated lymphatics in the tips of villi. Faecal fat was 11 g/day. ^{131}I-PVP excretion 7.8% (normal less than 1.5%).

Radiology of the hands and feet shows resorption of terminal phalanges with subcutaneous calcinosis. There are minor skeletal deformities with bowing of radii and ulnae, varus deformities of femoral necks and unusual modelling of humeri and fibulae. Skull X-ray shows flattening and asymmetry of the pituitary fossa.

Skin biopsy from a finger shows microscopic calcium deposits in the epidermis surrounded by histiocytes. There is no evidence of scleroderma. The patient has been treated with a low fat diet and remains well although the phalangeal resorption has progressed and the distal bones have disappeared completely. The general appearance was very similar to that of patients with metageria (Gilkes *et al.* 1974).

In primary intestinal lymphangiectasia there is evidence to suggest that the defect may be due to congenital malunion of lymphatics with impaired drainage of lacteals and of submucosal lymphatics. The affected channels are distended by hydrostatic pressure and electron microscopic studies show a more prominent supporting structure with an increase in intracellular fibrils, in surrounding collagen fibrils and in supporting cells. Lipid droplets are seen at the base of the absorptive cells, even after an overnight fast, and chylomicrons gather in the extracellular spaces and within the lumens of lymphatics (Dobbins 1966).

The distended lymphatic channels discharge their contents into the lumen of the intestine (Waldmann 1966): the protein is digested and resorbed via the portal system into the circulating pool of amino acids; the fat may also be absorbed if there are normal

Table 21.2. Secondary causes of intestinal lymphangiectasia.

Lymph channels obstructed
  Infection — TB peritonitis
  Acute inflammatory processes — SLE (Pachas et al. 1971), eosinophilic enteritis, mesenteric panniculitis (McDonagh et al. 1965)
  Fibrosis — non-specific fibrosis (Belaiche et al. 1980), radiation damage
  Intraluminal precipitates — hypobeta-lipoproteinaemia (Dobbins 1968)
  Extraluminal compression — pregnancy, malrotation (Iida et al. 1980, Case 1)

Lymph node infiltration
  Infection — TB, Whipple's disease (Laster et al. 1966)
  Inflammation — Crohn's disease
Neoplasm — carcinoma, lymphoma esp. macroglobulinaemia (Tubbs et al. 1977, Rogé et al. 1978)

Raised pressure in thoracic duct
  Constrictive pericarditis (Petersen & Hastrup 1963, Nelson et al. 1975)
  Right-sided heart disease — atrial septal defect (Davidson et al. 1961), pulmonary stenosis (Jeejeebhoy 1962), familial cardiomyopathy (Dolle et al. 1962), carcinoid disease (Waldmann et al. 1969)

---

lymphatics distally in the small intestine; the lymphocytes are probably irrevocably lost. Thus the degree of hypoproteinaemia will depend on the ability of body protein synthetic mechanisms to compensate for the excess loss of protein; the degree of steatorrhoea will depend on the site and degree of obstruction of lymphatics and the lymphocytopaenia may be related to compensatory mechanisms affecting the movement of lymphocytes through the intestinal mucosa.

Secondary intestinal lymphangiectasia

Intestinal lymphangiectasia secondary to lymphatic obstruction has been described in many neoplastic and infiltrative conditions (Table 21.2). Pathologists were aware of the disorder before clinicians had started to elucidate the many causes of 'sprue' syndromes. Indeed there is an early report of the pathology of the blockage of major abdominal lymphatics in the mid-nineteenth century (von Rokitansky 1855). Hamilton Fairley recognized the association in lymphomatous disorders but also described two cases in which the underlying mechanism was unclear (Fairley & Mackie 1937) and other such cases have also been described (Hill 1937, Glynn & Rosenheim 1938, Vaux 1943).

A case of transitory oedema due to intestinal lymphangiectasia possibly caused by filariasis is described below.

> J.W., a man born in 1922, worked in and around East Africa for 16 years. At age 42 he suffered recurrent attacks of fever with rigors and pain in the right groin. A year later he developed oedema of penis and legs and he was subsequently treated at the Hospital for Tropical Diseases with diethylcarbamazine as a case of possible filariasis. He was referred to Hammersmith Hospital for investigation of persistent hypoproteinaemia.
> Investigations showed: serum total protein 49 g/l (albumin 29 g/l, globulin 20 g/l, [IgG 1.7, IgA 1.75, IgM 0.2], no proteinuria, normal liver function (45-min BSP retention 3%), faecal fat 4–11 g/day, vitamin E absorption 30% (normal > 55%) (Fig. 21.4). Barium meal showed coarse folds in the small intestine and dilated lymphatics were found in a mucosal biopsy. Protein loss from the intestine: 6.3% of labelled chromium in 5 days. IgM turnover $T\frac{1}{2}$ = 3.0 days (normal 4.9–7.9 days) (Fig. 21.5). Lymphangiography revealed a probable block of retroperitoneal lymphatics at the level of the 2nd lumbar vertebra. Serology and skin tests for filariasis were negative.
> The patient was given a further course of diethylcarbamazine and prescribed a low fat diet. Over a period of 12 months the oedema resolved and serum total proteins increased to 60 g/l (albumen 30 g/l).

Natural history and clinical aspects

In its most obvious form the primary disorder affects children and young adults. The majority of reported cases are less than 30 years old at presentation. Males and

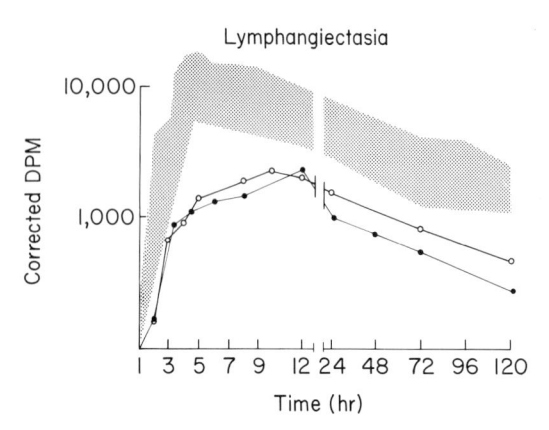

Fig. 21.4. Absorption of vitamin E in intestinal lymphangiectasia. Concentrations of ^{3}H-vitamin E in plasma in two patients (J.W. and B.M.) after oral ingestion of labelled vitamin compared with those in seven control subjects. The shaded area shows the normal range.

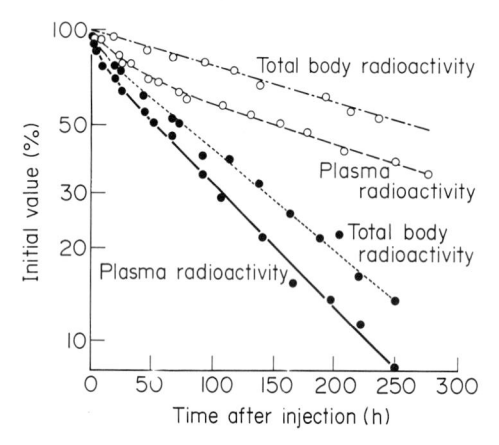

Fig. 21.5. Clearance of radiolabelled IgM in a patient with intestinal lymphangiectasia (●——●) (J.W.) compared with a normal subject 8 (○——○).

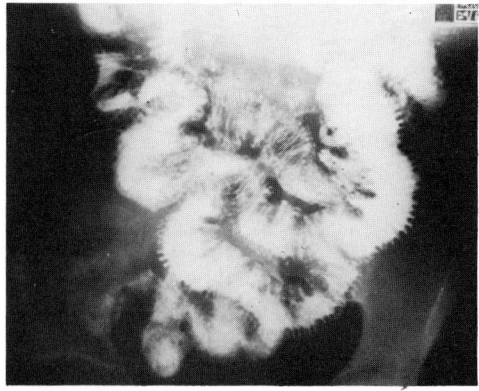

Fig. 21.6. Barium follow-through examination of small intestine in intestinal lymphangiectasia, showing oedematous mucosal folds giving a 'picket fence' appearance.

females are equally affected and although most cases are sporadic, familial clustering and association with other congenital disorders suggest a genetic aetiology. The more severely affected patients have marked reductions in circulating gamma globulins and low lymphocyte counts with evidence of impaired cell-mediated immunity; nevertheless susceptibility to infection is not a major problem.

The primary disorder may be more common than is generally believed (Vardy et al. 1975, Roberts & Douglas 1976). It has been shown that the clinical manifestations may be severe or mild, chronic or transitory, and in some cases only become manifest when there is an exacerbation of hypoproteinaemia or transient disturbance of gastrointestinal function (Kobayashi & Obe 1971, Szücs & Köves 1972).

The natural history of the secondary disorder is directly related to the causative disease process.

Clinical findings

Patients presenting shortly after birth usually have severe manifestations of disease with marked oedema, effusions (chylous in many cases), and failure to thrive with associated diarrhoea and steatorrhoea (Waldmann 1966). Children and young adults may be less severely affected and usually have asymmetrical oedema. Gastrointestinal symptoms are often mild although intermittent diarrhoea may be noted. Vomiting, growth retardation, anaemia, hypocalcaemic tetany, rickets and myopathy are less frequent manifestations (Vardy et al. 1975).

Establishing the diagnosis

In most cases hypoproteinaemic oedema in the absence of renal, hepatic and cardiac disease suggests loss of protein into the gut for which a cause must be sought. Ulcerative and neoplastic conditions of the gastro-

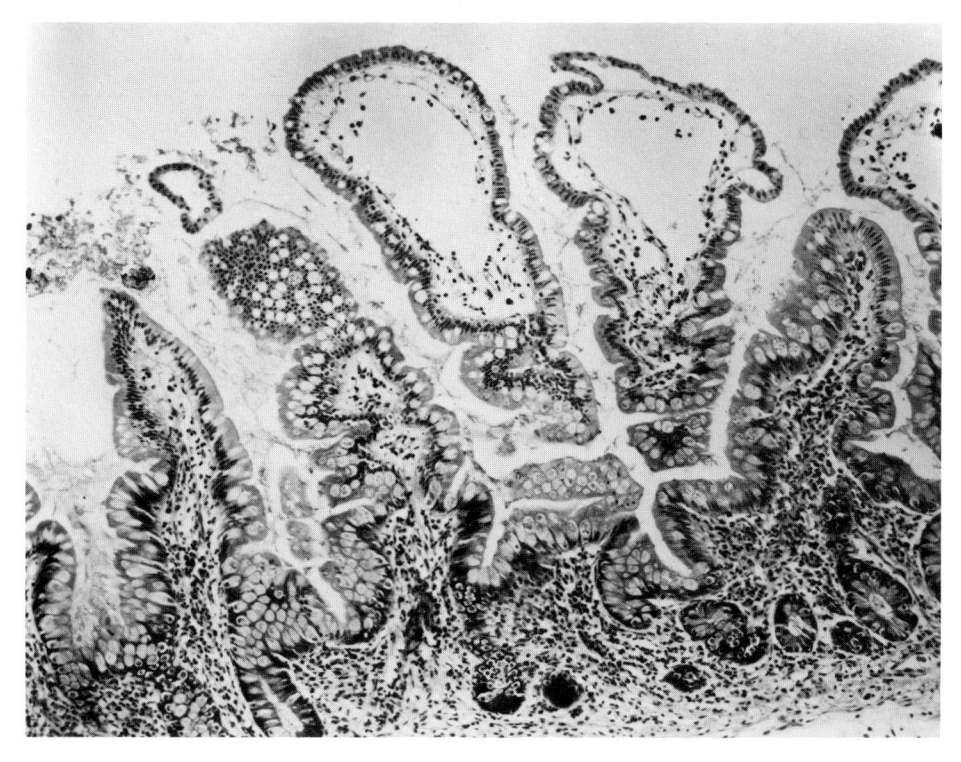

Fig. 21.7. Jejunal biopsy showing villus tip (H & E × 100). (Courtesy of Professor D.J. Evans.)

intestinal tract are usually identified by appropriate radiological and endoscopic investigations.

In patients with lymphangiectasia affecting the small intestine the radiographic findings are variable and non-specific. Diffuse symmetrical thickening of mucosal folds (Fig. 21.6) with evidence of increased secretion are commonly seen and nodular defects, segmentation and dilatation are usually minimal, or non-existent (Marshak & Lindner 1970, Olmsted & Madewell 1976).

The finding of lymphocytopenia is useful (usually between 500—1000 cells/mm^3) and is helpful in distinguishing the weeping of ruptured lymphatics from the loss of fluid through an ulcerated or neoplastic mucosa. Histological examination of one or more biopsies of the small intestine is the only certain means of confirming the suspected diagnosis. The finding of distended lymphatics in a jejunal biopsy taken after an overnight fast is diagnostic (Fig. 21.7). Nevertheless the lesion is often patchy.

The enteroscope and laparoscope are sometimes useful in achieving a diagnosis. The mucosa of the small intestine may show scattered white spots, bulbous white tips to the villi and chylous material sticking to the surface (Asakura et al. 1981). The serosal surface of small intestine is often brown from the deposition of ceroid and against this background the distended lymphatics show up clearly.

Usually it is not necessary to quantitate the loss of protein into the small intestine. If required it is most often done by collecting faeces after an intravenous injection of radio-chromium which labels circulating proteins *in vivo*. It is possible to get similar information from the intestinal clearance of alpha-1-antitrypsin (Crossley & Elliott 1977, Florent et al. 1981, Hill et al. 1981) or from scintigraphy (Soucy et al. 1983).

Lymphangiography may be helpful in diagnosis. There is often significant hypoplasia of peripheral lymphatics and apparent stasis in retroperitoneal channels. There may be

Table 21.3. Reversible causes of intestinal lymphangiectasia.

	Disorder	Treatment
Infective	Whipple's disease Tuberculosis	Antibiotics
Inflammatory	SLE (Pachas et al. 1971, Trentham & Masi 1976) Retroperitoneal inflammation (McDonagh et al. 1965, Fleischer et al. 1979)	Corticosteroids
Neoplastic	Lymphoma (Tubbs et al. 1977, Broder et al. 1981)	Chemotherapy
Mechanical	Dilated lymphatics due to high CVP (Nelson et al. 1975) Malrotation of the gut Megalymphatic with reflux (Mistilis & Skyring 1965)	Reduction of CVP Surgical correction Lymphatico-venous anastomosis
Segmental disease	Localized disorder demonstrated at laparotomy (Kinmonth 1982)	Resection of affected segment

absence of periaortic lymph nodes and obstruction to the thoracic duct (Bookstein et al. 1965; Shimkin et al. 1970) with extravasation of contrast medium into the gastrointestinal tract (Mihara et al. 1981). On the other hand, lymphangiography from the lower limbs may show normal retroperitoneal lymphatics. In such cases the abnormality presumably affects the smaller lymphatic channels. Chylous effusions may also be shown (Fig. 21.8).

Differential diagnosis

Children with intestinal lymphangiectasia are often diagnosed as suffering from coeliac disease or allergic gastroenteropathy (Waldmann et al. 1966). The histology of the jejunal mucosa usually provides the key to diagnosis although in a minority of cases the clinician may remain in doubt (Gorske et al. 1969). For example, primary hypogammaglobulinaemia may be associated with lymphocytopenia, hypoalbuminaemia and gastrointestinal disorders. The reduction in circulating immunoglobulins is usually disproportionately greater than that of albumin and dilated lymphatics will not be found in biopsies of the jejunum.

Intestinal lymphangiectasia is not a complete diagnosis. Sometimes it is an important indication of an unsuspected lesion as illustrated by the following report.

A.W. presented with swelling of the lower limbs at the age of 6 months. She appeared to be a normal infant at birth but suffered badly from infantile colic and episodes of diarrhoea. On examination she had a somewhat distended abdomen and peripheral oedema but otherwise appeared healthy. Investigations showed: Hb 11.7 g/100 ml, WCC 4000/mm^3 (lymphocytes 950), total protein 48 g/l (albumin 25, globulin 23) but otherwise no significant abnormalities. A jejunal biopsy showed dilated lacteals and a diagnosis of intestinal lymphangiectasia was made. A barium follow-through examination showed slightly dilated loops of small intestine with thickened folds. A month later the infant developed intestinal obstruction and underwent laparotomy. There was a volvulus involving the whole small intestine and the ascending colon which had a much thickened and congested mesentery. It was possible to relieve the obstruction without resecting small intestine and the infant made a good recovery. Six weeks later the concentration of circulating proteins had returned to normal.

Intestinal Lymphangiectasia

phatic channels provide a pathway for the absorption of fat.

On the other hand the hypoproteinaemic state, together with the functionally reduced lymphatic bed, may cause marked oedema of the wall of the intestine with associated attacks of nausea, vomiting and abdominal pain.

Disordered absorption

Most patients with intestinal lymphangiectasia are well nourished and well developed despite their hypoproteinaemic state. Steatorrhoea, when it occurs, is usually modest, faecal nitrogen is normal or slightly increased, and tests of absorption of carbohydrates and water-soluble vitamins are within normal limits. On the other hand the absorption of the fat-soluble vitamins D and E may be markedly impaired (Fig. 21.4). In

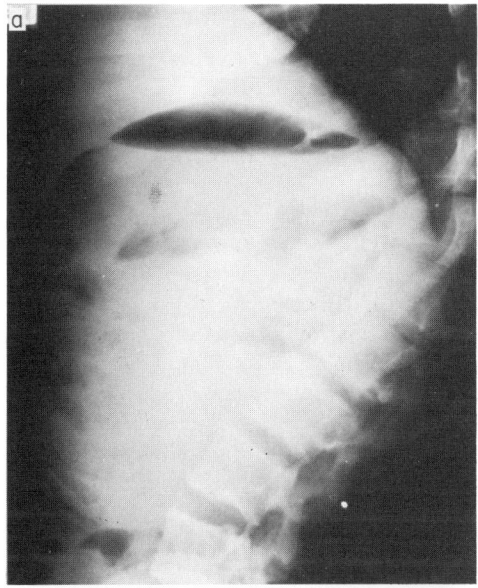

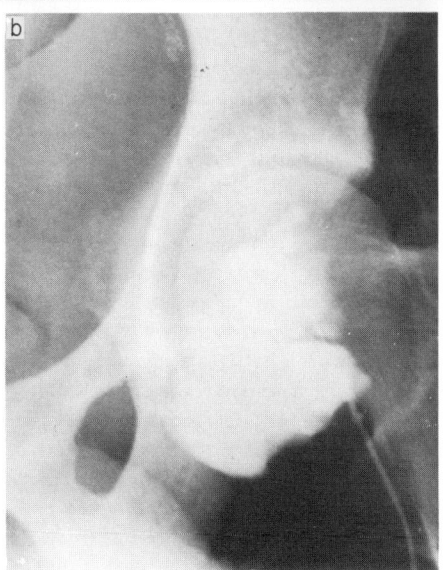

Fig. 21.8. Encysted chylous effusions in a patient with primary intestinal lymphangiectasia. (a) Left iliac fossa. (b) Left loin in retroperitoneal area.

Consequences

The leakage of lymph by patients with intestinal lymphangiectasia does not usually cause overt gastrointestinal dysfunction. Indeed most patients are symptom-free and have little or no diarrhoea or steatorrhoea. Presumably in such cases unaffected lym-

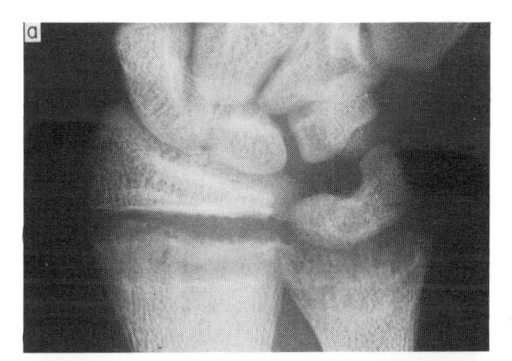

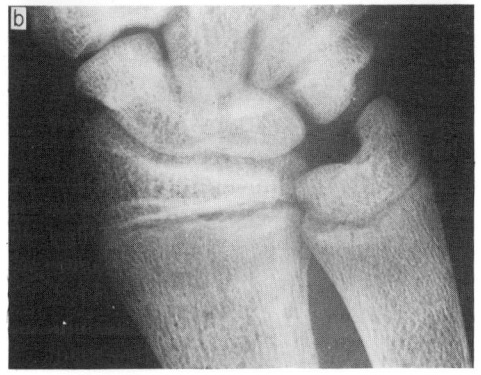

Fig. 21.9. (a) Rickets due to vitamin D deficiency in an adolescent patient with intestinal lymphangiectasia; there is undermineralization, tufting and splaying out of the epiphyses at the wrist. (b) Healing induced by ultraviolet light (5 min exposure twice a week).

most cases this does not give rise to overt disease but osteomalacia is probably common (Fig. 21.9) and will vary with the season of the year.

Vitamin E deficiency causes a deposit of ceroid pigment in the smooth muscle cells of the muscularis externa but there are no reports of more serious pathology in patients with intestinal lymphangiectasia.

Serious malnutrition with weight loss and inanition rarely occurs and is usually associated with profound hypoalbuminaemia, severe gut dysfunction (probably due to oedema) and a much reduced food intake (Waldmann et al. 1961, Mistilis et al. 1965).

Secondary effects of loss of lymph

The concentrations of circulating proteins in plasma will fall if the synthetic mechanisms are unable to compensate for losses into the intestine. Normally there is a marked reduction in albumin, IgA, IgG and IgM globulin with a moderate reduction in transferrin and caeruloplasmin and normal values for fibrinogen, α_2 macroglobulin and IgE (Waldmann 1966). Serum lipoproteins and consequently cholesterol are reduced in the more severely affected. In addition there is an enteric loss of lymphocytes with preferential depletion of thymus-dependent long-lived cells (Weiden et al. 1972, Douglas et al. 1976). These may decrease from 80% to less than 5% of the total lymphocyte pool. In spite of these remarkable changes the functional effect is often no more than peripheral oedema.

Patients with intestinal lymphangiectasia are able to make humoral antibodies when challenged with antigens in spite of the low concentration of circulating immunoglobulins and enhanced susceptibility to bacterial infection does not occur. On the other hand the reduced lymphocyte count is associated with a marked disturbance of cellular immunity. There is impaired *in vitro* transformation of lymphocytes challenged with non-specific mitogens, specific antigens and allogenic cells, absence of delayed hypersensitivity skin reactions, and an ability to accept skin grafts from unrelated donors. It is postulated that these changes are due to depletion of the pool of circulating long-lived T lymphocytes (Weiden et al. 1972) which may have been responsible for the extensive viral wart formation described in one patient with intestinal lymphangiectasia (Ward et al. 1977), and the apparently increased risk of lymphoreticular malignancy (Waldmann et al. 1972, Ward et al. 1977). It is suggested that malignant change is due to a defect in immune surveillance with impaired detection and destruction of neoplastic cells or to a defect in the physiological regulation of immunity with a loss of suppressor T-cells responsible for restraining the proliferation of B-cell clones (Broder et al. 1981). One patient who developed a monoclonal B-cell lymphoma localized to breast 15 years after the diagnosis of intestinal lymphangiectasia responded extraordinarily well to treatment with cytotoxic drugs and prednisolone. The lymphoma regressed completely, and so did the protein loss from the gut which did not appear to be involved in the lymphomatous process. The response of this patient indicates the possibility of resolving lymphangiectasia with anti-inflammatory drugs (see below).

In addition to lymphocytes and protein there may be losses of other endogenous material including fat (Mistilis et al. 1965), iron (Ulstrom & Krivit 1960) and calcium (Nicolaidou et al. 1980). One patient has been described as excreting 8–10 g fat/day after not taking any fat in the diet for a week. This fat-losing state may be associated with loss of circulating lipoproteins and marked hypocholesterolaemia.

The low value of circulating calcium in intestinal lymphangiectasia is usually secondary to hypoproteinaemia but in a proportion of patients the ionized fraction is also reduced, in some cases causing tetany. The loss of endogenous calcium in faeces may be markedly elevated (Milhaud & Vesin 1961, Nicolaidou et al. 1980) and it has been suggested that these losses are due to calcium carried into the gut bound to albumin. The kinetics of calcium and vitamin D in patients with intestinal lymphangiectasia have not been fully elucidated.

Treatment

Correction of lymphatic abnormalities

All patients with internal lymphangiectasia should be assessed carefully to determine whether or not it is possible to deal with the cause or to resect a localized segment of affected gut. The potentially reversible causes are listed in Table 21.3. It is important to identify the recently described group of patients with a non-specific inflammatory process. They have no readily discernible cause for lymphangiectasia but show rather variable signs of inflammatory disease, including a raised ESR, normal or elevated concentrations of circulating immunoglobulins and possibly a positive auto-antibody marker (such as ANF). Treatment with corticosteroids may lead to a remission (Fleischer et al. 1979).

In patients with primary lymphangiectasia it is usually difficult to determine the length of intestine involved even at laparotomy. Tests for gut protein loss are usually unhelpful in localizing the disease and mesenteric lymphangiography can only be undertaken at laparotomy (Kinmonth & Cox 1974). In one selected series a segment of small intestine was resected in five of six patients undergoing exploratory laparotomy with apparent benefit to three (Kinmonth 1982). It is unusual to find a distended large lymphatic channel. There is a report of a lymphatico-venous anastomosis performed to relieve intestinal lymphangiectasia (Mistilis & Skyring 1965) but although the mucosal changes appeared to regress the protein-losing state persisted (Skyring, pers. comm.).

Medical management of the disorders produced by intestinal lymphangiectasia

Most patients do well on a simple low fat diet which reduces the demands made on the intestinal lymphatic system and diminishes the postprandial flow of lymph. Patients may take fat in the form of medium-chain triglycerides which are absorbed via the portal vein, but the value of MCT preparations is limited by their low palatability. It is important to undertake checks of nutritional status from time to time because of the disease which may occur as a result of deficiencies of fat soluble vitamins, especially cholecalciferol, and of divalent cations lost via the gut, for example iron or calcium.

References

Albright F., Bartter F.C. & Forbes A.P. (1949) The fate of human serum albumin administered intravenously to a patient with idiopathic hypoalbuminaemia and hypoglobulinaemia. *Trans. Ass. Amer. Phys.* **62**, 204–210.

Asakura H., Miura S., Morishita T., Aiso S., Tanaka T., Kitahora T., Tsuchiya M., Enomoto Y. & Watanabe Y. (1981) Endoscopic and histopathological study on primary and secondary intestinal lymphangiectasia. *Dig. Dis. Sci.* **26**, 312–320.

Asellius G. (1627) *De Lactibus sive Lacteis Venis, Quarto Vasorum Mesaraicorum Genere Novo Invento.* J. Baptam Biddellium, Mediolani, Milan.

Belaiche J., Vesin P., Chaumette M.T., Julien M. & Cattan D. (1980) Lymphangiectasies intestinales et fibrose des ganglions mesenteriques. *Gastroenterol. Clin. Biol.* **4**, 52–58.

Bookstein J.J., French A.B. & Pollard H.M. (1965) Protein-losing gastroenteropathy, concept derived from lymphangiography. *Amer. J. Dig. Dis.* **10**, 573–581.

Broder S., Callihan T.R., Jaffe E.S., DeVita V.T., Strober W., Bartter F.C. & Waldmann T.A. (1981) Resolution of long-standing protein-losing enteropathy in a patient with intestinal lymphangiectasia after treatment for malignant lymphoma. *Gastroenterol.* **80**, 166–168.

Champion R.H. (1972) Disorders of lymphatics. In *Textbook of Dermatology*, Chapter 34, pp. 1017–1023. (Ed. by A. Rook, D.S. Wilkinson & F.J.G. Ebling). Blackwell Scientific Publications, Oxford.

Citrin Y., Sterling K. & Halsted J.A. (1957) The mechanism of hypoproteinaemia associated with giant hypertrophy of the gastric mucosa. *New Engl. J. Med.* **257**, 906–912.

Clark M.L. & Harries J.T. (1975) Absorption of the fat-soluble vitamins. In *Intestinal Absorption in Man.* pp. 207–211. (Ed. by I. McColl & G.E. Sladen). Academic Press, London.

Cope C.L. & Goadby H.K. (1935) Study of a case of idiopathic hypoproteinaemia *Lancet*, **i**, 1038–1040.

Corbeel L., Malbram H. & de Vischer M. (1954) L'hypoprotéinémie essentielle chez l'enfant. *Acta Pediat. Belg.* **8**, 337–350.

Crossley J.R. & Elliott R.B. (1977) Simple method for diagnosing protein-losing enteropathy. *Brit. Med. J.* **i**, 428–429.

Csépai K. (1923) Ueber isolierte Störung des

Salzstoffwechsels bei Fall von polyglandulärer Sklerose. *Klin. Wschr.* **2**, 1988.

Davidson J.D., Waldmann T.A., Goodman S.D. & Gordon R.S. (1961) Protein-losing gastroenteropathy in congestive heart failure. *Lancet*, i, 899–902.

Dobbins W.O. (1966) Electronmicroscopic study of the intestinal mucosa in intestinal lymphangiectasia. *Gastroenterol.* **51**, 1004–1017.

Dobbins W.O. (1968) Hypo-beta-lipoproteinemia and intestinal lymphangiectasia. *Arch. Intern. Med.* **122**, 31–38.

Dolle W., Martini G.A. & Peterson F. (1962) Idiopathic familial cardomegaly with intermittent loss of protein into the gastro-intestinal tract. *Germ. med. Mthly*, **7**, 300–306.

Douglas A.P., Weetman A.P. & Haggith J.W. (1976). The distribution and enteric loss of ^{51}Cr-labelled lymphocytes in normal subjects and in patients with coeliac disease and other disorders of the small intestine. *Digest.* **14**, 29–43.

Dummer, P.M.H. (1977). Severe enamel hypoplasia in a case of intestinal lymphangiectasia: a rare protein-losing enteropathy. *Oral Surgery, Oral Medicine, Oral Pathology*, **43**, 702–706.

Editorial (1959) Protein-losing gastro-enteropathy. *Lancet*, i, 351–352.

Esterly J.R. (1965) Congenital hereditary lymphoedema. *J. Med. Genet.* **2**, 93–98.

Fairley N. & Mackie F.P. (1937) The clinical and biochemical syndrome in lymphadenoma and allied diseases involving the mesenteric lymph glands. *Brit. Med. J.* i, 375–380.

Fleischer T.A., Strober W., Muchmore A.V., Broder S., Krawitt E.L. & Waldmann T.A. (1979) Corticosteroid-responsive intestinal lymphangiectasia secondary to an inflammatory process. *N. Eng. J. Med.* **300**, 605–606.

Florent C., L'Hirondel C., Desmazures C., Aymes C. & Bernier J.J. (1981) Intestinal clearance of alpha-1-antitrypsin. A sensitive method for the detection of protein-losing enteropathy. *Gastroenterol.* **81**, 777–780.

Gilkes J.J., Sharvill D.E. & Wells (1974) The premature aging syndromes. Report of eight cases and description of a new entity named metageria. *Brit. J. Dermatol.* **91**, 243–262.

Glynn L.E. & Rosenheim M.L. (1938) Mesenteric chyladenectasis with steatorrhoea and features of Addison's disease. *J. Path.* **47**, 285–290.

Gordon Jr R.S. (1958) Preparation of radio-active polyvinyl pyrrolidone for medical use. *J. Polymer Sci.* **31**, 191–192.

Gordon Jr R.S. (1959) Exudative enteropathy: abnormal permeability of the gastro-intestinal tract demonstrable with labelled polyvinyl pyrrolidone. *Lancet*, i, 325–326.

Gordon Jr R.S., F.C. Bartter & T. Waldmann (1959) Idiopathic hypoalbuminemias: Clinical Staff Conference at the National Institutes of Health. *Ann. Inter. Med.* **51**, 553–576.

Gorske K., Winchester P. & Grossman H. (1969) Unusual protein-losing enteropathies in children. *Radiol.* **92**, 739–744.

Herzog D.B., Logan R. & Kooistra J.B. (1976) The Noonan syndrome with intestinal lymphangiectasia. *J. Pediat.* **88**, 270–272.

Hill J.M. (1937) Mesenteric chyladenectasis: report of a case. *Amer. J. Path.* **13**, 267–276.

Hill R.E., Hercz A., Corey M.L., Gilday D.L. & Hamilton J.R. (1981) Fecal clearance of alpha-1-antitrypsin: a reliable measure of enteric protein loss in children. *J. Pediat.* **99**, 416–417.

Hunter W. (1784) *Two introductory Lectures to his last course of Anatomical Lectures at his theatre in Windmill Street.* J. Johnson, London.

Iida F., Wada R., Sato A. & Yamada T. (1980) Clinicopathologic consideration of protein-losing enteropathy due to lymphangiectasia of the intestine. *Surg. Gynecol. Obstet.* **151**, 391–395.

Jeejeebhoy K.N. (1962) Cause of hypoalbuminaemia in patients with gastrointestinal and cardiac disease. *Lancet*, i, 343–348.

Jungmann P. (1922) Ueber eine isolierte Störung des Salzstoffwechsels. Ein klinischer Beitrag zur Frage der Abhängigkeit der Salzausscheidung von Nervensystem. *Klin. Wschr.* **1**, 1546–1548.

Kay D. Robinson D.S. (1962) The structure of chylomicra obtained from the thoracic duct of the rat. *Quart J. Exp. Physiol.* **47**, 258–261.

Kingham J.G., Moriarty K.J., Furness M. & Levison D.A. (1982). Lymphangiectasia of the colon and small intestine. *Brit. J. Radiol.* **55**, 774–777.

Kinmonth J.B. (1982) Chylous diseases and syndromes. In *The Lymphatics*, Chapter 13. Edward Arnold, London.

Kinmonth J.B. & Cox S.J. (1974) Protein-losing enteropathy in primary lymphoedema: mesenteric lymphography and gut resection. *Brit. J. Surg.* **61**, 589–596.

Kinmonth J.B., Taylor G.W. & Jantet G.H. (1964) Chylous complications of primary lymphoedema. *J. Cardiovasc. Surg. (Torino)*, **5**, 327–333.

Kobayashi A. & Obe Y. (1971) Protein-losing enteropathy associated with arsenic poisoning. *Amer. J. Dis. Child.* **121**, 515–517.

Königes H.G. & Otto M. (1936) Studies on the filtration mechanism of the intestinal lymph and on the action of acetyl-choline on it and on the circulation of the intestinal villi. *Quart. J. Exp. Physiol.* **26**, 319–329.

Laster L.T., Waldmann T.A., Fenster L.F. & Singleton J.A. (1966) Albumin metabolism in patients with Whipple's disease. *J. Clin. Invest.* **45**, 637–644.

Luginbühl H., Chaeko S.K., Patterson D.F. & Medway W. (1967) Congenital hereditary lymphoedema in the dog. Part II. Pathological studies. *J. Med. Genet.* **4**, 153–165.

Marshak R.H. & Lindner A.E. (1970) *Radiology of the Small Intestine*, p. 69. W.B. Saunders Co., Philadelphia.

McDonagh T.J., Gueft B., Pym K. & Arias I.M.

(1965) Hypoproteinaemia, chylous ascites, steatorrhoea and protein-losing enteropathy due to chronic inflammatory obstruction of major intestinal lymph vessels. *Gastroenterol.* **48**, 642–647.

Meyer-Bisch R. (1925) Ueber isolierte Störungen des intermediären Salzstoffwechsels und ihre Klinische Bedeutung. *Klin. Wschr.* **4**, 588.

Mihara K., Koga K., Tsurudome H., Nakano T., Hoshi H., Yamada H. Kawahira K., Inakura M., Haraguchi Y. & Watanabe K. (1981) Extravasation of contrast medium into the gastrointestinal tract following lymphangiography: report of two cases. *Gastrointest. Radiol.* **6**, 239–242.

Milhaud G. & Vesin P. (1961) Calcium metabolism in man with Calcium-45. Malabsorption syndrome and exudative enteropathy. *Nature (Lond.)* **191**, 872–874.

Milroy W.F. (1892) An undescribed variety of hereditary oedema. *N.Y. Med. J.* **56**, 505–508.

Mistilis S.P. & Skyring A.P. (1965). Intestinal lymphangiectasia. Therepeutic effect of lymph venous anastomosis. *Amer. J. Med.* **40**, 634–641.

Mistilis S.P., Skyring A.P. & Stephen D.D. (1965) Intestinal lymphangiectasia. Mechanism of enteric loss of plasma protein and fat. *Lancet*, **i**, 77–81.

Myers W.K. & Taylor F.H.L. (1933) Hypoproteinaemia probably due to deficient formation of plasma proteins. *Amer. Med. Assoc.* **101**, 198–200.

Nelson D.L., Blaese R.M. & Strober W. (1975) Constrictive pericarditis, intestinal lymphangiectasia and reversible immunologic deficiency. *J. Pediat.* **86**, 548–554.

Nicolaidou P., Ladefoged K., Hylander E., Thale M. & Jarmion S. (1980) Endogenous faecal calcium in chronic malabsorption syndromes and intestinal lymphangiectasia. *Scand. J. Gastroenterol.* **15**, 587–592.

Olmsted W.W. & Madewell J.E. (1976) Lymphangiectasia of the small intestine: description and pathophysiology of the roentgenographic signs. *Gastrointest. Radiol.* **1**, 241–247.

Pachas W.N., Linscheer W.G., Pinals R.S. (1971) Protein-losing enteropathy in systemic lupus erythematosus. *Amer. J. Gastroenterol.* **55**, 162–167.

Petersen V.P. & Hastrup J. (1963) Protein-losing enteropathy in constrictive pericarditis. *Acta Med. Scand.* **173**, 401–410.

Pomerantz M. & Waldmann T.A. (1963) Systemic lymphatic abnormalities associated with gastro-intestinal protein loss secondary to intestinal lymphangiectasia. *Gastroenterol.* **45**, 703–711.

Roberts S.H. & Douglas A.P. (1976) Intestinal lymphangiectasia: the variability of presentation. A study of 5 cases. *Quart. J. Med.* **45**, 39–48.

Rogé J., Marche C., Camilleri J.P., Druet P., Silvéréano-Rogé F. & Vernier G. (1978) Enteropathie exsudative et macroglobulinemie. Presentation d'un cas suivi depuis 9 ans. Revue de la literature. *G. astroenterol. Clin. Biol.* **2**, 897–906.

von Rokitansky C. (1855) *Anomalien des Inhalts. Lehrbuch der pathologischen Anatomie (1855–1861).* 3rd. ed., Vol. ii, pp. 394–395, Vienna.

Royer P., Mathieu H., Habib R. & Vermeil G. (1963) Les syndromes nephrotiques de l'enfant. In *Des Syndromes Nephrotiques*, p. 265 Masson, Paris.

Salazar De Sousa K., Guerreiro O., Cunha A. & Aranjo J. (1968) Association of nephrotic syndrome with intestinal lymphangiectasia. *Arch. Dis. Child.* **43**, 245–250.

Schwartz M. & Thomsen B. (1957) Idiopathic hypercatabolic hypoproteinaemia. *Brit. Med. J.* **i**, 14–17.

Shani M., Theodor E., Fraud M. & Goldman B. (1974) A family with protein-losing enteropathy. *Gastroenterol.* **66**, 433–445.

Shimkin P.M., Waldmann T.A. & Drugman R.L. (1970) Intestinal lymphangiectasia. *Amer. J. Radiol.* **110**, 827–841.

Silver J., Brazenoer L.F. & Neale G. (1972) Acro-osteolysis and intestinal lymphangiectasia. *Proc. Roy. Soc. Med.* **65**, 723–724.

Simmonds W.J. (1955) Some observations on the increase in thoracic duct lymph flow during intestinal absorption of fat in unanaesthetized rats. *Aust. J. Exp. Biol. Med. Sci.* **33**, 305–314.

Soucy J.P., Eybalin M.C., Taillefer R., Levassewe A. & Jobin J. (1983). Lymphoscintigraphic demonstration of intestinal lymphangiectasia. *Clin. Nucl. Med.* **8**, 535–537.

Szücs J. & Köves P. (1972) Intestinalis lymphangiektasiás hypoproteinaemia decompensatiójá terhesség és hepatitis Következtében. *Orv. Hetil.* **113**, 2122–2124.

Trentham D.E. & Masi A.T. (1976) Systemic lupus erythematosus with a protein-losing enteropathy. *J. Amer. Med. Assoc.* **236**, 287–288.

Tubbs R.R., McLaughlin J.P. & Winkelman E.I. (1977) Macroglobulinemia and malabsorption. *Cleveland Clinic Q.* **44**, 189–197.

Ulstrom R.A. & Krivit W. (1960) Exudative enteropathy, hypoproteinaemia edema and iron deficiency anemia. *Amer. J. Dis. Child.* **100**, 509–512.

Vallet H.L., Holtzapple P.G., Eberlein W.R., Yakovac W.C., Moshang T. & Borgiowanni H.M. (1972) Noonan syndrome with intestinal lymphangiectasia. *J. Pediat.* **80**, 269–274.

Vardy P.A., Lebanthal E. & Schwachman H. (1975) Intestinal lymphangiectasia: a reappraisal. *Paediat.* **55**, 842–851.

Vaux D.M. (1943) Chyladenectasis with steatorrhoea. *J. Path. Bact.* **55**, 93–99.

Waldmann T.A. (1966) Protein-losing enteropathy. *Gastroenterol.* **50**, 422–443.

Waldmann T.A., Steinfeld J.L., Dutcher T.F., Davidson J.O. & Gordon Jr R.S. (1961) The role of the gastro-intestinal system in 'idiopathic hypoproteinaemia'. *Gastroenterol.* **41**, 197−207.

Waldmann T.A., Wochner R.D. & Strober W. (1969) The role of the gastrointestinal tract in plasma protein metabolism. *Amer. J. Med.* **46**, 275−285.

Waldmann T.A., Strober W. & Blaese R.M. (1972) Immunodeficiency disease and malignancy; various immunological deficiencies of man and the role of the immune process in the control of malignant disease. *Ann. Intern. Med.* **77**, 605−628.

Ward M., Roux A.L., Small W.P. & Sircus W. (1977) Malignant lymphoma and extensive viral wart formation in a patient with intestinal lymphangiectasia and lymphocyte depletion. *Postgrad. Med. J.* **53**, 753−757.

Warshaw A.L. & Walker W.A. (1974) Intestinal absorption of intact antigenic protein. *Surgery*, **76**, 495−499.

Weiden P.L., Blaese R.M., Strober W., Block J.B. & Waldmann T.A. (1972) Impaired lymphocyte transformation in intestinal lymphangiectasia: evidence for at least two functionally distinct lymphocyte population in man. *J. Clin. Invest.* **51**, 1319−1325.

Wells H.S. & Johnson R.G. (1934) The intestinal villi and their circulation in relation to absorption and secretion of fluid. *Amer. J. Physiol.* **109**, 387−402.

Chapter 22
Tumours and Tumour-like Conditions

GERARD SLAVIN

Introduction 363
Epithelial tumours 363
Secondary carcinoma 365
Non-epithelial tumours 366
Tumour-like lesions 368
Inflammatory and hyperplastic lesions 371

Introduction

Primary tumours of all types are uncommon in the small intestine. Adenocarcinoma, malignant lymphoma, carcinoid tumour and leiomyosarcoma are well recognized but the incidence of these malignant tumours is difficult to determine. Even in large institutions experience is limited and there is no agreement amongst authors whether to include tumours of the ampullary region. The frequency of benign tumours is even more difficult to determine: in many reports the pathology is incompletely described and represented at best by the descriptive term 'polyp' which may be applied to many lesions. Moreover, it is clear that there is much confusion between neoplasms, hamartomas and heteroplasias and indeed in some cases the distinction is not clear.

In this review, primary tumours of the small bowel are considered, together with those non-neoplastic conditions which clinically simulate neoplasia. Malignant tumours of lymphoid tissue and endocrine tumours of the bowel are dealt with elsewhere (cf. Chapters 10 and 23).

Epithelial tumours

Adenomas

Adenomas of the small intestine have been reported to account for up to 20% of benign small intestinal neoplasms (Garvin et al. 1979) Nevertheless, when non-neoplastic lesions are critically excluded, it is probable that true benign epithelial neoplasms are rare. For example, the apparent macroscopic extension of familial polyposis coli into the small bowel is misleading (Fig. 22.1). Almost all such lesions are due to associated lymphoid hyperplasia (Bussey 1975). In contrast true adenomas occur in the small bowel in Gardner's syndrome (Bussey 1970, Gorlin & Chaudhry 1960); most patients with multiple adenomas of colon and small bowel have this syndrome.

Adenomas of the small bowel are histologically similar to those in the colon. Tubular adenomas are seen most often in the ileum, characteristically as small stalked or sessile polyps 1–3 cm in diameter. They are usually single but occasionally multiple. Villous tumours are sessile and generally more extensive (Mir-Madjlessi et al. 1973, Cooperman et al. 1978). They occur predominantly in the duodenum and upper jejunum and may surround the bowel wall but are soft so that they are impalpable through the unopened wall and their true extent underestimated.

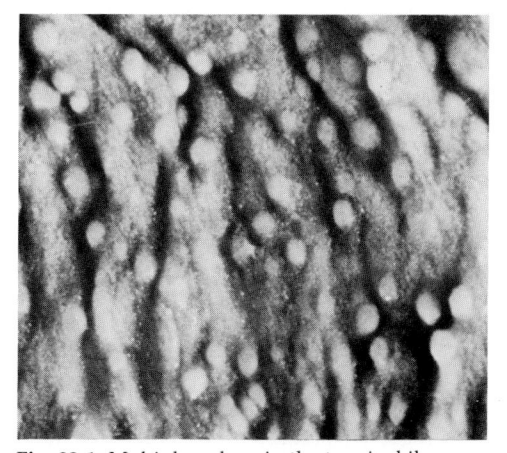

Fig. 22.1. Multiple polyps in the terminal ileum associated with familial polyposis. The polyps are due to lymphoid hyperplasia and not to epithelial proliferation. (Courtesy of Dr A.B. Price.)

Many adenomas are symptomless and may be incidental findings. They can, however, present with bleeding, intussusception and intestinal obstruction. Adenomas at the ampulla of Vater may produce obstructive jaundice.

It has become clear that villous tumours in the small intestine have the same propensity for malignant change as colonic villous tumours. Mir-Madjlessi *et al.* (1973) reviewed twenty-seven small intestinal villous adenomas: twenty lesions occurred in the duodenum, five contained invasive carcinoma and three focal or carcinoma *in situ*. Of seven villous tumours in the jejunum, two showed invasive carcinoma and one *in situ* change.

Adenocarcinoma

Adenocarcinomas occur in the small intestine forty to sixty-five times less frequently than in the colon and rectum. Nevertheless, large series have been collected from within single services or from the literature (Bernstein & Chey 1958, Brooks *et al.* 1968, Bridge & Perzin 1975). They are most common in the age group 50–60 years and are seen equally in males and females. The distribution within the bowel varies in different reports depending on whether or not lesions in the region of the ampulla of Vater are classified as a duodenal or biliary tumours (Table 22.1). Carcinomas are most frequent in the duodenum, upper jejunum and terminal ileum. In the duodenum, carcinomas of the peri-ampullary region predominate; when these are excluded there is no difference in the frequency of supra-papillary and infra-papillary tumours.

Macroscopically, small intestinal carcinomas are usually ulcerating and infiltrative producing a sharply localized 'napkin ring' structure (Wood 1967), but larger polypoidal, exophytic lesions are seen. The size varies from 1–10 cm in diameter. Some however, may be occult and difficult to see even on examination after fixation (Thompson *et al.* 1983). Histologically, they are usually of moderate differentiation and at the time of diagnosis have extended through the full thickness of the bowel wall to involve the peritoneum with transperitoneal spread and seeding. Occasionally enterocolic fistulae occur; perforation is rare. Spread to lymph nodes is initially to regional nodes and then to the para-aortic nodes. The 5-year survival rate after operation varies from 5–25% (Bridge & Perzin 1975, Brooks *et al.* 1968, Darling & Welch 1959). These data include patients undergoing both palliative and curative procedures. Too few cases have been studied systematically to relate histological features to the outcome of the disease. Superficial invasion limited to the mucosa or submucosa is a good prognostic feature but tumours are rarely seen at this stage. The presence of regional node involvement is important. In the study of Bridge & Perzin (1975), 88% of patients with nodal metastases died from the tumour whereas the corresponding figure for those with nodes free of tumour was 45%.

The rarity of small intestinal adenocarcinoma, especially when contrasted with the colon, is unexplained. Nevertheless, there are certain conditions with which it is associated. There is evidence that a number of carcinomas arise from pre-existing adenomatous polyps (Gannon *et al.* 1962, Johansen & Larsen 1969). Bridge & Perzin (1975) reported that five of forty-three jejunal and ileal adenocarcinomas had originated in adenomas and in Gardner's syndrome adenomas of the small intestine and peri-ampullary carcinoma may both occur.

Patients with coeliac disease are at greater risk than the general population for the development of malignant neoplasms, especially malignant lymphoma, but also including adenocarcinoma of small bowel (Saverymuttu *et al.* 1983). In the series reported by Swinson *et al.* (1983), nineteen cases of small intestinal adenocarcinoma occurred amongst 259 neoplasms complicating coeliac disease, compared with 0.23 expected from national cancer registration (Fig. 22.2).

There is an association between Crohn's disease and gastrointestinal carcinoma which is best established for the colon. The link is less well established in the small bowel but Thompson *et al.* (1983) were able to collect sixty-six cases from the literature of

Table 22.1. Distribution of small bowel adenocarcinoma.

Authors	Total number	Duodenum	Jejunum	Ileum	Multi-centric
Darling & Welch (1959)	33*	10	19	4	—
Rochlin & Longmire (1961)	321	113	108	98	—
Pagtalunan et al. (1964)	128*	41	65	22	—
Brooks et al. (1968)	53	20	18	11	—
Bridge & Perzin (1975)	122	79	32	11	2

*Excludes carcinomas arising in the ampullary region.

small intestinal carcinoma complicating Crohn's disease. Fifty-one cases occurred in the ileum matching the site of the primary inflammatory process which is in contrast to the usual distribution. This report is of importance in stressing the possible occult nature of the carcinoma complicating Crohn's disease and the need for close scrutiny of the specimen by the pathologist if it is not to be missed.

Carcinoma of the peri-ampullary region

Most patients with carcinoma of the peri-ampullary region are between 50 and 70. Weight loss, obstructive jaundice and abdominal pain are common clinical features. Carcinomas in this region may arise from bile ducts, pancreatic ducts or from the ampulla and adjacent duodenal mucosa. Rarely carcinomas may arise from Brunner's glands (Christie 1953). Exact definition of the site of origin may be difficult and Baggenstoss (1938) has indicated the difficulties in distinguishing the various epithelia in the ampullary region so that the histological appearances may be of little help. Macroscopic appearances of fungating or ulcerating duodenal mucosa may be a pointer to an ampullary origin.

It has been stated that there is little evidence of antecedent lesions preceding the development of carcinoma (Wood 1967) but they do appear to arise from pre-existing polyps (Cattell & Pyrtek 1950). Moreover, peri-ampullary carcinoma is increasingly recognized as a complication of Gardner's syndrome (McDonald et al. 1967, Capps et al. 1968), and this may develop on the basis of existing polyps or because of a predisposi-

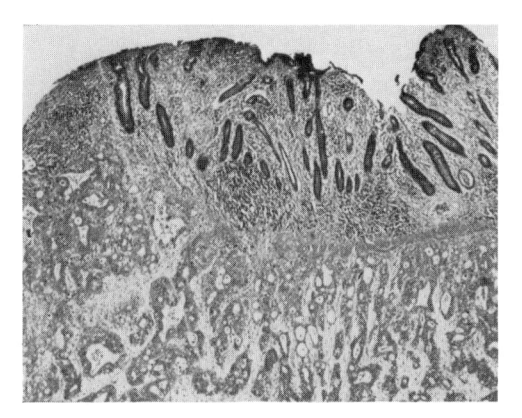

Fig. 22.2. Jejunal adenocarcinoma infiltrating through the bowel wall in a patient with coeliac disease. He had been treated with a gluten-free diet for 3 years before development of the carcinoma.

tion to malignant change in other local tissue. Carcinoma of the duodenum in this group of patients is more common in males and occurs in a younger age group. Bussey (1975) reported that the interval of time between colectomy and diagnosis of ampullary carcinoma varied between 1 and 25 years, averaging about 12 years.

Secondary carcinoma

True metastatic deposits of tumour in the small intestine are infrequent. More often there is involvement of a loop of intestine by direct spread from a contiguous primary tumour. Secondary spread from skin (melanoma) lung, adrenal, ovary, stomach, large intestine, uterus and kidney have been recorded (De Castro et al. 1957). Metastatic adenocarcinoma may spread in the mucosa and may histologically simulate a primary tumour. Rarely spread from a diffuse linitis plastica involves the small bowel wall with marked fibrosis and producing segmental stricturing to simulate Crohn's disease (Correia et al. 1968). Metastases from malignant melanoma produce a very characteristic gross appearance with multiple polypoidal and mushroom-like mucosal lesions (Fraser-Moodie et al. 1976).

Non-epithelial tumours

Smooth muscle tumours

Leiomyomas and leiomyosarcomas (Starr et al. 1955, Akwari et al. 1978) are less common in the small intestine than in the stomach. They are seen most commonly in the jejunum and ileum and less frequently in the duodenum. They may originate in any of the muscle layers and may grow into the lumen or through the wall towards the mesentery. Small tumours may be found incidentally at necropsy but larger tumours present as a mass with intussusception and obstruction, pain and intestinal bleeding.

Grossly smooth muscle tumours are lobulated and sharply delineated. Large size, greater than 5 cm diameter, multiple nodules and areas of macroscopic haemorrhage and necrosis are pointers towards malignancy. However, the microscopic identification of malignancy may be difficult (Ranchod & Kempson 1977). The frequency of mitoses is important: more than 5 mitoses/10 HP fields indicates malignancy but some leiomyosarcomas may show fewer mitoses than this (Akwari et al. 1978). Malignancy should be suspected with highly cellular lesions even if mitoses are not identified.

The histologically distinct leiomyoblastoma may also occur in the small bowel and is characterized by a predominance of large clear cells as well as more typical spindle cell areas. Most of these tumours are benign.

Neurogenic tumours

Neurilemmomas (Schwannomas) may arise in the bowel wall either as *de novo* lesions or as a complication of the hamartomatous von Recklinghausen's syndrome. They involve the submucosa or muscularis and may ulcerate the overlying mucosa. Grossly and histologically they may be difficult to distinguish from muscle tumours. Malignant Schwannomas and ganglioneuromas have been reported (Sivak et al. 1975, Haff & San Diego 1972). Multi-focal ganglioneuromatosis may occur in the submucosal and myenteric plexuses in association with phaeochromocytoma and medullary carcinoma of the thyroid (Williams & Pollock 1966).

Gangliocytic para-ganglioma, a benign tumour of uncertain histogenesis, occurs almost always in the second part of the duodenum adjacent to the ampulla of Vater (Taylor & Helwig 1962, Kepes & Zaccharias 1970, Reed et al. 1977). It presents as a small pedunculated polyp and frequently ulcerates. The histological appearances are complex but distinctive with epithelioid cells in a ribbon pattern, some in a rather radial distribution, set in juxtaposition to more solid areas of spindle and compact cells. Large ganglion-like cells are also seen. The exact nature of the tumour is unknown but argyrophilic granules are found in the cytoplasm and electron microscopy shows dense core granules of neuroendocrine type. Amyloid may be found in the stroma (Reed et al. 1977).

Haemangiomas

Haemangiomas are probably vascular malformations rather than true neoplasms and occur only infrequently in the gastrointestinal tract either as independent lesions or as part of a generalized vascular disorder such as the Parkes–Weber–Klippel or Rendu–Osler–Weber syndromes (Hansen 1948, Gentry et al. 1949, Shepherd 1953). They may be found at any age from early childhood to senescence, and account for 3–4% of all tumours of the small bowel. It is likely that this figure is an underestimate of the true frequency for many remain asymptomatic.

Haemangiomas in the small bowel are single or multiple and occur as cavernous or capillary haemangiomas either infiltrating diffusely in the submucosa or as circumscribed vascular polyps protruding into the lumen. They produce mechanical symptoms of intestinal obstruction and intussusception or of bleeding with overt melaena and anaemia; perforation rarely occurs. Malignant change in haemangiomas is rare (Murray-Lyon *et al.* 1971) and multiple, simple haemangiomas must be distinguished from true vascular metastasis.

Bandler (1960) reported multiple areas of phlebectasia in the submucosa of the bowel associated with mucocutaneous pigmentation and similar multiple small bowel involvement in relatives. It is not clear whether this lesion is a hamartoma or a vascular degeneration in normally formed vessels.

Malignant vascular tumours

Malignant vascular tumours are rare in the alimentary tract and probably arise *de novo* (Stout 1943). There are a few reports of angiosarcoma of the small bowel which have usually presented as solitary tumours though Murray-Lyon *et al.* (1971) reported a patient in whom malignant change supervened as a complication of haemangiomatosis of the small and large bowel.

Kaposi's sarcoma is predominantly a disease of the skin but may present in a systematized form involving lymph nodes and other organs including gut (Slavin *et al.* 1969). It may be seen in the small intestine as multiple haemorrhagic polyps, but also as a more circumscribed thickening of the wall (Fig. 22.3). Occasionally Kaposi's sarcoma may initially present within or be confined to the gut. The histological appearances in the intestine are identical to those found in the more common skin nodules.

Lipoma and liposarcoma

Lipomas are well recognized as submucosal tumours throughout the alimentary tract. Most are found in the ileum and they are commoner in the duodenum than the jejunum. Macroscopically they arise from the submucosal fat, protruding into the lumen as small yellowish nodules which may become pedunculated. They are usually asymptomatic incidental findings but they may ulcerate and bleed. They may form a

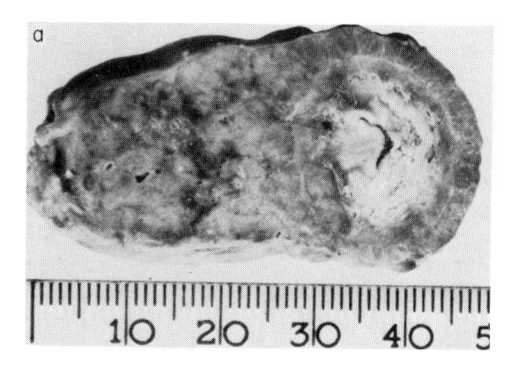

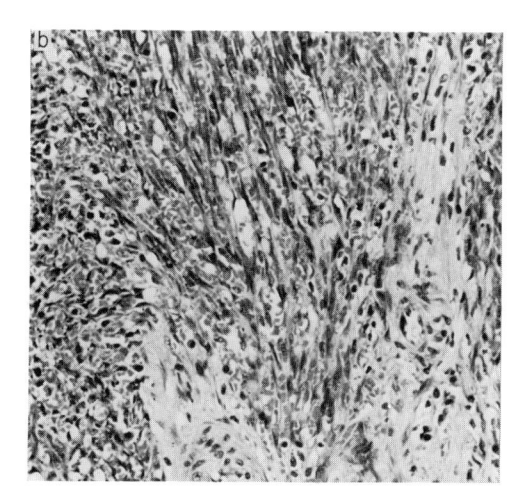

Fig. 22.3. (a) Small bowel in an African male who presented with intestinal obstruction. The submucosa is infiltrated with a haemorrhagic mass which extends into the mesentery. (b) Histology shows the characteristic features of Kaposi's sarcoma. No cutaneous lesions were found.

focus for intussusception and rarely a large lipomatous mass may compress the lumen. They are not distinctive histologically and resemble lipomas seen at other sites, being composed of mature adipose tissue with a variable mixture of fibrous tissue.

Most lipomas are probably not true neoplasms but represent local hyperplasia and, in keeping with this view, a diffuse lipomatosis affecting the ileocaecal valve has been described (Hopkins & Deaver 1963). Lipomas are benign and not prone to malignant change, though a true metastasizing liposarcoma of the ileum has been described (Mohandas *et al.* 1972).

Tumour-like lesions

Hamartomas

A hamartoma is a tumour-like but non-neoplastic malformation of tissue, 'characterized by an abnormal mixture of tissues indigenous to the part with an excess of one or more of these tissues and with evidence of an underlying developmental abnormality which may show itself at birth or by excessive growth in the postnatal period' (Willis 1958). Hamartomas may affect either epithelial or connective tissues and involve either a single organ or many organs in a complex syndrome. They are common in the gastrointestinal tract (Dawson 1969).

It is necessary to stress that hamartomas are not neoplastic though clinically they may present as tumour-like masses. However, hamartomatous malformations may undergo malignant change with the development of true neoplasms. The separation of some hamartomas from neoplasms is difficult and in some cases there may be real doubt as to the nature of the process. It is clear that many lesions commonly described as 'benign tumours', e.g. angiomas and neurofibromas, are tissue malformations rather than tumours.

Peutz–Jeghers syndrome

The Peutz–Jeghers syndrome is a hamartomatous complex characterized by oral and subcutaneous pigmentation with polyps in the gastrointestinal tract. Though the eponym acknowledges Peutz's report of the lesion in three members of a family (Peutz 1921), the buccal pigmentation was initially described by Hutchinson in twins (Willis 1958). Most reports are of single cases but Jeghers et al. (1949) described ten patients with a detailed review of the clinical features.

Males and females are equally affected and the most common presentation is in children and adolescents with colic and intestinal obstruction due to intussusception. This may resolve spontaneously and then recur. Haemorrhage from the polyps is frequent and anaemia is a prominent feature. The pigmentation is due to melanin deposition

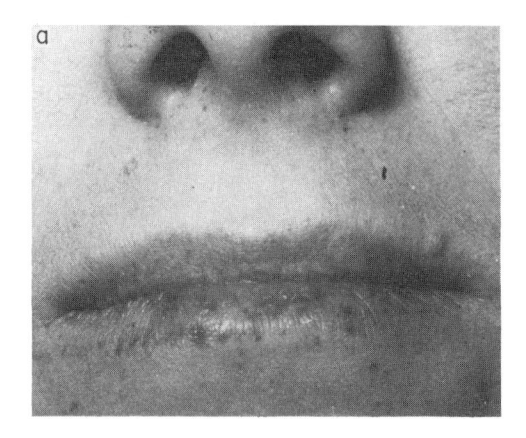

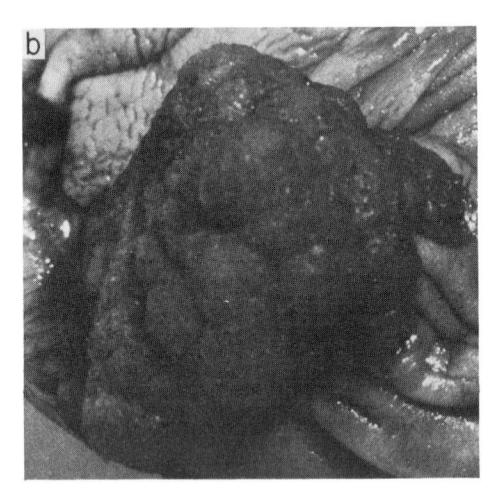

Fig. 22.4. (a) Pigmentation of lips and buccal mucosa in a patient with Peutz–Jeghers syndrome. (b) A resected polyp from the jejunum shows the characteristic coarsely lobulated pattern on the surface. In this patient invasive carcinoma developed in a duodenal polyp and at necropsy metastatic adenocarcinoma was found in regional lymph nodes and lungs. (Unpublished case of Dr A.H. James and Dr A Davey.)

and affects the buccal mucosa, skin of face and sometimes of the hands and feet. It is seen at birth or appears shortly afterwards as numerous small freckles about the eyes, nose and lips. On the mucosa of the lips the pigmentation shows as bluish, oval rather ill-defined areas of pigment (Fig. 22.4a).

Polyps in the Peutz–Jeghers syndrome occur in the stomach and colon but are most frequent in the small intestine where they are multiple and especially affect the jejunum. Most are small, 0.5–1 cm diameter; occasional large forms, 4–5 cm in diameter, are seen. The surface of the polyps is lobulated and similar to that of an adenomatous polyp though rather coarser. It does not have the smooth surface of the so-called juvenile polyp. They may be sessile or pedunculated though the stalk is broad and poorly defined (Fig. 22.4b).

The polyposis may progress by intermittent periods of growth with development of new polyps in areas of mucosa previously unaffected or by enlargement of previously noted polyps. There may then appear to be 'crops' of polyps occurring simultaneously in different parts of the bowel.

Microscopically Peutz–Jeghers polyps show a characteristic structure with arborescent proliferation of the muscularis mucosae: the branches of the muscularis become progressively finer and disappear at the surface. Each branch is covered by mucosa with normal epithelium and lamina propria. In small intestinal polyps the epithelial layer contains Paneth cells and endocrine cells in their normal crypt situation and in their normal number. In the body and fundus of the stomach the epithelium includes normal pepsin and oxyntic cells. The epithelium adjacent to the polyp is usually normal but may show mild villiform change.

Peutz–Jeghers polyps are hamartomatous and non-neoplastic. The epithelium covering them shows none of the stigmata of malignancy. This is of importance where mucus secretion is trapped and surrounding epithelial cells may simulate invasion. The normality of the epithelial cells will indicate the true nature of the lesion. Nevertheless in occasional cases the syndrome is complicated by the development of malignancy with metastasis to lymph nodes (Bussey 1970). Dozois et al. (1969) reviewed the literature concerning Peutz–Jeghers syndrome and recorded 321 cases in which 11 developed carcinoma: stomach 4, duodenum 3, colon and rectum 3, and ileum 1. In only three patients did the carcinoma appear to arise in a pre-existing polyp and some of the malignancies were in areas of mucosa lacking polyps. They concluded that these polyps do not predispose to malignant change. Bussey, however, is more cautious and concludes that the malignant potential of the Peutz-Jeghers syndrome cannot be considered negligible.

Inheritance of the syndrome is by an autosomal dominant gene (Dormandy 1957). Some members of affected families show the characteristic pigmentation without clinical evidence of polyps. Polyposis without pigmentation also occurs. Other abnormalities noted in association with the Peutz–Jeghers syndrome include carcinoma of stomach and colon, granulosa cell tumours of the ovary, vesical papillomas, amenorrhagoea and some of the cutaneous and skeletal hamartomas associated with Gardner's syndrome. The significance of these associations is not known and some at least may represent mere coincidence.

Juvenile polyposis

Juvenile polyps are found most frequently in the rectum and colon of children and adolescents but also in adults (Morson 1962, Roth & Helwig 1963). Rarely multiple juvenile polyps may be found throughout the gastrointestinal tract involving the stomach and small intestine as part of the juvenile polyposis syndrome (Veale et al. 1966). In the small bowel the polyps appear macroscopically similar to those in the colon: a smooth-surfaced polyp, 1–2 cm diameter with a thin pedicle. Surface ulceration and haemorrhage is common. On the cut surface, cysts with mucoid contents are apparent and it is this appearance which has given rise to the alternative title of 'retention polyp'.

Microscopically epithelial crypts and tubules, often dilated and cystic, are surrounded by an increased loose lamina propria. The inflammatory component is variable but may be marked, especially if there is ulceration. The crypts are lined by essentially normal cells though there may be flattening and degeneration. The epithelium does not show the proliferative pattern of an adenoma but when there is surface ulceration there may be reactive hyperplasia. This should not cause confusion; muscularis mucosae is not included which aids separation from Peutz–Jeghers polyps.

Juvenile polyps are not neoplastic. Their nature, however, is in doubt. They may be inflammatory but Morson & Dawson (1979) regard them as hamartomatous malformations of the lamina propria. They have been said to have no malignant potential but Stemper et al. (1975) described a remarkable kindred of twenty-one which contained ten members with single or multiple juvenile polyposis. Eleven of the kindred developed carcinomas of the stomach, duodenum and pancreas. The distribution of lesions within the kindred suggested a single, or two closely linked autosomal dominant inheritances for the polyp and development of carcinoma.

Bussey (1970) has distinguished two groups of juvenile polyposis: one is non-familial but is associated with other anomalies including congenital heart disease, hydrocephalus and visceral malrotations; the second is familial but without associated congenital anomalies.

Hamartomas of Brunner's glands

Proliferation of Brunner's glands may occur as single, sometimes multiple polyps on the posterior wall of the first and second parts of the duodenum and may be found incidentally or present clinically with melaena or obstruction. They have been described as adenomas but probably are non-neoplastic hamartomas or hyperplasias (Re Mine et al. 1970, Silverman et al. 1961, Buchanan 1961). They vary in size from a few millimetres to several centimetres and may be pedunculated. Histologically they show nodular or diffuse hyperplasia of Brunner's glands deep to the muscularis mucosae and lobulated by a connective tissue stroma. The epithelial cells are normal with basal nuclei lacking atypia; Paneth cells may be present. The cytological features exclude malignancy. However, the intimate mixture of normal epithelium, stroma and an associated proliferation of muscularis mucosae may suggest a Peutz–Jegher polyp, but a true tree-like structure is absent and the other cutaneous components of the syndrome are lacking. Rarely there may be cystic degeneration in a polyp which suggests an enterogenous cyst but these remain small in comparison to true enterogenous cysts which are more common in the ileal region (Booher & Pack 1946).

Cronkhite–Canada syndrome

This is a rare syndrome of widespread gastrointestinal polyposis associated with ectodermal changes characterized by alopecia, cutaneous pigmentation and atrophy of the nails (Manousos & Webster 1966). The mucosa throughout the gut shows marked polypoidal hypertrophy. The epithelial tubules are distended and cystic with flattened epithelium and the lamina propria shows marked oedema. These changes are associated with diarrhoea and malabsorption which may be severe.

The appearance of the oedematous stroma, lacking significant inflammation, resembles juvenile polyposis and Ruymann (1969) has suggested that these conditions may be related.

Multiple neurofibromatosis

Multiple neurofibromatosis is a hamartomatous syndrome usually presenting with subcutaneous nodules. These are characterized by an overgrowth of nerve sheath tissue. Gastrointestinal lesions are not uncommon and may affect about 10% of patients with the syndrome (Hochberg et al. 1974). Besides the hamartomatous nodules true neoplasms may develop, including neurilemmomas and malignant Schwannomas (Sivak et al. 1975).

Heterotopia

Heterotopia is the development of a particular tissue in a site where it is not normally found (Willis 1958). This may include the formation of a supernumerary organ or its transfer to an abnormal site, but it includes also dislocation of part of an organ rudiment and this may affect the bowel with the formation of sequestration cysts. Included in heterotopia is heteroplasia which is the anomalous differentiation of a developing epithelium such as the development of gastric mucosa in a Meckel's diverticulum. It is important that heterotopia and heteroplasia are distinguished from metaplasia, a reactive change of one mature epithelial cell type to another in response to inflammation or irritation.

Heterotopic tissue is well known to occur in the gastrointestinal tract. Heterotopic pancreas is most common in the duodenum and upper jejunum (Barbosa et al. 1946). It normally presents as a well-circumscribed nodule protruding into the lumen but it may extend through the wall into the mesentery. In the wall of the bowel the ectopic pancreas mixes intricately with the muscle fibres; acinar and endocrine tissue may be present and one or more accessory ducts seen. When the acinar component is scanty with dilated ducts and surrounded by the smooth muscle of the bowel, the appearances have given rise to the term 'myoepithelial hamartoma' of the duodenum.

Heterotopic gastric mucosa occurs in Meckel's diverticulum where it may produce ulceration, haemorrhage and perforation. However, with use of endoscopy it is increasingly recognized in the proximal duodenum where it may produce distortion with nodules up to 1 cm in diameter (Fig. 22.5). The incidence of the condition is probably much higher than the reported frequency and may be present in up to 2% of the population. Lessels & Martin (1982) identified thirteen cases in one endoscopy clinic over an 18-month period. Isolated case reports of polypoidal masses up to 2.5 cm in diameter have been described in the duodenum at the ampulla of Vater and in the jejunum (Gore & Williams 1953). As yet gastric heteroplasia in the duodenum appears to have little clinical significance and there is no evidence of an association with peptic ulceration.

Inflammatory and hyperplastic lesions

Inflammatory fibroid polyps

Inflammatory fibroid polyps of the gastrointestinal tract are localized non-neoplastic lesions which occur usually in the stomach

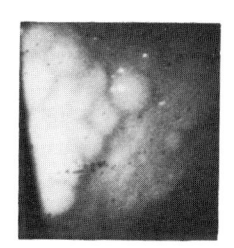

Fig. 22.5. Endoscopic appearance as seen through the pylorus of heterotopic gastric mucosa in the duodenum with multiple mucosal nodules protruding into the lumen. (Courtesy of Dr A.M. Lessels.)

but also in the small intestine. Initially reported by Vanek (1949) as gastric submucosal lesions with eosinophilic infiltration, they have been described by many other names. These include eosinophilic granulomas, haemangiopericytoma, inflammatory pseudo-tumour, fibroma with eosinophilic infiltration and eosinophilic gastroenteritis. The multiplicity of names and relatively infrequent occurrence within a single pathologist's experience have led to confusion with other entities including neoplasms.

Inflammatory fibroid polyps are nearly always solitary and occur most frequently in the stomach. McGee (1960) described similar lesions in the ileum. Johnstone & Morson (1978) reviewed seventy-six cases and added thirteen of their own; nine cases were ileal polyps presenting as intussusception. The infrequency of the lesion may be more apparent than real. Nkanga et al. (1980) were able to describe a further twelve cases of ileal intussusception due to inflammatory fibroid polyps in Africans from Malawi.

When removed at operation the lesions are sessile or stalked polypoidal masses localized in the bowel wall and protruding into the lumen (Fig. 22.6). They are variable in size, usually 2–4 cm in diameter but larger masses may occur. They arise in the submucosa and the overlying mucosa is frequently ulcerated at the polyp tip. On the cut surface the polyps have a homogeneous, somewhat translucent, appearance.

Microscopically the polyps consist of a mass of loose connective tissue arising in the submucosa and projecting into the lumen. The tissue is vascular with proliferating capillaries in a loose stroma and little collagen formation. Thick-walled vessels are prominent and ectatic vascular channels at the base are a constant feature. There is a variable inflammatory infiltrate with lymphocytes and plasma cells and in ulcerated lesions an admixture of acute inflammatory cells. Eosinophils are usually seen but the degree of tissue eosinophilia, both between lesions and within a single polyp, ranges from normal to those in which it is a predominant and striking feature.

At the base the loose connective tissue of the stalk extends into and separates the muscle layers. There may be apparent destruction of the muscle with extension of the lesion to the serosa. There is no sharp line of distinction of the polyp at its base from the adjacent normal tissues and there is no encapsulation.

Vanek (1949) considered such polyps as inflammatory and this is now generally agreed. Johnstone & Morson (1978) have speculated that the condition is an uncontrolled mesenchymal proliferation occurring as a result of minor trauma.

Previous reports that the lesion is a neoplasm of neural origin, neurofibroma and Schwannoma or a vascular tumour (Stout 1949), now hold little attraction. Recurrence after incomplete excision has been reported but malignant change has not been described (McGreevy et al. 1967).

There is still some confusion between inflammatory fibroid polyps and eosinophilic gastroenteritis. This was partly because of the frequency of tissue eosinophilia in each and also because of confused nomenclature compounded by a lack of understanding of the aetiology of either condition. Johnstone & Morson (1978) reviewed the literature on eosinophilic gastroenteritis and clearly distinguished it from inflammatory fibroid polyps so that the entities should not now be confused (Table 22.2).

Lymphoid hyperplasia

Peyer's patches may clearly be seen on the mucosal surface of the small intestine. In

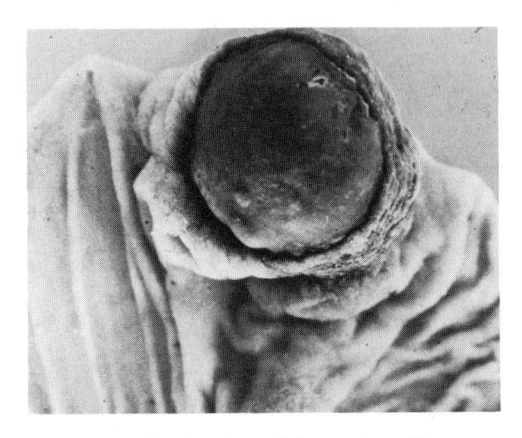

Fig. 22.6. Stalked, polypoidal mass 2 cm diameter protruding into the lumen of the ileum. The mass is composed of a vascular connective tissue with a marked inflammatory component.

young children and adults there may be lymphoid hyperplasia which forms polypoid tumour-like masses. These may be of such an extent that intestinal obstruction occurs either directly or because of intussusception. The remaining small bowel is normal. Microscopically, the lesions are characterized by lymphoid hyperplasia with active germinal centres. There is no relationship with malignant lymphoma.

In adults and children with hypogammaglobulinaemia the small bowel mucosa may show a generalized lymphoid hyperplasia producing small lymphoid polyps. This may be associated with giardiasis. It is considered fully in Chapter 8.

Endometriosis

Endometriosis may involve the small intestine producing an intramural mass with distortion and occasional obstruction (Rio et al. 1970). Microscopically, however, the diagnosis is straightforward with endometrial glands and stroma clearly separating the lesion from carcinoma.

References

Akwari O.E., Dozois R.R. & Weilland L.H. (1978) Leiomyosarcoma of small and large bowel. *Cancer*, **42**, 1375–1384.

Baggenstoss A.H. (1938) Major duodenal papilla.

Table 22.2. Inflammatory fibroid polyp and eosinophilic gastroenteritis (after Johnstone & Morson 1978).

	Inflammatory fibroid polyp	Eosinophilic gastroenteritis
Main age group	6–7th decades	5–4th decades
M : F	1.3 : 1.0	2.0 : 1.0
Allergic history	Absent	Present in 25%
Blood eosinophilia	Absent	Present in 80%
Tissue eosinophilia	Present	Present
Site	Stomach (small intestine)	Stomach (small intestine)
Gross appearance	Localized : Solitary	Diffuse : Multiple
Microscopy	Fibroblastic, granulation-like tissue	Oedematous tissue
Recurrence	None	Common

Variations of pathologic interest and lesions of the mucosa. *Arch. Path.* **26**, 853–868.
Bandler M. (1960) Haemangiomas of the small intestine associated with mucocutaneous pigmentation. *Gastroenterol.* **38**, 641–645.
Barbosa J.J. de C., Dockerty M.B. & Waugh J.M. (1946) Pancreatic heterotopia. *Surg. Gynae. Obstet.* **82**, 527–542.
Bernstein H.S. & Chey W.Y. (1958) Small bowel tumours — a clinical study of 109 cases. *Mt. Sinai J. Med.* **25**, 1–28.
Booher R.J. & Pack G.T. (1946) Cysts of the duodenum. *Arch. Surg.* **53**, 588–602.
Bridge M.F. & Perzin K.H. (1975) Primary adenocarcinoma of the jejunum and ileum. *Cancer*, **36**, 1876–1887.
Brooks J.S., Waterhouse J.A.H. & Powell D.J. (1968) Malignant lesions of the small intestine — A 10-year survey. *Brit. J. Surg.* **55**, 405–410.
Buchanan E.B. (1961) Nodular hyperplasia of Brunner's glands of the duodenum. *Amer. J. Surg.* **101**, 253–257.
Bussey H.J.R. (1970) Gastrointestinal polyposis. *Gut*, **11**, 970–978.
Bussey H.J.R. (1975) *Familial Polyposis Coli.* Johns Hopkins University Press, Baltimore.
Capps W.F., Lewis M.I. & Gazzaniga D.A. (1968) Carcinoma of the colon, ampulla of Vater and urinary bladder associated with familial multiple polyposis. *Dis. Colon Rect.* **11**, 298–305.
Cattel R.B. & Pyrtek L.J. (1950) Premalignant lesions of the ampulla of Vater. *Surg. Gynae. Obstet.* **90**, 21–30.
Christie A.C. (1953) Duodenal carcinoma with neoplastic transformation of the underlying Brunner's glands. *Brit. J. Cancer*, **7**, 65–67.
Cooperman M., Clausen K.P., Hecht C., Lucas J.G. & Keith, L.M. (1978) Villous adenomas of the duodenum. *Gastroenterol.* **74**, 1295–1297.

Correia J.P., Baptista A.S. & António J.P. (1968) Slowly evolving widespread diffuse alimentary tract carcinoma. *Gut*, **9**, 485–488.
Darling R.C. & Welch C.E. (1959) Tumours of the small intestine. *New Engl. J. Med.* **260**, 397–408.
Dawson I.M.P. (1969) Hamartomas in the alimentary tract. *Gut*, **10**, 691–694.
De Castro C.A., Dockerty M.B. & Mayo C.W. (1957) Metastatic tumours of the small intestines. *Surg. Gynae. Obstet.* **105**, 159–165.
Dormandy T.L. (1957) Gastrointestinal polyposis with mucocutaneous pigmentation (Peutz–Jeghers syndrome). *New Eng. J. Med.* **256**, 1093–1103.
Dozois R.R., Judd E.S., Dahlin D.C. & Bartholomew L.G. (1969) The Peutz–Jeghers syndrome: is there a predisposition to the development of intestinal malignancy? *Arch. Surg.* **98**, 509–517.
Fraser-Moodie A., Hughes R.G., Jones S.M., Storey B.A. & Sharp L. (1976) Malignant melanoma metastasic to the alimentary tract. *Gut*, **17**, 206–209.
Gannon P.G., Dahlin D.C., Bartholomew L.G. & Beahrs O.H. (1962) Polypoid glandular tumours of the small intestine. *Surg. Gynec. Obstet.* **114**, 666–672.
Garvin P.J., Herrmann V., Kaminski D.L. & Willman V.L. (1979) Benign and malignant tumours of the small intestine. *Curr. Prob. Cancer*, **3**, 1–46.
Gentry R.N., Dockerty M.B. & Clagget O.T. (1949) Collective Review. Vascular tumours and vascular malformation of the gastrointestinal tract. *Int. Abstr. Surg.* **88**, 281–323.
Gore I. & Williams W.J. (1953) Adenomatous polyp of the jejunum composed of gastric mucosa. *Cancer*, **6**, 164–166.
Gorlin R.J. & Chaudhry A.P. (1960) Multiple osteomatosis, fibromas, lipomas and fibrosarcomas

of skin and mesentery, epidermoid inclusion cysts of skin, leiomyomas and multiple intestinal polyposis. (1960). *New Engl. J. Med.* **263**, 1151–1158.

Haff R.C. & San Diego A.G. (1972) Ganglioneuroma of the ileocaecal valve. *Arch. Pathol.* **93**, 549–551.

Hansen P.S. (1948) Haemangioma of the small intestine. With special reference to intussusception. Review of the literature and report of 3 new cases. *Amer. J. Clin. Path.* **18**, 14–42.

Hochberg, F.H., Da Silva A.B., Galdabini J. & Richardson E.P. (1974) Gastrointestinal involvement in von Recklinghausen's neurofibromatosis. *Neurology (Minneapolis)*, **24**, 1144–1151.

Hopkins J.E. & Deaver J.M. (1963) Lipomatosis of the ileocaecal valve. *Dis. Colon Rect.* **6**, 215–218.

Jeghers H., McKusick V.A. & Katz K.H. (1949) Generalised intestinal polyposis and melanin spots on the oral mucosa, lips and digits. *New Engl. J. Med.* **241**, 993–1005.

Johansen A. & Larsen E. (1969) Adenomas of the small intestine. A report of four cases with special reference to their relationship to carcinoma. *Acta Path. Microbiol. Scand.* **75**, 247–253.

Johnstone J.M. & Morson B.C. (1978) Eosinophilic gastroenteritis. *Histopath.* **2**, 335–348.

Johnstone J.M. & Morson B.C. (1978) Inflammatory fibroid polyp of gastrointestinal tract. *Histopath.* **2**, 349–361.

Kepes J.J. & Zaccharias D.L. (1970) Gangliocytic paraganglioma of the duodenum. Report of two cases with light and electron microscopic examination. *Lancet*, **27**, 61–70.

Knox W.G., Miller R.E., Begg C.F. & Harold A.Z. (1960) Juvenile polyposis of the colon. A clinico-pathological analysis of 75 polyps in 43 patients. *Surg. St. Louis*, **48**, 201–210.

Lessels A.M. & Martin D.F. (1982) Heterotopic gastric mucosa in the duodenum. *J. Clin. Path.* **35**, 591–598.

McDonald J.M., Davis W.C., Crago H.R. & Berk A.D. (1967) Gardner's syndrome and periampullary malignancy. *Amer. J. Surg.* **113**, 425–430.

McFarland P.H., Scheetz W.L. & Knisley R.E. (1968) Gardner's syndrome: Report of two families. *J. Oral Surg.* **26**, 632–638.

McGee Jr H.J. (1960) Inflammatory fibroid polyps of the ileum and caecum. *Arch. Path.* **70**, 203–207.

McGreevy P., Doberneck R.C., McLeay J.M. & Miller F.A. (1967) Recurrent eosinophilic infiltrate (granuloma) of the ileum causing intussusception in a 2-year-old child. *Surg.* **61**, 280–284.

Manousos O. & Webster C.U. (1966) Diffuse gastrointestinal polyposis with ectodermal changes. *Gut*, **7**, 375–379.

Mir-Madjlessi S., Farmer A.G. & Hawk W.A. (1973) Villous tumours of the duodenum and jejunum: report of 4 cases and review of the literature. *Amer. J. Dig. Dis.* **18**, 467–476.

Mohandas D., Chandra R.S., Srinivasan V. & Bhaskar A.G. (1972) Liposarcoma of the ileum with secondaries in the liver. *Amer. J. Gastroenterol.* **58**, 172–176.

Morson B.C. (1962) Some peculiarities in the histology of the intestinal polyps. *Dis. Colon Rect.* **5**, 337–344.

Morson B.C. & Dawson I.M.P. (1979) *Gastrointestinal Pathology*. 2nd ed., p. 254. Blackwell Scientific Publications, Oxford.

Murray-Lyon I.M., Doyle D., Philpott R.M. & Porter N.H. (1971) Haemangiomatosis of the small and large bowel with histological malignant change. *J. Path.* **105**, 295–297.

Nkanga N.K., King M.H. & Hutt M.S.R. (1980). Intussusception due to inflammatory fibroid polyps of the ileum: a report of 12 cases from Africa. *Brit. J. Surg.* **67**, 271–274.

Pagtalunan R.J.G., Mayo C.W. & Dockerty M.B. (1964) Primary malignant tumours of the small intestine. *Amer. J. Surg.* **108**, 13–18.

Peutz J.D.A. (1921) Over een zeer Merkwendige, gecombineerde familiare polyposis van der sylijmueligen van den tractus intestinalis met die van deu neuskeelhotte engepaard met eigenaardige pigmentaties van huid en slijmuliegen. *Ned. Tijdschr. Geneeskd.* **10**, 134–146.

Ranchod M., French T.J., Novis B.H., Banks E. & Marks I.M. (1972) Diffuse nodular lipomatosis and diverticulosis of the small intestine. *Gastroenterol.*, **63**, 667–671.

Ranchod M. & Kempson R.L. (1977) Smooth muscle tumours of the gastrointestinal tract and retroperitoneum. *Cancer*, **39**, 255–262.

Reed R.J., Daroca P.J. & Harkin J.C. (1977) Gangliocytic paraganglioma. *Amer. J. Surg. Pathol.* **1**, 207–216.

Re Mine W.H., Brown Jr. P.W., Gomes M.N.R. & Harrison Jr E. (1970) Polypoid hamartomas of Brunner's glands. Report of six surgical cases. *Arch. Surg.* **100**, 313–316.

Rio F.W., Edwards D.L., Regan J.F. & Schmutzer K.J. (1970) Endometriosis of the small bowel. *Arch. Surg.* **101**, 403–405.

Rochlin D.B. & Longmire W.P. (1961) Primary tumours of the small intestine. *Surg.* **50**, 586–592.

Roth S.I. & Helwig E.B. (1963) Juvenile polyps of the colon and rectum. *Canc. N.Y.* **16**, 468–479.

Ruymann F.B. (1969) Juvenile polyps with cachexia; report of an infant and comparison with Cronkite–Canada syndrome in adults. *Gastroenterol.* **57**, 431–438.

Saverymuttu S., Hodgson H.U.F. & Evans D.J. (1983) Coeliac disease, adenocarcinoma of jejunum and *in situ* squamous carcinoma of oesophagus. *J. Clin. Path.* **36**, 62–68.

Shepherd J.A. (1953) Angiomatous conditions of the gastrointestinal tract. *Brit. J. Surg.* **40**, 409–421.

Silverman L., Waugh J.M., Huizenga K. & Harrison Jr E.G. (1961) Large adenomatous polyp of Brunner's gland. *Amer. J. Clin. Path.* **36**, 438–443.

Sivak M.V., Sullivan B.H. & Farmer R.G. (1975) Neurogenic tumours of the small intestine. *Gastroenterol.* **68**, 374–380.

Slavin G., Cameron H. & Singh H. (1969) Kaposi's sarcoma in mainland Tanzania. *Brit. J. Canc.* **23**, 349–357.

Starr G.F. & Dockerty M.B. (1955) Leiomyomas and leiomyosarcomas of the small intestine. *Cancer,* **8**, 101–111.

Stemper T.J., Kent T.H. & Summers R.W. (1975) Juvenile polyposis and gastrointestinal cancer. A study of a kindred. *Ann. Int. Med.* **83**, 639–646.

Stout A.P. (1943) Haemangioendothelioma: a tumour of blood vessels featuring vascular endothelial cells. *Ann. Surg.* **129**, 538–547.

Stout A.P. (1949) Haemangiopericytoma, a study of 25 new cases. *Cancer,* **2**, 1027–1054.

Swinson C.M., Slavin G., Coles E.C. & Booth C.C. (1983) Coeliac disease and malignancy. *Lancet,* **i**, 111–115.

Taylor H.B. & Helwig E.B. (1962) Benign non-chromaffin para-gangliomas of the duodenum. *Virchow. Arch. Path. Anat.* **335**, 356–366.

Thompson E.M., Clayden G. & Price A.B. (1983) Cancer in Crohn's disease — an 'occult' malignancy. *Histopath.* **7**, 365–377.

Vanek J. (1949) Gastric submucosal granuloma with eosinophilic infiltration. *Amer. J. Path.* **25**, 397–411.

Veale A.M.O., McColl I., Bussey H.J.R. & Morson B.C. (1966) Juvenile polyposis coli. *J. Med. Genet.* **3**, 5–16.

Williams E.D. & Pollock D. (1966) Mucosal neuromata with endocrine tumours: a syndrome allied to von Recklinghausen's disease. *J. Path. Bact.* **91**, 71–80.

Willis R.A. (1958) *The Borderland of Embryology and Pathology.* Butterworth & Co., London.

Wood D.A. (1967) *Tumours of the Intestines.* Armed Forces Institute of Pathology, Washington.

Chapter 23
Regulatory Peptides and Hormone-secreting Tumours

S.R. BLOOM AND JULIA M. POLAK

Regulatory peptides 377
Endocrine cells 377
Functions of individual peptides 378
Intestinal disease 383
Endocrine tumours 388

It is more than 80 years since secretin was discovered by Bayliss & Starling, the first demonstration of a hormone and the first recognition that hormonal substances are present in the gastrointestinal tract. Subsequent progress was inhibited, however, by the technical difficulties involved in isolating the gastrointestinal hormones. Unlike other endocrine systems in the body, where cells producing a hormone are present in specific and defined endocrine glands, the endocrine cells of the gut are scattered diffusely throughout a mass of tissue containing a wide variety of cell types. Furthermore, the gastrointestinal tract contains digestive enzymes capable of rapidly destroying hormones and it was therefore necessary to develop isolation techniques which inhibited enzyme activity without destroying the elusive hormone. In recent years, the successful development of such techniques (Mutt 1980) has led to the isolation of a wide variety of peptides from the gastrointestinal tract. Whilst some of these substances undoubtedly act as hormones, or as neurotransmitters, the precise role of other gastrointestinal peptides in human physiology and disease requires further elucidation.

Understanding of the relationship between the endocrine and nervous systems has developed rapidly during the past decade. The same substances that function as gut hormones may also be present in the nervous system where they may act as neurotransmitters or neuromodulators. Cholecystokinin, for example, is present in greater quantities in the brain than in the intestine. There is clearly a close integration of neural and endocrine activity. In the adrenergic system, the circulating levels of noradrenaline may rise to act in a hormonal manner throughout the body if sufficient peripheral adrenergic activity is stimulated. This system, furthermore, has developed a specific endocrine component, the adrenal gland.

In the gut, the neural and endocrine systems should be considered as an integrated whole. The intestine has two major neural plexi, the myenteric and the submucous, both of which have distinct populations of neurones which produce different neurotransmitters, many of which are peptides. This system constantly interacts with the endocrine cells of the gut which are localized in the mucosa (Ferri *et al.* 1983). It is a finely balanced system with a *sensory component* capable of recognizing the nature of the substances present within the lumen of the gastrointestinal tract, and an *effector component* comprising the endocrine and neural response to these intraluminal substances. The appropriate reactions of the gut to ingested food are therefore determined by this neuroendocrine system. Various types of food stimulate the production of hormones which then act upon organs such as stomach and pancreas to produce appropriate secretions. Whilst there is now abundant evidence to indicate how the hormones stimulate secretor responses, their precise role in the control of intestinal motility is less clearly defined.

The endocrine cells may release their products not only into the bloodstream but also locally to diffuse throughout local tissue and act in a paracrine manner. It is thought, for example, that cholecystokinin may influence the production of succus entericus by local release in this way. The peptidergic nervous system within the bowel wall does not demonstrate point innervation (the type of innervation seen in the small muscles of the hand, where a single nerve fibre controls a single muscle fibre). By contrast, peptidergic intestinal nerves are relatively sparse but their product diffuses over some distance to exert a wide influence. When these neuropeptides are particularly active, significant escape can occur into the bloodstream and then produce hormonal effects. This is seen, for example, after bowel ischaemia when neuronal vasoactive intestinal peptide (VIP) in the bowel may escape into the general circulation in considerable quantities (Modlin et al. 1978b).

Recent advances in intestinal endocrinology rest on the success of biochemists in isolating each of the regulatory peptides and then manufacturing large quantities of the pure material by means of synthetic chemistry. If antibodies are then raised to these substances, individual cells producing each peptide can be localized by immunocytochemistry and the concentrations of these peptides may be measured by radioimmunoassay in tissue or body fluids.

Regulatory peptides

Table 23.1 lists the regulatory peptides that have so far been isolated from the gastrointestinal tract. Of these, gastrin, secretin, cholecystokinin, pancreatic polypeptide, motilin, neurotensin and somatostatin act physiologically as hormones. Gastric inhibitory polypeptide and PYY are putative hormones but their precise function is not yet established. The actions of the remaining peptides, located to nerves, is probably as neurotransmitters or neuromodulators.

Their distribution in the gastrointestinal tract varies. Some peptides, such as gastrin and secretin, are present only in the stomach or proximal small intestine. Others are proximal small intestinal peptides and yet others are associated with the distal small intestine.

Endocrine cells

The endocrine cells of the gastrointestinal tract were originally recognized as enterochromaffin cells. In 1938, Feyrter first suggested that there was a group of cells diffusely distributed throughout the gastrointestinal tract which could be characterized as a 'diffuse endocrine epitheliala Organa' in the epithelium. The cells had faintly stained cytoplasm and he called these clear cells 'helle Zellen'. Ultrastructural studies have shown that these cells are typical endocrine cells, containing characteristic secretory granules. These features, together with their histochemical properties (Amine Precursor Uptake and Decarboxylation) led Pearse to develop the concept that there is a specific family of cells, which he termed APUD cells, which are responsible for the secretion of low molecular weight polypeptide hormones. The endocrine and enterochromaffin cells of the gut epithelium belong to the APUD series, as well as the pancreatic islet cells, the adrenal medulla, the calcitonin-producing cells of the thyroid gland, carotid body cells and some cells of the anterior pituitary.

On conventional histological staining the endocrine cells of the gut appear more lightly stained than the non-endocrine mucosal cells. The cells are pear-shaped or triangular in section, the narrower portion facing the lumen and the broader part, sometimes showing a basal extension, resting on the basement membrane, frequently in close association with a capillary (Fig. 23.1). There are microvilli on the luminal side of the cell (Fig. 23.1b), where they are presumed to be involved in the sensory component of the gut neuroendocrine system. The cytoplasm contains numerous electron-dense secretory granules of typical shape, density, size and limiting membrane which permit the characterization of individual endocrine cell types. Classification of endocrine cells on purely ultrastructural characterization has gradually given place to a more 'functional' classification in parallel with the association of particular types of secretory granule with the production of specific peptides established by means of combined immunocytochemistry and electron microscopy (Table 23.2).

Since the first characterization of antral endocrine cells containing gastrin by means

Table 23.1. Regulatory peptides isolated from the gastrointestinal tract.

Peptide	Probable mode of action	Distribution
Gastrin	Hormone	Antral cells
Secretin	Hormone	Upper small intestinal cells
Cholecystokinin	Hormone, paracrine (neurotransmitter in brain)	Upper small intestinal cells
Pancreatic, polypeptide	Hormone	Pancreatic cells (including islets)
Motilin	Hormone	Small intestinal cells
Glucose-dependent insulinotropic peptide (GIP)	Hormone	Small intestinal cells
Neurotensin	Hormone	Lower small intestinal cells
Enteroglucagon	Hormone	Lower small intestinal and colonic cells
Peptide Tyrosine Tyrosine (PYY)	Hormone	Lower small intestinal and colonic cells
Somatostatin	Hormone, paracrine (neurotransmitter)	Entire GI tract
Neuropeptide Y (NPY)	Neurotransmitter	Upper GI tract nerves
Vasoactive intestinal peptide (VIP) including peptide histidine isoleucine (PHI) which is co-secreted	Neurotransmitter	Entire GI tract nerves
Substance P	Neurotransmitter	Entire GI tract nerves
Enkephalin	Neurotransmitter	Entire GI tract nerves
Bombesin	Neurotransmitter	Entire GI tract nerves
Calcitonin gene-related peptide (CGPR)	Proposed neurotransmitter	Probably entire GI tract
Galanin	Proposed neurotransmitter	Probably entire GI tract

of immunocytochemistry (McGuigan 1968), the use of immunocytochemistry for the visualization of gut endocrine cells has continued to increase (Fig. 23.2), supplemented by combining immunocytochemistry with electron microscopy in the sequential semi-thin/thin method (Busolati & Canese 1972, Polak et al. 1975) and lately by the use of direct electron microscopical immunocytochemistry and the use of region-specific antibodies (Varndell et al. 1983). This approach has led to a reclassification of the endocrine cells of the gut based on the addition of immunocytochemical findings to the ultrastructural features obtained by using conventional electron microscopy (Fig. 23.3) (Solcia et al. 1981).

Functions of individual peptides

Gastrin

In man, while most gastrin is synthesized in G cells of the antrum of the stomach, a few gastrin cells are also found in the mucosa of the upper small intestine. Gastrin has an active core, this being the last four amino acids, but has a beginning section of variable length, referred to by the total amino acid number (G-34, G-17, G-14 and so on). The larger form (G-34) is cleared more slowly from the circulation, having a half-life in man of about 40 min (Walsh et al. 1976) while the small G-17, although released in larger quantities, has a half-life of only 5 min. This

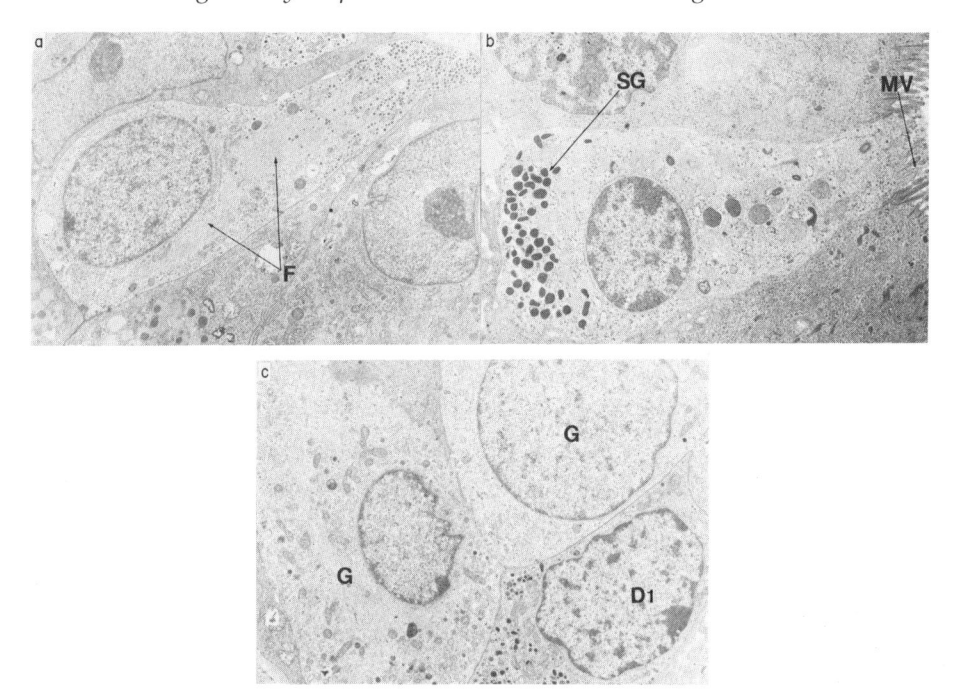

Fig. 23.1. (a) Somatostatin-containing cell from human gastric antrum. Numerous secretory granules are observed in the distal cytoplasm. The remaining cytoplasm has a central bundle of fibrils (F) running from the granules to a perinuclear termination. Glutaraldehyde/uranyl acetate-lead citrate (× 9500).
(b) Endocrine cell from ileal mucosa exhibiting apical microvilli (MV) and distal secretory granules (SG). The secretory granules are slightly pleomorphic. Glutaraldehyde/uranyl acetate−lead citrate (× 12,000).
(c) Cluster of endocrine cells from human gastric antrum exhibiting gastrin-containing (G) and an unknowning peptide (D_1)-containing cells. Glutaraldehyde/uranyl acetate-lead citrate (× 12,600).

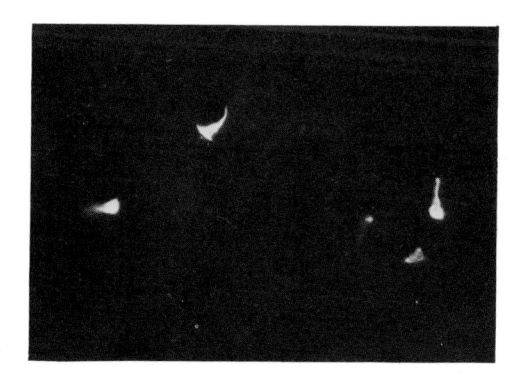

Fig. 23.2. A section of human colon, including mucosa, cut longitudinally. Enteroglucagon-containing cells can be seen with luminal elongations. Indirect immunofluorescence (× 450).

illustrates a general principle, that the smaller forms of the regulatory peptides are more rapidly destroyed, and where such multiple forms are produced, the endocrine cell tends to secrete the bigger form, while the neuronally produced regulatory peptide is more usually the smaller form, more rapid destruction perhaps being favoured for a neurotransmitter role. Gastrin has three major biological activities, stimulation of acid secretion, stimulation of gastric mucosal growth and enhancement of gastric motor activity.

Pancreatic polypeptide

Pancreatic polypeptide (PP) was isolated as a contaminant of insulin and only subsequently was its biological role investigated. This thirty-six amino acid polypeptide is synthesized by particular small granule endocrine cells of the pancreas which are most commonly found in the islets but also seen scattered throughout the substance of the exocrine pancreas. Both PP and gastrin

Table 23.2. Human gastroenteropancreatic endocrine cells.

Cell	Main product	Pancreas	Stomach Oxyntic	Stomach Antral	Small intestine Upper	Small intestine Lower	Large
P	Peptides?	a	+	+	+		
D₁	Peptides?	f	+	f	f	f	f
EC	5HT peptides	r,b	+	+	+	+	+
D	Somatostatin	+	+	+	+	f	f
B	Insulin	+					
PP(F)	Pancreatic polypeptide	+					
A	Glucagon	+	a,b				
X	Unknown		+				
ECL	Unknown (b, histamine)		+				
G	Gastrin			+	f		
IG	Gastrin			b	+		
TG	C-terminal gastrin/CCK			b	+	b	
I	CCK				+	f	
S	Secretin				+	f	
K	GIP				+	f	
Mo	Motilin				+	f	
N	Neurotensin			r	+	r	
L	GLI			f	+	+	

a = fetus or newborn; b = animals; f = few; r = rare (Solcia *et al.* 1981).

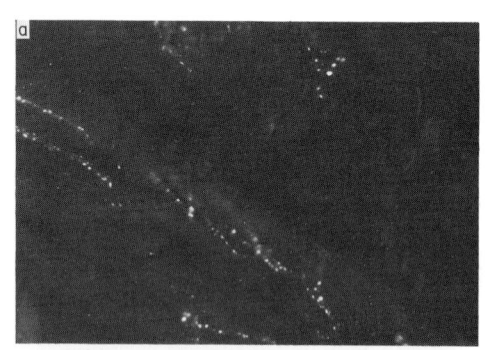

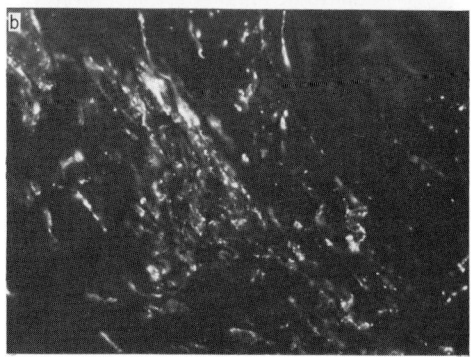

Fig. 23.3. Vasoactive intestinal polypeptide (VIP) nerves, stained using the indirect immunofluorescence technique in human colon from: (a) normal colon, and (b) Crohn's disease with colonic involvement (× 500).

are released by food, especially by protein and its constituents, but both can be released by vagal activation alone (for example during insulin-induced hypoglycaemia). PP is a weak inhibitor of gall bladder contraction and pancreatic enzyme secretion but whether these actions are its sole physiological role is unknown.

Secretin

Secretin is produced by a small number of endocrine cells in the duodenal mucosa. It is released by acid, when duodenal pH falls below 4 (Greenberg *et al.* 1982). The sole physiological action of secretin is the stimulation of pancreatic bicarbonate juice production. Plasma secretin, however, does not usually rise postprandially in man, and present evidence suggests that the release of secretin by low duodenal pH, which causes alkaline juice secretion from the pancreas, is a safety mechanism which only comes into play physiologically if the duodenal pH falls excessively.

Cholecystokinin

The last five amino acids of CCK are identical to those of gastrin and in both hormones this sequence composes the active site necessary for biological activity. Relative specificity of CCK for the pancreas and gallbladder is achieved by the three amino acids adjacent to the terminal pentapeptide as they differ from the sequence seen in gastrin. This octapeptide of cholecystokinin is the main form in the brain. In the gut, several larger forms are released with longer half lives in the circulation. Release of circulating cholecystokinin is stimulated by luminal long-chain fatty acids and amino acids. The extent of the rise in human plasma after a meal is still undecided but is only a few picomoles per litre and some authors conclude that CCK-8, though present in the mucosa, is not normally released (Dockray 1982). Cholecystokinin not only causes gallbladder contraction and pancreatic enzyme secretion, but also stimulates pancreatic growth. It may also have a role in stimulating local secretions in the intestine. Although cholecystokinin is a central neurotransmitter, most cholecystokinin-like immunoreactivity in the gut is localized in a specific mucosal endocrine cell, the I cell.

Motilin

Motilin is a peptide produced by endocrine cells scattered throughout the mucosa of the duodenum and jejunum. High concentrations are found in fasting human plasma but little change occurs after a mixed meal. Pharmacological studies show that it is active in causing contraction of smooth muscle of several areas of the gastrointestinal tract. When sequential measurements have been carried out at the same time as studies of motility using multi-luminal tubes inserted for the detection of the interdigestive myoelectric complex, motilin is found to be highest just before, or at the same time as initiation of the complex, and lowest immediately after a complex has occurred. Furthermore, infusion of motilin in fasting volunteers can induce the formation of a new complex even in the refractory period immediately following a previous complex. The motilin levels necessary to achieve this effect are, however, some two-to three-fold greater than those seen under physiological circumstances (Vantrappen et al. 1979). By contrast, only a small increment in plasma motilin is necessary to accelerate gastric emptying, suggesting that this effect may be physiologically significant (Christofides et al. 1979). Motilin has also been shown to induce colonic motor activity. Physiologically, therefore, motilin seems to act as a general stimulus to intestinal contractility.

Gastric inhibitory peptide

Gastric inhibitory peptide (GIP) is also produced by endocrine cells in the mucosa of the duodenum and jejunum, as well as the ileum. Its sequence is similar to that of secretin and glucagon. It therefore belongs to the same family, perhaps being the result of gene reduplication early in evolution. Although this peptide was discovered because of its inhibitory effect on gastric acid secretion, it was later found to be much more potent in stimulating insulin release from the beta cell of the pancreas. It has thus been re-named glucose-dependent insulinotropic peptide (GIP). It is now thought to be one of the mediators of the enteroinsular axis, the mechanism by which food taken by mouth is more effective in stimulating insulin release than substances given intravenously.

Neurotensin

Neurotensin was first isolated from the hypothalamus and later found to be produced by endocrine cells of the ileum. In man only a small rise of neurotensin occurs after a meal and its physiological role is still uncertain. Infusion experiments producing near physiological blood levels demonstrate a weak effect in inhibiting gastric acid secretion, slowing the rate of gastric emptying and stimulating pancreatic bicarbonate secretion.

Enteroglucagon

Enteroglucagon is a large peptide which contains within it the sequence of pancreatic glucagon. Its structure is such, however, that part of the pancreatic glucagon sequence is covered by a molecular fold so that the molecule does not activate pancreatic glucagon receptors, neither does it influence hepatic glycogenolysis. Enteroglucagon is released from EG cells found in the mucosa of the small and large intestine by two stimuli, long-chain fatty acids and carbohydrate. By contrast, both these stimuli suppress the release of pancreatic glucagon which, in man, is found only in the alpha cells of the islets of Langerhans. These two hormones, whose structure puts them in the same family as GIP and secretin, therefore play quite separate physiological roles. Animal experiments demonstrate a correlation between enterocyte production rate and plasma enteroglucagon concentrations. Pure enteroglucagon is not yet available but crude purified enteroglucagon stimulates the incorporation of labelled nucleic acids into the DNA of cultured enterocytes. This observation, together with studies in patients with small intestinal resection (cf. Chapter 6), lends support to the theory that enteroglucagon may be a 'growth hormone of the gut'. The association of villous hyperplasia with a tumour secreting enteroglucagon is described later in this chapter.

PYY

One of the regulatory peptides most recently isolated from the intestine is a 36 amino acid moiety with a tyrosine at either end. The symbol for tyrosine is Y and so it has been given the name PYY. This material inhibits gastric acid and pancreatic enzyme secretion and it may be the active component of Harper's pancreatone. Since it cannot yet be assayed in plasma, nothing is known of its physiological role.

Somatostatin

Somatostatin is interesting because it is present in the gut, both in endocrine cells and in nerves. Several molecular forms are known. The smallest, a 14 amino acid cyclic peptide, has full biological activity and this sequence is present in all the larger forms. Its name was originally invented to describe the inhibition of release of growth hormone from pituitary somatotrophs but it was subsequently found to be one of the most potent inhibitors known of all endocrine functions. In addition it also acts on the various hormone receptor tissues so that it blocks the effect of even an exogenous infusion of hormone. For example, it not only blocks gastrin release completely but also, if exogenous gastrin is infused, the actions of gastrin on the gastric parietal cell. It is therefore the most powerful known inhibitor of gastric acid secretion. Somatostatin also inhibits the release of motilin, secretin, cholecystokinin, GIP, neurotensin and enteroglucagon. It is thus a regulator of regulators. During infusion of somatostatin, absorption of nutrients in the small intestine is inhibited. Somatostatin also blocks the effect of intestinal secretagogues but, surprisingly, appears to enhance the frequency of interdigestive myoelectric complex-formation. The amount of somatostatin released after a meal is small, only producing a rise in the order of 2 or 3 pmol/1. This may, however, be enough to have physiological effects. The very large quantities of somatostatin locally within the bowel wall suggest that its major actions are probably paracrine and local. It is thus conceivable that the rise in concentration in the peripheral circulation is merely an overflow phenomenon. Cysteamine, an agent which depletes somatostatin, results in excessive acid secretion and ulcer formation. Animals given somatostatin antibodies also have augmented gastric acid secretion.

Vasoactive intestinal peptide

Vasoactive intestinal peptide (VIP) is a peptide neurotransmitter found throughout the body. The gut contains relatively large amounts, where it is produced by neurons of both the myenteric and submucous plexus (Fig. 23.3). It is present throughout the alimentary tract from the oesophagus to the rectum, including salivary glands and pancreas. This peptide, another member of the secretin/glucagon family, is a potent vasodilator and also acts to relax smooth muscle on the one hand and to stimulate many types of glandular secretions on the other. Systemic infusion in man produces mild flushing, hypotension and inhibition of intestinal absorption of fluid and electrolytes. More prolonged administration in animals results in watery diarrhoea. It is also a potent stimulator of pancreatic bicarbonate secretion, and of bile production, while it inhibits gall-bladder contraction and inhibits gastric acid secretion. In addition, it has been shown to relax the lower oesophageal sphincter and it presumably inhibits intestinal motor activity in general. As mentioned in the introduction, the physiological role of neurotransmitters in the gut is extremely difficult to study. VIP is thought to be important because of the large number of VIP-containing nerves present in the intestinal tract and in the central nervous system, but its precise role remains conjectural.

Peptide histidine isoleucine

Peptide histidine isoleucine (PHI) is a newly found member of the secretin/glucagon family and has the greatest similarity to VIP (Agnostides et al. 1984). Like VIP, it relaxes smooth muscle and stimulates secretion but it appears to have only a weak vasodilatory effect. Its distribution appears to mimic that of VIP and tissues examined by immunocytochemistry demonstrate co-localization with VIP. It has been suggested that VIP and PHI may be co-synthesized (Christofides et al. 1982). It is in fact possible that co-synthesis of more than one active peptide is a common phenomenon. Such a mechanism might increase specificity of action as both peptides would need to activate two separate receptors for the full biological effect to be seen. Since PHI has only recently been discovered, its physiological role and involvement in human disease is as yet unknown.

Substance P

Though substance P, an 11 amino acid peptide, is found in sensory neurones and the dorsal horn of the spinal cord, and has therefore been proposed as a sensory neurotransmitter, its role in the gut is more enigmatic. Most of the substance P is produced locally by neurones in the two neural plexi. It is not affected by agents such as capsaicin which, elsewhere, produces substance P depletion and loss of pain sensation. Substance P produces vasodilation and causes spasm of smooth muscle, for example in isolated guinea pig ileum. There seem, however, to be several different substance P receptors and C- and N-terminal fragments of the peptide appear to have different effects. Despite substance P being one of the earliest regulatory peptides to be found, its physiological role in the gut is uncertain.

Bombesin

Bombesin, so called because a similar peptide was first extracted from the skin of the frog *Bombina bombina*, is produced by intestinal neurones. It is a potent stimulant of the release of many other regulatory peptides and therefore has the opposite action to that of somatostatin. In addition, it stimulates pancreatic enzyme secretion and gastric acid secretion. Since it is present in considerable quantities and the peptide is freely available, it presumably has physiological effects but these are yet to be defined.

Enkephalin

Enkephalin is a member of the endogenous morphia-like peptide family (endorphins). A large number of similar, and potently active, peptides with the same active sequence, have now been isolated. The known effects of substances such as codeine which act through enkephalin receptors, suggest an important role in intestinal physiology.

Intestinal disease

A comprehensive survey of a wide variety of conditions has been carried out using a uniform stimulus (a 530 kcal normal test breakfast of two eggs, toast, marmalade, orange and coffee) and using standardized immunoassay techniques. These radioimmunoassay techniques have been described in detail by Bloom & Long (1982).

Obesity

While there has been much speculation that a hormone released from the gut might feed back on the brain to diminish appetite, there is little evidence for this. Many claims have been made but none substantiated. In a study of nineteen obese patients and age-matched controls, we could detect no difference in the release of gastrointestinal hormones, with the sole exception of insulin (Fig. 23.4) which showed a greater rise in the obese, inadequate, however, to deal with the greater postprandial hyperglycaemia (Bloom 1980).

Bypass procedures

Ileal bypass

This operation is carried out in patients with familial hypercholesterolaemia in order to reduce serum cholesterol by causing bile salt malabsorption. In a study of six patients with heterozygote familial hypercholesteremia, studied at least a year after bypass of the distal third of the ileum, cholecystokinin showed an excessive rise so that 1 h and 2 h after the meal CCK concentrations were more than twice those seen in the control group. Other hormones, including the ileal hormone neurotensin, were not strikingly affected (Allen et al. 1983).

Jejunoileal bypass

In twenty patients studied between 6 months and 1 year following a 7-inch proximal jejunum to 7-inch distal ileum anastomosis, with the intervening portion of bowel left *in situ* as a self-emptying loop, mean weight had fallen from 225% of ideal to 181%. In spite of the persistence of obesity in these patients, glucose tolerance greatly improved and the postprandial release of insulin fell to well below that seen in an age- and sex-matched group of healthy controls (Fig. 23.4). Postprandial release of enteroglucagon in the bypass patients was sixteen-fold elevated (Fig. 23.5), neurotensin eight-fold elevated (Fig. 23.6) and gastrin moderately elevated, while the release of GIP was greatly reduced.

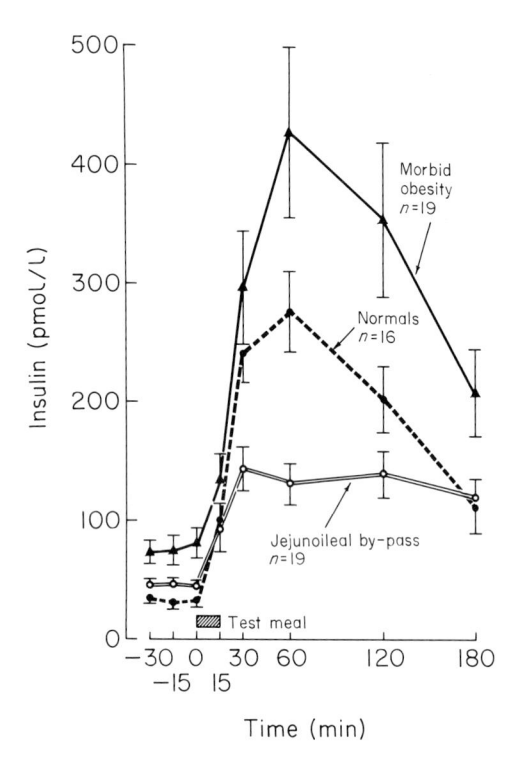

Fig. 23.4. Plasma insulin following a 530 calorie test breakfast in a group of non-diabetic morbidly obese subjects of more than 200% ideal body weight, a series of age- and sex-matched healthy subjects and patients who had undergone a 7-inch jejunum to 7-inch ileum small intestinal bypass procedure at least 6 months earlier and were now of steady weight and in good health.

These changes can be explained by the bypass of the area of the bowel bearing GIP cells with food passing unduly rapidly to the terminal ileum, where enteroglucagon and neurotensin cells are found. The slight increase of gastrin may be due to loss of an as yet unknown intestinal inhibitor of gastrin release. If the theory that enteroglucagon is trophic to the gut is true, then the large rise in the postprandial concentrations of this hormone may be responsible for the considerable growth of the bowel left in continuity. The operation, as described in Chapter 6, has a significant immediate mortility and subsequent substantial morbidity. Since it is also relatively unsuccessful in producing weight loss in the long term (Jewell et al. 1975, McLean et al. 1980), it has largely been abandoned.

fold elevated and GIP four-fold reduced following the same standard test meal as was used in the jejunal ileal bypass study mentioned above (Sarson et al. 1981).

Intestinal resection

Small intestinal resection in man might be expected to cause an elevation of enteroglucagon if the theory of its association with mucosal growth is correct. In a series of eighteen patients studied after partial resection of the ileum (0.4–2 m) the postprandial rise of enteroglucagon was more than doubled. Pancreatic glucagon, insulin, GIP and neurotensin release were unaffected but there was an approximately three-fold rise of postprandial gastrin, PP and motilin by comparison with an age-matched control group (Besterman et al. 1982). These hormonal changes are clearly part of the adaptive response but their precise significance is still uncertain. In contrast, in a group of nine patients who had undergone total or partial colectomy, although PP and gastrin were approximately two-fold elevated, other hormones were not significantly different from the control group. In particular, the postprandial response of enteroglucagon was actually lower than that of the controls (Besterman et al. 1982). A series of ten patients, who had had a proctocolectomy and formation of ileostomy for ulcerative colitis at least 18 months previously and were now in excellent general health, were studied. The basal enteroglucagon concentration was found to be significantly depressed in these ileostomists and while there was a slight elevation of basal motilin and postprandial neurotensin, other hormones were unchanged (Kennedy et al. 1982). Thus the large bowel has little influence on small intestinal gut hormone release.

Acute infective diarrhoea

A group of twelve patients were studied who, although previously completely healthy, had developed acute severe diarrhoea (at least eight motions a day) and required admission to hospital for treatment with intravenous fluid and electrolyte re-

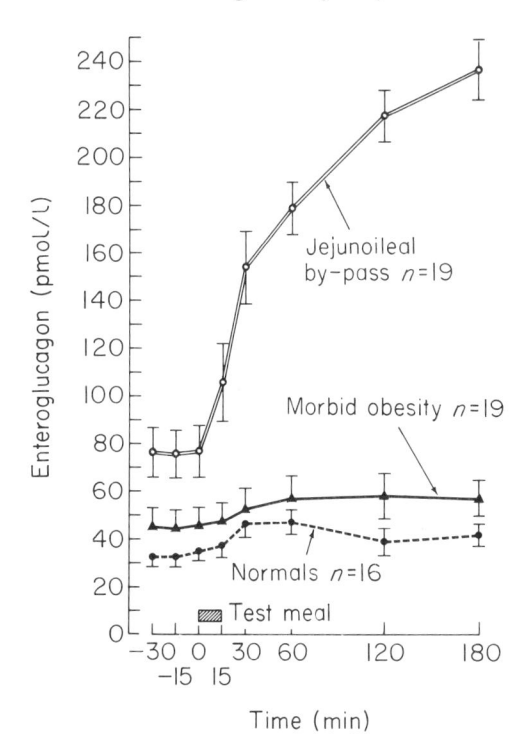

Fig. 23.5. Plasma enteroglucagon following a 530 calorie test breakfast in a group of non-diabetic morbidly obese subjects of more than 200% ideal body weight, a series of age- and sex-matched healthy subjects and patients who had undergone a 7-inch jejunum to 7-inch ileum small intestinal bypass procedure at least 6 months earlier and were now of steady weight and in good health.

Biliopancreatic bypass

This operation was evolved as a means for producing a more permanent but less drastic weight loss in the treatment of obesity (Scopinaro et al. 1980). In this procedure, the bypassed loop of intestine drains biliary and pancreatic secretions directly into the terminal ileum. Compensatory hypertrophy is a less marked feature of this procedure and weight loss is more permanent. Following both this procedure and jejunoileal bypass, weight loss is predominatly due to a reduced food intake rather than overt malabsorption. It is conceivable that this is due to an elevated hormone concentration, for example enteroglucagon, affecting appetite. In the biliopancreatic bypass enteroglucagon is about five-fold elevated, neurotensin four-

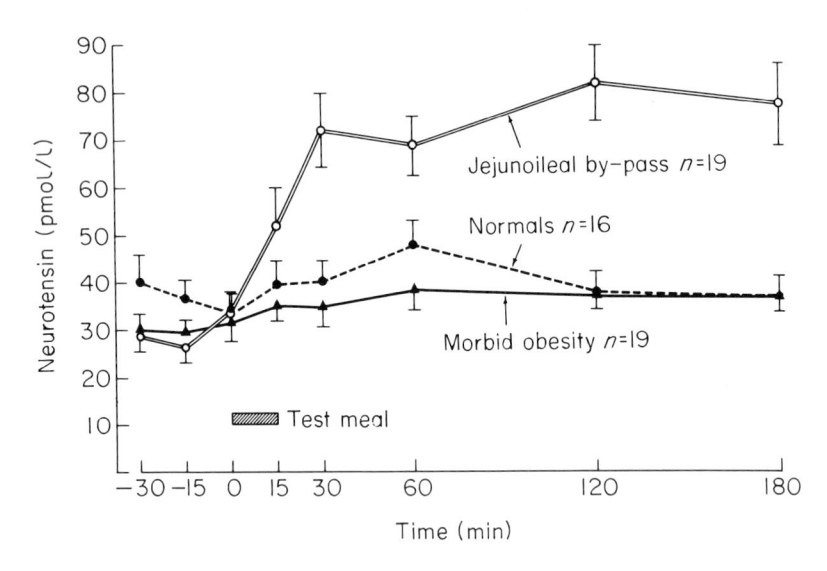

Fig. 23.6. Plasma neurotensin following a 530 calorie test breakfast in a group of non-diabetic morbidly obese subjects of more than 200% ideal body weight, a series of age- and sex-matched healthy subjects and patients who had undergone a 7-inch jejunum to 7-inch ileum small intestinal bypass procedure at least 6 months earlier and were now of steady weight and in good health.

placement. In only four patients was the aetiology found (two Salmonella and two Entamoeba coli). All patients made a complete recovery. Following a test breakfast, the patients were found to have a three-fold increased release of motilin (Fig. 23.7) and enteroglucagon (Fig. 23.8) and also slightly raised circulating gastrin and VIP concentrations. GIP, PP and pancreatic glucagon levels were normal (Besterman et al. 1983a).

Inflammatory bowel disease

Comparing fourteen healthy age-matched control subjects with fourteen patients with active Crohn's disease, the Crohn's disease patients were found to have increased fasting and postprandial levels of GIP, motilin and enteroglucagon (Besterman et al. 1983b). Further, they had a greater postprandial pancreatic polypeptide release. Levels of other hormones, including insulin, pancreatic glucagon, neurotensin and plasma VIP were normal. Since in exogenous motilin infusion studies with normal healthy volunteers, doubling the plasma motilin concentration causes a similar increase in the rate of gastric emptying, the more than twofold elevation of motilin in the Crohn's patients suggests that it may play a role in the induction of symptoms. The doubling of the plasma enteroglucagon concentration may relate to mucosal damage and the need for increased enterocyte turnover. By contrast, studies of intestine resected from Crohn's patients shows in both the area of active disease and in distal and apparently unaffected bowel, a gross alteration in the VIP-containing nerves (Fig. 23.3). Not only is the VIP content of the bowel wall increased, but the nerves themselves are distorted and dilated (Bishop et al. 1980). The significance of this change in the VIPergic innervation of the bowel is unknown. It may be of diagnostic value if it can be detected in rectal biopsies (O'Morain et al. 1984).

Coeliac disease

Eleven patients with untreated coeliac disease were compared with thirteen healthy age-matched control subjects and thirteen coeliac patients in remission following treatment with a gluten-free diet. After the standard meal, the enteroglucagon concen-

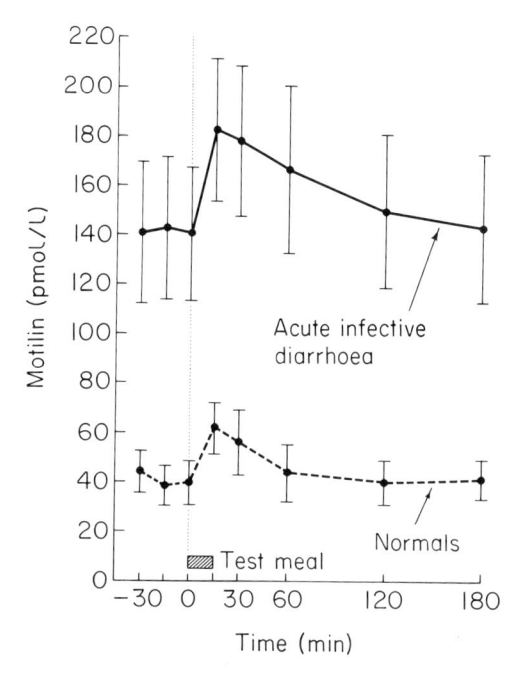

Fig. 23.7. Plasma motilin concentrations in twelve previously healthy subjects hospitalized for acute infective diarrhoea and thirteen age- and sex-matched healthy controls following a 530 calorie test breakfast.

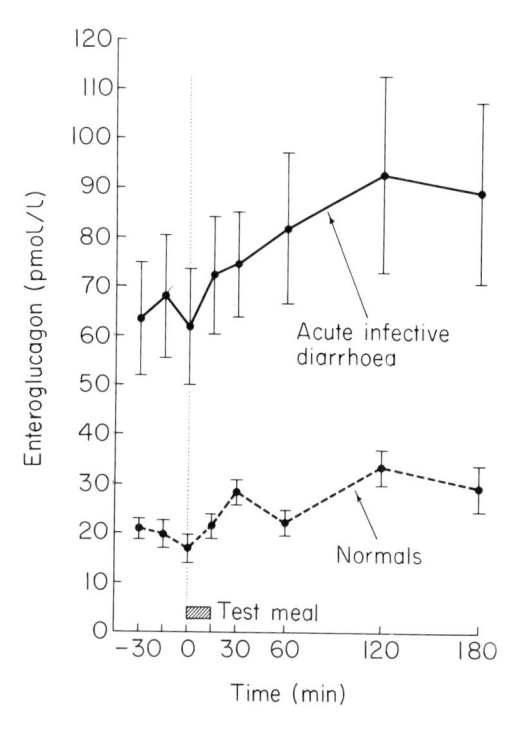

Fig. 23.8. Plasma enteroglucagon concentrations in twelve previously healthy subjects hospitalized for acute infective diarrhoea and thirteen age- and sex-matched healthy controls following a 530 calorie test breakfast.

tration was grossly elevated in the subjects with active coeliac disease but within the expected normal range in the controls and in the coeliacs after treatment. Neurotensin was elevated and GIP depressed, giving a similar picture to that seen after jejunoileal bypass.

The two conditions are comparable in that the upper small intestine is either diseased, as in coeliac disease, or bypassed, so that the upper intestine is unable to respond to nutrients normally. In the untreated coeliac group, secretin release, following intraduodenal acid was greatly reduced (Besterman et al. 1978). Pancreatic polypeptide and gastrin, both hormones released from unaffected organs, were normal. The profile of hormone change therefore accurately reflects the area of bowel affected by the disease. Upper small intestinal hormone release is reduced and the failure of pancreatic exocrine secretion to respond to luminal stimuli such as the Lundh test meal in coeliac disease, while being normal to intravenous secretin and cholecystokinin infusion, suggests failure of release of these hormones by normal luminal stimuli. Lower small intestinal hormone release, however, is increased. Furthermore, the elevated enteroglucagon levels of the coeliac patients may be related to the increased jejunal enterocyte turnover characteristic of this condition, and to the adaptive changes which enhance absorption in the ileum (cf. Chapter 9).

Tropical malabsorption

Six men and two women aged 19–57, normally dwelling in temperate climates, returned from periods in Afghanistan, Nepal, Thailand, Indonesia, Brazil or India and were found to have features of tropical sprue. There was raised faecal fat excretion, elevated breath hydrogen, abnormal jejunal biopsy, xylose malabsorption and reduced absorption of vitamin B_{12}. They were given the standard test breakfast and were found to have a grossly raised basal and postprandial plasma motilin and enteroglucagon. GIP and insulin, however, were significantly reduced. The pattern differed from that seen in active coeliac patients and subjects with jejunoileal bypass in that the basal values were grossly elevated, and there was little further rise occurring postprandially in the subjects with tropical malabsorption. The elevation of enteroglucagon in each individual correlated with the time to breath hydrogen appearance (Besterman et al. 1979). The same subjects were re-studied 4 years after treatment, at a time when they had fully recovered. The fasting and postprandial hormone values were now normal (Cook et al., unpubl. observ.).

Dumping syndrome after partial gastrectomy

The dumping syndrome, referred to in Chapter 5, illustrates the changes in hormone pattern that occur in individuals where unduly rapid gastric emptying results in postprandial symptoms. Such symptoms have been attributed in the past to postprandial hypoglycaemia, but it can be shown that simultaneous intravenous infusion of glucose does not relieve symptoms. In dumping a number of gastrointestinal hormones have an unduly rapid and large rise. The peak enteroglucagon concentration is very high, which would be expected if undigested food is carried distally by rapid intestinal transport (Bloom et al. 1972, Thomson & Bloom 1976) to the ileum and colon where enteroglucagon is released. Neurotensin, another hormone found in the lower small intestine, also shows an abnormally large rise (Blackburn et al. 1980). VIP, a neurotransmitter, not usually affected by gastrointestinal stimuli, also shows a significant postprandial elevation in the dumping syndrome (Sagor et al. 1981). Methods to slow down rapid gastric emptying and intestinal transport, such as addition of viscous fibre (Jenkins et al. 1980), or agents which prevent the osmotic pressure of glucose by inhibiting digestion of complex carbohydrate, such as the alpha glucosidase inhibitor, acarbose (McLoughlin et al. 1979) improve symptoms and reduce the abnormal hormone release. Although the excessive hormone release is clearly a secondary phenomenon, both neurotensin and VIP are vasodilatory, and they may, therefore, exacerbate the tendency to hypotension.

Gut hormones in the neonate

In the new-born infant fed parenterally, gut hormones remain at a low level. Oral feeding, however, results in a dramatic rise with subsequent maturation of the response to a nutrient load (Lucas et al. 1981). Since the cells capable of producing the regulatory peptides of the gut develop early during fetal maturation (Bryant et al. 1982), the defect in parenterally fed infants appears to be due to a lack of luminal stimulus. The development of the gut is clearly influenced by oral feeding, as is the case in the development of the immunocytes of the small intestine (cf. Chapter 8). Continuous parenteral feeding may cause difficulties in establishing oral feeding at a later stage.

The question whether artificial formula feeding of infants is different from natural breast-milk feeding has been difficult to answer. The gut hormone profile, however, was significantly different with different types of food. Infants given 'Cow & Gate Premium' had significantly higher concentrations of almost all hormones, particularly neurotensin and motilin, than breast-fed babies (Lucas et al. 1980).

Endocrine tumours

In general, endocrine disorders may be classified according to whether there is failure of production of the relevant hormone, as in myxoedema or Addison's disease, or excessive production due to either hyperplasia of the relevant endocrine cell type or tumour. So far as the diffuse endocrine system of the gut is concerned, no instance of absolute failure of production of any hormone has yet been described. Hyperplasia of pancreatic islet cells is, however, well recognized as a cause of the hypergastrinaemia of the Zollinger–Ellison syndrome. Tumours have now been described producing not only gastrin but also VIP, neurotensin, pancreatic polypeptide and glucagon. In the carcinoid syndrome, the secretory product is not a regulatory peptide but is predominantly 5-hydroxytryptamine.

In all patients with gut endocrine tumours, the syndrome associated with the tumour is usually due to one particular hormone; other hormones, however, may be secreted simultaneously.

Endocrine cholera

In 1958, Verner and Morrison described a syndrome of refractory and severe watery diarrhoea with marked hypokalaemia that was found to be associated with an islet cell tumour. It seemed likely that the tumour was producing a hormonal substance that caused an inhibition of fluid and electrolyte transport in the gastrointestinal tract. Subsequent reports established that the main features of the syndrome are severe secretory diarrhoea, stool volumes of more than 2–4 l/day being common, weight loss, dehydration, hypokalaemic acidosis and sometimes mild uraemia. There was also reduced gastric acid secretion in two-thirds of the patients. Approximately half the patients have metastasis at the time of diagnosis.

Pathology

The tumours associated with this endocrine cholera are principally of two types. One is the classical pancreatic endocrine tumour composed of characteristic cuboidal or round, regular cells arranged in ribbons, irregular masses or glandular structures separated by bands of connective tissue and blood vessels. The other type is a classical ganglioneuroma with cells of two types — some round with a small hyperchromatic nucleus arranged in irregular masses or whirls, and others elongated with abundant irregular cytoplasm sometimes arranged in

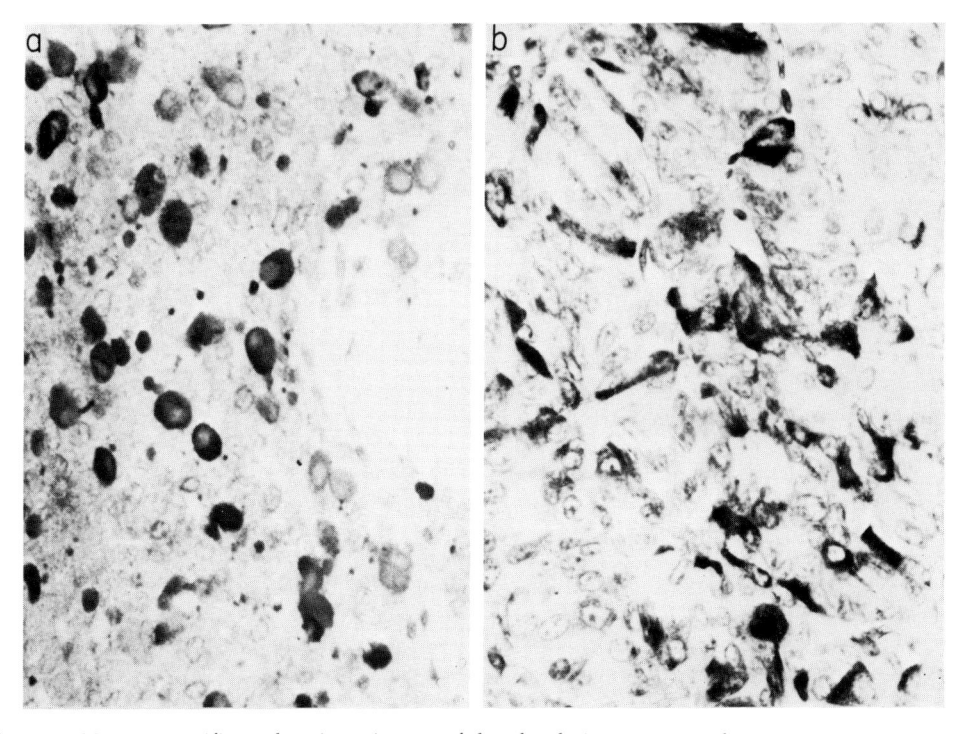

Fig. 23.9. Neuron-specific enolase is an isomer of the glycolytic enzyme enolase present in neurons and in nerve components of the diffuse neuroendocrine system. Their use for the demonstration of the neuroendocrine nature of tumours has recently been proposed (Tapia *et al.* 1981). (a) Neuron-specific enolase; (b) vasoactive intestinal polypeptide (VIP) (PAP, × 450).

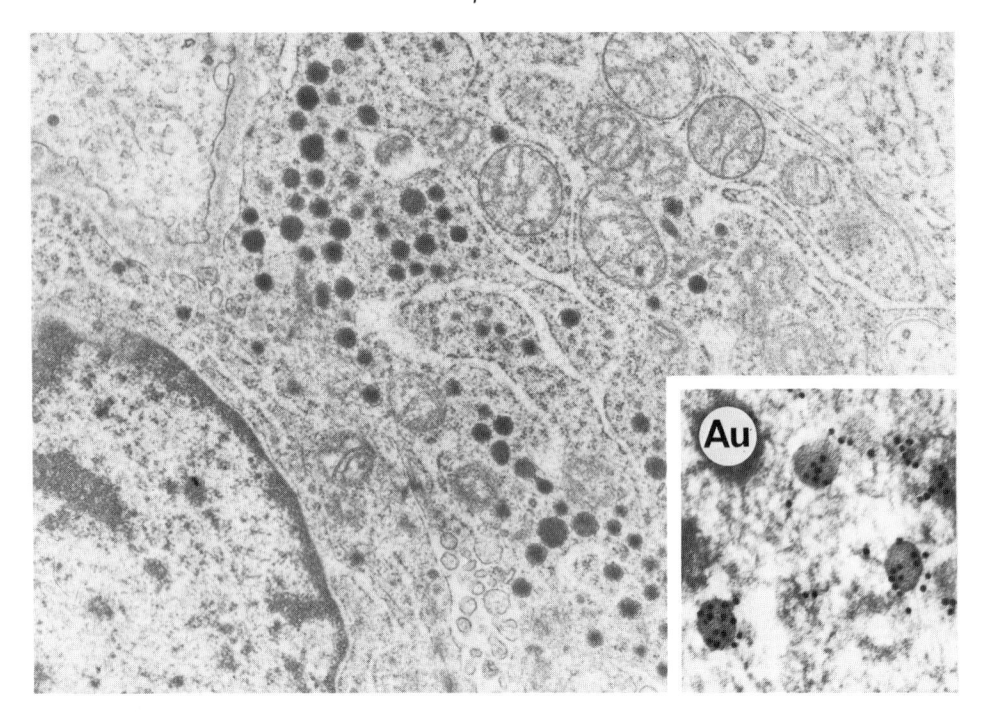

Fig. 23.10. Electron micrograph of a vasoactive intestinal polypeptide (VIP) producing tumour of the pancreas showing characteristic small electron-dense granules (× 25,000). Inset: vasoactive intestinal polypeptide (VIP) like immunoreactivity in secretory granules of a pancreatic vipoma, using gold-labelled antibodies (× 78,500). Gold particles, which are electron-dense, can produce gold particles of different sizes. These separate sized gold particles can be used to label different antibodies to demonstrate two or more antigens in a single tissue section (Varndell et al. 1982).

palisades (Swift et al. 1975, Tiedman et al. 1981). Both classes of tumour react with antibodies to neuron-specific enolase (Fig. 23.9), a glycolytic enzyme first found in central neurons and later found in normal and tumour APUD cells (Tapia et al. 1981). All tumours are furnished with characteristic round, small, electron-dense secretory granules (Fig. 23.10) (Capella et al. 1983).

Implications of VIP

Following considerable speculation as to the humoral mechanisms involved in pancreatic endocrine cholera, Elias et al. (1972) investigated a single patient and suggested that the syndrome was due to the production of gastric inhibitory polypeptide. This report was based on an immunofluorescent study of the tumour obtained from the liver at autopsy. Subsequently, sensitive immunoassays were developed for both GIP and for VIP and Bloom et al. (1973) were able to show a year later that in this first patient and in five others, there was elevation of the level of VIP in the plasma, as well as a positive immunofluorescence for VIP in the tumour. Plasma levels of GIP were normal in the two patients in whom measurements were made. In sixty-two patients with VIP-producing tumours (Fig. 23.11), there was a good correlation between symptoms and VIP concentration in the plasma (Long et al. 1981, Editorial 1984). Furthermore, experimental infusion of VIP in animals reproduced the syndrome (Modlin et al. 1978a). The newly discovered peptide histidine isoleucine (PHI) may well be co-synthetized with VIP. Thus all patients with VIPomas have also been found to be secreting PHI (Christofides et al. 1982). Furthermore, PHI appears equipotent in stimulating fluid secretion in the bowel (Ghiglione et al. 1982). It is therefore possible that the effect of VIPomas on

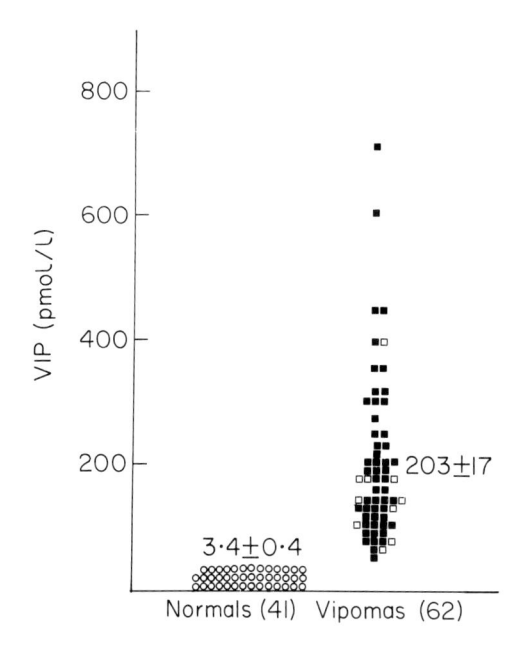

Fig. 23.11. Plasma VIP concentrations in the first received samples from sixty-two patients with the VIPoma syndrome and forty-one age-matched healthy controls. ■, Pancreatic tumours; □, ganglioneuroblastoma.

the bowel is partly mediated by PHI.

Diagnosis

The measurement of plasma VIP is the single most useful test if diarrhoea due to a secretory tumour is suspected. VIP is a labile substance and precautions to prevent degradation are essential if the measurement of plasma level of VIP is to be reliable. When samples of blood are taken, it is essential to add the enzyme inhibitor aprotinin and to deep-freeze the plasma immediately.

Other conditions causing endocrine diarrohoea

Although VIP is the hormone incriminated in the pathogenesis of endocrine cholera in most cases, there are other hormonal abnormalities associated with diarrhoea which may be severe. Approximately 30% of patients with medullary carcinoma of the thyroid develop diarrhoea (Hill et al. 1973) and this may be severe. Thyrocalcitonin has a clear-cut secretory effect on the human jejunum and ileum. Prostaglandins have also been suggested as mediators of diarrhoea in the syndrome of medullary carcinoma of the thyroid (Field 1974) and there may be other unknown substances involved (Modigliani & Bernier 1982).

Other conditions associated with diarrhoea include somatostatinoma and pancreatic glucagonoma, when diarrhoea is thought to be due to pancreatic insufficiency. No clear instance of a secretin-producing tumour has yet been described.

Hyperthyroidism is also associated with diarrhoea in approximately 10% of cases. Rapid transit through the gastrointestinal tract is probably the mechanism.

Pancreatic VIPomas are usually easily localized by angiography but if no pancreatic tumour is found, and especially in children, selective venous sampling may be required to find the location of an extra pancreatic ganglioneuroma.

Treatment

If surgical resection is not possible, these tumours may be extremely sensitive to the cytotoxic agent streptozotocin (Weiss 1982). The major problem with this agent is renal toxicity and it should be used with care if there is impaired renal function. As with all slow-growing pancreatic endocrine tumours, where the main symptoms are due to hormone secretion, it is often worthwhile to attempt palliative tumour bulk reduction, either surgically or by hepatic artery embolization (Irving & Mallinson 1981).

Gastrinomas

The Zollinger–Ellison syndrome is usually due to a pancreatic gastrinoma stimulating excessive acid secretion by the stomach. Rarely the tumours arise from the upper small intestine itself. Whereas it is probable that all pancreatic gastrinomas are malignant, upper small intestinal tumours may well be curable by resection (McCarthy 1980). Approximately one-third of gastrinomas are associated with diarrhoea, probably due to inactivation of pancreatic enzymes by the low duodenal pH. There may also be a direct effect of low pH on the intestinal mucosa stimulating secretion. The diarrhoea associated with the Zollinger–Ellison syndrome rapidly remits with successful inhibition of acid secretion following gastrectomy, removal of the tumour, or potent acid inhibitors (Omeprazole, Ranitidine etc.). Indeed some now recommend that all patients with Zollinger–Ellison syndrome be treated with pharmacological agents, as when the recurrence of tumour is plotted against years after apparent successful resection the line appears to reach 100% recurrence at about 30 years. This suggests that unlike, for example, insulinomas, 80% of which are benign, all gastrinomas are malignant. Our own policy is to attempt to localize the tumour and if operative removal is straightforward to undertake this. A significant proportion of gastrinomas are multiple, however, and the gastrin levels do not fall to normal postoperatively. Gastrinomas infrequently respond to the cytotoxic agent, streptozotocin.

Neurotensinomas and PPomas

Approximately 10% of VIPomas and a smaller percentage of other types of pancreatic tumour are also found to secrete neurotensin. There is no clinical consequence yet discovered of permanently elevated circulating neurotensin concentrations. Column chromatography demonstrates the molecular form to be closely similar to that normally secreted from the ileum and so presumably biologically active. Approximately 50% of pancreatic endocrine tumours produce considerable quantities of PP in addition to their named hormone, i.e. that giving the clinical diagnosis. Again no clinical symptoms are attributable to the sometimes massive secretion of PP. The high incidence of PP production, however, makes PP measurement diagnostically useful (Polak et al. 1976). Unfortunately PP is raised in a variety of other conditions where cholinergic tone is high. This necessitates a rather high cut-off point before high plasma PP concentrations can be considered to indicate the presence of a tumour. In order to increase diagnostic sensitivity the atropine test has been introduced (Adrian et al. 1982). Thus we have so far always found atropine suppression of PP in circumstances where the elevation is not associated with a tumour and conversely never found tumour PP production to be affected by atropine. Further experience with this test is required.

Pancreatic glucagonoma

Tumours of the pancreas producing pancreatic glucagon have been recognized for some years. The glucagonoma syndrome comprises a necrolytic migratory erythematous rash, weight loss, normochromic normocytic anaemia, angular stomatitis, painful glossitis, glucose intolerance and possibly symptoms referrable to an abdominal pancreatic tumour (Mallinson et al. 1974). Many of the features appear to be due to excessive uptake of amino acids by the liver to fuel excessive glucagoneogenesis. Thus the mean plasma amino acid concentration is approximately half normal. These tumours are frequently malignant but very slow growing. Palliative measures will often allow the patient to survive many years. The rash is particularly helped by zinc therapy. Some of the tumours produce large molecular forms of glucagon.

Somatostatinoma

Tumours secreting somatostatin have been described in the pancreas. Recently carcinoid tumours of the duodenum strongly positive to immunolocalization with an antibody to somatostatin have been reported in association with von Recklinghausen's disease or phaeochromocytoma (Griffiths et al. 1983).

Enteroglucagon-producing tumour

In 1971 Gleeson and his colleagues described a single patient with an endocrine tumour of the kidney associated with villous hyperplasia and abnormalities of small intestinal motility and function which reverted to normal following removal of the tumour. Their observations suggested the possibility that enteroglucagon may be trophic to the small intestine.

The patient was a 44-year-old woman who was referred to Hammersmith Hospital for investigation of polyuria and nocturia, and there had been increasing constipation in recent months. She had noticed generalized oedema. For 3 weeks she had been nauseated and had occasionally vomited. She developed amenorrhoea and loss of scalp hair. There was also a transient erythematous skin rash. The abdomen was markedly distended and a barium meal revealed grossly dilated small intestine with thickened mucosal folds. Jejunal biopsy showed markedly enlarged villi on dissecting microscopy and there was villous hyperplasia on histological examination. Subsequent investigation revealed a tumour in the right kidney which was removed surgically. Histological examination of the tumour strongly suggested an endocrine tumour (Fig. 23.12) and on electron microscopy there were distinctive electron-dense secretory granules within the cells (Fig. 23.13). Histochemical examination fulfilled the criteria for APUD cells and immunocytochemical studies demonstrated the presence of enteroglucagon. This was confirmed by the demonstration of large amounts of enteroglucagon in the tumour by radioimmunoassay (Bloom 1972).

Although this is the only instance of an enteroglucagon-producing tumour yet described, some patients with pancreatic glucagonoma may also have hypertrophy of the small intestinal mucosa, possibly because these tumours produce the pro-hormone for pancreatic glucagon which is identical to that for enteroglucagon (Stevens *et al.* 1984).

Carcinoid syndrome

These tumours, commonest in the small intestine, were originally distinguished by their biological behaviour, being less malignant than true carcinomas. They frequently

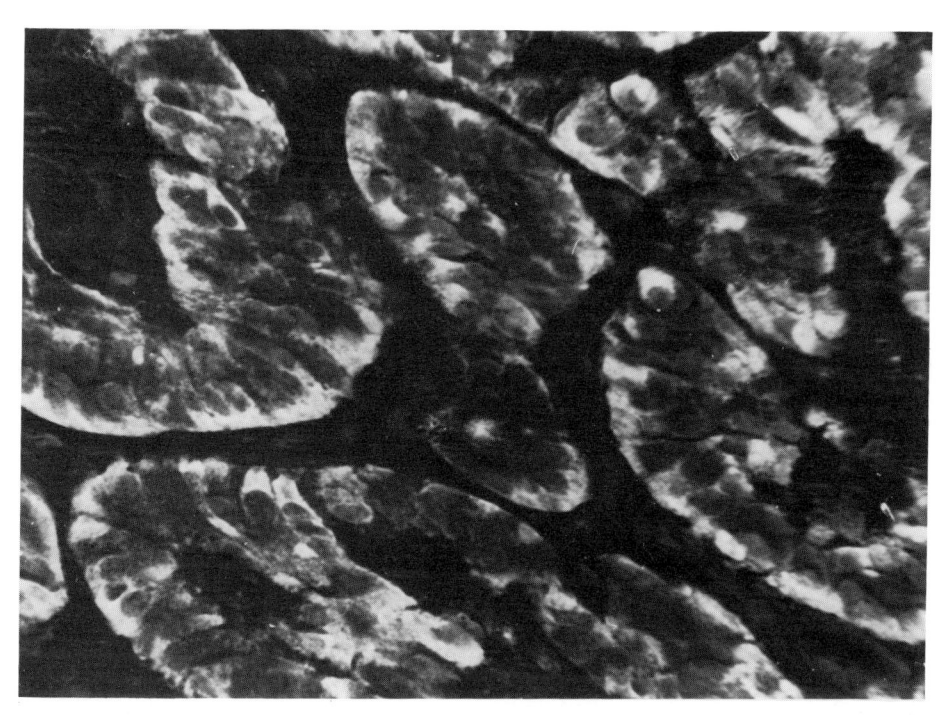

Fig. 23.12. Enteroglucagon-like immunoreactivity in tumour cells of an enteroglucagonoma. Formalin fixation, wax embedding, 5 μm section. Indirect immunofluorescence method (× 450).

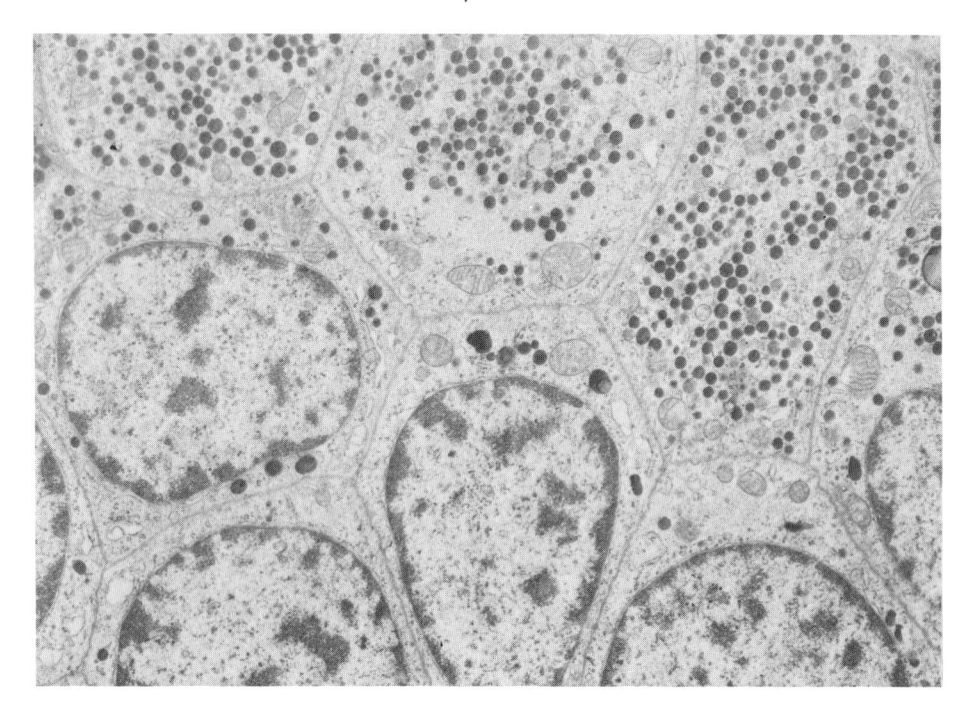

Fig. 23.13. Cluster of enteroglucagon-containing tumour cells from an enteroglucagonoma. Glutaraldehyde fixation, ultrathin Araldite section. Uranyl acetate and lead citrate counterstains ($\times$ 14,000).

store 5-hydroxytryptamine, the basis for the 5-hydroxyindole histochemical stains. It is now thought probable that several different sub-types exist with different secretory products and biological behaviour. Co-production of histamine, vasoactive kinins and prostaglandins can occur as well as the more classical 5-hydroxytryptamine and 5-hydroxy tryptophan. Appendiceal tumours are usually benign and ileal tumours (the commonest site) usually produce symptoms only after extensive metastases develop. Symptoms include hepatic flushing, diarrhoea and abdominal pain, subsequently leading to cachexia, small bowel obstruction and right-sided endomyocardial fibrosis. Diagnosis is usually made by the clinical picture, urinary 5-hydroxyl indole acetic acid elevation and biopsy of hepatic metastases. Therapy is usually just supportive and cytotoxics are not helpful but tumour debulking or hepatic artery emboilization can give significant relief (Allison et al. 1977). Drug therapy is idiosyncratic and often unrewarding. Antihistamines, chlorpromazine, phenoxybenzamine and indomethacin may be useful.

Methysergide or cyproheptadine should not be used for more than a few months because of the danger of retroperitoneal fibrosis. Parachlorphenylalanine specifically inhibits tryptophan hydroxylase and produces good remission of symptoms but most patients quickly develop allergy to this agent. An interesting new development is the use of long-acting somatostatin (Long et al. 1981) and preparations are now being developed which would only require a single daily injection.

References

Adrian T.E., Wood S.M. & Bloom S.R. (1982) Atropine suppression of pancreatic polypeptide (PP) completely distinguishes tumour PP production from other rises. Gut, 23, A905.

Agnostides A.A., Christofides N.D., Tatemoto K., Chadwick V.S. & Bloom S.R. (1984) Peptide histidine isoleucine, a secretagogue in human intestine. Gut, 25, 381–385.

Allen J.M., Sarson D.L., Arian T.E., Wood C., Thompson G.R. & Bloom S.R. (1983) Effect of partial ileal bypass on the gut hormone responses to food in man. Digest., 28, 191–196.

Allison D.J., Modlin I.M. & Jenkins W.J. (1977) Treatment of carcinoid liver metastases by hepatic artery embolisation. *Lancet* ii, 1323–1325.

Besterman H.S., Adrian T.E., Mallinson C.N., Christofides N.D., Sarson D.L. Pera A., Lombardo L., Modigliani R. & Bloom S.R. (1982) Gut hormone release after intestinal resection. *Gut,* 23, 854–861.

Besterman H.S., Bloom S.R., Sarson D.L., Blackburn A.M., Johnston D.I., Patel H.R., Stewart J.S., Modigliani R., Guerin S. & Mallinson C.N. (1978) Gut-hormone profile in coeliac disease. *Lancet,* i, 785–788.

Besterman H.S., Christofides N.D., Welsby P.D., Adrian T.E., Sarson D.L. & Bloom S.R. (1983a) Gut hormones in acute diarrhoea. *Gut,* 24, 665–671.

Besterman H.S., Cook G.C., Sarson D.L., Christofides N.D., Bryant M.G., Gregor M. & Bloom S.R. (1979) Gut hormones in tropical malabsorption. *Brit. Med. J.* 2, 1252–1255.

Besterman H.S., Mallinson C.N., Modigliani R., Christofides N.D., Piera A., Ponti V., Sarson D.L. & Bloom S.R. (1983b) Gut hormones in inflammatory bowel disease. *Scand. J. Gastroenterol.,* 18, 1845–1852.

Bishop A.G., Polak J.M., Bryant M.G., Bloom S.R. & Hamilton S. (1980) Abnormalities of vasoactive intestinal polypeptide-containing nerves in Crohn's disease. *Gastroenterol.* 79, 853–860.

Blackburn A.M., Christofides N.D., Ghatei M.A., Sarson D.L., Ebeid F.H., Ralphs D.N.L. & Bloom S.R. (1980) Elevation of plasma neurotensin in the dumping syndrome. *Clin. Sci.* 59, 237–243.

Bloom S.R. (1972) An enteroglucagon tumour. *Gut,* 13, 520–523.

Bloom S.R. (1980) Hormonal changes after jejunoileal bypass and their physiological significance. In *Surgical Management of Obesity,* pp. 115–123. (Ed. by J.D. Maxwell, J.-C. Gazet & T.R. Pilkington. Academic Press, London.

Bloom S.R. & Long R.G. (1982) *Radioimmunoassay of Gut Regulatory Peptides.* W.B. Saunders Co., London.

Bloom S.R., Polak J.M. & Pearse A.G.E. (1973) Vasoactive intestinal peptide and watery diarrhoea syndrome. *Lancet,* ii, 14–16.

Bloom S.R., Royston C.M.S. & Thomson J.P.S. (1972) Enteroglucagon release in the dumping syndrome. *Lancet,* ii, 789–791.

Bloom S.R. & Ward A.S. Failure of secretin release in patients with duodenal ulcer. *Brit. Med. J.* i, 126–127.

Bryant M.G., Buchan A.M.J., Gregor M., Ghatei M.A., Polak J.M. & Bloom S.R. (1982) Development of intestinal regulatory peptides in the human fetus. *Gastroenterol.,* 83, 47–54.

Busolati G. & Canese M. (1972) Electron microscopical identification of the immunofluorescent gastrin cells in the cat pyloric mucosa. *Histochem.* 29, 198–206.

Capella C., Polak J.M., Buffa R., Tapia F.J., Heitz Ph. Usellini, L., Bloom S.R. & Solcia E. (1983) Morphologic patterns and diagnostic criteria of VIP-producing endocrine tumours. *Cancer* 52, 1860–1814.

Christofides N.D., Modlin I.M., Fitzpatrick M.L. & Bloom S.R. (1974) Effect of motilin on the rate of gastric emptying and gut hormone release during breakfast. *Gastroenterol.* 76, 903–907.

Christofides N.D., Yiangou Y., Blank M.A., Tatemoto K., Polak J.M. & Bloom S.R. (1982) Are peptide histidine isoleucine and vasoactive intestinal peptide co-synthesized in the same pro-hormones? *Lancet,* ii, 1398.

Dockray G.J. (1982) The physiology of cholecystokinin in brain and gut. *Brit. Med. Bull.* 38, 253–258.

Editorial (1984) VIP and diarrhoea. *Lancet,* i, 202.

Elias E., Polak J.M., Bloom S.R., Pearse A.G.E., Welbourn R.B., Booth C.C., Kuzi M. & Brown J.C. (1972) Pancreatic cholera due to production of gastric inhibitory polypeptide. *Lancet* ii, 791–793.

Ferri G.-L., Adrian T.E., Ghatei M.A., O'Shaughnessy D.J. Probert L., Lee Y.C. Buchan A.M.J., Polak J.M. & Bloom S.R. (1983) Tissue localization and relative distribution of regulatory peptides in separated layers from the human bowel. *Gastroenterol.* 84, 777–786.

Field M. (1974) Intestinal secretion. *Gastroenterol.* 66, 1063–1084.

Ghiglione M., Christofides N.D., Yiangou Y., Uttenthal L.O. & Bloom S.R. (1982) PHI stimulates intestinal fluid secretion. *Neuropept.* 3, 79–82.

Gleeson M.H., Bloom S.R., Polak J.M., Henry K. & Dowling R.M. (1971) An endocrine tumour in kidney affecting small bowel structure, motility and absorptive function. *Gut,* 12, 733–782.

Greenberg G.R., McCloy R.F., Baron J.H., Bryant M.G. & Bloom S.R. (1982) Gastric acid regulates the release of plasma secretin in man. *Eur. J. Clin. Invest.* 12, 361–372.

Griffiths D.F.R., Williams G.T. & Williams E.D. (1983) Multiple endocrine neoplasia associated with von Recklinghausen's disease. *Brit. Med. J.* ii, 1341.

Hill C.S., Hibanes M.L., Somarn N.A., Ahearn M.J. & Clark R.L. (1973) Medullary carcinoma of the thyroid gland: analysis of the MD Anderson Hospital experience with patients with a tumour, its special features and its histogenesis. *Med.* 52, 141–145.

Irving D. & Mallinson C.N. (1981) Interventional radiology. In *Gastrointestinal and Hepatobiliary Cancer.* (Ed. by H.J.F. Hodgson & S.R. Bloom). Chapman and Hall, London.

Jenkins D.J.A., Bloom S.R., Albuquerque R.H., Leeds A.R., Sarson D.L., Metz G.L. & Alberti K.G.M.M. (1980) Pectin and complications after gastric surgery: normalisation of postprandial glucose and endocrine responses. *Gut,* 21, 574–579.

Jewell W.R., Hermreck A.S. & Harding C.A. (1975) Complications of jejuno-ileal bypass for morbid obesity. *Arch. Surg.* **110**, 1039–1042.

Kennedy H.J., Sarson D.L., Bloom S.R. & Truelove S.C. (1982) Gut hormone responses in subjects with a permanent ileostomy. *Digest.* **24**, 133–136.

Long R.G., Bryant M.G., Mitchell S.J., Adrian T.E., Polak J.M. & Bloom S.R. (1981) Clinicopathological study of pancreatic and ganglioneuroblastoma tumours secreting vasoactive intestinal polypeptide (VIPomas). *Brit. Med. J.* **282**, 1767–1771.

Long R.G., Peters J.R., Bloom S.R., Brown M.R., Vale W., Rivier J.E. & Grahame-Smith D.G. (1981) Somatostatin, gastrointestinal peptides, and the carcinoid syndrome. *Gut*, **22**, 549–553.

Lucas A., Aynsley-Green A. & Bloom S.R. (1981) Gut hormones and the first meals. *Clin. Sci.* **60**, 349–353.

Lucas A., Sarson D.L., Blackburn A.M., Adrian T.E., Aynsley-Green A. & Bloom S.R. (1980) Breast vs bottle: endocrine responses are different with formula feeding. *Lancet*, **i**, 1267–1269.

McCarthy D.M. (1980) The place of surgery in the Zollinger–Ellison syndrome. *N. Engl. J. Med.* **302**, 1344–1347.

McGuigan J.E. (1968) Gastric mucosal intracellular localization of gastrin by immunofluorescence. *Gastroenterol.* **55**, 315–327.

McLean L.D., Rochon G., Munro M., Watson K.E.L. & Chizal H.M. (1980) Intestinal bypass for morbid obesity. *Can. J. Surg.* **23**, 54–59.

McLoughlin J.C., Buchanan K.D. & Alam M.J. (1979) A glycoiside-hydrolase inhibition in treatment of dumping syndrome. *Lancet*, **ii**, 603–605.

Mallinson C.N., Bloom S.R., Warin A.P., Salmon P.R. & Cox B. (1974) A glucagonoma syndrome. *Lancet*, **ii**, 1–4.

Modigliani R. & Bernier J.J. (1982) Pathophysiology of hormonal diarrhoea. In *Butterworths International Medical Reviews: Gastroenterology*, vol. 2, pp. 265–279. (Ed. by V.S. Chadwick & S. Phillips). Butterworths, London.

Modlin I.M., Bloom S.R. & Mitchell S.J. (1978a) Experimental evidence for vasoactive intestinal peptide as the cause of the watery diarrhoea syndrome. *Gastroenterol.* **75**, 1051–1054.

Modlin I.M., Bloom S.R. & Mitchell S.J. (1978b) Plasma vasoactive intestinal polypeptide (VIP) levels and intestinal ischaemia. *Experient.* **34**, 535–536.

O'Morain C., Bishop A.E., McGregor G.P., Levi A.J., Bloom S.R., Polak J.M. & Peters T.J. (1984) Vasoactive intestinal peptide levels and immunocytochemical studies in rectal biopsies from patients with inflammatory bowel disease. *Gut* **25**, 57–61.

Mutt V. (1980) Gastrointestinal hormones. *Biochem. Soc. Trans.* **8**, 11–14.

Polak J.M. & Bloom S.R. (1982) Regulatory peptides in the gut and their relevance to disease In *Disorders of Neurohumoural Transmission* pp. 83–104. (Ed. by T.J. Crow. Academic Press, London.

Polak J.M., Bloom S.R., Adrian T.E. Heitz. Ph., Bryant M.G. & Pearse A.G.E. (1976) Pancreatic polypeptide in insulinomas, gastrinomas, VIPomas and glucagonomas. *Lancet*, **i**, 328–330.

Polak J.M., Pearse A.G.E., Heath C.M. (1975) Complete identification of endocrine cells in the gastrointestinal tract using semithin-thin sections to identify motilin cells in human and animal intestine. *Gut*, **16**, 225–229.

Sagor G.R. Bryant M.G., Ghatei M.A., Kirk R.M. & Bloom S.R. (1981) Release of vasoactive intestinal peptide in the dumping syndrome. *Brit. Med. J.* **282**, 507–510.

Sarson D.L., Scopinaro N. & Bloom S.R. (1981) Gut hormone changes after jejunoileal (JIB) or biliopancreatic (BPB) bypass surgery for morbid obesity. *Int. J. Obestet.* **5**, 471–480.

Scopinaro N., Gianetti E., Kivaleri D., Bonalumi U. & Bachi V. (1980) Two years of clinical experience with bilio-pancreatic bypass for obesity. *Amer. J. Clin. Nutr.* **33**, 506–514.

Solcia E., Polak J.M., Larsson L.-I., Buchan A.M.J. & Capella C. (1981) Update on Lausanne classification of endocrine cells. In *Gut Hormones*, 2nd ed., pp. 96–106. (Ed. by S.R. Bloom and J.M. Polak.) Churchill Livingstone, Edinburgh.

Stevens F.M., Flanagan R.W., O'Gorman D. & Buchanan K.D. (1984). Glucagonoma syndrome demonstrating giant duodenal villi. *Gut* **25**, 784–791.

Swift P.G.F., S.R. Bloom & F. Harris (1975) Watery diarrhoea and ganglioneuroma with secretion of vasoactive intestinal peptide. *Arch. Dis. Child.* **50**, 896–899.

Tapia F.J., Polak J.M., Barbosa A.J.A., Bloom S.R., Marangos P.J., Dermody C. & Pearse A.G.E. (1981) Neuron-specific enolase is produced by neuroendocrine tumours. *Lancet*, **i**, 808–811.

Tiedmann K., Long R.G., Pritchard J. & Bloom S.R. (1981) Plasma vasoactive intestinal polypeptide and other regulatory peptides in children with neurogenic tumours. *Eur. J. Pediatr.* **137**, 147–150.

Thomson J.P.S. & Bloom S.R. (1976) Plasma enteroglucagon and plasma volume change after gastric surgery. *Clin. Sci.* **51**, 177–183.

Vantrappen G., Janssens J., Peeters T.L., Bloom S.R., Christofides N.D. & Hellemans J. (1979) Motilin and the interdigestive migrating motor complex in man *Dig. Dis. Sci.* **24**, 497–500.

Varndell I.M., Tapid F.J., Probert L., Buchan A.M.J., Gu J., De Mey J., Bloom S.R. Papia, D. & Polak J.M. (1982) Immunogold-staining procedure for the localization of regulatory peptides. *Peptides*, **3**, 259–272.

Verner J.V. & Morrison A.B. (1958) Islet cell tumour and a syndrome of refractory watery diarrhea and hypolcalaemid. *Amer. J. Med.* **25**,

374–380.

Walsh J.H. & Grossman M.I. (1975) Gastrin. *N. Engl. J. Med.* **292**, 1324–1332, 1377–1384.

Walsh J.H., Isenberg J.I., Ansfield J. & Maxwell V. (1976) Clearance and acid-stimulating action of human big and little gastrins in duodenal ulcer subjects. *J. Clin. Invest.* **57**, 1125–1131.

Weiss R.B. (1982) Streptozotocin: a review of its pharmacology, efficacy and toxicity. *Cancer Treat Rep.* **66**, 427–438.

Chapter 24
Drug-induced Disorders

CHARLES F. GEORGE AND GREG E. HOLDSTOCK

Drugs with a direct toxic effect on the mucosa	398
Drugs which inhibit mucosal transport	403
Binding and precipitation of micellar components	405
Submucosal haemorrhage of the small intestine	406
Practolol-induced oculomucocutaneous syndrome	407
Interference with the vascular supply	407
Other drugs	407
Purgative abuse (contributed by Dr. G. Neale)	408

Drugs may affect the structure and function of the small intestine in several different ways (Table 24.1). First, they may have a direct toxic effect on the morphology of the mucosa of the small intestine. Second, they may inhibit mucosal enzymes and in some cases this is associated with mucosal damage. Third, drugs may interfere with micelle formation in the lumen of the intestine. Fourth, drugs may alter the physicochemical state of dietary ions or other drugs. Examples of this include chelation of tetracyclines with divalent or trivalent cations such as iron, calcium and magnesium. Fifth, alterations of motility can occur due to interference with nerve transmission or blockade of receptor sites. This subject has been covered in a previous review (George 1980). Next, drugs may produce profound structural alteration: examples include submucosal haemorrhage associated with the use of oral anticoagulants and hypertrophy of the serosal membrane associated with practolol usage. Finally, drugs may be associated with alterations in either the blood supply or venous drainage of the intestine.

In addition, it should be remembered that most medicines are given by mouth in tablet form and that lactose represents an important ingredient. Ingestion of large numbers of tablets can occasionally represent a significant load of lactose and provoke diarrhoea in patients with a previous disaccharidase deficiency.

Drugs with a direct toxic effect on the mucosa

Drugs which have a direct toxic effect on the intestinal mucosa include neomycin (and certain other broad spectrum antimicrobials), colchicine, other cytotoxic agents used in cancer chemotherapy, alcohol and, possibly, mefenamic acid. Certain laxatives, such as ricinoleic acid and magnesium sulphate, may cause a shedding of cells by the jejunal mucosa, as measured by the rate of DNA loss in a perfused segment of small intestine (Bretagne *et al.* 1981).

Neomycin

Neomycin (B) was first isolated from a soil organism in 1949. It has since been used in the preoperative preparation for bowel surgery and to reduce bacterial colonization of the bowel in patients suffering from porto-systemic encephalopathy associated with liver disease. Neomycin is an aminoglycoside which inhibits protein synthesis within the bacterial ribosomes. Normally it is poorly absorbed from the gastrointestinal tract so that damage to the hair cells in the labyrinth and nephrotoxicity are rare. However, a common adverse effect is the development of malabsorption. Furthermore, when the dose exceeds 4–6 g/day a sprue-like syndrome can occur. The causes of this have been studied thoroughly and are complex (Longstreth & Newcomer 1975).

Histologically (Fig. 24.1), neomycin causes a reduction in the height of the intestinal villi, infiltration of the submucosa with

Table 24.1. Drugs affecting small intestinal structure and function.

Mechanism/Effect	Examples
Direct toxicity on the mucosa	Neomycin Colchicine Cytotoxics Alcohol Mefenamic acid Some laxatives
Inhibition of mucosal enzyme transport	Laxatives P.A.S. Biguanides
Binding and precipitation of micellar components	Cholestyramine
Chelation	Tetracyclines
Submucosal haemorrhage	Warfarin
The oculomucocutaneous syndrome	Practolol
Interference with vascular supply or drainage	Potassium salts Contraceptive pill Corticosteroids
Others	See Table 24.2

oedema formation and changes in the morphology of the mucosal cells (Rogers et al. 1966, Dobbins et al. 1968). Examination under the electron microscope has shown ballooning, fragmentation and loss of the microvilli (Cain et al. 1968). Disaccharidase deficiency may occur (Cain et al. 1968) and there is reduced intraluminal hydrolysis of long-chain triglycerides. Next, and perhaps most important, there is precipitation of bile salts, the cationic amino groups of neomycin binding and precipitating the fatty acid and bile acid anions of the micelles (Thompson et al. 1971). This disruption of the micelle leads to faulty absorption of its components which include monoglycerides, fatty acids, cholesterol and the fat-soluble vitamins, especially vitamin A. However, vitamin B_{12}, calcium and iron malabsorption have also been reported (Dobbins 1968). Because of these problems neomycin is rarely used in long term treatment. However, even short-term therapy has been shown to reduce dramatically the absorption of digoxin (Lindenbaum et al. 1976). Furthermore, it is likely that the absorption of other drugs will be reduced by neomycin therapy. However, not all instances of diarrhoea following neomycin therapy can be attributed to the effects described above since this drug can also cause pseudomembranous colitis (Weiderma et al. 1980).

Although neomycin is the best known and most thoroughly studied of the various antimicrobials that cause malabsorption, similar problems have been described for kanamycin, polymyxins and bacitracin, as well as with tetracyclines (Dobbins 1968, Mitchell et al. 1982).

Colchicine

Colchicine is an alkaloid derived from the autumn crocus plant which has a unique action in acute gout. The pharmacologic basis of this remains uncertain but appears to involve an action on the neutrophil leucocyte after the latter has ingested urate crystals. The latter event is associated with the release of glycoprotein from the leucocyte and it is either the synthesis or release of the latter which is prevented by colchicine treatment. Since this drug binds to micro-tubular protein to cause metaphase arrest and inhibition of secretion from other cells, this may be the most relevant effect in gout (cf. Wallace 1961, Wallace et al. 1970). Its use as a treatment for an acute attack of gouty arthritis is frequently associated with gastrointestinal problems. These include nausea, colicky abdominal pain, repeated vomiting and diarrhoea. Although it has been suggested (Butt et al. 1974) that these symptoms may reflect increased intestinal prostaglandin biosynthesis, morphological changes have been reported, involving particularly the differentiating cells of the villi. Furthermore, at high doses, metaphase arrest can occur and lead to severe villous atrophy (Longstreth & Newcomer 1975). Normally, there is a cessation of the gastrointestinal problems within hours of discontinuing treatment with colchicine but occasional fatalities have been reported from repeated diarrhoea leading to hypovolaemic shock and coma (Macleod & Phillips 1947).

Colchicine is used comparatively infrequently as a long-term treatment for gout. However, small doses given regularly can lead to steatorrhoea, megaloblastic anaemia (secondary to vitamin B_{12} malabsorption) as well as to abnormal absorption of xylose and carotene (Longstreth & Newcomer 1975). These changes are rare and in twelve patients with familial Mediterranean fever who received the drug for at least 3 years only three had proven (but mild) steatorrhoea and none had any clinical evidence of malnutrition (Ehrenfeld et al. 1982). Furthermore, jejunal histology was normal in all but in four cases Na/K-ATPase activity was reduced.

Other cytotoxic agents

It is well recognized that malignant tumours, both of the gastrointestinal tract and elsewhere, are associated with marked weight loss and in some patients with evidence of malnutrition (Deller et al. 1967, Dymock et al. 1967). Often these symptoms can be explained by a fall in caloric intake, secondary to nausea and vomiting. However, villous atrophy has been reported and is particularly common in patients with gastrointestinal lymphoma (Isaacson & Wright 1978). It has also been reported to occur in up to 30% of non-gastrointestinal tumours (Dymock et al. 1967, Klipstein & Smarth 1969). In addition, the treatments used for malignant disease can themselves affect gastrointestinal function.

Radiotherapy of the small gut has been demonstrated to result in transient villous atrophy, reduced enzymic activity and in electron microscopic abnormalities (Trier & Browning 1966, Weirnik 1966, Tarpila 1971). These effects occur with radiation dosages above 2500 rads and tend to be transitory. Clinically, the diarrhoea rarely persists but occasionally ulceration and/or perforation may occur (Duncan & Leonard 1965). Patients exposed to very high doses of radiation may occasionally develop chronic malabsorption and in such patients lymphatic obstruction or secondary bacterial overgrowth should be considered.

Because of their rapid turnover rate, small intestinal epithelial cells are susceptible to damage from cytotoxic drugs. These may have a variety of different pharmacologic actions as shown in Fig. 24.2. They will be considered here under the main groups of drugs used, but only those drugs which cause problems are discussed here. For further details readers are referred to a review by Shaw and colleagues (1979).

Alkylating agents

The most commonly used drugs of this group include nitrogen mustard, cyclophosphamide and lomustine. Animal studies have shown that lethal doses cause intestinal abnormalities, including reduced villus height and an inflammatory infiltrate (Ecknauer & Lohrs 1976). In addition, functionally there is a reduction in the absorption of glucose. No changes have been demonstrated in man given usual therapeutic doses, and diarrhoea is a rare complication of treatment with these drugs. In all probability this reflects limited access of the drugs to the enterocyte, nitrogen mustard being administered intravenously and cyclophosphamide requiring metabolic activation within the microsomal system of the liver.

Antimetabolites

By contrast, the antimetabolites such as methotrexate, aminopterin, 5-fluorouracil (5FU), cytosine arabinoside and 6-mercaptopurine more frequently affect the gastrointestinal tract. Both aminopterin and methotrexate are folate antagonists and have been shown to reduce xylose absorption and produce histological abnormalities similar to those seen in patients with gluten sensitivity (Small et al. 1959). Less severe changes occur in man at therapeutic doses (Trier 1962a & b) and these may be clinically important in two respects. First, in children methotrexate produces sub-clinical malabsorption (Craft et al. 1977) and, second, such treatment may delay the absorption of other drugs.

5-Fluorouracil, which acts by interfering with the synthesis of DNA, produces the side-effects of nausea, vomiting, stomatitis and diarrhoea. Experimentally, 5FU produces widespread mucosal abnormalities in both mice and rats. In the mouse both atrophy and severe proliferative lesions resembling carcinoma *in situ* have been reported

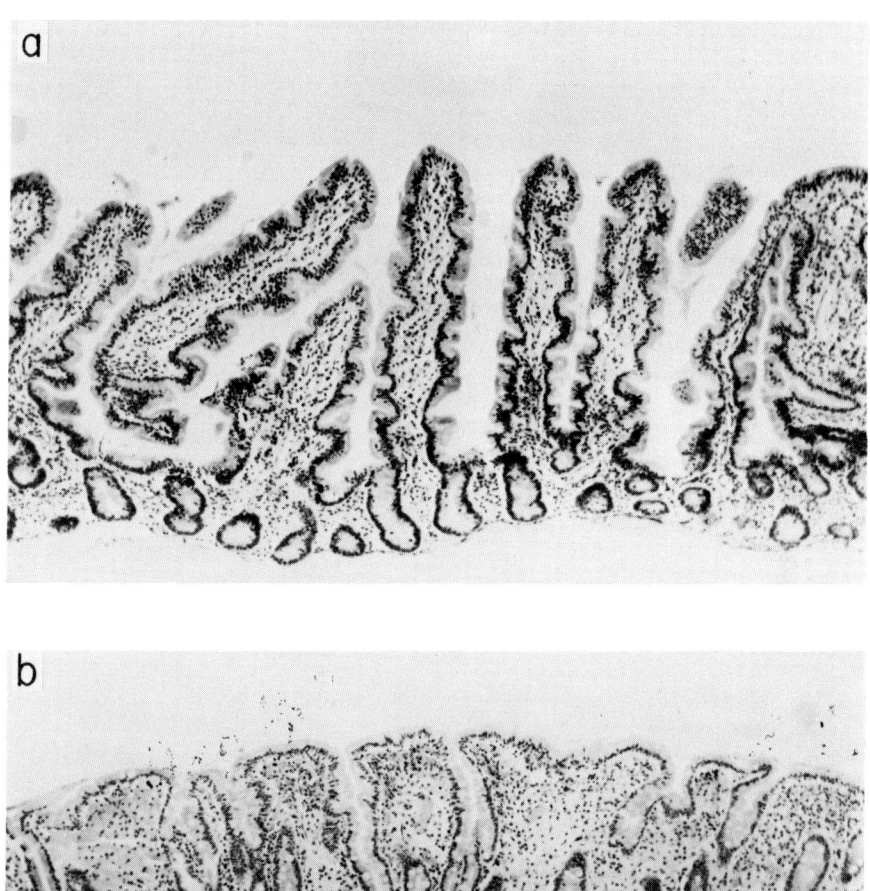

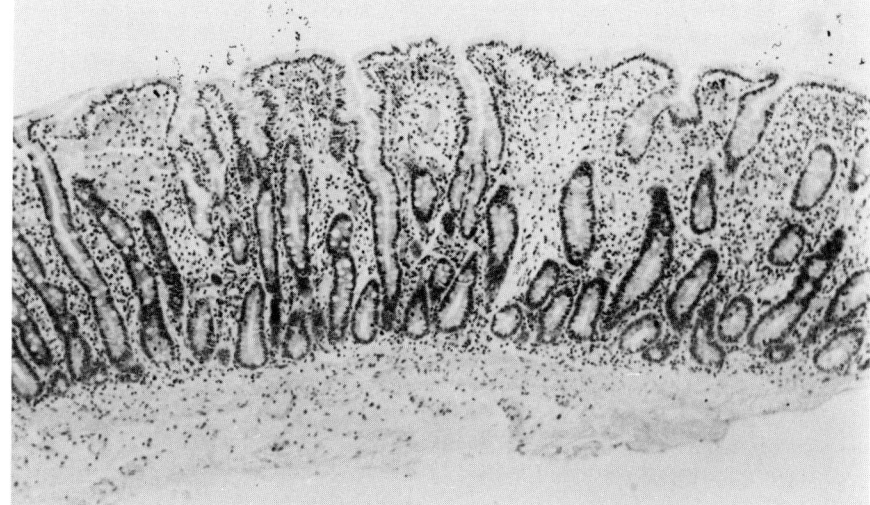

Fig. 24.1. Jejunal biopsies taken from a patient before (a) and after (b) taking neomycin. (a) Normal; (b) Partial villous atrophy with excess of intraepithelial lymphocytes (H & E, × 100).

(Muggia et al. 1963) and in the rat there is malabsorption of both glucose and other sugars (Levin 1968). Bounous et al. (1971) have shown that this drug can produce histological abnormalities in the small intestine of both man and rat: however, small intestinal changes are confined to the rat. These changes can be prevented by an elemental diet containing amino acids.

The use of 6-mercaptopurine is occasionally associated with diarrhoea which presumably has a similar basis to that produced by 5FU. Cytosine arabinoside, a pyrimidine analogue which inhibits DNA polymerase, is used in the treatment of acute myeloblastic leukaemia. Patients who have received this drug in combination with various others may show focal loss or shortening of the jejunal villi, as well as destruction of the crypts (Slavin et al. 1978).

Vinca alkaloids

Vincristine can cause both intestinal ulceration and adynamic ileus (Kingry et al. 1973). Morphological changes similar to those seen in gluten enteropathy and glucose malabsorption may be produced in rats, but the significance of these findings has been questioned (Shaw et al. 1979).

Alcohol

The effects of alcohol on the gastrointestinal tract have been reviewed recently by Langman & Bell (1982) and by Burbage et al. (1984). Although it is clear that ethanol can have major effects on the morphology of the duodenum and upper jejunum as well as the function of the enterocyte, interpretation of many studies which have been reported is difficult because of the complex effects of this drug and co-existent hepatic and/or pancreatic damage plus poor dietary intake. Nevertheless, the main effect would appear to be a general depression of transport mechanisms which can contribute to malnourishment and produce diarrhoea.

Alcohol has been shown to have a direct effect on the lipoprotein membrane of the enterocyte (Wilson & Hoyumpa 1979) and long-term administration produces ultrastructural changes involving the mitochondria, endoplasmic reticulum and the Golgi

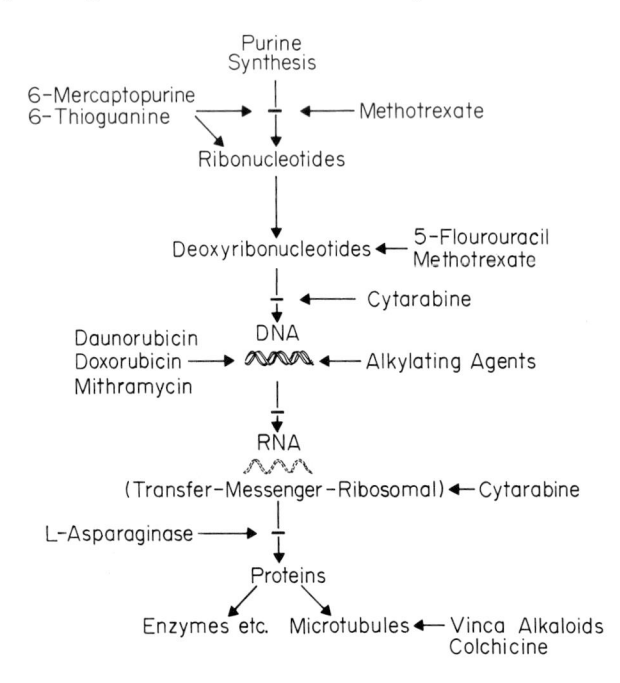

Fig. 24.2. Sites of action of some of the main cytotoxic agents used in cancer chemotherapy.

apparatus (Garcia-Paredes 1979). Functionally, there is reduced oxygen utilization and activity of the enzymes located in the brush border including lactase, sucrase, maltase. Perhaps more significantly, Na/K ATPase activity is reduced.

The effects of these enzyme systems are particularly important as they are involved in the carrier-mediated transport of a variety of nutrients including sugars, amino acids, water, electrolytes and thiamine (vitamin B_1). Depressed Na/K ATPase activity, coupled with a net secretion of intestinal fluid, secondary to stimulation of adenylate cyclase, may account for the diarrhoea which is seen in many alcoholics. In addition, alcohol has an effect on small bowel motility. Withdrawal of alcohol is frequently associated with cessation of diarrhoea. If this is not the case, it is more likely that chronic pancreatitis is present.

Mefenamic acid

Mefenamic acid is a non-steroidal anti-inflammatory drug derived by N-substitution of phenylanthranilic acid. Like aspirin, it is an inhibitor of prostaglandin synthetase and is used in patients with rheumatoid arthritis, as well as to relieve pain from other conditions. Adverse effects include gastritis, duodenitis and bleeding peptic ulcers (Wolfe et al. 1976). However, unlike most other non-steroidal anti-inflammatory agents, profuse steatorrhoea can occur. The first such report was by Marks & Gleeson (1975) of a 65-year-old man receiving mefenamic acid in a dose of 250 mg three times daily. Gross steatorrhoea was demonstrated which responded to withdrawal of the drug. Subsequently, Chadwick et al. (1976) reported two patients with a similar problem. However, unlike the previous authors, they found intestinal abnormalities on biopsy. These included irregular villous processes with leaf forms and an infiltration by chronic inflammatory cells. These abnormalities disappeared on stopping mefenamic acid.

Drugs which inhibit mucosal transport

Drugs which inhibit the mucosal transport systemsm include laxatives, para-aminosalycylic acid, alcohol and biguanides.

Laxatives

Traditionally, laxatives have been classified into several groups including osmotic, lubricant, wetting and stimulant. However, the validity of these sub-groups (apart from osmotic) has been questioned (Fingl & Preston 1979, Fingl 1980). While it is true that some of the laxative substances do have 'stimulant' properties, e.g. the anthraquinones, and that dioctylsulphosuccinate has surfactant/wetting properties, their other actions are probably more important.

The major action of laxative drugs is to increase the water content of the stool and this is achieved in one of several ways. First, electrolyte (and water) absorption is dependent upon the enzyme, Na/K ATPase. Secondly, the integrity of the mucosal surface and the 'tight junctions' between epithelial cells are important in determining the permeability of the mucosa. Fluid resorption is influenced also by the secretion of gastrointestinal hormones and by the activity of adenylate cyclase. Thus, reduced absorption of electrolytes and water, and even fluid secretion can occur if one or more of these structures/activities is disrupted. In recent years, laxatives have been demonstrated to have an action on one or more of these functions (Fingl & Preston 1979, Fingl 1980).

Bisacodyl

The effects of bisacodyl on the structure and function of both rodent and human intestine have been studied by Saunders et al. (1977). Water absorption from the jejunum and to a greater extent the ileum and colon, was inhibited in a dose-dependent fashion. Patients with an established ileostomy showed a 15% increase in fluid output from the stoma when receiving this drug in a dose of 5 mg 6-hourly. Ultra-structural changes were demonstrated in the mucosal cells: in particular, there was an alteration in the apparent density of both the cytoplasm and nucleus.

Castor oil

Castor oil is an extract of plant seeds that is hydrolysed by pancreatic lipase to liberate glycerol and the laxative ricinoleic acid, an unsaturated, monohydroxy fatty acid. Perfusion of the rabbit colon with this agent has been shown to produce dose-related mucosal changes (Gaginella et al. 1977). The morphologic damage was associated with increased mucosal permeability and net secretion of fluid.

Dioctyl sulphosuccinate

Although regarded widely as altering the wetting characteristics of the stool by its detergent action, Gullikson et al. (1977) have shown that it produces changes in the microstructure of the hamster small intestinal membrane. The villi become shortened and there is exfoliation of cells, together with increased permeability and a net secretion of water.

Thus, it seems likely that the common mechanism of action of laxatives is their ability to prevent fluid resorption and increase the stool wet weight. A similar mechanism is thought to be important for the anthraquinones (Fingl 1980), e.g. senna and cascara, which are glycosides that are subject to breakdown by the intestinal microflora. These substances also affect the activity of the intramural parasympathetic plexuses and long-term use can give rise to melanosis coli with degeneration of the ganglion cells (Steer & Colin-Jones 1975).

Ethacrynic acid

The use of ethacrynic acid is frequently associated with watery diarrhoea (Binder et al. 1966). The precise aetiology of this problem is uncertain, but the drug is known to affect prostaglandin synthesis or breakdown, thereby increasing concentrations of cyclic AMP (Williamson et al. 1976). Since cholera toxin has a similar pharmacologic action in inhibiting electrolyte and water resorption (Field 1971), it may be that the potential of ethacrynic acid for causing this problem has a similar basis.

p-Amino salicylic acid (PAS)

This anti-tubercular drug is now rarely used in the Western hemisphere (indeed the last preparation was withdrawn in September 1982). This is partly because of the availability of more effective agents, such as rifampicin, but also because these other agents have fewer unwanted effects. Nevertheless, PAS is still used in developing countries and gastrointestinal side-effects occur commonly. These have been reviewed by Longstreth & Newcomer (1975) and include steatorrhoea (despite normal jejunal histology) as well as malabsorption of vitamin B_{12}. However, the latter is sub-clinical as there are no reported cases of megaloblastic anaemia occurring. A more important finding is that administration of PAS with rifampicin results in reduced absorption of the rifampicin (Boman et al. 1971).

Biguanides

The biguanide drugs, which include metformin and phenformin, are oral hypoglycaemic agents which cause malabsorption of glucose. In addition, there is a reduced absorption of xylose, amino acids and particularly of vitamin B_{12} (Tomkin et al. 1971). Arvanitakis et al. (1973) have demonstrated changes in the jejunal mucosa seen with the electron microscope but not with light microscopy. Decreased disaccharidase activity has been demonstrated in these patients but the reduction in glucose absorption is thought to be the result of a direct action of biguanides on the active transport of the sugar.

Other substances

Antacids, particularly aluminium hydroxide, reduce phosphate absorption and rarely may produce phosphorus depletion in patients who are on a long-term therapy. Eventually severe debility with anorexia, muscle weakness and osteomalacia may occur. Antacids can also interfere with the absorption of tetracyclines from the gastrointestinal tract.

Oral anticonvulsants have complex effects on folate metabolism. These have been reviewed by Longstreth & Newcomer (1975) and by Dobbins (1968) and the reader is referred to these publications for further details.

Cimetidine, the histamine H_2 antagonist, can cause moderately severe diarrhoea which stops on withdrawal and can be reproduced with a further challenge (Field & Meyer 1978, Ruddell & Losowsky 1980). The diarrhoea is thought to result either from overgrowth of bacteria consequent to reduced gastric acidity or from a secondary intolerance of lactose. The following case history illustrates how the failure to appreciate the possible role of drugs in causing intestinal symptoms may lead to unnecessary investigation.

> A 74-year-old man, hospitalized because of rheumatoid arthritis, complained that he had suffered moderately severe diarrhoea for the previous 3 months with bowel frequency of between six and eight times daily. There was no blood or mucus and no history of recent antibiotic use. Apart from anti-inflammatory agents (aspirin and indomethacin), he had taken Tagamet (cimetidine) for about 6 months for a presumed duodenal ulcer. He was slightly anaemic (Hb 10.8) and had an elevated ESR (48 mm/h). Sigmoidoscopy was considered normal but a rectal biopsy revealed 'slight excess of inflammatory cells of uncertain significance'. This led to radiological assessment of his upper and lower gut and both barium meal and follow-through and barium enema were normal. He was started on sulphasalazine as it was thought that the rectal biopsy might indicate inflammatory bowel disease. However, on review of his records, there was no good evidence of peptic ulcer disease and the cimetidine was discontinued. Almost immediately his diarrhoea stopped and his bowel function returned to normal. Rechallenge with cimetidine led to a recurrence of his symptoms.

Binding and precipitation of micellar components

This is an important cause of diarrhoea and steatorrhoea, particularly that associated with the use of neomycin. It is also an important effect of cholestyramine.

Cholestyramine

This anion exchange resin binds bile acids and increases their faecal excretion. As such it has a role in the treatment of pruritis associated with liver disease (Van Itallie et al. 1961). In addition, the drug is widely used in the treatment of certain forms of hyperlipidaemia — especially Friedrikson type II (Levy et al. 1973). Finally, it has been used to control cholereic diarrhoea resulting from disease or resection of the ileum (Hofmann & Poley 1969).

Its use is frequently associated with a slight increase in faecal fat excretion (Longstreth & Newcomer 1975) but when used in patients with ileal resections, malabsorption of fat-soluble vitamins may occur (Heaton et al. 1972). Green & Tall (1979) have put forward an hypothesis to explain why malabsorption occurs. They suggest that, under normal circumstances, pancreatic lipase hydrolyses the triglyceride core of fat emulsion droplets, producing amphipathic lipids. This results in the apolar core shrinking and the surface lipid expanding, possibly folding into bi-layer lamellar structures. These are normally removed by bile salts forming mixed micelles. Neomycin and cholestyramine bind bile acids in the jejunum and may cause diarrhoea and steatorrhoea by preventing this last stage.

Cholestyramine binds other substances within the gastrointestinal tract, including oxalate and drug molecules, especially the digitalis glycoside, digitoxin, thereby interfering with its enterohepatic recirculation. By contrast, cholestyramine has little effect on the absorption of digoxin (Hall et al. 1977), although the absorption of warfarin from the gastrointestinal tract is reduced.

Submucosal haemorrhage of the small intestine

This condition was reviewed by George (1980). Most commonly it follows blunt trauma to the abdomen but may be a feature of the haemorrhagic diatheses and of Schönlein–Henoch purpura. However, its occurrence during anticoagulant therapy has been well documented. Typical features include the sudden onset of cramping abdominal pain, nausea and vomiting in a patient on oral anticoagulants (Senturia et al. 1961). Examination reveals a low grade fever, a distended abdomen, which is tender on palpation and rebound, with hypoactive or absent bowel sounds. Laboratory investigations may show a fall in the haemoglobin level, a leucocytosis and a very prolonged prothrombin time. Once suspected, the diagnosis is relatively simple and is based on barium follow-through examination which shows a rigid, narrow bowel segment often with a coarse mucosal pattern and spikey or 'picket fence' projections (Fig. 24.3). Medical treatment includes nasogastric suction, intravenous fluids plus transfusion if necessary. The haemorrhagic diathesis should be corrected with fresh plasma and the efficacy of this procedure can be checked by frequent prothrombin times or thrombotest estimations. Vitamin K is often given in addition to encourage the synthesis of new clotting factors.

Submucosal haematoma is a rare condition: by 1968, Herbert found eighty-eight cases in the world literature. Furthermore, although haemorrhagic complications occurred in 5.3% of 1029 patients receiving anticoagulants, only four patients developed submucosal haematomas (Lawson 1976). Most cases involve warfarin because it is by far the most widely used drug of this type. Inter-individual differences in sensitivity occur (Breckenridge 1977, 1978) and undue sensitivity may occur because of poor diet or malabsorption (George 1980). Haemorrhagic complications are most common in the elderly and increased sensitivity of the vitamin K_1 receptor is the likely cause (Shepherd et al. 1977). Finally, bleeding may occur due to inhibition of the metabolism of

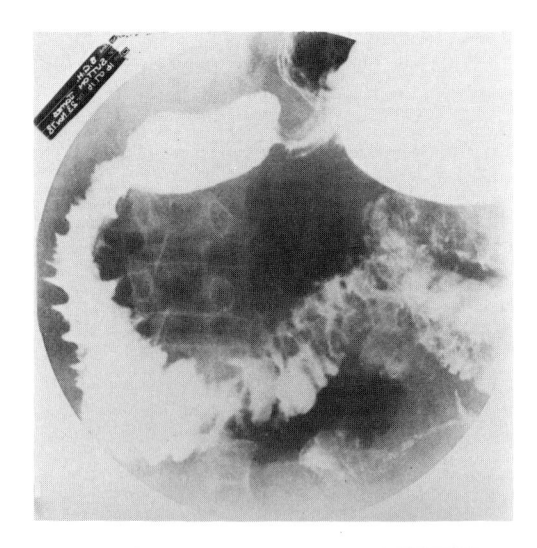

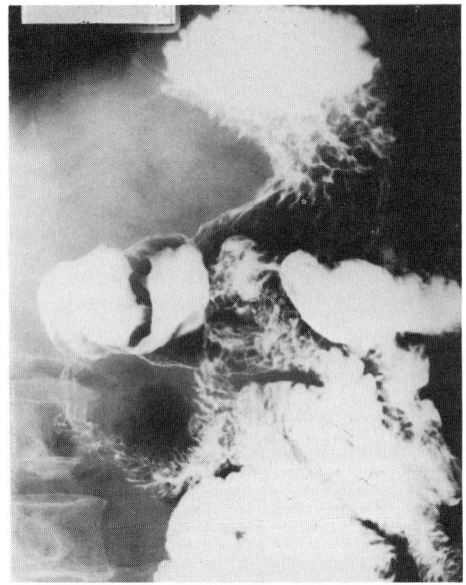

Fig. 24.3. *Top*: Barium meal examination showing submucosal haemorrhage of the duodenal loop during anticoagulent therapy; *bottom*: after recovery.

warfarin by drugs which include phenylbutazone, chloramphenicol and phenyramidol (Breckenridge 1977). Inhibition of warfarin metabolism has also been reported following the use of distalgesic which contains dextropropoxyphene. Orme et al. (1976) have described two patients who developed haematuria following the use of distalgesic whilst receiving warfarin. One of us (C.G.) had personal experience of the first of these two patients who also had a submucosal haemorrhage of the small intestine. A full list of drugs which can interact with oral anticoagulants has been published recently (Standing Advisory Committee for Haematology 1982).

Practolol-induced oculomucocutaneous syndrome

The features of this syndrome were reviewed by Marshall et al. (1977) and by George (1980). Symptoms include colicky abdominal pain and diarrhoea because of subacute obstruction of the small intestine. This is due to overgrowth of collagen in the serosa which has the effect of compressing and truncating the small intestine within a 'plastic cocoon'. Although the precise aetiology of this condition remains uncertain, it was clearly associated with the use of practolol and should no longer occur following the withdrawal of this beta-adrenoceptor antagonist from the market.

Interference with the vascular supply

Potassium supplements

Potassium salts in high concentration can cause spasm of smooth muscle, particularly in the veins. This can lead to ischaemic ulceration of the intestinal mucosa. Occasionally this may lead to haemorrhage at the site but it is more likely that healing will occur and the subsequent fibrosis can lead to stricture formation. Oral potassium supplements can be given in several different forms. Ideally, they should be given in the diet or in liquid form. However, potassium chloride solution is unpalatable and tends to cause nausea and/or vomiting in some patients. One way of circumventing the problem was to use enteric-coated potassium chloride which ensured that the tablet did not dissolve until the alkaline contents of the small intestine were reached. However, when such tablets did release their contents within the gut they tended to produce high potassium concentrations locally and this favoured the ischaemic ulceration of the bowel. Such preparations are no longer available in the UK. An alternative tablet preparation, slow-K, is still used. Normally, this formulation (which consists of potassium chloride in a wax matrix) releases its contents slowly throughout the gastrointestinal tract. But, if intestinal transit is delayed by general debility, poor diet or concurrent drug therapy, potassium ulceration and stricture formation can occur (Farquharson-Roberts et al. 1975). Nevertheless, potassium-induced ulceration of the small intestine is now very rare and accounts for only a small proportion of non-specific ulcers of this organ (Boydstun et al. 1981).

The contraceptive pill

Superior mesenteric vein thrombosis most commonly affects the middle-aged and elderly, males being more frequently affected than females. However, since the use of oral contraceptives became widespread, an increasing number of young females with mesenteric thrombosis have been identified. The association between the use of oral contraceptives and mesenteric thrombosis remains unproven but the circumstantial evidence is strong and many patients who were affected gave a past history of thrombosis elsewhere. The typical features are of severe abdominal pain and symptoms and signs of intestinal obstruction (Rose 1972). On laboratory testing there is often a leucocytosis in excess of $20 \times 16^6/l$ and plain radiographs show fluid levels. The diagnosis is usually made at laparotomy and the majority of patients will need excision with an end-to-end anastomosis as well as anticoagulation during the recovery period. Occasionally, reversal of the vascular problem has followed the withdrawal of oral contraceptives (Northmann et al. 1973).

Other drugs

A number of other drugs have been reported to affect small intestinal function. In general, these changes have been mild and have little clinical significance. They are summarized in Table 24.2.

There is also evidence that intestinal per-

Table 24.2. Other drugs which may affect small bowel function, modified from Longstreth & Newcomer (1975) and Losowsky *et al.* (1974).

Drug implicated	Absorption defect	Possible mechanism involved
Aspirin	Glucose, amino acids, xylose	Active transport
Amphetamine	Anticonvulsants	Reduced gut motility
Cellulose phosphate	Calcium	Intraluminal binding
Chloramphenicol	Lactose	Disaccharidase inhibition
Chlorothiazide	Water, sodium	?Active transport
Clofibrate	Sterols	Decreased glycolytic enzyme activity
Corticosteroids	Calcium, iron, electrolytes	Active transport
Cyclamates	Lincomycin	?
Cycloserine	Folic acid	?
Indomethacin	Xylose	Active transport
Kanamycin (polymixin, paramycin, bacitracin)	Fat and protein	?
Penicillamine	?Digoxin	Reduced enterohepatic recycling
Phenylbutazone	Amino acids	?
Phenytoin (and phenobarbitone)	Xylose, folic acid	?Inhibition of folate conjugase
Potassium chloride	Vitamin B_{12}	Ileal acidification
Probenecid	Amino acids	?
Pyrimethamine	Folic acid	Dihydrofolate reductase inhibition
Quinacrine	Fat	?
Sulphasalazine	Folic acid	Decreased folate transport
Sulphonamides	Oxacillin	?
Tricyclic antidepressants	Phenylbutazone	Reduced gut motility
Triparanol	Fat, protein, carotene	Abnormal morphology

meability may be increased in chronic alcoholism, providing a possible route of entry for toxic compounds (Bjarnason *et al.* 1984).

Purgative abuse (Contributed by Dr Graham Neale)

Like fasting and bleeding, purgation is recorded in man's earliest writings as a means of relieving mental and physical distress. Purgation calendars are among the first printed documents of medicine (Witts 1937) and psychiatrists have spent much time analysing the popular concept that emptying the intestine is not only beneficial but, in children at least, worthy of praise. Thus, perhaps, it is not surprising that laxatives have been abused not only by subjects with chronic constipation but also by those who have the need to create the appearance of being unwell.

Clinical features

Laxative-induced diarrhoea occurs primarily in adult women of any age. It is characteristically associated with complaints of abdominal pain, thirst and generalized weakness. Diarrhoea is not always a prominent symptom. Indeed some patients go to extraordinary lengths to conceal their bowel disturbance

(Love et al. 1971). Diagnosis is nearly always delayed especially if there are features suggesting organic disease such as nausea and vomiting, weight loss, fever, skin pigmentation, finger clubbing (Silk et al. 1975), fatty stools (Coghill et al. 1959) and metabolic bone disease (Frame et al. 1971). The physician is then lured into a cycle of investigation which may reveal anaemia, electrolyte disturbances, steatorrhoea, impaired absorption of glucose and xylose, gastrointestinal protein loss and hormonal disorders. Repeated admissions to hospital are common and often patients end up by being submitted to laparotomy (Cummings 1976).

Diagnosis

Suspicion is the key to diagnosis. The clinician is faced with a female patient with diarrhoea (sometimes concealed as indeterminate bowel symptoms), weakness, tiredness and often with abnormal values for circulating urea and electrolytes (especially a low serum potassium). At this point the astute clinician may recognize that the patient has an odd personality or evidence of a psychiatric disorder usually with features of depression. A history of recurrent gastrointestinal upsets in childhood (anorexia, 'difficult to feed', vomiting, constipation) and some links with hospital personnel either by job or by association appear to be much more common in those abusing laxatives than in the general population.

Investigations

Simple investigation is usually not very helpful. Sigmoidoscopy and rectal biopsy are useful in identifying the melanosis caused by anthracene derivatives. Barium studies may also be helpful but only in a small proportion of cases. In these the terminal ileum is tube-like, the ileocaecal valve is incompetent and the colon featureless except for the occasional smooth, tapering pseudostricture (Le Maitre et al. 1970).

In the majority of cases, however, anatomical studies are unrewarding. Admission to hospital becomes necessary in order to achieve a diagnosis. The patient is usually very co-operative but is sometimes quite devious in trying to create the impression of serious organic disease. Few, however, have the knowledge and skill to outwit an alert, well-informed and vigilant ward team.

In most reported cases the patient is taking either a drug of the anthracene group (e.g. senna, cascara, danthron) or a phenylmethane derivative (e.g. phenolphthalein, bisacodyl). These substances are fairly easily detected in urine or faeces (Cummings 1976). The taking of aperient salts or poorly absorbed sugars (e.g. lactulose) presents a more difficult challenge which may be solved by balance studies or by detecting the effects of excessive fermentation in the colon. If suspicions are supported by the results of investigation then most clinicians are prepared to authorize a search of the patient's bedside locker. This unpleasant action requires the exercise of the utmost discretion.

Treatment

The management of purgative abuse is difficult and there are no reports of long-term follow-up. Confronting the patient with the evidence usually leads to denial followed by hostility. The problem is then how best to give continued care and support. The patient may be prepared to discuss her habit and to seek means of relief. Often, however, the outcome is less satisfactory. Self-discharge from hospital is common. Depression may become overt and occasionally leads to an attempt to commit suicide.

Thus the physician may prefer to seek the support and advice of a psychiatrist in assessing the patient's problem. An indirect approach to the underlying disorder may offer a better means of providing help without the patient losing face in an unacceptable way. In many cases, however, the habit persists or the problem shows itself in another way. Most case reports indicate the difficulty in helping such patients adjust to life in a more satisfactory way, as is illustrated by the following case report.

> E.A., unmarried daughter of a hospital architect, had a humdrum clerical job. She presented with diarrhoea at the age

of 40 and, after fruitless investigation as an out-patient, was admitted to hospital. She was found to have mild diabetes, severe diarrhoea (stool volume up to 11/day) and mild steatorrhoea. After many special studies and trials of treatment she was submitted to laparotomy to exclude pancreatic disease. No pathology was discovered. The patient was given intravenous fluids to counter dehydration and spent nearly 9 months in the private wing of the hospital. Sympathetic nursing staff stayed with her at home during long weekend leaves.

She was referred to the Metabolic Unit at Hammersmith Hospital for balance studies. On examination she was found to be well-nourished. There were no signs of organic disease and despite the complaint of a 'glove and stocking' anaesthesia, there was no objective evidence of either a peripheral or an autonomic neuropathy. The patient seemed totally unconcerned about the diarrhoea except that she indicated that she would never be able to leave hospital.

The stools were watery and although negative to tests for anthracenes and phenylmethanes they were noted to smell of hydrogen sulphide. They contained 52 mmol magnesium ions/24 h. A locker search revealed nothing, but an observant ward sister then reported that the patient's bath salts were white and unscented. Analysis showed these to be Epsom salts.

The patient was confronted with the evidence. After a vigorous denial she became agitated and withdrawn. The following day she attempted to throw herself out of the ward window. Subsequently she accepted a short spell of care from a psychiatrist but was then lost to follow-up.

References

Arvanitakis C., Lorenzsonn V. & Olsen W.A. (1973) Phenformin-induced alteration of small intestinal function and mitochondrial structure in man. *J. Lab. Clin. Med.* **82**, 195–200.

Barr W.H., Adir J. & Garrettson L. (1971) Decrease of tetracycline absorption in man by sodium bicarbonate. *Clin. Pharmacol. Therapeut.* **12**, 779–784.

Binder H.J., Katz L.A., Spencer R.P. & Spiro H. (1966) The effect of inhibition of renal transport on the small intestine. *J. Clin. Investig.* **45**, 1854–1858.

Bjarnason I., Ward K. & Peters T.J. (1984) The leaky gut of alcoholism: possible route of entry for toxic compounds. *Lancet*, **i**, 179–182.

Boman G., Hanngren A. & Malmborg A.S. (1971) Drug interaction: decreased serum concentrations of rifampicin when given with PAS. *Lancet*, **i**, 800.

Bounous G. (1971) Elemental diet in the management of the intestinal lesion produced by 5-fluorouracil in man. *Can. J. Surg.* **14**, 132–134.

Boydstun J.S., Gaffey T. & Bartholomew L.G. (1981) Clinico-pathologic study of nonspecific ulcers of the small intestine. *Dig. Dis. Sci.* **26**, 911–916.

Breckenridge A.M. (1977) Interindividual differences in the response to oral anticoagulants. *Drugs*, **14**, 367–375.

Breckenridge A. (1978) Oral anticoagulant drugs: pharmacokinetic aspects. *Sem. Hematol.* **15**, 19–26.

Bretagne J.F., Vidon N, L'Hirondel C. & Bernier J.J. (1981) Increased cell loss in the human jejunum induced by laxatives (ricinoleic acid, dioctyl sodium sulphosuccinate, magnesium sulphate, bile salts). *Gut*, **22**, 264–269.

Burbage E.J., Lewes D.R.Jr. & Halsted, C.H. (1984). Alcohol and the gastrointestinal tract. *Med. Clin. N. Amer.* **68**, 77–89.

Butt A.A., Collier H.O.J., Gardiner P.J. & Saeed S.A. (1974) Effects of prostaglandin biosynthesis of drugs affecting gastrointestinal function. *Gut*, **15**, 344.

Cain G.D., Reiner E.B. & Patterson M. (1968) Effects of neomycin on disaccharidase activity of the small bowel. *Arch. Inter. Med.* **122**, 311–314.

Chadwick R.G., Hossenbocus A. & Colin-Jones D.G. (1976) Steatorrhoea complicating therapy with mefenamic acid. *Brit. Med. J.* **i**, 397.

Craft A.W., Kay H.E.M., Lawson D.N. & McElwain T.J. (1977) Methotrexate-induced malabsorption in children with acute lymphoblastic leukaemia. *Brit. Med. J.* **ii**, 1511–1512.

Coghill N.F., McAllen P.M. & Edwards F. (1959) Electrolyte losses associated with the taking of purgatives investigated with the aid of sodium and potassium radio-isotopes. *Brit. Med. J.* **i**, 14–19.

Cummings J.H. (1976) The use and abuse of laxatives. In *Recent Advances in Gastroenterology*, Chapter 6. (Ed. by I.A.D. Bouchier). Churchill Livingstone, Edinburgh.

Deller D.J., Murrel T.G.C. & Blowes R. (1967) Jejunal biopsy in malignant disease. *Aust. Ann.*

Med. 16, 236–241.
Dobbins W.O., Herrero B.A. & Mansbach C.M. (1968) Morphologic alterations associated with neomycin induced malabsorption. *Amer. J. Med. Sci.* **255**, 63–77.
Dobbins W.O. (1968) Drug-induced steatorrhoea. *Gastroenterol.* **54**, 1193–1195.
Duncan W. & Leonard J.C. (1965) The malabsorption syndrome following radiotherapy. *Quart. J. Med.* **34**, 319–329.
Dymock I.W., Mackay N., Miller V., Thomson T.J., Gray B., Kennedy E.H. & Adams J.F. (1967) Small intestinal function in neoplastic disease. *Brit. J. Canc.* **21**, 505–511.
Ecknauer R. & Lohrs U. (1976) The effect of a single dose of cyclophosphamide on the jejunum of specified pathogen-free and germ-free rats. *Dig.* **14**, 269–280.
Ehrenfeld M., Levy M., Sharon P., Rachmilewitz D. & Eliakim M. (1982) Gastrointestinal effects of long-term colchicine therapy in patients with recurrent polyserositis (familial Mediterranean fever). *Dig. Dis. Sci.* **27**, 723–727.
Farquharson-Roberts M.A., Giddings A.E.B. & Nunn A.J. (1975) Perforation of small bowel due to slow release potassium chloride. *Brit. Med. J.* **iii**, 206.
Field M. (1971) Intestinal secretion: effect of cyclic AMP and its role in cholera. *N. Engl. J. Med.* **284**, 1137–1144.
Field R. & Meyer G.W. (1978) Diarrhoea from cimetidine. *N. Engl. J. Med.* **299**, 262.
Fingl E. (1980) Laxatives and cathartics. In *The Pharmacological Basis of Therapeutics*, 6th ed. pp. 1002–1012. (Ed. by A.G. Gilman, C.S. Goodman & A. Gilman). New York, Macmillan.
Fingl E. & Preston J.W. (1979) Antidiarrhoeal agents and laxatives: changing concepts. *Clin. in Gastroenterol.* **8**, 161–186.
Frame B., Guiang H.L., Frost H.M. & Reynolds W.A. (1971) Osteomalacia induced by laxative (phenolphthalein) ingestion. *Arch. Int. Med.* **128**, 794–796.
Gaginella T.S., Chadwick V.S., Debongnie J.C., Lewis J.C. & Phillips S.F. (1977) Perfusion of rabbit colon with ricinoleic acid: dose-related mucosal injury, fluid-secretion, and increased permeability. *Gastroenterol.* **73**, 95–101.
Garcia-Paredes J. (1979) Some effects of alcohol on jejunal mucosa. *Topics in Gastroenterology*, 7th ed. pp. 291–302. (Ed. by S.C. Truelove & C.P. Willoughby). Blackwell Scientific Publications, Oxford.
George C.F. (1980) Drugs causing intestinal obstruction: a review. *J. Roy. Soc. Med.* **73**, 200–204.
Green P.H.R. & Tall A.R. (1979) Drugs, alcohol and malabsorption. *Amer. J. Med.* **67**, 1066–1076.
Greenberger N.J., Ruppert R.D. & Cuppage F.E. (1967) Inhibition of intestinal ion transport induced by tetracycline. *Gastroenterol.* **53**, 590–599.
Gullikson G.W. Cline W.S., Lorenzsonn V., Benz L., Olsen W.A. & Bass P. (1977) Effects of anionic surfactants on hamster small intestinal membrane structure and function: relationship to surface activity. *Gastroenterol.* **73**, 501–511.
Hall W.H., Shappers S.M. & Doherty J.E. (1977) Effect of cholestyramine on digoxin absorption and excretion in man. *Amer. J. Cardiol.* **39**, 213–216.
Heaton K.W., Lever J.V. & Barnard D. (1972) Osteomalacia associated with cholestyramine therapy for postileectomy diarrhoea. *Gastroenterol.* **62**, 642–646.
Herbert D.C. (1968) Anticoagulant therapy and the acute abdomen. *Brit. J. Surg.* **55**, 353–357.
Hoffman A.F. & Poley J.R. (1969) Cholestyramine treatment of diarrhoea associated with ileal resection. *N. Engl. J. Med.* **281**, 397–402.
Isaacson P. & Wright D.H. (1978) Intestinal lymphoma associated with malabsorption. *Lancet*, **i**, 67–70.
Kingry R.L., Hobson R. & Muir R.W. (1973) Cecal necrosis and perforation with systemic chemotherapy. *Amer. Surg.* **39**, 129–133.
Klipstein F.A. & Smarth G. (1969) Intestinal structure and function in neoplastic disease. *Amer. J. Dig. Dis.* **14**, 887–899.
Langman M.J.S. & Bell G.D. (1982) Alcohol and the gastrointestinal tract. *Brit. Med. Bull.* **38**, 71–75.
Lawson D.H. (1976) Anticoagulants and haemostatics. In *Drug Effects in Hospitalized Patients*, Chapter 12, pp. 101–108. (Ed. by R.R. Miller & D.J. Greenblatt). John Wiley & Sons, New York.
Le Maitre G., L'Hermine C., Decoulx M., Houcke M. & Linquetti M. (1970) Aspect radiologique des colites chronique par abus de laxatif. A propos quatre observations. *J. Bel. Radiol.* **53**, 339–348.
Levy R.I., Fredrickson D.S., Stone N.J., Bilheimes D.W., Brown W.V., Glueck C.J., Gotto A.M., Herbert P.N., Kwiterovich P.O., Lauger J., La Rosa J., Lux S.E., Rider A.K., Shulman R.S. & Sloan H.R. (1973) Cholestyramine in type II hyperlipoproteinemia. *Ann. Intern. Med.* **79**, 51–58.
Levin R.J. (1968) Anatomical and functional changes of the small intestine induced by 5-fluorouracil. *J. Physiol.* **197**, 73–74.
Lindenbaum J., Maulitz R.M. & Butler V.P. (1976) Inhibition of digoxin absorption by neomycin. *Gastroenterol.* **71**, 399–404.
Longstreth G.F. & Newcomer A.D. (1975) Drug-induced malabsorption. *Mayo Clin. Proc.* **50**, 284–293.
Losowsky M.S., Walker B.E. & Kelleher J. (1974) Causes of steatorrhoea. 3 Pharmacological. In *Malabsorption in Clinical Practice*, pp. 160–168. (Ed. by M.S. Losowsky, B.E. Walker & J. Kelleher). Churchill Livingstone, London.
Love D.R., Brown J.J., Fraser R., Lever A.F., Robertson J.I.S., Timbury G.C., Thompson S. & Tree M. (1971) An unusual case of self-induced electrolyte depletion. *Gut*, **12**, 284–290.
Macleod J.G. & Phillips L. (1947) Hypersensitivity

to colchicine. *Ann. Rheum. Dis.* **6**, 224−229.

Marks J.S. & Gleeson M.H. (1975) Steatorrhoea complicating therapy with mefenamic acid. *Brit. Med. J.* **4**, 442.

Marshall A.J., Badderley H., Barritt D.W., Davies J.D., Lee R.E., Low-Beer T.S. & Read A.E. (1977) Practolol peritonitis: a study of 16 cases and a survey of small bowel function in patients taking beta-adrenergic blockers. *Quart. J. Med.* **46**, 135−149.

Mitchell T.H., Stamp T.C.B. & Jenkins M.V. (1982) Steatorrhoea after tetracycline. *Brit. Med. J.* **285**, 780.

Muggia A.L., Wagman S.S. Milles S.G. & Spiro H. (1963) Response of the gastrointestinal tract of the mouse to 5-fluorouracil. *Amer. J. Pathol.* **43**, 407−414.

Northmann B.J., Chittinand S. & Schuster M.M. (1973) Reversible mesenteric vascular occlusion associated with oral contraception. *Amer. J. Dig. Dis.* **18**, 361−368.

Orme M. L'E., Breckenridge A. & Cook P. (1976) Warfarin and distalgesic interaction. *Brit. Med. J.* **i**, 200.

Rogers A.I., Vloedman D.A., Bloom E.C. & Kalser M.H. (1966) Neomycin-induced steatorrhoea. *J. Amer. Med. Assoc.* **197**, 185−190.

Rose M.B. (1972) Superior mesenteric vein thrombosis and oral contraception. *Postgrad. Med. J.* **48**, 430−433.

Ruddell W.S.J. & Losowsky M.S. (1980) Severe diarrhoea due to small intestinal colonisation during cimetidine treatment. *Brit. Med. J.* **281**, 273.

Saunders D.R., Sillery J., Rachmilewitz D., Rubin C.E. & Tytgat G.N. (1977) Effect of bisacodyl on the structure and function of the rodent and human intestine. *Gastroenterol.* **72**, 849−856.

Senturia H.R., Susman N. & Shyken H. (1961) The Roentgen appearance of spontaneous intramural hemorrhage of the small intestine associated with anticoagulant therapy. *Amer. J. Roentgenol. Rad. Ther. Nucl. Med.* **86**, 62−69.

Shaw M.T., Spector M.H. & Ladman A.J. (1979) Effect of cancer, radiotherapy and cytotoxic drugs on intestinal structure and function. *Canc. Treat. Rev.* **6**, 141−151.

Shepherd A.M.M., Hewick D.S., Moreland T.A. & Stevenson I.H. (1977) Age as a determinant of sensitivity to warfarin. *Brit. J. Clin. Pharmacol.* **4**, 315−320.

Silk D.B.A., Gibson J.A. & Murray C.R.H. (1975) Reversible finger clubbing in a case of purgative abuse. *Gastroenterol.* **68**, 790−794.

Slavin R.E., Dias M.A., & Saral R. (1978) Cytosine arabinoside-induced gastrointestinal toxic alteration in sequential chemotherapeutic protocol. *Canc.* **42**, 1747−1759.

Small M.D., Cavanagh R.L., Gottlieb L., Colon P.L. & Zamcheck N. (1959) The effect of aminopterin on the absorption of xylose from the rat small intestine. *Amer. J. Dig. Dis.* **4**, 700−705.

Standing Advisory Committee for Haematology of the Royal College of Pathologists (1982) Drug interaction with coumarin-derivative anticoagulants. *Brit. Med. J.*, **285**, 274−275.

Steer H.W. & Colin-Jones D.G. (1975) Melanosis coli: studies of the toxic effects of irritant purgatives. *J. Pathol.* **115**, 199−205.

Tarpila S. (1971) Morphological and functional response of human small intestine to ionising irradiation. *Scand. J. Gastroenterol.* **6**, Supp. 12, 9−52.

Thompson G.R., Barrowman J., Gutierrez L. & Hermon Dowling R. (1971) Action of neomycin on intraluminal phase of lipid absorption. *J. Clin. Invest.* **50**, 319−323.

Tomkin G.H., Hadden D.R., Weaver J.A. & Montgomery D.A.D. (1971) Vitamin B_{12} status of patients on long-term metformin therapy. *Brit. Med. J.* **ii**, 685−687.

Trier J.S. (1962a) Morphologic alterations induced by methotrexate in the mucosa of human proximal intestine. *Gastroenterol.* **42**, 295−305.

Trier J.S. (1962b) Morphologic alterations induced by methotrexate in the mucosa of human proximal intestine (II) Electron microscopic observations. *Gastroenterol.* **43**, 407−424.

Trier J.S. & Browning T.H. (1966) Morphologic response of the mucosa of human small intestine to X-ray exposure. *J. Clin. Invest.* **45**, 194−204.

Van Itallie T.B., Hashim S.A., Crampton R.S. & Tennant D.M. (1961) The treatment of pruritis and hypercholesteremia of primary biliary cirrhosis with cholestyramine. *N. Engl. J. Med.* **265**, 469−474.

Wallace S.L. (1961) Colchicine. Clinical pharmacology in acute gouty arthritis. *Amer. J. Med.* **30**, 439−448.

Wallace S.L., Omokuku B. & Ertel N.H. (1970) Colchicine plasma levels. Implications as to pharmacology and mechanisms of action. *Amer. J. Med.* **48**, 443−448.

Weiderma W.F., von Meyenfeldt M.F., Soeters P.B., Wesdorp R.I.C. & Greep J.M. (1980) Pseudomembranous colitis after whole gut irrigation with neomycin and erythromycin base. *Brit. J. Surg.* **67**, 895−896.

Weirnik G. (1966) Changes in the villous pattern of the human jejunum associated with heavy radiation damage. *Gut* **7**, 149−153.

Williamson H.E., Marchand G.R., Bourland W.A., Farley D.B. & Van Orden D.E. (1976) Ethacrynic acid induced release of prostaglandin E to increase renal blood flow. *Prostaglandins*, **II**, 519−522.

Wilson F.A. & Hoyumpa A.M. (1979) Ethanol and small intestinal transport. *Gastroenterol.* **76**, 388−403.

Witts L.J. (1937) Ritual purgation in modern medicine. *Lancet*, **i**, 427−430.

Wolfe J.A., Plotzker R., Safina F.J., Ross M., Popky G. & Rubin W. (1976) Gastritis, duodenitis and bleeding duodenal ulcer following mefenamic acid therapy. *Arch. Intern. Med.* **136**, 923−925.

Chapter 25
Radiation Enteritis

BARRY T. JACKSON

Pathological effects of radiation on the
    intestine 413
Aetiology of chronic radiation enteritis 415
Clinical features 416
Investigations 418
Malabsorption 418
Management 420
Prevention 422

Wilhelm Roentgen discovered X-rays in November 1895. Less than 2 years later, Walsh (1897) recorded the first known case of radiation damage to the small intestine.

> 'A practical worker, Mr Greenhill, was carrying out a series of experiments including exposure of the region of the stomach for a period of about 2 h daily. After some weeks he complained of gastric symptoms, such as pain, tenderness on pressure, flatulence, colic and diarrhoea. He went away into the country for a fortnight and got well. On his return he resumed his experiments, and after a fortnight experienced a similar attack. He subsequently shielded his stomach with a thin sheet of lead and his symptoms finally disappeared. This history certainly suggests that in his case the rays of the focus tube caused a direct inflammation of the gastrointestinal mucous membranes.'

In 1898 the Curies discovered radium. During the first two decades of the twentieth century the use of radiation as a treatment for cancer was extensively studied and the condition of roentgen-ray cachexia, sometimes called roentgen-ray intoxication, became a well-recognized side-effect of treatment. This was investigated in animals by Warren & Whipple (1922) who suggested that the symptoms were caused by an acute radiation injury to the small intestine. This suggestion was confirmed by Martin & Rogers (1924) who irradiated exteriorized small bowel in dogs and noted anorexia, weight loss and cachexia with ulcers and strictures of the bowel developing up to 6 months after irradiation. Desjardins (1931) and Jones (1939) both reported small series of intestinal radiation injury in humans and Warren & Friedman (1942) reported a much larger series of thirty-eight patients. Eleven of their patients had injury to the small bowel, two to the stomach and twenty-five to the rectosigmoid. Most were acute injuries, developing within a few weeks of irradiation but two patients developed ileal strictures 7 years after treatment. Succeeding accounts of radiation injuries remained infrequent until the introduction of supervoltage therapy into clinical practice some 30 years ago. Since then there have been many accounts of radiation injury to the intestine and the pathology and clinical manifestations have become well defined. Even so, the diagnosis of chronic radiation enteritis is still often not made for an excessively long period, the management is both controversial and difficult and the morbidity and mortality rates are high. Although any part of the intestine may be damaged from the duodenum (Burn 1971) to the anus (Wellwood & Jackson 1973), the following account relates to chronic injury of the small bowel. The pathology and clinical manifestations of large bowel injuries are essentially similar, although the detail of surgical management is different (Smith & Milford 1976, Cooke & De Moor 1981, Ledda *et al.* 1981).

Pathological effects of radiation on the intestine

Ionizing radiation preferentially affects inter-mitotic cells with short reproductive cycles. The small bowel is therefore highly sensitive, more so than the colon or rectum, because of the very rapid normal mucosal cell turnover cycle that occurs in the enteron (Rubin & Casarett 1968).

Acute radiation effects

These may range from minimal degenerative changes in the epithelium of the mucosa to massive necrosis of the bowel wall depending on the total dose of radiation and the way in which it is fractionated. Major early complications are rare, but symptoms of nausea, vomiting, abdominal cramps and diarrhoea are often encountered during or immediately after irradiation. Acute radiation enteritis is normally self-limited because the mucosa regenerates rapidly. The morphological changes that cause these symptoms have been studied by direct observation in animals (Friedman & Warren 1942, Withers 1971) and by examining serial peroral small bowel biopsies in humans (Trier & Browning 1966, Wiernik 1966). There is rapid epithelial cell death in the walls of the crypts of Lieberkühn leading to mucosal denudation as cells in the upper crypts and villi are not replaced. There follows a progressive shortening of the villi leading to a flattened surface, disintegration of the crypts, mucosal oedema, focal ulceration, infiltration of the lamina propria by inflammatory cells and capillary endothelial swelling. Although structural recovery is usually complete within 2 or 3 weeks of completion of treatment, this is not invariable and in the symptom-free patient there may be long term persistence of villous atrophy and abnormal crypts. This accounts for the sub-clinical malabsorption that can be demonstrated by bile acid breath tests in patients who have undergone therapeutic irradiation (Kinsella & Bloomer 1980).

Late effects of radiation

The major feature is due to vascular damage which may take several years to develop. Complications include stricture formation, necrosis leading either to perforation or fistula formation and malabsorption. The intestinal ischaemia, which is often widespread, also accounts for many of the problems encountered by the surgeon when operating on these unfortunate patients.

The macroscopic changes in radiation-damaged small bowel vary somewhat according to the interval after exposure. There is more oedema and fibrinous peritonitis in cases of early onset and more fibrosis and rigidity in those of late onset. In general, however, there is an obvious colour change in the bowel which has a matt white appearance in contrast to the normal pink sheen and the bowel is markedly thickened and indurated. A mottled red and white roughened appearance of the serosa may also be seen. Narrowing of the lumen is usual and frank stenosis may occur, in which case there will be distension of the bowel proximal to the stricture. Adherence to adjacent structures is common, especially in the pelvis, and fistulae may be present. Mucosal ulceration may be observed within the lumen of the bowel. The macroscopic abnormalities are rarely discrete and almost always merge surreptitiously into the non-injured bowel, making it difficult or impossible to tell with certainty where the junction lies. This causes difficulty to the surgeon for anastomosis of occult-damaged intestine is likely to result in anastomotic leakage. An added complication, not infrequently observed, is the presence of multiple damaged segments of bowel with relatively normal segments interposed.

There is a wide variety of microscopic abnormalities (Berthrong & Fajardo 1981). Consistently, the submucosa is severely damaged showing gross thickening by fibrosis in which there are scattered bizarre fibroblasts with abnormal nuclei. Venous and lymphatic ectasia is prominent. Throughout the bowel wall arterioles and small arteries show an obliterative vasculitis leading on to sclerosis. Venules also may show obliterative changes. The mucosa is usually flat and often ulcerated while the muscularis mucosa is thicker than normal as a result of both muscular hyperplasia and fibrosis. The serosa is always thickened by collagen and is usually infiltrated with lymphocytes and bizarre fibroblasts.

It is generally agreed that the effect of radiation on the intestinal arterioles resulting in progressive ischaemia is the cardinal factor in the development of chronic radiation enteritis. This has been studied experimentally in dogs by Bosniak et al. (1969), using angiographic techniques, and Fonkalsrud et al. (1977), using electron micrsocopy. They have shown that an early effect of radiation on the intestine is a reversible arteriolar spasm which is later replaced by irreversible thrombosis and narrowing of the vessel lumen.

Aetiology of chronic radiation enteritis

Although it is known that the clinical manifestations of chronic radiation enteritis are caused by an ischaemic injury to the bowel, the reasons why only a small minority of patients undergoing therapeutic radiation develop these serious complications are unclear. There is a loose association between severe acute radiation enteritis and the late development of chronic symptoms but the absence of acute effects gives no assurance that late complications will not develop. Kline et al. (1972), in a study of 410 patients receiving pelvic irradiation, showed that 41% of the thirty-four patients developing late bowel complications had been without acute symptoms during treatment.

The incidence is difficult to assess as many studies do not distinguish between large and small bowel disease, while other papers give an incidence relating only to complications requiring surgical operation. The reported overall incidence of surgically treated chronic radiation enteritis varies considerably. For example, while Requarth & Roberts (1956) suggest that 2% of patients at risk may develop severe intestinal complications, De Cosse et al. (1969) suggest the figure is nearer 12%. The incidence of severe radiation injury confined to the small bowel is generally reported as around 3% or less (Aune & White 1951). Such figures are not strictly comparable, however, as radiotherapeutic regimens differ in different centres.

There is considerable evidence that the likelihood of chronic intestinal injury is directly related to the total radiation dose and the volume of bowel irradiated (Rubin 1974). Strockbine et al. (1970) studied a series of 831 patients with carcinoma of the cervix and found the incidence of bowel complications to increase in a linear fashion with higher doses of irradiation. Similar observations have been reported for colonic injuries sustained after radiotherapy given for carcinoma of the cervix (Gray & Kottmeier 1957). The association between late bowel complications and the volume of bowel irradiated has been shown by Wharton et al. (1977). Piver & Barlow (1977) and Withers & Romsdahl (1977), all of whom reported a much higher incidence of chronic radiation enteritis when patients with pelvic malignancy underwent irradiation to the para-aortic lymph nodes in addition to the pelvis.

It is thus accepted that if a very high dose of radiotherapy is given, either calculatingly for advanced disease or in error, intestinal complications may result and many published series include a small number of patients who fall into this category. Radiotherapy given in association with hyperbaric oxygen may also place patients at special risk (Wellwood & Jackson 1973). As a result, radiotherapists are exceedingly conscious of the possibility of bowel complications resulting from their treatment and take great care with dose calculation, fractionation and shielding so as to minimize the risk. Green et al. (1975) suggest that all patients undergoing pelvic radiotherapy should undergo pre-treatment barium studies of the small bowel in order to define any mobile intestinal loops that may enter the treatment field. The patients should then be positioned in such a way as to make the mobile loops fall away from the radiation beam. Many radiotherapists recommend that irradiation of the pelvis should be performed routinely with the patient in a head down position so as to displace the small bowel as far away from the pelvis as possible. Computer-controlled treatment designed to minimize the irradiation of normal tissues is being developed (Levene et al. 1978). Despite this care, a minority of patients still develop late radiation injury of the bowel while the majority, treated in identical fashion, do not.

Graham & Villalba (1963) suggested that patients with a history of previous abdominal operation or pelvic sepsis are at special risk because they are likely to have adhesions anchoring loops of small bowel in the pelvis and thus within the irradiated field. Although both Joelsson & Raf (1973) and Schmitz et al. (1974) confirmed these associations, Maruyama et al. (1974) were unable to demonstrate any association with previous abdominal operations but agreed that sepsis might be important. DeCosse et al. (1969) found the opposite in that, whereas previous abdominal hysterectomy seemed to be a factor in their series, there was no association with pelvic sepsis.

Similarly, some have suggested both hypertension and diabetes mellitus as factors (Van Nagell et al. 1974, Maruyama et al. 1974) but these are denied by others (Galland & Spencer 1979, Jackson 1982). Arteriosclerosis was considered important by DeCosse et al. (1969) but not by Galland & Spencer (1979) and, whereas somatotype was incriminated by Graham & Villalba (1963), it was denied by DeCosse et al. (1969). Unconfirmed reports suggest that concomitant chemotherapy at the time of irradiation may increase the risk of late bowel complications. Actinomycin-D (Donaldson et al. 1975), 5-fluouracil (Moertel et al. 1969) and adriamycin (Byfield et al. 1975) have all been implicated, but the majority of patients with radiation enteritis have not had chemotherapy.

In summary, not one of these factors can confidently be asserted as the cause of chronic radiation enteritis; the aetiology in most patients remains elusive.

Clinical features

The great majority of patients who present with chronic radiation enteritis will be young or middle-aged women who have been treated for pelvic malignancy. DeCosse et al. (1969) in an unusually large series of 100 patients reported a mean age of 52 years; 95% of the patients were women and 84% had been treated for carcinoma of the cervix or endometrium. Other authors have recorded similar findings (Deveney et al. 1976, Deitel & Vasic 1979, Galland & Spencer 1979). It should be stressed, however, that radiation injury may occur in any patient who has undergone abdominal or pelvic radiotherapy and radiation enteritis in elderly men who have undergone treatment for carcinoma of the prostate (Duggan et al. 1975) is as well recognized as it is in adolescents treated for testicular tumours (Roswit et al. 1972).

The time interval between radiotherapy and the onset of symptoms is widely variable and is of no guide on diagnosis. DeCosse et al. (1969) reported a mean of 6.5 years (range 1 month to 31 years) and the present author's experience is similar (Jackson 1976).

The presenting symptoms and physical signs will depend upon the underlying pathology. *Strictures* will cause partial intestinal obstruction with colicky abdominal pain associated with abdominal distension, nausea and occasional vomiting. Characteristically, these symptoms are intermittent, a feature which leads to delay in diagnosis. *Necrosis* of the intestine may cause free perforation into the peritoneal cavity with sudden onset of peritonitis but, alternatively, may cause a fistula especially to the vagina. A localized perforation of the terminal ileum sometimes becomes sealed by omentum with resulting symptoms and signs similar to those of an appendix mass. Mucosal damage may cause *malabsorption* presenting in a variety of ways. Diarrhoea and steatorrhoea are the most common features together with nutritional disturbances such as megaloblastic anaemia, hypocalcaemia, hypomagnesaemia and hypoproteinaemia. Weight loss and clinical evidence of malnutrition are also typical features which must not be ascribed to recurrence of malignant disease.

Commonly, these various presentations are not clear-cut and many patients will not fall into a clearly defined category. Additionally, concurrent radiation damage to the rectosigmoid area of the large intestine is often present and symptoms such as rectal haemorrhage or tenesmus may mask the features of involvement of the small bowel. A combination of small and large bowel obstruction may occur and if the patient has radiation cystitis urinary symptoms such as frequency, dysuria or haematuria may also be present. The pelvis may become grossly indurated with radiation fibrosis and a frozen pelvis suggestive of widespread malignancy may be palpated on rectal or vaginal examination.

A high index of suspicion that radiation damage is a possible explanation of the patient's symptoms is the key to diagnosis. All too often the diagnosis is delayed for many months as a result of the clinician wrongly ascribing the clinical features to an alternative cause, especially that of recurrent tumour. Regrettably, the diagnosis is sometimes not made until the bowel perforates and laparotomy is undertaken. The following case history is illustrative:

> Mrs T.D., aged 43, presented in 1971 with a Stage II squamous carcinoma of the cervix. This was treated by intracavity radiation and external radiotherapy. Twelve treatments were given over 28 days with 4200 rads (42 Grays) being the maximum dose to the pelvis. She had undergone no previous abdominal operation, but 15 years earlier had severe depression treated in a mental hospital. She was neither hypertensive nor diabetic.
> Eight months after treatment, while symptom-free, she was diagnosed by a gynaecologist as having 'firm recurrence of the left pelvic wall'. This was on the basis of a vaginal examination performed at a routine follow-up appointment. She was admitted for consideration of hysterectomy, but when examined under anaesthetic, this diagnosis was found to be incorrect and biopsies showed radiation fibrosis only.
> One year after treatment she began to complain of recurrent attacks of nausea, diarrhoea and abdominal discomfort. In a letter from the hospital to the general practitioner, it was written 'we are satisfied that the recent attacks of nausea, diarrhoea and abdominal discomfort are due to chronic constipation'. Two months later, however, the patient was referred to a psychiatrist. This was her first psychiatric attendance for 16 years.
> A consultant psychiatrist diagnosed depression and wrote to her general practitioner 'I would regard her reaction as a physiological depressive state. This would explain the long duration of her illness and the perpetuation of abdominal pain'.
> During the next 2 years she continued to have increasingly severe bouts of abdominal colic associated with diarrhoea and intermittent vomiting. She was treated with anti-emetics and analgesics whilst attending simultaneously the psychiatric, radiotherapy and gynaecological clinics. In April 1974, the general practitioner wrote 'I am becoming increasingly worried about these attacks of nausea, vomiting and abdominal pain which are more frequent and more severe'. The hospital reply was 'as you will know, her abdominal symptoms have been recurring for over 3 years now and this goes a long way to precluding any serious disease. I could not find any evidence of an organic basis for this and thought it secondary to her psychiatric state. I have left her on her previous dose of Surmontil and Ativan'.
> In March 1975 she was admitted as an emergency with generalized peritonitis and diagnosed by both the casualty officer and duty registrar as having a perforated duodenal ulcer. At laparotomy, however, she was found to have a perforated radiation stricture of her terminal ileum, 20 cm proximal to the ileocaecal valve. There was macroscopic radiation damage of the terminal 1 m of ileum, but laparotomy was otherwise normal. An extended right hemicolectomy was performed with primary anastomosis and a covering loop ileostomy. This was closed 1 month later after a gastrografin enema had shown integrity of the anastomosis.

It is by no means unusual for one complication to be followed by another some months or years later (Haddad et al. 1983). Radiation enteritis is classically a progressive disease and no patient who develops it can be considered permanently cured by either medical or surgical treatment.

Investigations

The diagnosis of radiation enteritis should be considered in all patients who present with abdominal symptoms and give a past history of pelvic or abdominal irradiation. In many instances this diagnosis will prove to be wrong but unless a radiation-damaged bowel is suspected, and appropriate investigations performed, the true explanation of the patient's symptoms may be missed.

Radiographic examination of the abdomen is the mainstay of diagnosis. A plain radiograph may show dilated loops of intestine with or without multiple fluid levels. Barium contrast studies may show a range of abnormality such as single or multiple strictures, widening of the bowel with transverse barring, rosethorn fissures, nodular filling defects and fistulae (Figs 25.1, 25.2 and 25.3). It has been suggested that these radiographic abnormalities are specific for radiation-damaged bowel but this is not so. In fact, the radiographic appearances are non-specific and compatible with any chronic inflammatory disease of the small bowel. Sometimes they may be indistinguishable from Crohn's disease or coeliac disease (Goldstein 1979).

Misleadingly, contrast studies of the damaged bowel are sometimes normal. This is especially so if the symptoms are intermittent and the examination is performed at a time of quiescence. In such cases repeat examinations should unhesitatingly be performed when symptoms recur. Sigmoidoscopy and barium enema studies should always be performed in addition to small bowel contrast studies in order to exclude concurrent rectal or colonic disease. Fibre-optic colonoscopy also may be helpful in the diagnosis both of colonic and terminal ileal disease. Cystoscopy and intravenous urography should be performed if urinary symptoms are present and investigation into the possibility of malabsorption should always be carried out.

Malabsorption

Selvesan & Kobro (1939) appear to be the first

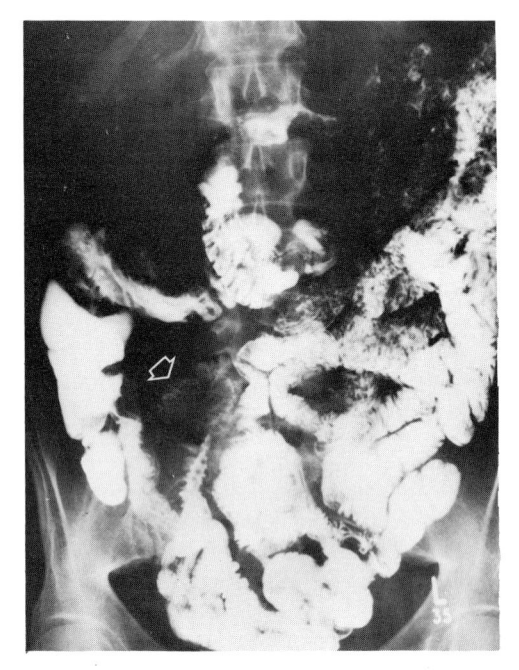

Fig. 25.1. Mrs S.P., *aet* 48. Carcinoma of ovary treated by excision and radiotherapy. Three years later she developed recurring bouts of subacute intestinal obstruction. Small bowel barium meal shows a long stricture of terminal ileum (arrowed). Radiation enteritis confirmed at laparotomy.

authors to report an established malabsorption syndrome caused by radiation enteritis. Their patient had steatorrhoea associated with a radiation stricture of the ileum. No further case was described for 20 years until Scudamore & Green (1959) and Sauer (1959) reported single case histories of steatorrhoea. Wood et al. (1963) and Greenberger & Isselbacher (1964) also reported cases of steatorrhoea, while Tankel et al. (1965) reported malabsorption of fat, iron, vitamin B_{12} and an impaired xylose excretion test developing in a patient with a radiation-damaged small intestine. Duncan & Leonard (1965) described six patients with malabsorption syndrome in whom diarrhoea, wasting, steatorrhoea and megaloblastic anaemia caused by vitamin B_{12} deficiency were the main clinical features. One of their patients had subacute combined degeneration of the spinal cord. Wellwood & Jackson (1973) reported two cases of severe calcium deficiency, one patient presenting with tetany. The up-to-date history of this patient nicely

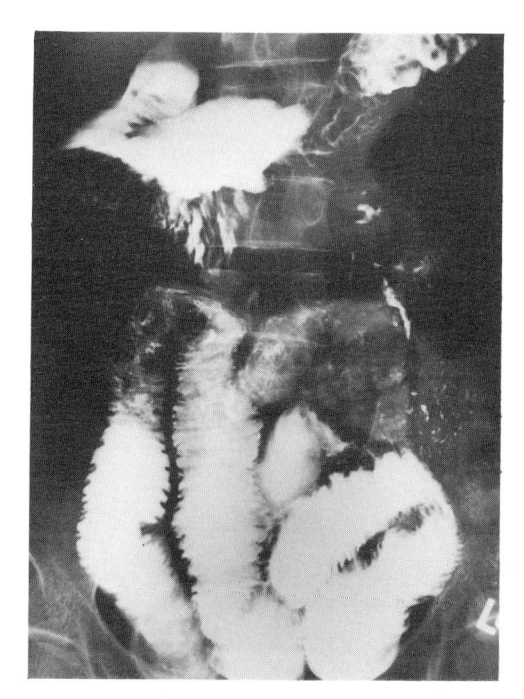

Fig. 25.2. Mrs. J.T., *aet* 33. Carcinoma of ovary treated by excision and radiotherapy. Four years later she developed recurring bouts of abdominal pain that remained undiagnosed for 15 years before a small bowel barium meal was performed. This shows dilated ileum with transverse barring and irregular outline of bowel. Radiation enteritis confirmed at laparotomy. Fifteen months earlier a normal gall bladder had been removed through a sub-costal incision for a mistaken diagnosis of gall bladder dyspepsia.

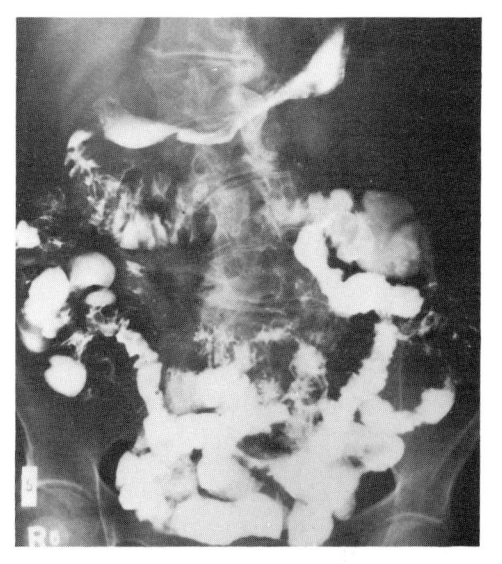

Fig. 25.3. Mrs A.O., *aet* 70. Carcinoma of endometrium treated by excision and radiotherapy. Three years later she developed chronic diarrhoea and steatorrhoea with malabsorption of vitamin B_{12} and calcium. Small bowel barium meal shows diffuse abnormality with a rigid and largely featureless bowel. She was treated medically but 6 months later emergency laparotomy was necessary for acute intestinal obstruction caused by the impaction of a plum stone in the most proximal of four separate strictures.

demonstrates that radiation enteritis is a continued and progressive disease:

> Miss C.B., aged 48, presented in 1970 with a papillary cyst-adenocarcinoma of the ovary. A hysterectomy and bilateral salpingo-oophorectomy was performed followed by a course of external radiotherapy. Ten treatments were given over 26 days with 4750 rads (47.5 Grays) given to the pelvis. Severe diarrhoea was noted as a side-effect but this subsided over 2 months. The patient was neither diabetic nor hypertensive. Eight months after treatment she complained of colicky abdominal pain and vomiting, and was thought to have recurrent tumour accounting for her symptoms. Vaginal examination revealed 'almost certain recurrence at the top of the vagina'. The patient's abdominal symptoms continued but it was not until 3 months later that she was referred for consideration of laparotomy with a clinical diagnosis of subacute intestinal obstruction.
> At laparotomy there was no evidence of recurrent tumour, the symptoms being caused by a short radiation stricture of the terminal ileum. The rest of the small intestine and the large intestine appeared normal. A right hemicolectomy was performed, removing 8 inches of the ileum including the stricture. Recovery was straightforward and the patient was discharged home after 10 days.
> One month later she complained of paraesthesiae in hands and feet, together with weakness and dizziness; 2 months later she had a *grand mal* attack and was admitted with a diagnosis of probable cerebral secondaries. Almost

immediately after admission she developed severe tetany with carpopedal spasm, a clenched jaw and positive Chvostek's and Trousseau's signs. She also complained of seeing stars in front of her eyes. Her serum calcium was found to be 2.6 mEq/l (1.3 mmol/l) and her serum potassium 2.1 mEq/l (2.1 mmol/l). She was treated energetically with infusion of the appropriate ions and the tetany resolved rapidly. A small bowel barium meal showed abnormality throughout the small intestine compatible with widespread radiation damage.

Two years later, in 1973, she again presented with nutritional deficiency. Her haemoglobin was 7.3 g/100 ml (7.3 g/dl), serum calcium 4.2 mEq/l (2.1 mmol/l), serum magnesium 1.2 mEq/l (0.6 mmol/l) and serum iron 25 µg/dl (4.5 µmol/l). Radiographic studies with barium showed diffuse abnormality of the small intestine. Routine investigation of the large bowel by contrast radiography and fibre-optic colonoscopy showed no abnormality. After correction of the nutritional deficiencies the patient remained well on treatment until 1978 when, 8 years after treatment with radiotherapy, she developed subacute small bowel obstruction. At laparotomy she was found not only to have a tight stricture both at and proximal to the site of the previous anastomosis with macroscopic radiation damage over much of the ileum, but also a radiation stricture of the rectosigmoid. The jejunum, surprisingly, appeared normal. A staged resection of both large and small bowel disease was performed with restoration of continuity. Histology of the resected specimens confirmed diffuse radiation damage. The patient made a good recovery and has since remained well on regular vitamin B_{12} injections, cholestyramine sachets and codeine phosphate tablets to slow her bowel frequency.

Malabsorption after radiotherapy, however, may be sub-clinical. McBrien (1973) showed by means of the Schilling test that vitamin B_{12} absorption may be impaired in symptomless patients without anaemia several years after irradiation of the pelvis. Newman et al. (1973) showed that a majority of symptom-free patients who had received pelvic irradiation for gynaecological malignancy at least 1 year earlier had an abnormal cholylglycine-1-[^{14}C] breath test, indicating an impaired enterohepatic circulation of bile salts. They suggested that this was caused by sub-clinical ileal damage. Although their data were not confirmed by Stryker et al. (1977) a study by Kinsella & Bloomer (1980) suggested that bile acid breath testing is a highly sensitive indicator of sub-clinical radiation damage to the small intestine in the first few weeks after radiotherapy and may even predict for late bowel damage. This suggestion has not been confirmed.

Management

The management of radiation enteritis is difficult, protracted and often dangerous. The outcome in many reported cases is either death or, at best, chronic disability. All too frequently complication follows upon complication, especially after surgical operation, and long-term follow-up is essential. Although the mainstay of treatment is surgical resection of the diseased intestine, meticulous supportive medical treatment is also necessary and this may need to be long continued.

Many patients will present with subacute intestinal obstruction and be in reasonably good fluid and electrolyte balance. Others will present with a small bowel fistula and accompanying electrolyte deficiency and dehydration. Yet others will present with a perforated intestine, peritonitis and profound shock while all may have varying degrees of malabsorption. Clearly, the management will vary in detail from patient to patient and only general principles can be outlined here.

Preoperative

Rehydration, correction of electrolyte imbalance and correction of malabsorption is necessary for many patients. Energetic parenteral nutrition using a tunnelled central venous catheter is indicated if the patient is chronically malnourished. Blood transfusion is given if the patient is anaemic. Sometimes pre-operative antibiotics are indicated for the treatment of toxaemia, but more usually these are started at the time of operation. A preoperative sigmoidoscopy is essential to assess any radiation changes that may be present in the rectum or lower sigmoid. Great care should be taken not to attempt to force the instrument around the rectosigmoid junction because of the risk of perforating friable bowel.

Surgical

Intravenous metronidazole and a broad spectrum antibiotic are given at the time of induction. Prophylaxis against deep vein thrombosis is given routinely and a generous incision is made so as to effect good exposure and access to the entire peritoneal cavity. The incision should avoid any skin which has obviously been damaged by irradiation (Girvan et al. 1971). A full laparotomy is performed in order to exclude the presence of metastatic tumour or local tumour recurrence. Not infrequently the irradiated pelvic contents are hard and fixed but these changes should not be mistaken for infiltrating tumour. If in doubt a biopsy and frozen tissue section may be performed in order to confirm or refute this diagnosis. Deep pelvic dissection must be avoided at all costs for the risk of damage to surrounding organs is considerable. The urinary bladder and ureters are particularly at risk as they will have been rendered partially ischaemic by the radiotherapy. Attention is then turned to the damaged intestine.

Both the small and large bowel are carefully examined throughout with special reference to the ileum and rectosigmoid junction. Occasionally the radiation damage will appear to be confined to a small segment of the small intestine. This should be resected, together with a generous length of normal bowel on either side. Usually, however, there is no clear line of demarcation between normal and abnormal intestine and the surgeon is faced with uncertainty as to how much bowel to resect in order to effect a safe anastomosis, while at the same time avoiding an overgenerous resection which may lead to the development of the 'short bowel syndrome'. This dilemma has led to difference of opinion as to whether resection and anastomosis is always the correct treatment. Several authors have suggested that side-to-side bypass of the damaged area is less dangerous than resection in that anastomotic leakage is less likely to occur and postoperative short bowel problems will not result (Dencker et al. 1971, Swan et al. 1976 Lillemoe et al. 1983, Wobbes et al. 1984). This view is challenged by others (Localio et al. 1969, Deveney et al. 1976, Palmer & Bush 1976). Sterns et al. (1964) stressed that bypass operations do not prevent perforation of the bypassed bowel and reported this complication with death of the patient. Schmitt & Symmonds (1981) reported massive haemorrhage occurring from bypassed intestine 6 years later.

That there are risks from resection and anastomosis of irradiated small intestine cannot be denied. Wellwood et al. (1974) report a retrospective review of five patients with radiation enteritis who underwent a total of eleven small bowel anastomoses with a leakage rate of 100%. All five patients died. Swan et al. (1976) report a mortality rate of 53% and an anastomotic leak rate of 65% in a series of seventeen patients. Even so, a majority of writers believe resection to be the treatment of choice. Some authors have suggested that frozen tissue section examination of the cut ends of the bowel should be performed before anastomosis in order to exclude radiation changes (Localio et al. 1979), but sound surgical principles are probably of more importance. Meticulous attention to surgical detail is essential. The anastomosis should be performed without clamps so as to avoid jeopardizing an already precarious blood supply; the anastomosis should be tension-free; a pulsatile blood supply should be visible at the cut ends of the bowel; small bits of tissue should be taken and the sutures should not be inserted too tightly; the anastomosis should be wrapped in omentum; if there is any vestige of doubt about the viability of the anastomosis, a temporary loop stoma above the anastomosis should be performed.

Medical

Not all patients with radiation-damaged intestine are sufficiently ill to require surgical treatment and many who have undergone surgical operation require active and long-lasting medical care. Watery diarrhoea may be associated with both chronic inflammatory disease of the ileum and surgical resection, especially if the ileocaecal valve is removed. This, in part, is caused by bile salts entering the colon. Vitamin B_{12} malabsorption may also occur. Large resections of the ileum may be associated with steatorrhoea, while diffuse disease or removal of the jejunum may cause deficiency of folate, iron, calcium and magnesium. Medical treatment is therefore directed principally towards the correction of these abnormalities.

A low-fat diet, sometimes lactose-free, should be encouraged, although compliance may be poor as the fare is unappetizing. Diarrhoea induced by the spillage of bile salts into the colon may be controlled with cholestyramine and intestinal transit time may be slowed by giving drugs such as codeine phosphate, diphenoxylate or loperamide. Regular vitamin B_{12} injections should be given if the terminal ileum is diseased or has been resected, and care must be taken that the patient does not insidiously develop folate, calcium or other deficiency. Smooth muscle relaxants are often prescribed but are of uncertain value.

Other suggested but less widely accepted medical measures include the prescription of a medium-chain-triglyceride diet (Haddad et al. 1974), a gluten-free diet (Donaldson et al. 1975), sulphonamides (Goldstein et al. 1976) and steroids (Morgenstern et al. 1977).

Prevention

The radiotherapist faces a dilemma when planning the treatment of pelvic or abdominal malignancy. On the one horn is optimal cancer treatment which may well include a high radiation dose and on the other horn is the presence of a limited intestinal tolerance to radiation. Obviously, these two factors must be balanced as a conscious exercise for each and every patient treated. Nevertheless, apart from avoiding an excessive radiation dose, identifying possible high risk patients and taking those few mechanical preventative measures already described, there is currently no satisfactory prophylaxis. Experimentally, the use of sulphonamides (Spratt et al. 1961), salicylates (Mennie et al. 1975) and antiproteases (Rachootin et al. 1972) have been shown to reduce acute radiation enteritis but none of these agents has found a place in clinical practice and there is no evidence that they reduce the likelihood of late complications. For patient, radiotherapist and clinician alike, the enigma of chronic radiation enteritis remains.

References

Aune E.F. & White B.V. (1951) Gastrointestinal complications of irradiation for carcinoma of uterine cervix. *J. Amer. Med. Assoc.* **147**, 831–834.

Berthrong M. & Fajardo L.F. (1981) Radiation injury in surgical pathology. *Amer. J. Surg. Pathol.* **5**, 153–178.

Bosniak M.A., Hardy M.A., Quint J. & Ghossein N.A. (1969) Demonstration of the effect of irradiation on canine bowel using *in vivo* photographic magnification angiography. *Radiol.* **93**, 1361–1368.

Burn J.I. (1971) Radiation duodenitis. *Proc. Roy. Soc. Med.* **64**, 395–396.

Byfield J.E., Watring W.G., Lemkin S.R., Juillard G.J., Hauskins L.A., Smith M.L., & Lagasse L.D. (1975) Adriamycin; a useful drug for combination with radiation therapy. *Proc. Amer. Assoc. Canc. Res.* **16**, 253.

Cooke S.A.R. & De Moor N.G. (1981) The surgical treatment of the radiation-damaged rectum. *Brit. J. Surg.* **68**, 488–492.

DeCosse J.J., Rhodes R.S., Wentz W.B., Reagan J.W., Dworken H.J. & Holden W.D. (1969) The natural history and management of radiation induced injury of the gastrointestinal tract. *Ann. Surg.* **170**, 369–384.

Deitel M. & Vasic V. (1979) Major intestinal complications of radiotherapy. *Amer. J. Gastroenterol.* **72**, 65–70.

Dencker H., Johnsson J.E., Liedberg G. & Tibblin S. (1971) Surgical aspects of radiation injury to the small and large intestines. *Acta Chirurg. Scand.* **137**, 692–695.

Desjardins A.U. (1931) Action of Roentgen rays and radium on the gastrointestinal tract. *Amer. J. Roentgenol.* **26**, 337–370.

Deveney C.W., Lewis F.R. & Shrock T.R. (1976) Surgical management of radiation injury of the small and large intestine. *Dis. Col. Rect.* **19**, 25–29.

Donaldson S.S., Jundt S., Ricour C., Sarrazin D., Lemerle J. & Schweisguth O. (1975) Radiation enteritis in children. *Canc.* **35**, 1167–1178.

Duggan F.J., Sanford E.J. & Rohner T.J. (1975) Radiation enteritis following radiotherapy for prostatic carcinoma. *Brit. J. Urol.* **47**, 441–444.

Duncan W. & Leonard J.C. (1965) The malabsorption syndrome following radiotherapy. *Quart. J. Med.* **34**, 319–329.

Fonkalsrud E.W., Sanchez M., Zerubavel R. & Mahoney A. (1977) Serial changes in arterial structure following radiation therapy. *Surg. Gynecol. Obstet.* **145**, 395–400.

Friedman N.B. & Warren S. (1942) Evolution of experimental radiation ulcers of the intestine. *Arch. Pathol.* **33**, 326–333.

Galland R.B. & Spencer J. (1979) Surgical aspects of radiation injury to the intestine. *Brit. J. Surg.* **66**, 135–138.

Girvin G.W., Schnug G.E., Cavenaugh C.R. & McGonigle D.J. (1971) Complications of abdominal irradiation. *Amer. Surg.* **37**, 498–502.

Goldstein F., Khoury J. & Thornton J.J. (1976) Treatment of chronic radiation enteritis and colitis with salicylazo-sulfapyridine and systemic corticosteroids. *Amer. J. Gastroenterol.* **65**, 201–208.

Goldstein H.M. (1979) Small bowel and colon. In *Diagnostic Roentgenology of Radiotherapy Change*, pp. 85–100. (Ed. by H.I. Libschitz). Williams and Wilkins Company, Baltimore.

Graham J.B. & Villalba R.J. (1963) Damage to the small intestine by radiotherapy. *Surg. Gynecol. Obstet.* **116**, 665–668.

Gray M.J. & Kottmeier H.L. (1957) Rectal and bladder injuries following radium therapy for carcinoma of the cervix at the Radiumhemmet. *Amer. J. Obstet. Gynecol.* **74**, 1294–1303.

Green N., Iba G. & Smith W.R. (1975) Measures to minimise small intestine injury in the irradiated pelvis. *Canc.* **35**, 1633–1640.

Greenberger N.J. & Isselbacher K.J. (1964) Malabsorption following radiation injury to the gastrointestinal tract. *Amer. J. Med.* **36**, 450–456.

Haddad H., Bounos G., Tahan W.T., Devroede G., Beaudry R. & Lafond R. (1974) Long-term nutrition with an elemental diet following intensive abdominal irradiation. *Dis. Col. Rect.* **17**, 373–376.

Haddad G.K., Grodsinsky C. & Allen H. (1983). The spectrum of radiation enteritis. *Dis. Col. Rect.* **26**, 590–594.

Jackson B.T. (1976) Bowel damage from radiation. *Proc. Roy. Soc. Med.* **69**, 683–686.

Joelsson I. & Raf L. (1973) Late injuries of the small intestine following radiotherapy for uterine carcinoma. *Acta Chirurg. Scand.* **139**, 194–200.

Jones T.E. (1939) Benign strictures of the intestine due to irradiation. *Surg. Clin. N. Amer.* **19**, 1185–1194.

Kinsella T.J. & Bloomer W.D. (1980) Tolerance of the intestine to radiation therapy. *Surg. Gynecol. Obstet.* **151**, 273–284.

Kline J.C., Buchler D.A., Boone M.L., Peckham B.M. & Carr W.F. (1972) The relationship of reactions to complications in the radiation therapy of cancer of the cervix. *Radiol.* **105**, 413–416.

Ledda P., Shaw J.F.L. & Everett W.G. (1981) Surgical treatment of irradiation injury to the large bowel. *J. Roy. Coll. Surg. Edin.* **26**, 348–356.

Levene M.B., Kijewski P.K., Chin L.M., Bjarngard B.E. & Hellman S. (1978) Computer-controlled radiation therapy. *Radiol.* **129**, 769–775.

Lillemoe K.D., Brigham R.A., Harmou J.W., Feaster M.M., Saunders J.R. & d'Avis J.A. (1983). Surgical management of small bowel radiation enteritis. *Arch. Surg.* **118**, 905–907.

Localio S.A., Stone A. & Friedman M. (1969) Surgical aspects of radiation enteritis. *Surg. Gynecol. Obstet.* **129**, 1163–1172.

Localio S.A., Pachter H.L. & Gouge T.H. (1979) The radiation-injured bowel. In *Surgery Annual*, pp. 181–205. (Ed. by L.M. Nyhus). Appleton-Century-Crofts, New York.

McBrien M.P. (1973) Vitamin B_{12} malabsorption after cobalt teletherapy for carcinoma of the bladder. *Brit. Med. J.* **i**, 648–650.

Martin C.L. & Rogers F.T. (1924) Roentgen-ray cachexia. *Amer. J. Roentgenol.* **11**, 280–286.

Maruyama Y., Van Nagell J.R., Utley J., Vider M.L. & Parker J.C. (1974) Radiation and small bowel complications in cervical carcinoma therapy. *Radiol.* **112**, 699–703.

Mennie A.T., Dalley V.M., Dineen L.C. & Collier H.O.J. (1975) Treatment of radiation-induced gastrointestinal distress with acetysalicylate. *Lancet*, **ii**, 942–943.

Moertel C.G., Childs D.S., Reitemeier R.J., Colby M.Y. & Holbrook M.A. (1969) Combined 5-fluorouracil and supervoltage radiation therapy of locally unresectable gastrointestinal cancer. *Lancet*, **ii**, 865–867.

Morgenstern L., Thompson R. & Friedman N.B. (1977) The modern enigma of radiation enteropathy: sequelae and solutions. *Amer. J. Surg.* **134**, 166–172.

Newman A., Katsaris J., Blendis L.M., Charlesworth M. & Walter L.H. (1973) Small intestinal injury in women who have had pelvic radiotherapy. *Lancet*, **ii**, 1471–1473.

Palmer J.A., & Bush R.S. (1976) Radiation injuries to the bowel associated with the treatment of carcinoma of the cervix. *Surg.* **80**, 458–464.

Piver M.S. & Barlow J.J. (1977) High dose irradiation to biopsy confirmed aortic node metastases from carcinoma of the uterine cervix. *Canc.* **39**, 1243–1246.

Rachootin S., Shapiro S., Yamakawa T., Goldman L., Patin S. & Morgenstern L. (1972) Potent anti-proteases derived from *Ascaris lumbricoides*: efficacy in amelioration of post-radiation enteropathy. *Gastroenterol.*, **62**, 796.

Requarth W. & Roberts S. (1956) Intestinal injuries following irradiation of pelvic viscera for malignancy. *Arch. Surg.* **43**, 682–688.

Roswit B., Malsky S.J. & Reid C.B. (1972) Severe radiation injuries of the stomach, small intestine, colon and rectum. *Amer. J. Roentgenol.* **114**, 460–475.

Rubin P. (1974) The radiographic expression of radiotherapeutic injury: an overview. *Seminars Roentgenol.* **9**, 5–13.

Rubin P. & Casarett G.W. (1968) Clinical radiation pathology as applied to curative radiotherapy. *Canc.* **22**, 767–778.

Sauer W.G. (1959) Actinic or factitial enteritis: an unusual cause of the malabsorption syndrome. *Postgrad. Med.* **26**, 352–355.

Schmitt F.H. & Symmonds R.E. (1981) Surgical treatment of radiation-induced injuries of the intestine. *Surg. Gynecol. Obstet.* **153**, 896–900.

Schmitz R.L., Chao J.H. & Bartolome J.S. (1974) Intestinal injuries incidental to irradiation of the cervix of the uterus. *Surg. Gynecol. Obstet.* **138**, 29–32.

Scudamore H.H. & Green P.A. (1959) Secondary malabsorption syndromes of intestinal origin. *Postgrad. Med.* **26**, 340–351.

Selvesan H.A. & Kobro M. (1939) Symptomatic sprue. *Acta Med. Scand.* **102**, 277–294.

Smith J.S. & Milford H.E. (1976) Management of colitis caused by irradiation. *Surg. Gynecol. Obstet.* **142**, 569–572.

Spratt J.S., Heinbecker P. & Slatzstein S.L. (1961) The influence of succinylsulfathiazole (sulfasuxidine) upon the response of canine small intestine to irradiation. *Canc.* **14**, 862–874.

Sterns E.E., Palmer J.A. & Kergin F.G. (1964) The surgical significance of radiation injuries to bowel. *Can. J. Surg.* **7**, 407–413.

Strockbine M.F., Hancock J.E. & Fletcher G.H. (1970) Complications in 831 patients with squamous cell carcinoma of the intact uterine cervix treated with 3000 rad or more whole pelvis irradiation. *Amer. J. Roentgenol.* **108**, 293–304.

Stryker J.A., Hepner G.W. & Mortel R. (1977) The effect of pelvic irradiation on ileal function. *Radiol.* **124**, 213–216.

Swan R.W., Fowler W.C. & Boronow R.C. (1976) Surgical management of radiation injury to the small intestine. *Surg. Gynecol. Obstet.* **142**, 325–327.

Tankel H.I., Clark D.H. & Lee F.D. (1965) Radiation enteritis with malabsorption. *Gut*, **6**, 560–569.

Trier J.S. & Browning T.H. (1966) Morphologic response of the mucosa of human small intestine to X-ray exposure. *J. Clin. Invest.* **45**, 194–204.

Van Nagell J.R., Maruyama Y., Parker J.C. & Dalton W.L. (1974) Small bowel injury following radiation therapy for cervical cancer. *Amer. J. Obstet. Gynecol.* **118**, 163–167.

Walsh D. (1897) Deep tissue traumatism from Roentgen ray exposure. *Brit. Med. J.*, **ii**, 272–273.

Warren S.L. & Whipple G.H. (1922) Roentgen ray intoxication. *J. Exp. Med.* **35**, 187–202.

Warren S. & Friedman N.B. (1942) Pathology and pathologic diagnosis of radiation lesions in the gastrointestinal tract. *Amer. J. Pathol.* **18**, 499–513.

Wellwood J.M. & Jackson B.T. (1973) The intestinal complications of radiotherapy. *Brit. J. Surg.* **60**, 814–818.

Wellwood J.M., Jackson B.T. & Bates T.D. (1974) Breakdown of small bowel anastomoses after pelvic radiotherapy. *Ann. Roy. Coll. Surg. Engl.* **54**, 306–308.

Wharton J.T., Jones H.W., Day T.G., Rutledge F.N. & Fletcher G.H. (1977) Preirradiation celiotomy and extended field irradiation for invasive carcinoma of the cervix. *Obstet. Gynecol.* **49**, 333–338.

Wiernik G. (1966) Radiation damage and repair in the human jejunal mucosa. *J. Pathol.* **91**, 389–393.

Withers H.R. (1971) Regeneration of intestinal mucosa after irradiation. *Canc.* **28**, 75–81.

Withers H.R. & Romsdahl M.M. (1977) Postoperative radiotherapy for adenocarcinoma of the rectum and rectosigmoid. *Internat. J. Rad. Oncol. Biol. Phys.* **2**, 1069–1076.

Wobbes T., Verschuereu R.C.J., Lubbers E-J.C., Jansen W. & Paping R.H.L. (1984) Surgical aspects of radiation enteritis of small bowel. *Dis. Col. Rect.* **27**, 89–92.

Wood I.J., Ralston M. & Kurrle G.R. (1963) Irradiation injury to the gastrointestinal tract: clinical features, management and pathogenesis. *Austr. Ann. Med.* **12**, 143–152.

Index

Abdomen, examination 4
Abdominal pain 1
　episodic functional 86, 88
Abetalipoproteinaemia 56–9
　clinical and biochemical features 56–7
　diagnosis 57
　enterocyte defects 56
　gastrointestinal symptoms 56
　pathogenesis 56
　steatorrhoea, age effects 57
　treatment 57–9
Absorption, small intestinal sites 105–7
　see also Malabsorption; *various substances and sites*
Acanthocytosis, abetalipoproteinaemia 56
Acrodermatitis enteropathica 69–71
　Paneth cells 18
Actinomycin-D, radiation enteritis 416
Adenocarcinomas
　intestinal 364–5
　pre-existing disorders 364–5
Adenomas, intestinal 363–4
Adenoviruses 243
Adipose tissue, skinfold thickness 31–2, 33
Adriamycin, radiation enteritis 416
AIDS 145
　cryptosporidiosis 140, 294
　giardiasis 289
Albendazole, parasitic diseases 285, 286, 293
Albumin
　catabolism, intestinal lymphangiectasia 348
　chromium-labelled 26–7
　circulating levels 34
Alcohol, gastrointestinal effects 402–3
Alkaline phosphatase
　coeliac disease 167
　post-gastrectomy serum levels 99
Alkylating agents, gastrointestinal cytotoxicity 400
Allergic disorders, IgA deficiency 137–8
Allergy, definition 118
Alpha-lipoprotein deficiency 227
Aluminium hydroxide, gastrointestinal side-effects 404–5
Alveolitis, fibrosing, coeliac disease 168
Amino acids
　absorption, protein–calorie malnutrition 304
　essential
　　bacterial overgrowth 261
　　post-resection deficiency 112–13
　malabsorption 62–5
　plasma levels 34
　transport 61
　　defects 62

　tropical sprue 319
Aminopterin, xylose absorption effects 400
Amyloid 218
Amyloidosis 218–21
　bleeding and protein loss 220
　classification 218–19
　Crohn's disease 200
　heredofamilial 219
　lamina propria 19
　localized 219
　primary 218–19
　prognosis 221
　radiology and clinical features 219–21
　secondary 219
　Whipple's disease 274
Anaemia, post-gastrectomy 98
Anaerobes, bile salt deconjugation 256
Aneurysms, superior mesenteric 8
Angiodysplasias 8, 344–5
Angioedema, hereditary 147–8
Angiography 8–10
　therapeutic 9–10
Angiokeratoma corporis diffusum 342
Anisakis infections 286
Ankylosing spondylitis
　Crohn's disease association 196, 201
　HLA-B27 association 196, 201
Ankylostoma duodenale 283–5
　larvae development stages 284
Ankylostomiasis 283–5
Antacids, gastrointestinal side-effects 404–5
Anthropometry, nutrition assessment 29–31
Antibody deficiency disorders 136–44
Anticoagulants, intestinal haemorrhage 406–7
Anticonvulsants, folate metabolism effects 405
Antigen–antibody reactions, Crohn's disease 197
Antigens
　intestinal permeability 120–1
　see also *various types*
Antimetabolites, gastrointestinal cytotoxicity 400
Antiperistaltic loops, bacterial overgrowth 263–4
Antispasmodics, intestinal motility disorders 90
α1-antitrypsin, faecal measurement 27
Aphthoid ulcers, Crohn's disease 198
Apoprotein B, synthesis, chylomicron formation 56, 57
APUD cells 377
Argyrophil ganglion cells, small intestine 50
Arterial thrombosis, precipitating disorders 335
Arterio-venous malformations 344–5
Arterioles, intestinal, radiation effects 414–15
Arteritis, necrotizing 341–2
Arthritis

coeliac disease 167
  post-bypass surgery 114
  Whipple's disease 274−5
Arthropathy 4
  Crohn's disease 200−1
Ascariasis 285−6
Ascaris lumbricoides 285−6
Astroviruses 243
Atheroma, mesenteric 335
Atopic disease, food allergy effects 127−8
Atresia 44−6
  aetiology 44
  associated abnormalities 44
  clinical features 45
  congenital 45
  definition 44
  diagnosis 45
  ileal duplication 46
  management 45−6
Autoimmune disorders, primary lymphoma association 183
Autonomic neuropathy, secondary 89

Backward pacing, intestinal motility disorders 90
Backwash, bacterial, post-resection 265
Bacteria, intestinal
  normal 249−50
  role 250
Bacterial diarrhoea 232−40
  diagnostic features 245−6
  invasive infections 236−40
  stool microscopy 245
  toxigenic infections 232−6
  toxin classification 232, 233
  see also Cholera
Bacterial overgrowth 249−69
  absorption effects 254−60
  antibiotic regimen 266−7
  associated clinical disorders 261−6
  bacteria types 251−2, 253
  clinical assessment 260−1
  coeliac disease 167
  Crohn's disease 201, 264
  deleterious effects 252−60
  IgA deficiency 95
  intestinal motility effects 85, 250
  IPSID 186
  mucosal abnormalities 252, 254
  postoperative 46, 95, 112, 251, 265−6, 261−12
  treatment 266−7
  xylose breath test 22, 260
  see also Stagnant loop syndrome
Barium enema 8
Barium examination 5−8
Behçet's syndrome 209−12
  clinical features 210
  HLA association 210
  intestinal ulcers 210−12
  prevalence 210
Bephenium hydroxynapthoate, hookworm infections 284
Biguanides, gastrointestinal side-effects 404
Bile acids
  bacterial overgrowth effects 255−7, 262−3

breath test, bacterial overgrowth 260
  malabsorption, post-resection 108, 109−11
  serum, bacterial overgrowth 256−7
  steatorrhoea 256
  tropical sprue 321−2
Bile salts
  bacterial deconjugation 255−6
  bacterial dehydroxylation 255−6
  breath test 25
  ileal absorption 25−6
  malabsorption 60
Biliopancreatic bypass, gastrointestinal peptides 385
Billroth II gastrectomy
  bacterial overgrowth 95
  fat malabsorption 96
  rapid gastric emptying 93
  rapid jejunal emptying 94
Biopsy
  assessment 15−19
  handling 13
  morphometry 19
  small intestinal 4−5, 12−21
  Whipple's disease 277
Bisacodyl, intestinal transport effects 403−4
Blind loops, bacterial overgrowth 263−4
Blood flow, mesenteric 333−4
Blue diaper syndrome 64−5
Body composition 31−2, 33
Body lean mass 32, 33
Body weight/height, healthy adults 30−1
Bombesin, functions and distribution 378, 383
Bone, biopsies 35
Bone disease, post-gastrectomy 98−9
  see also Osteomalacia; Osteoporosis
Bone marrow, sternal 33
Brunner's glands, hamartomas 370
Brush border
  enzymes, intestinal ischaemia 334
  glucose and galactose binding sites 53
  membrane abnormalities 52, 254
  sodium and potassium binding sites 53
Bruton's agammaglobulinaemia 139
Buerger's disease 342
Bypass surgery 113−14
  adaptive response 113
  complications 114, 263−4
  hepatic changes 114
  hormonal aspects 384−5
  mortality 114
  postoperative function 113−14
  pyschiatric complications 114
  types 113

C1-esterase inhibitor (C1-INH) deficiency 3, 147−8
Caeruloplasmin, copper-labelled 26
Calcitonin gene-related peptide 378
Calcium
  body levels 35−6
  loss, intestinal lymphangiectasia 358
Caliciviruses 243
Cambendazole, parasitic infection 293
Campylobacter infections, hypogammaglobulinaemia 141−2

Index

Capillaria philippinensis, infections 294
Carbohydrates
  absorption 22–3
    post-gastrectomy 96
    protein–calorie malnutrition 302–4
  hydrolysis 52
  intolerance 54
  malabsorption 53–5
  metabolism, bacterial overgrowth 254
  transport 52–3
Carcinoid syndrome 393–4
  5-hydroxytryptamine 389, 394
Carcinoma, intestinal metastases 365–6
Cardiac disorders, Whipple's disease 273, 275
Cardiac valvular disorders, Whipple's disease 273, 275
Cardiovascular disorders 4
β-Carotene, serum levels, bacterial overgrowth 260
Castor oil, mucosal damage 404
Cell-mediated immunity
  food-allergic disorders 121
  foods 127
Cervical carcinoma, radiation enteritis 416
Chagas' disease, intestinal motility 84, 88
α-Chain disease *see* Immunoproliferative small intestinal disease
Children, anthropometry 29
Chloridorrhoea
  clinical aspects 66–7
  congenital 22, 66–8
  fetal ultrasound 66
Cholecystokinin
  coeliac disease 166
  functions and distribution 378, 380–1
  levels, ileal bypass 384
  succus entericus production 376
Cholera 233–4
  endocrine 389–91
  intestinal motility 88
  vaccine 234
Cholesterol ester storage disease 227
Cholestyramine
  drug interactions 405
  micellar component binding 405
Cholinergics, intestinal motility disorders 90
Chromosome abormalities, IPSID 190
Chvostek's sign 4
Chylous ascites, Whipple's disease 273
Cimetidine, diarrhoea induction 405
Clostridium difficile, stool microscopy 245
Clostridium welchii, type C 343
CNS, Whipple's disease 273–4, 275–6
Coeliac axis compression 338
Coeliac disease 153–78
  adult 162–7
  aetiology 159–61
  associated conditions 167–8
  autoantibodies 164
  childhood 161–2
  clinical features 161–7
  complications 169–70
  cytokinetics 156
  definition and terminology 153
  dietary antibodies 164
  enzyme deficiency 159
  epithelial lymphocytes 17
  flat mucosa 154, 156
  gastrointestinal function tests 165–6
  gastrointestinal peptides 396–7
  genetic and geographic aspects 156–7
  histology 154–6
  history 153
  hypogammaglobulinaemia 142
  IgA deficiency 138
  immunological aspects 159–61, 168
  intestinal abnormalities 164–5
  intestinal permeability decrease 23–4
  latent, partial gastrectomy effects 84–5
  lymphocyte/epithelial cell ratio 155
  lymphoma association 180–2
  lymphoreticular dysfunction 164
  malignancy association 169–70, 364
  neurological disorders 167–8
  non-responsive 213–16
  pancreatic function 166
  pathology 153–6
  scanning electron microscopy 154
  serum immunoglobulins 164
  stereomicroscopy 154
  teenagers 162
  ulceration and strictures 170
Colchicine, gastrointestinal effects 399–400
Collagen diseases 340
Collagenous sprue 19, 169
Complement components, Crohn's disease 196
Contraceptives, oral, mesenteric thrombosis 407
Copper
  caeruloplasmin binding 36
  deficiency 36
Coronaviruses 243
  tropical sprue 320
Cow's milk intolerance 128
Coxsackie viruses 243
Creatinine-height index (CHI) 32–3
Creeping eruption, strongyloidiasis 291
Crohn's colitis, differences from ileitis 199–200
Crohn's disease 195–208
  activated T cells 197
  aetiology 196
  clinical examination 199–200
  complications 199, 200–1
  diagnosis 201–3
  differential diagnosis 202–3
  disease activity assessment 203
  enterocyte abnormalities 17
  epidemiology 195
  gastrointestinal peptides 386
  history and terminology 19
  immunological aspects 196–7
  incidence 195
    increase 3
  infective agent aetiology 196
  intestinal adenocarcinoma 364–5
  intestinal motility 89
  joint pain 2
  magnesium deficiency 36
  mortality 206
  pathology 197, 198–9

Peyer's patches, micro-ulceration 198
  prognosis 206
  proximal intestine enzymes 199
  strictures, bacterial overgrowth 264
  surgery 205
  symptoms 199
  treatment 204–5
Cronkhite–Canada syndrome 370
Crosby biopsy capsule 5
Cryptosporidiosis 288, 294
  hypogammaglobulinaemia 140–1
Crypts of Lieberkühn, radiation effects 414
CSF, PAS-positive cells, Whipple's disease 274, 276
Cyclic AMP, salmonellosis 237
Cystic fibrosis
  bile acid malabsorption 60
  intestinal atresia therapy 46
Cysticercosis 287
Cystinuria 63–4
  incidence 63
  treatment 63–4
  types 63
Cytomegaloviruses 243
Cytosine arabinoside, jejunal effects 402
Cytotonic toxins 232
Cytotoxic toxins 232

Danazol, C1-INH deficiency 148
Darmbrand 343
Deoxycholic acid, mucosal toxicity 256
Dermatitis herpetiformis 3, 170–1
  cytokinetics 156
  lymphoma association 180
Dermatomyositis 340
Diabetes mellitus
  pseudo-obstruction 89
  radiation enteritis and 416
Diarrhoea 1–2
  acute undifferentiated, ETEC 236
  autoimmunity 118
  bacterial 232–40
  bile acid malabsorption 109
  endocrine 389–91
  familial protracted 67–8
    associated anomalies 68
  idiopathic, food allergy 128–9
  infective, gastrointestinal peptides 385–6
  laxative-induced 408–10
  post-vagotomy, IgA deficiency 138–9
  viral 240–6
Diarrhoea alba 311
Dichlorophen, tapeworm infections 287
Di George's syndrome 144
Digestion, post-gastrectomy 95–7
Digestive hyperaemia, mesenteric 333
Dihydroxy bile acids, post-vagotomy diarrhoea 93
Diodoquin, acrodermatitis enteropathica 70
Dioctyl sulphosuccinate, gastrointestinal effects 404
Diphyllobothrium latum, malabsorption association 288
Disaccharidase, mucosal, assay 23
Disaccharides, absorption 22–3

protein–calorie malnutrition 303
Dissecting microscopy, biopsies 13–14
Diverticulosis
  bacterial overgrowth 262–3
  jejunal, bacterial overgrowth 252
DNA
  loss, idiopathic mucosal enteropathy 215
  synthesis, enteroglucagon effects 104
Dopamine antagonists, intestinal motility disorders 89
D-penicillamine, cystinuria 63
Drugs
  absorption, intestinal motility effects 83
  intestinal disorder induction 398–412
Dumping syndrome, postoperative 93–4
  gastrointestinal hormones 388
Duodenal diverticulosis 262
Duodenal ulcer, intestinal motility 87, 88
Duodenocolic fistulae, bacterial overgrowth 265
Duodenum, intrinsic obstruction, associated disorders 45
Dysphagia, scleroderma 1

Echoviruses 243
Ehlers–Danlos synrome 344
Elderly
  bacterial overgrowth 250–1
  necrotizing enteritis 342–3
Electrolytes
  absorption, post-vagotomy 96
  deficiencies, post-resection 110
  stool 21–2
  transport, defects 65–8
Electron microscopy
  scanning 20–1
  transmission 19–20
Elemental diets, food allergy 131
ELISA test
  strongyloidiasis 292
  tapeworm infections 287
Embolism, mesenteric occlusion 335–6
Embonate, parasitic diseases 284–5
Emetic mechanism, retroperistalsis 80
Empirical diets, food allergy 132
Endemic diarrhoea, childhood, rotaviruses 240–2
Endocarditis, Whipple's disease 273, 275
Endocrine cells
  functional classification 377, 380
  gastropancreatic 377–8, 379, 380
Endocrine cholera 389–91
  associated tumours 389–90
  regulatory peptide associations 390–1
Endocrine tumours 388–94
Endometrial carcinoma, radiation enteritis 416
Endorphins 383
Endoscopy, Whipple's disease 277
Enkephalin
  functions and distribution 378, 383
  small bowel motility effects 83
Enteric antigens, immune responses 121–2
Enteritis
  necrotizing 342–3
  radiation 400, 413–24

Enterobacter cloacae, tropical sprue 319
Enteroblasts, hyperplasia, idiopathic mucosal enteropathy 215
Enterochromaffin cells, gut epithelium 377
Enteroclysis 6–7
  double contrast 6–7
Enterocolic fistulae
  adenocarcinoma 364
  bacterial overgrowth 265
Enterocytes
  brush border membrane abnormalities 52
  coeliac disease 154, 160–1
  defects 17–18, 52–77, 160–1
  intra-cell metabolic disorders 52
  lipid absorption and handling 55–6
  membrane defects, coeliac disease 159
Enteroglucagon
  DNA synthesis effects 104
  functions and distribution 378, 381–2
  levels 319
Enteroglucagonomas 392–3
Enterokinase deficiency 62
Enterolithiasis, Crohn's disease 199, 200
Enteropathy, mucosal idiopathic 213–16
Enzymes
  autodigestion, trypsin 95–6
  bacterial overgrowth effects 254
  brush border, intestinal ischaemia 334
  mucosal, coeliac disease 154
Eosinophilia, peripheral, ascariasis 286
Eosinophilic gastroenteritis 222–5, 288
  differential diagnosis 223
  inflammatory fibroid polyps 372, 373
  mucosal involvement 223, 224
  muscle involvement 223–4
  serosal involvement 224
  terminology 222–23
Eosinophilic granuloma, localized 224–5
Eosinophilic pseudo-tumoral enterocolitis 224
Epithelial tumours 363–5
Erythema multiforme, Behçet's syndrome 210
Escherichia coli
  enteropathogenetic 234, 235
  enterotoxigenic 235–6
  pathogen types 235
  tropical sprue 319
Essential amino acids, bacterial overgrowth 261
Essential fatty acids
  levels 37
  post-resection deficiency 112–13
C1-esterase inhibitor (C1-INH) deficiency 3, 147–8
Ethacrynic acid, prostaglandin synthesis effects 404
Eustoma rotundum 286

Fabry's disease 342
Fasciolopsis buski 287
Fat
  absorption 24–5
    neomycin effects 399
    postoperative 96
    protein–calorie malnutrition 304
  balance 24–5

dietary, bacterial metabolism 255
faecal excretion, tropical sprue 321
malabsorption
  bacterial overgrowth 255
  bile acid malabsorption 60
Fatty acids, essential
  levels 37
  post-resection deficiency 112–13
Fibro-elastic hyperplasia 339
Fibroid polyps, inflammatory 224–5, 371–2
  differences from eosinophilic gastroenteritis 372, 373
Finger clubbing 4
Flubendazole, parasitic diseases 285, 286
Fluke infections 287–8
5–Fluorouracil
  mucosal abnormality induction 400, 402
  radiation enteritis 416
Folic acid
  absorption
    postoperative 97
    tests 28
  deficiency 33–4
    bacterial overgrowth 257–9
    post-gastrectomy 98
  malabsorption
    congenital 69
    tropical sprue 322
  metabolism, oral anticonvulsants 405
Food-allergic disorders 118–34
  definitions 118–19
  diagnosis 131–2
  management 132
  oral tolerance and 122
  symptom provocation 132
Food allergy, atopic disease effects 127–8
Food idiosyncrasy 118
Food intolerance 118–19
  diagnosis 126–7
  food types 130–1
  general malaise 130
  management 132
Fructose, absorption 53
Function tests, intestinal 21–9
Functional reserve, intestinal 106–7

Galactose
  malabsorption 52, 55
  transport 52–3
Galanin, functions and distribution 378
Gallstones
  bile acid malabsorption 110
  Crohn's disease 201
  post-bypass surgery 114
Gangliocytic paragangliomas 366
Ganglioneuromatosis, myenteric plexuses 366
Gardner's syndrome
  hamartomas 369
  intestinal adenocarcinoma 364
Gastrectomy, partial
  bacterial overgrowth 46, 261–2
  dumping syndrome 93–4
    regulatory peptides 388

effects 93–100
 intestinal morphology effects 94–5
 intestinal motility effects 93–4
 latent coeliac disease 84–5
 parasitic infection risk 95
 see also Billroth and Polya
Gastric abnormalities, bacterial overgrowth 261–2
Gastric acidity, infection control 231
Gastric hypersecretion, post-resection 112
Gastric inhibitory peptide, functions and distribution 378, 381
Gastrin, functions 378–9
Gastrinomas 391–2
Gastrocolic fistulae, bacterial overgrowth 264–5
Gastrointestinal tract, duplication 46–7
Giardia lamblia 288
Giardiasis 288–91
 abdominal discomfort 1
 HLA association 290
 hypogammaglobulinaemia 139–40, 142
 parasitology 289–90
 post-gastrectomy 95
 predisposing factors 290–1
 protein–calorie malnutrition 307
 treatment 291
Gliadin 158, 159
Glucagon, barium enema reflux 8
 see also Enteroglucagon
Glucagonomas, pancreatic 391, 392
Glucose
 absorption 22
 malabsorption 52, 55
 transport 52–3
Gluten
 fraction test systems 158–9
 role in coeliac disease 157–9
Gluten-free diet, coeliac disease 166–7
Gluten-sensitive enteropathy, saccharide urinary excretion 24
Glutenin 158
Glycine malabsorption
 tropical enteropathy 329
 tropical sprue 321
Glycyl-glycine malabsorption
 tropical enteropathy 329
 tropical sprue 321
Gnathostoma spinigerum 286
Graft-versus-host diseases (GVHD) 145–6
Grahini ryadhi 311
Granulomas
 Crohn's disease 198–9
 malignant 339
Granulomatous disease, chronic 146–7
Ground itch, hookworm infection 283
Gut
 developing, rotation and fixation 44–5
 peptides, action modes 82–3

Haemangiomas, intestinal 366–7
Haematology, nutrition assessment 33–4
Haematomas, submucosal, warfarin-associated 406–7
Haemochromatosis, idiopathic primary 71

Haemoglobin measurement 33
Haemoglobinuria, paroxysmal nocturnal 343
Haemolytic-uraemic syndrome 341
Haemorrhage
 acute, isotope scanning 11
 chronic, isotope scanning 11
 gastrointestinal 8–9
 submucosal, drug-induced 406–7
Haemorrhagic telangiectasia, hereditary 343–5
Hamartomas
 intestinal 367, 368, 370
 myoepithelial 371
Haptens 120
Harper's pancreatone 382
Hartnup disease 52, 62
'Healthy weight', young adults 30–1
Height/body weight, healthy adults 30–1
Henoch–Schönlein purpura 340, 406
Hepatic failure, post-resection 111
Hepatobiliary complications, Crohn's disease 201
Herxheimer reaction, Whipple's disease 277
Heteroplasia 370–1
Heterotopia 370–1
Hill station diarrhoea 311
Histiocytosis, malignant, 184
HLA
 Behçet's syndrome 210
 coeliac disease associations 157, 159
 giardiasis associations 290
HLA-B27
 Crohn's disease 196, 201
 Whipple's disease 279–80
 Yersinia enterocolitica 240
HLA-DR3, IgA deficiency association 138, 142
Hookworm infection 283–5
 blood loss 283
Hydrogen breath test 23
 bacterial overgrowth 260
25-Hydroxycalciferol, post-gastrectomy levels 99
5-Hydroxytryptamine, carcinoid syndrome 389, 394
Hymenolopis spp. 287
Hyperoxaluria
 Crohn's disease 200
 post-bypass surgery 114
 post-resection 112
Hypersensitivity, definition 118
Hypersensitivity reactions 123–5
Hypertension
 malignant 341–2
 radiation enteritis and 416
Hypoaldosteronism, secondary, chloridorrhoea 67
Hypobetalipoproteinaemia 60
Hypocalcaemia, post-resection 110
Hypochlorhydria, tropical sprue 320
Hypocholesterolaemia, intestinal lymphangiectasia 358
Hypogammaglobulinaemia
 commensal bacteria 142–3
 differences from protein-losing enteropathy 148–9
 parasitic diseases 139–40, 142
 primary 139–43
 secondary 148–9

see also Immunodeficiency
Hypolactasia *see* Lactase deficiency
Hypomagnesaemia
 post-resection 110
 primary 71–2
Hypoproteinaemia
 hypercatabolic, idiopathic 348
 post-gastrectomy 97–8
Hypothalamus, Whipple's disease 276

IgA
 helper T cells 121
 incomplete heavy chains 185, 186–7
 monoclonal gammopathy, IPSID 188
 secretory (S-IgA) 232
IgA deficiency 136–9
 allergic disease 137–8
 coeliac disease 138
 jejunal biopsy 136
 post-vagotomy
  bacterial overgrowth 95
  diarrhoea 138–9
 protein–calorie malnutrition 305
IgE anti-food antibodies 126–7
IgG deficiency 148
Ileal bypass, cholecystokinin release 384
Ileitis, pre-stomal 216
Ileocolitis, Behçet's syndrome 210
Ileum
 conjugated bile salt transport 105
 tropical sprue 318
 vitamin B_{12} receptors 105
IME *see* Mucosal enteropathy, idiopathic
Imerslund–Grasbeck syndrome 68–9
Iminoglycinuria 65
Immune complex hypersensitivity 124–5
Immune status, systemic 125
Immune system, intestinal 119–23
Immune tolerance, food allergic disorders 122
Immunity, intestinal
 infection control 231–2
 investigation techniques 125–6
Immunocyte development, intestinal flora role 250
Immunodeficiency
 cellular 144–7
 primary, classification 137
 see also Hypogammaglobulinaemia
Immunodeficiency syndrome 18
Immunoproliferative small intestinal disease 18, 179, 185–91
 clinical features 185–6
 clinical variants 188–9
 disease course 189–91
 histopathology 187–8
 immunoelectrophoresis 187
 non-secretory 189
 parasitic infection 186, 190
 plasma cells 187
 premalignant stage 187, 189, 191
 predisposing factors 191
 prognosis and therapy 191
 protein studies 186–7
 tissue karyotyping 189–90

Immunosuppression, strongyloidiasis hyperinfection 292
Indicanuria 27
Infantilism, intestinal, bacterial overgrowth 259–60
Infarction, intestinal, non-obstructive 335
Infections
 control mechanisms 231–2
 intestinal motility 88
Infective diarrhoea, gastrointestinal peptides 385–6
 see also Bacterial diarrhoea; Cholera
Infertility, coeliac disease 167
Inflammatory bowel disease, idiopathic 129–30
Inflammatory masses, gallium-67 imaging 12
Innocent bystander effect 118
Intrinsic factor deficiency, postoperative 97
Intestinal development, peri-natal, PCM 304–5
Intestinal muscle, congenital absence 50
Intestinal resection
 absorption changes 103
 distal, malabsorption 107–11
 enterocyte hyperplasia 102
 enzyme changes 103
 epithelial cell proliferation 102–3
 functional adaptation 103–4, 105
 gastrointestinal peptides 385
 indications 101
 morphological adaptation 102, 105
 morphological and functional response 101–5
 proximal 111–12
Intestinal stasis, bacterial overgrowth 262–4
Intra-uterine growth retardation, intestinal effects 308
Iron absorption 29
 postoperative 96
Iron deficiency 307–8
 anaemia, hookworm infection 283
 bacterial overgrowth 259
 post-cricoid web 1
 post-gastrectomy 98
 sternal marrow 33
Iron metabolism, inborn error 71
Irradiation
 acute effects 414
 concomitant chemotherapy, enteritis and 416
 late effects 414–15
 pathological effects 413–15
 urinary symptoms 416
 vascular damage 414–15
 see also Radiation enteritis
Ischaemia, intestinal
 acute 336–7
 amyloidosis 221
 chronic 335, 337–8
 clinical features 336–8
 experimental 334–5
 focal 338
 intestinal motility 88
 mortality 337
 VIP loss 377
Islet cell hyperplasia, hypergastrinaemia 388
Isomaltase deficiency 54–5

Isospora belli 294
Isosporiasis 288, 294
   post-gastrectomy 95
Isotope imaging 11–12

Jejunitis
   acute 212–13
   necrotizing 343
   ulcerative, lymphoma association 182
Jejunoileal bypass, gastrointestinal peptides 384–5
Jejunoileum, intrinsic obstruction 46
   associated disorders 45
Jejunum
   absorption sites 105
   diverticulosis 262
   tropical sprue 315–18
   water and electrolyte absorption 21
Joint disorders
   coeliac disease 167
   post-bypass surgery 114
   Whipple's disease 274–5
Juvenile polyposis 369–70

Kaposi's sarcoma 145, 367
Klebsiella pneumoniae, tropical sprue 319
Köhlmeier–Degos syndrome 339
Kwashiorkor 299
   disaccharidase activity 303
   intestinal recovery 307
   mucosal appearances 302
Kynurenine–nicotinamide pathway inhibition 62

Lactase deficiency
   acquired 54
   congenital 53–4
   Crohn's disease 200
   hydrogen breath tests 23
   postoperative 96
Lactase, types 52
Lactic acidosis, post-resection 112
Lactose
   absorption 22
     tropical sprue 321
   intolerance
     giardiasis 289
     protein–calorie malnutrition 303
   malabsorption 54
   tolerance, hypolactasia 54
Ladd's bands 48
Ladd's operation, malrotation 49
Lamina propria
   biopsy studies 18–19
   coeliac disease 154, 155–6
Laxatives
   diarrhoea induction 408–10
   intestinal transport effects 403
   see also Purgative abuse
Leiomyoblastomas, intestinal 366
Leiomyomas, intestinal 366
Leiomyosarcomas, intestinal 366
Leucocytes, faecal, intestinal infections 245
Leukaemia, intestinal 226

Levamisole, ascariasis 286
Lieberkühn crypts, biopsy studies 18
Lipid storage disease 226–7
Lipids
   digestion and solubilization 55
   enterocyte handling 55–6
   malabsorption 56–60
Lipodystrophy, intestinal *see* Whipple's disease
Lipomas, intestinal 367
Liposarcomas, intestinal 367
Loperamide, indigenous tropical sprue 328
Lowe's syndrome 65
Lungs, Whipple's disease 273, 275
Lymph loss effects, intestinal lymphangiectasia 357, 358
Lymphangiectasia, intestinal 148, 348–62
   age at presentation 353
   clinical findings 354
   congenital anomalies 351–3
   diagnosis 355–7
   differential diagnosis 356–7
   early terminology 348–50
   familial 351–3
   histopathology 349–50, 355
   natural history 353–4
   pathology 350–3
   primary 351–3
   reversible causes 356
   secondary 353
   treatment 359
Lymphangiography, intestinal lymphangiectasia 355–6
Lymphatic channels, intestinal, anatomy and physiology 350
Lymphocytes
   gluten-sensitive, lamina propria 160
   intraepithelial 17
Lymphoid tissue, gut-associated (GALT)
   hyperplasia 143–4
   immunoglobulins 135–6
   role 135
Lymphokines, gluten effects 161
Lymphoma
   definition 179
   secondary 184–5
   villous atrophy 400
   see also Mediterranean lymphoma; Western primary lymphoma
Lysinuric protein intolerance 52, 64
Lysosomal acid esterase deficiency 227

M cells 14
   Peyer's patches 136
Macrophages, PAS-positive, Whipple's disease 270–1
Magnesium, body levels 36
Malabsorption
   amyloidosis 220
   bacterial overgrowth 254–60
   gluten-free diet non-responsive 168–9
   intestinal lymphangiectasia 357–8
   post-gastrectomy 95–7
   radiation enteritis 418–20

sub-clinical 284
   radiation-induced 414, 420
  tropical
   differential diagnosis 288
   gastrointestinal peptides 387–8
  type 1 resection 108
  type 2 resection 108–10
  type 3 resection 111
Malabsorption syndromes, food intolerance 128
Malnutrition, ascariasis 286
Malrotation
  aetiology 47–8
  clinical features 48
  diagnosis 48–9
  management 49
  small intestine 47–9
Marasmus 299
  fat malabsorption 304
  mucosal appearances 301–2
Mast cell degranulation, food-allergic disorders 127
Mastocytosis, systemic 225–6
Mean corpuscular haemoglobin concentration (MCHV) 33
Mean corpuscular volume (MCV) 33
Mebendazole, parasitic diseases 284–5, 286, 293
Meckel's diverticulitis 50
Meckel's diverticulum 8, 49–50
  diagnosis and managment 50
  haemorrhage 11–12
Mediterranean lymphoma 179, 185–91
Mefenamic acid, gastrointestinal side-effects 403
Megaloblastic anaemia, bacterial overgrowth 257–8
  see also Vitamin B$_{12}$
Melaena, Meckel's diverticulum 49
Membrane reactive hypersensitivity 124
Meningitis, Whipple's disease 276
6-Mercaptopurine, diarrhoea association 402
Mesenteric arteries, compression 335
Mesenteric circulation 333–4
  anatomy and physiology 333–4
Mesenteric lymph nodes, Whipple's disease 272
Mesenteric occlusion, acute 10
Mesenteric thrombosis, oral contraceptives 407
Mesenteric varices 345
Metageria, intestinal lymphangiectasia 351, 352
Methionine malabsorption 65
Methotrexate, xylose absorption effects 400
Metronidazole
  Crohn's disease 204–5
  giardiasis 291
Microflora
  faecal, tropical sprue 320
  tropical sprue 319–20
  see also Bacteria; and under Bacterial and Viral
Microthrombosis, intestinal 341
Migrating myoelectric complex (MMC), intestinal motility 79
Milk intolerance, post-gastrectomy 96
Minerals, body levels 35–6
Monkey hookworm infection 285
Morphology, intestinal, protein–calorie
   malnutrition 299–302
Motilin 82
  functions and distribution 378, 381
  levels, tropical sprue 319
  release, infective diarrhoea 386
Motility, intestinal
  amyloidosis 219–20
  bacterial overgrowth 264
  control 80–3
  disorders 83–90
   treatment 89–90
  extrinsic nervous control 83, 84
  fasted pattern 78–9
  fasting abnormal effects 84–5
  fed pattern 80
  gut peptide effects 82–3, 383–8
  infection control 231
  intrinsic nervous control 81, 84
  normal 78–80
  partial gastrectomy effects 93–4
  post-resection 107
  tropical sprue 318–19
Mouth, examination 3
Mucosa
  adult protein–calorie malnutrition 300–1
  intestinal
   drug toxic effects 398–403
   growth, intestinal flora role 250
   normal 14–15
Mucosal enteropathy, idiopathic 213–16
  aetiology 214
  clinical findings 214
  disease progression 214
  jejunal biopsy 214–15
  nomenclature 213–14
  treatment 215–16
Mushroom ingestion, trehalase deficiency effects 55
Mycobacterium bovis 244
Mycobacterium tuberculosis 244
Myenteric plexus, intestinal motility control 81–2, 84
Myocarditis, Whipple's disease 275

Necator americanus 283–5
Necrosis, intestinal, radiation-induced 416
Necrotizing arteritis 341–2
Necrotizing enteritis 342–3
  elderly 342–3
  tropical 343
Neomycin
  drug absorption interactions 399
  fat absorption effects 399
  malabsorption induction 398–9, 401, 405
  vitamin absorption effects 399
Neonates
  diarrhoea, enteropathogenetic *E. coli* 234, 235
  gastrointestinal peptides 388
Nephrolithiasis
  Crohn's disease 200
  cystinuria 63
  post-bypass surgery 114
  post-resection 112

Neurilemmomas, intestinal wall 366
Neuroendocrine system, intestinal 376–7
Neurofibromatosis, multiple 370
Neurogenic tumours, intestinal 366
Neuromyeloradiculitis, progressive 168
Neuropeptide, functions and distribution 378
Neurotensin, functions and distribution 378, 381
Neurotensinomas 392
Neutropenia, primary 146–7
Niclosamide, tapeworm infections 287
Nicotinic acid deficiency, bacterial overgrowth 260
Nimorazole, giardiasis 291
Nippostrongylus brasiliensis 293
Nitrogen
  absorption, protein–calorie malnutrition 304
  whole body neutron activation analysis 33
Nodular lymphoid hyperplasia (NLH) 143–4
Norwalk virus 242–3
  clinical and laboratory characteristics 241
Notochordal theory, intestinal duplication 46
Nutrition
  assessment 29–37
  deficiency 299–310
    clinical features 29, 30
  see also Malnutrition

Oast-house syndrome 65
Obesity
  bypass surgery 113–14
    hormonal aspects 384–5
  gastrointestinal hormones 384–5
Obstruction, partial, Crohn's disease 89
Ocular lesions 4
Ocular manifestations, Whipple's disease 275
Oedema, hypoproteinaemic, bacterial overgrowth 261
Oligoallergenic diets 132
Oligosaccharidases, surface 52
Opiates, intestinal motility disorders 89–90
Opioids, small bowel motility effects 83
Ornidazole, giardiasis 291
Osteomalacia 35
  post-gastrectomy 96
  post-resection 110
Osteoporosis 35
  bacterial overgrowth 260
  post-resection 110

Pancreatic enzymes, protein–calorie malnutrition 304
Pancreatic polypeptide
  functions 378, 379–80
  pancreatic tumours 392
Pancreaticocibal asynchrony 95
Pancreatitis, chronic, alcohol-induced 403
Paneth cells, abnormalities 18
Paracrine system, intestinal motility control 82–3
Paralytic ileus 89
Parasitic diseases
  differentiation from eosinophilic gastroenteritis 223
  hypogammaglobulinaemia 139–41, 142
  protein–calorie malnutrition 307
  see also various diseases
Paratyphoid fever 240
Parkes–Weber–Klippel syndrome 366
Paroxysmal nocturnal haemoglobinuria 343
Particulate embolization 10
PAS, gastrointestinal side-effects 404
PAS-positive cells, CSF, Whipple's disease 274, 276
PCM *see* Protein–calorie malnutrition
Pellagra, Hartnup disease 62
Peptide histidine isoleucine, functions and distributions 383
Peptide tyrosine tyrosine 378, 382
Peptides
  absorption 61
  malabsorption 62–5
  see also Regulatory peptides
Perforation, typhoid fever 239
Peri-ampullary carcinoma 365
Pericarditis, fibrous, Whipple's disease 273, 275
Peripheral neuropathy, post-bypass surgery 114
Peritoneal adhesions, Whipple's disease 273
Permeability, intestinal, tests 23–4
Pernicious anaemia, bacterial overgrowth 261
Pertechnetate imaging 11–12
Peutz–Jeghers syndrome 368–9
Peyer's patches 119, 135–6
  micro-ulceration 198
  suppressor T cells 121
  typhoid fever 238, 239
Phaeochromocytomas, anti-somatostatin antibodies 392
Phocanema infections 286
Phosphorus, body levels 36
Pig bel 343
Piperazine, ascariasis 286
Plasmacytoid lymphoma 18
Plasmacytomas, intestinal 184
Plasmodium falciparium, malabsorption association 288
Pleural adhesions, Whipple's disease 273
Pneumatosis cystoides intestinalis 227–8
  post-bypass surgery 114
Polyarteritis nodosa, intestinal 339–40
Polyarthropathy 4
Polymorphonuclear leucocytes, intestinal infections 245
Polyposis
  intestinal 368–72
  juvenile 369–70
Porphyria, acute intermittent, pseudo-obstruction 89
Potassium
  total body 35
  vascular smooth muscle effects 407
Practolol, side-effects 407
Praziquantel, tapeworm infections 287
Pre-stomal ileitis 216
Prednisone, Crohn's disease 204–5
Primary ulcers 212
Prognostic indices 37
Prostaglandins
  systemic mastocytosis 226

thyroid medullary carcinoma 391
Prostate carcinoma, radiation enteritis 416
Protein
  absorption 26–7, 60–1
    bacterial overgrowth 257
  deficiency, bacterial overgrowth 259
  digestion 60–1
  intolerance 128
  metabolism, bacterial overgrowth 257
  total concentration 34
Protein–calorie malnutrition 299–307
  bacterial overgrowth 261
  immunology 305–6
  intestinal physiology 302–4
  intestinal size and villus height 300
  microflora changes 306–7
  recovery 307
  small intestinal changes 300
Protein-losing enteropathy
  bacterial overgrowth 257, 259
  immunodeficiency differences 148–9
  isotope imaging 12
  tests 26–7
Protein-losing gastroenteropathy 349
Pseudo-obstruction
  Chagas' disease 88
  colonic, post-bypass surgery 114
  intestinal 85–6, 88, 89
  metabolic disorders 89
Pseudomembranous colitis, stool microscopy 245
Pseudotabes, coeliac disease 168
Pseudoxanthoma elasticum 344
Purgative abuse 408–10
  psychological aspects 409–10
Purine nucleoside phosphorylase deficiency 144
Pyrantel embonate, ascariasis 286
PYY, functions and distribution 378, 382

Radiation enteritis 400, 413–24
  aetiology 415–16
  clinical features 416–18
  incidence 415
  investigations 418
  low-fat diet 422
  management 420–2
  medical care 422
  preoperative care 420–1
  prevention 422
  radiation dose association 415
  radiography 418, 419
  risk after surgery 415–16
  surgery 421–2
  see also Irradiation
Radiological examination 5–12
Radionuclide scanning 11–12
Reaginic hypersensitivity 124
Receptors, intestinal cell, infection control 231
Regional enteritis see Crohn's disease
Regulatory peptides 377
  endocrine cholera 390–1
  endocrine tumours 388–94
  intestinal disease 383–8
  types and distribution 378

Rendu–Osler–Weber disease 343–5, 366
Respiratory system, examination 4
Retention polyps 369–70
Reticuloendothelial system, Whipple's disease 275
Reticulosis, intestinal lymphangiectasia 358
Retinol binding protein, levels 36–7
Retroperistalsis 80
Rheumatoid disease 340
Rice water stools 234
Rickets
  hypophosphataemic familial 72
  intestinal lymphangiectasia 357
  vitamin D resistant 72
Rotaviruses
  childhood endemic diarrhoea 240–2
  clinical and laboratory characteristics 241
Roundworm infections 285–6

Sarcocystis hominis 288, 294
Sarcocystosis 294
Salmonella paratyphi 240
Salmonella typhi 238
Salmonellosis 236–8
  bacteraemia 238
  clinical syndromes 237
  predisposing conditions 237
Schwannomas, intestinal wall 366
Schwartzmann reaction 341
Scleroderma 221–2
  intestinal smooth muscle lesions 84
  see also Systemic sclerosis
Secretin, functions and distribution 378, 380
Secretory antibodies, intestinal 121
SeHCAT clearance test 25–6
Short intestine
  absorption effects 46
  congenital 50
Sickle-form-particle containing (SPC) cells 271
Skeletal structure, assessment 35
Skin
  examination 3
  Whipple's disease effects 274
Skinfold thicknesses, adipose tissue 31–2, 33
Small bowel barium meal 6
Small intestinal disease
  assessment 1–41
  clinical assessment 1–5
  clinical history 1–2
  investigations 4
  physical examination 3–4
  previous history 2
  social history 2
Small intestine, embryology 43–4
  Gut; and under Intestinal
Smooth muscle
  intestinal 80–1
  lesions, intestinal motility effects 84
  tumours 366
Sodium cromoglycate, food allergy 128, 129, 132
Sodium, total body 35
Somatostatin 82
  functions and distribution 378, 382
Somatostatinomas, 391, 392

Soya protein, intolerance to 128
Sprue, unclassified 213–16
Stagnant loop syndrome 98
  bacterial overgrowth 251
  growth failure 31
  intestinal infantilism 259–60
  megaloblastic anaemia 249
  see also Bacterial overgrowth
Stanazol, C1-INH deficiency 148
Steatorrhoea
  Crohn's disease 201
  hypogammaglobulinaemia 142
  see also Fat, absorption
Stenosis 45–7
  aetiology 45
  clinical features 46
  definition 45
  diagnosis 46
  management 46–7
Strictures
  bacterial overgrowth 264
  radiation-induced 416
  tuberculous 264
Strongyloides fuelleborni 293
Strongyloides stercoralis 291
Strongyloidiasis 3, 291–4
  hyperinfection 292–3
Strontium excretion measurement 36
Substance P. functions and distribution 378, 383
Succus entericus, cholecystokinin 376
Sucrase deficiency 54–5
Sucrose absorption 22–3
Superior mesenteric artery
  acute occlusion 10
  angiography 8–10
Systemic lupus erythematosus 340
Systemic sclerosis 221–2
  gastrointestinal effects 86
  see also Scleroderma

Taenia saginatum 286
Taenia solium 286–7
Takayashu's disease 339
Tangier disease 227
Tapeworm infections 286–7
T-cell hypersensitivity 125
T cells
  immunoregulation 123–4
  mitogenesis, giardiasis 289
Telangiectasia, haemorrhagic, hereditary 343–5
Ternidens diminutus 285
Tetany
  intestinal lymphangiectasia 358
  iodiopathic mucosal enteropathy 214
Thiabendazole, parasitic infection 293
Thrombophlebitis migrans, Behçet's syndrome 210
Thrombophlebitis obliterans 342
Thrombotic thrombocytopenic purpura 335, 341
Thymic aplasia 144
Thyrocalcitonin, diarrhoea association 391
Thyroid medullary carcinoma, endocrine cholera 391
Tinidazole, giardiasis 291

T-lymphocyte defects 144
Trace elements, body levels 36–7
Transcobalamin II deficiency 69
Transit time, intestinal, post-resection 107
Transport inhibition, drug-induced 403–5
Traveller's diarrhoea, ETEC 236
Trehalase deficiency 55
Trichiniasis 286
Trichostrongyliasis 286
Triolein breath test 25
Trophozoites, *Giardia lamblia* 290
Tropical enteropathy 314, 329–30
  geographical distribution 329–30
  hookworm infection 284
  intestinal structure and absorption 329
  tropical sprue relations 329–30
  see also Malabsorption, tropical; Tropical sprue
Tropical sprue 311–32
  absorption tests 320–2
  acute 323–4
    differential diagnosis 324
  aetiology 328–9
  chronic 317, 324–7
    Schilling tests 323
  definition 314
  epidemiology 314, 315
  gastrointestinal peptides 319, 387–8
  geographical distribution 314, 315
  historical aspects 311–15
  indigenous 327–8
  latent 327
  microbiology 319–20
  pathology 315–18
  seasonality 315
  tropical enteropathy, relationship 329–30
  uncertain aetiology 313
Trousseau's sign 4
Trypsin, enzyme autodigestion, post-gastrectomy 95–6
Tryptophan
  dietary, nicotinamide synthesis 62
  malabsorption 64–5
Tuberculosis
  differentiation from Crohn's disease 203
  intestinal 243–4
    forms 244
  strictures, bacterial overgrowth 264
Tuft cells 14–15
Turner's syndrome, hereditary haemorrhagic telangiectasia 343
Typhoid fever 238–9
  relapses 239

Ubbumariyayae 311
Ulceration, intestinal
  causes 209
  primary 212
Ulcerative enteritis, chronic idiopathic 213–16
Ulcerative jejunoileitis, non-granulomatous 213–16
Ulcers, primary 212
Unclassified sprue 213–16
Urea, blood and urine levels 35

Index

Vagotomy, truncal
　intestinal motility 87, 88
　rapid gastric emptying 93
　bacterial flora changes 262
Vascular malformations 343–5
Vascular occlusion, acute 334
Vascular tumours, malignant 367
Vasoactive intestinal polypeptide
　functions and distribution 378, 380, 382–3
　immunofluorescence staining 380
　loss in ischaemia 377
Venous occlusion, intestinal 342
Viability, intestinal, radionuclide scans 12
Vibrio cholerae 232, 233
Villi
　biopsy assessment 16–17
　leaf, tropical climates 15–16
Villous atrophy
　hyoplastic 16–17
　hyperplastic 16
Villous hypertrophy 17
Villus hyperplasia, intestinal resection 102, 103
Vincristine, ulceration and ileus induction 402
VIP *see* Vasoactive intestinal polypeptide
VIPomas 390–1
Viral diarrhoea 240–6
　diagnostic features 245–6
Vitamin A
　liver tissue levels 36–7
　serum levels, bacterial overgrowth 260
Vitamin A absorption
　fat absorption test 29
　postoperative 96
Vitamin A deficiency 308
　abetalipoproteinaemia 58
Vitamin B_{12}
　congenital malabsorption 68–9
　ileal receptors 105
Vitamin B_{12} absorption
　postoperative 96–7
　protein–calorie malnutrition 304
　tests, 20–1, 27–8
Vitamin B_{12} deficiency 34, 307
　bacterial overgrowth 257–9, 263
　Crohn's disease 201
　post-gastrectomy 98
Vitamin B_{12} malabsorption
　congenital 68–9
　post-resection 108–9, 111
　tropical sprue 322
Vitamin B complex, deficiencies 36
Vitamin D absorption, postoperative 96
Vitamin D deficiency 4
　bacterial overgrowth 260
　intestinal lymphangiectasia 357–8
　post-gastrectomy 98–9
Vitamin D metabolism 37
Vitamin E deficiency
　abetalipoproteinaemia 58
　intestinal lymphangiectasia 353–4, 357, 358
Vitamin E levels 37
Vitamin K deficiency 3
　Crohn's disease 201
Vitamin K levels 37
Vitamins
　absorption, neomycin effects 399
　deficiencies, coeliac disease 163
　fat-soluble 36–7
　　absorption 28–9
　　bacterial overgrowth effects 257
　　postoperative absorption 96
　water-soluble 36
　　absorption 27–8
Vitello-intestinal duct patency 50
Volvulus 48–51
von Recklinghausen's disease, anti-somatostatin antibodies 392
von Willebrand's disease, hereditary haemorrhagic telangiectasia 343

Waldenström's macroglobulinaemia 226
　lamina propria 19
Warfarin
　metabolism inhibition, drug-induced 406–7
　submucosal haematomas 406–7
Water absorption, post-vagotomy 96
Water and electrolyte balance 21–2
Water and electrolyte transport
　protein–calorie malnutrition 304
　tropical sprue 320–1
Watson biopsy technique 5
Weanling diarrhoea 306
Wegener's granuloma 339
Weight loss, post-gastrectomy 97
Western primary lymphoma 179–85
　autoimmune disorders 183
　classification 183
　clinical features 179–80
　course and treatment 184
　histopathology 183–4
　immonodeficiency 182–3
　predisposing factors 180–3
　prognosis 184
Whipple's disease 270–82
　aetiology 277–80
　arthritis 274–5
　bacteria 278–9
　　culture and serology 278–9
　clinical features 274–6
　Herxheimer reaction 277
　HLA-B27 association 279–80
　immunological aspects 279–80
　investigations and diagnosis 276–7
　patient age 274
　relapse 277
　small intestinal 271–2, 276
　TEM studies 19
　treatment 277
White flux 311
Wilson's disease 36
Wolman's disease 227

Xylose
　breath test, bacterial overgrowth 22, 260
　catabolism, bacterial overgrowth 254
Xylose malabsorption

anti-metabolite-induced 400
protein–calorie malnutrition 302–4
tropical sprue 321

Yersinia enterocolitica 240

Zinc, defective intestinal absorption 69–71

Zinc deficiency 36
   immunity effects 70
   iodiopathic mucosal enteropathy 214
Zollinger–Ellison syndrome 226, 388
   pancreatic gastrinoma 391–2
Zymogen activation test, enterokinase defiency 62